Diabetes and Ocular Disease

Ophthalmology Monographs

A series published by Oxford University Press
in cooperation with the American Academy of Ophthalmology

Series Editor: Richard K. Parrish, II, MD, Bascom Palmer Eye Institute

American Academy of Ophthalmology Clinical Education Secretariat:
Louis B. Cantor, MD, Indiana University School of Medicine
Gregory L. Skuta, MD, Dean A. McGee Eye Institute

DIABETES AND OCULAR DISEASE

Past, Present, and Future Therapies, Second Edition

Edited by
Ingrid U. Scott, MD, MPH
Harry W. Flynn, Jr., MD
William E. Smiddy, MD

Published by Oxford University Press
in cooperation with
the American Academy of Ophthalmology

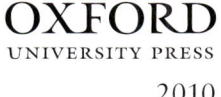

OXFORD
UNIVERSITY PRESS
2010

OXFORD
UNIVERSITY PRESS

Oxford University Press, Inc., publishes works that further
Oxford University's objective of excellence
in research, scholarship, and education.

Oxford New York
Auckland Cape Town Dar es Salaam Hong Kong Karachi
Kuala Lumpur Madrid Melbourne Mexico City Nairobi
New Delhi Shanghai Taipei Toronto

With offices in
Argentina Austria Brazil Chile Czech Republic France Greece
Guatemala Hungary Italy Japan Poland Portugal Singapore
South Korea Switzerland Thailand Turkey Ukraine Vietnam

Published by Oxford University Press, Inc.
198 Madison Avenue, New York, New York 10016
www.oup.com

Oxford is a registered trademark of Oxford University Press

Library of Congress Cataloging-in-Publication Data

Diabetes and ocular disease : past, present, and future therapies / edited by
Ingrid U. Scott, Harry W. Flynn Jr., William E. Smiddy.—2nd ed.
p. ; cm.—
(Ophthalmology monographs ; 14)
Includes bibliographical references and index.
ISBN 978-0-19-534023-5
1. Diabetic retinopathy. 2. Cataract. I. Scott, Ingrid U.
II. Flynn, Harry W. III. Smiddy, William E. IV. American Academy of Ophthalmology. V. Series.
[DNLM: 1. Diabetic Retinopathy—therapy. 2. Diabetic Retinopathy—diagnosis.
W1 OP372L v.14 2008 / WK 835 D5337 2008]
RE661.D5D46 2008
617.7'35—dc22
2008028396

9 8 7 6 5 4 3 2 1

Printed in China
on acid-free paper

Legal Notice

The American Academy of Ophthalmology provides the opportunity for material to be presented for educational purposes only. The material represents the approach, ideas, statement, or opinion of the author, not necessarily the only or best method or procedure in every case, nor the position of the Academy. Unless specifically stated otherwise, the opinions expressed and statements made by various authors in this monograph reflect the author's observations and do not imply endorsement by the Academy. The material is not intended to replace a physician's own judgment or give specific advice for case management. The Academy does not endorse any of the products or companies, if any, mentioned in this monograph.

Some material on recent developments may include information on drug or device applications that are not considered community standard, that reflect indications not included in approved FDA labeling, or that are approved for use only in restricted research settings. This information is provided as education only so physicians may be aware of alternative methods of the practice of medicine, and should not be considered endorsement, promotion, or in any way encouragement to use such applications. The FDA has stated that it is the responsibility of the physician to determine the FDA status of each drug or device he or she wishes to use in clinical practice, and to use these products with appropriate patient consent and in compliance with applicable law.

The Academy and Oxford University Press (OUP) do not make any warranties, as to the accuracy, adequacy, or completeness of any material presented here, which is provided on an "as is" basis. The Academy and OUP are not liable to anyone for any errors, inaccuracies, omissions obtained here. The Academy specifically disclaims any and all liability for injury or other damages of any kind for any and all claims that may arise out of the use of any practice, technique, or drug described in any material by any author, whether such claims are asserted by a physician or any other person.

DISCLOSURE STATEMENT

Acknowledgments

The authors gratefully acknowledge the contributions of all the chapter authors, who are experts in their fields and who generously share their expertise with all of our readers.

Preface

Diabetes mellitus is a complex, multifactorial disease often associated with progressive retinopathy and visual loss. This monograph compiles current information from leading authorities regarding treatment strategies for diabetic eye disease. The emphasis of the chapter authors has been to provide practitioners of ophthalmology with an up-to-date, practical reference for the diagnosis and management of ocular disease in diabetic patients. The contributors have assimilated pertinent basic science and clinical information comprehensively, yet concisely, to include not only the guidelines established by the collaborative studies but also the concepts of disease mechanisms and clinical management that have evolved subsequently.

In 1989, the American Academy of Ophthalmology initiated the Diabetes 2000® project with the mission of eliminating preventable blindness from diabetic retinopathy. Over the decade of the 1990s, Diabetes 2000® encouraged collaboration among primary care physicians, allied health professionals, and ophthalmologists to ensure early detection and appropriate management of diabetic retinopathy. Diabetes 2000® initiatives included instructional courses and symposia at the Annual Meeting of the American Academy of Ophthalmology, state and local seminars on diabetic management, and literature through pharmacists and package inserts for raising awareness of diabetic eye disease among patients. Federally funded economic studies show that detection and treatment of diabetic eye disease saves, even at suboptimal care, $250,000,000 annually. The Diabetes 2000® project has achieved its goal of informing medical care providers and patients that diabetic retinopathy screening and appropriate treatment are an essential part of medical care for persons with diabetes. In January 2000, the Foundation of the Academy assumed responsibility under a new name: EyeCare America℠ Diabetes Project. The program built on the success of the Diabetes 2000® project by focusing on the patient, as well as educating primary care physicians. The first edition of Monograph 14 was completed in 1999 and published in 2000 to coincide with a symposium entitled Diabetes 2000 at the AAO annual meeting. The second edition of Monograph 14 represents an additional 10 years of publications in the field of diabetes and ocular disease. Of particular note is the Diabetic Retinopathy Clinic Research Network, which has provided significant new information regarding the treatment of diabetic retinopathy. Additional chapters have been added on pharmacotherapies, optical coherence tomography, evidence-based medicine, evolving management strategies, telemedicine, and histopathology of diabetic retinopathy. We believe the current edition will serve as a valuable resource for ophthalmologists, researchers, as well as residents and medical students.

The educational objectives of this monograph follow:

- Provide an overview of the worldwide diabetes epidemic
- Review the classification of diabetic retinopathy
- Describe the histopathological manifestations of diabetic retinopathy
- Describe the pathogenesis of diabetic retinopathy
- Review the epidemiology and risk factors of diabetic retinopathy
- Summarize the history of evolving treatments for diabetic retinopathy
- Assess the use of photography, angiography, and ultrasonography in diabetic retinopathy
- Assess the use of optical coherence tomography in diabetic retinopathy
- Outline the clinical studies on treatment for diabetic retinopathy
- Explain the photocoagulation techniques for diabetic macular edema and diabetic retinopathy
- Analyze the use of vitrectomy for diabetic retinopathy
- Provide information on intravitreal pharmacotherapies for diabetic retinopathy
- Present evolving algorithms for managing diabetic macular edema
- Provide an evidence–based systematic review of the management of diabetic retinopathy
- Describe how cataract is managed in diabetes
- Identify nonretinal ocular abnormalities in diabetes
- Discuss the effect of systemic conditions on diabetic retinopathy
- Discuss medical management of the diabetic patient
- Describe telemedicine for diabetic retinopathy
- Explore future therapies for diabetic retinopathy
- Familiarize the reader with the major clinical trials for diabetic retinopathy

Ingrid U. Scott, MD, MPH
Harry W. Flynn, Jr., MD
William E. Smiddy, MD

Contents

Contributors

Everett Ai, MD
Pacific Vision Foundation
California Pacific Medical Center
San Francisco, California

Lloyd M. Aiello, MD
Beetham Eye Institute
Joslin Diabetes Center
Harvard Medical School
Boston, Massachusetts

Lloyd Paul Aiello, MD, PhD
Department of Ophthalmology
Joslin Diabetes Center
Harvard Medical School
Boston, Massachusetts

Nicholas G. Anderson, MD
Southeastern Retina Associates
Associate Clinical Professor
Department of Surgery
University of Tennessee
Knoxville, Tennessee

Sophie J. Bakri, MD
Associate Professor of Ophthalmology
Vitreoretinal Diseases and Surgery
Mayo Clinic
Rochester, Minnesota

William E. Benson, MD
Retina Service
Wills Eye Institute
Philadelphia, Pennsylvania

George W. Blankenship, MD
Former Chairman of the
  Department of Ophthalmology
Penn State College of Medicine
Hershey, Pennsylvania

Gary C. Brown, MD, MBA
Retina Service
Wills Eye Institute
Philadelphia, Pennsylvania

Jerry Cavallerano, OD, PhD
Beetham Eye Institute
Joslin Diabetes Center
Harvard Medical School
Boston, Massachusetts

Nauman A. Chaudhry, MD
Department of Ophthalmology
Bascom Palmer Eye Institute
University of Miami School of Medicine
Miami, Florida

Emily Y. Chew, MD
National Eye Institute
National Institutes of Health
Bethesda, Maryland

Matthew D. Davis, MD
Department of Ophthalmology
  and Visual Sciences
University of Wisconsin-Madison
Medical School
Madison, Wisconsin

Diana V. Do, MD
Wilmer Eye Institute
Johns Hopkins University School
  of Medicine
Baltimore, Maryland

Sander R. Dubovy, MD
Department of Ophthalmology
Bascom Palmer Eye Institute
University of Miami School
  of Medicine
Miami, Florida

Frederick L. Ferris III, MD
National Eye Institute
National Institutes of Health
Bethesda, Maryland

Mitchell S. Fineman, MD
Retina Service
Wills Eye Institute
Philadelphia, Pennsylvania

Harry W. Flynn, Jr., MD
Department of Ophthalmology
Bascom Palmer Eye Institute
University of Miami School of Medicine
Miami, Florida

Thomas W. Gardner, MD, MS
Departments of Ophthalmology and
  Cellular and Molecular Physiology
Penn State University
College of Medicine
Hershey, Pennsylvania

Mitchell J. Goff, MD
Brooke Army Medical Center
San Antonio, Texas

Matthew Guess, MD
Department of Ophthalmology
Indiana University School of Medicine
Indianapolis, Indiana

Julia A. Haller, MD
Wills Eye Institute
Jefferson Medical College of Thomas
  Jefferson University
Philadelphia, Pennsylvania

Peter K. Kaiser, MD
Cole Eye Institute
Cleveland Clinic Foundation
Cleveland, Ohio

Barbara E. K. Klein, MD, MPH
Department of Ophthalmology
  and Visual Sciences
University of Wisconsin-Madison
Medical School
Madison, Wisconsin

Ronald Klein, MD, MPH
Department of Ophthalmology
  and Visual Sciences
University of Wisconsin-Madison
Medical School
Madison, Wisconsin

Andrew Lam, MD
New England Retina Consultants
Springfield, Massachusetts

Robert E. Leonard II, MD
Dean A. McGee Eye Institute
Oklahoma City, Oklahoma

Helen K. Li, MD
Department of Ophthalmology
 and Visual Sciences
University of Texas Medical Branch
Galveston, Texas

H. Richard McDonald, MD
Pacific Vision Foundation
California Pacific Medical Center
San Francisco, California

Quresh Mohamed, MD
Cheltenham General Hospital
Cheltenham, Gloucestershire, United
Kingdom

Andrew A. Moshfeghi, MD
Department of Ophthalmology
Bascom Palmer Eye Institute
University of Miami Miller School
 of Medicine
Miami, Florida

David W. Parke II, MD
Dean A. McGee Eye Institute
Oklahoma City, Oklahoma

Carmen A. Puliafito, MD, MBA
Dean
University of Southern California
 Keck School of Medicine
Los Angeles, California

Carl D. Regillo, MD
Director, Clinical Retina Research
Wills Eye Institute
Professor of Ophthalmology
Thomas Jefferson University
Philadelphia, Pennsylvania

Ingrid U. Scott, MD, MPH
Professor of Ophthalmology and Public
 Health Sciences
Departments of Ophthalmology
 and Public Health Sciences
Penn State Hershey Eye Center
Penn State College of Medicine
Hershey, Pennsylvania

Jay S. Skyler, MD
Department of Medicine
University of Miami School
 of Medicine
Miami, Florida

William E. Smiddy, MD
Department of Ophthalmology
Bascom Palmer Eye Institute
University of Miami School
 of Medicine
Miami, Florida

Jennifer K. Sun, MD
Beetham Eye Institute
Joslin Diabetes Center
Harvard Medical School
Boston, Massachusetts

Matthew T. S. Tennant, MD, FRCSC
Department of Ophthalmology
University of Alberta
Edmonton, Alberta, Canada

Nigel H. Timothy, MD
Department of Ophthalmology
Joslin Diabetes Center
Harvard Medical School
Boston, Massachusetts

Charles P. Wilkinson, MD
Greater Baltimore Medical Center
Towson, Maryland

Tien Y. Wong, MD, PhD
Department of Ophthalmology
Centre for Eye Research Australia
University of Melbourne
East Melbourne, Victoria,
Australia

Diabetes and Ocular Disease

1

Medical Overview of the Worldwide Diabetes Epidemic

ROBERT E. LEONARD II, MD,
AND DAVID W. PARKE II, MD

CORE MESSAGES

- Diabetes is a worldwide epidemic.
- Most of the increase in total numbers of diabetic patients is expected to occur in developing nations.
- Changing dietary and exercise trends appear to play a major role in the increasing prevalence of diabetes mellitus.

In recent decades, diabetes mellitus has progressed from a disease affecting primarily people in developed countries into a true worldwide epidemic. The World Health Organization (WHO) in 1999 defined diabetes mellitus as "a state of absolute or relative insulin deficiency, characterized by hyperglycemia and the risk of microvascular and macrovascular complications." The purpose of this chapter is to emphasize the magnitude and impact of diabetes on developing nations and its implications for global health. The association of diabetes, pre-diabetes, and the metabolic syndrome will be discussed. By the end of this chapter, the reader should have a clear understanding of the demands that will be placed on health care providers around the world to cope with this looming healthcare crisis.

DIABETES: A WORLDWIDE EPIDEMIC

It is estimated that in 2005 nearly 200 million people worldwide had diabetes mellitus. Most of these patients are classified as having type 2 diabetes mellitus and the metabolic syndrome. The WHO data estimate the number of diabetic patients in Asia and India alone to be 52.4 million [1]: this number is expected to

3

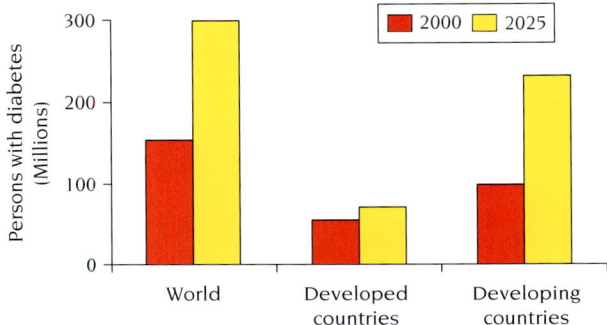

Figure 1.1. Global prevalence of diabetes 2000–2025. (Source: King H. *Diabetes Care.* 1998;21:1414–1431.)

skyrocket to approximately 121.8 million over the next 25 years [2]. Most of the increase in total numbers of diabetic patients is expected to occur in developing countries. Worldwide, about 300 million people are expected to have diabetes by 2025, affecting 5.4% of the world's population [3]. Changing dietary and exercise trends appear to play a major role in the increasing prevalence of diabetes mellitus. Figure 1.1 summarizes the changing prevalence of diabetes worldwide.

In the United States, diabetes mellitus has increased at a staggering rate. While in 1990, only 5 states reported an incidence of diabetes exceeding 6% of the population, by 1998, a total of 22 states reported an incidence of diabetes greater than 6% of the population (Fig. 1.2) [4]. In the United States, there are 18.2 million people (6.3% of the population) with diabetes [5]. The prevalence of diabetes in African Americans has doubled in slightly more than a decade to 18.2%, with type 2 accounting for nearly 95% of cases [6] as per estimates of 2002.

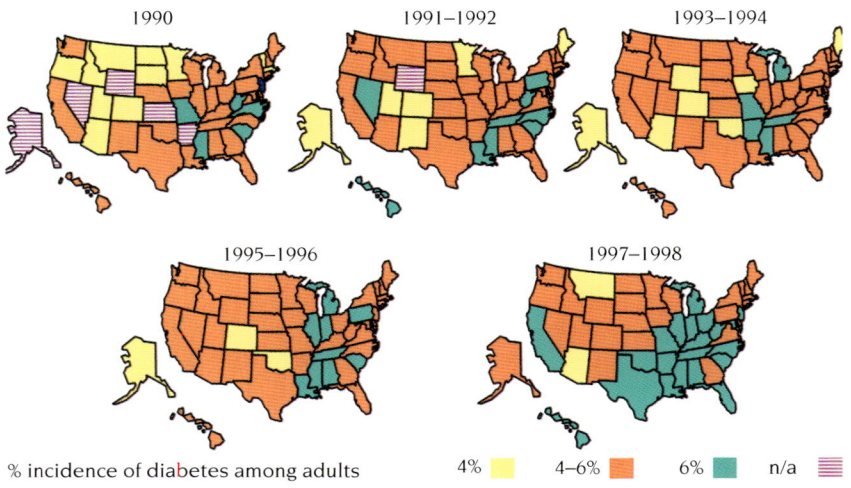

Figure 1.2. Diabetes trends in the United States: 1990–1998. (Source: Mokdad AH et al. *Diabetes Care.* 2000;23:1278–1283.)

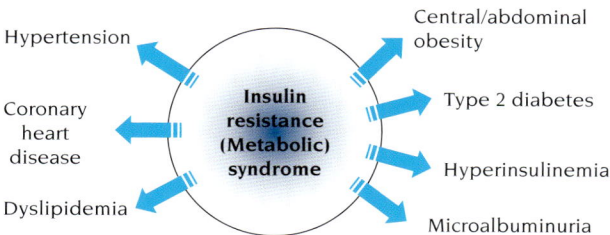

Figure 1.3. The insulin resistance (metabolic) syndrome and its components. (Source: Groop et al. *Front Horm Res.* 1997;22:131–156.)

DIABESITY: THE METABOLIC SYNDROME

The increasing prevalence of obesity is a critical factor associated with the growing numbers of people with diabetes, particularly type 2 diabetes. The WHO has recognized what it refers to as a "global epidemic of obesity" that is emerging in developing nations. In the United States, the Centers for Disease Control estimates that about 65% of Americans are either overweight or obese with about 23% characterized as "obese" [7]. The prevalence of type 2 diabetes appears to be rising in parallel with the global trend towards obesity [8]. It has been estimated that a weight gain of 11 to 15 pounds increases the risk of diabetes by 50% [9]. Data suggest that this increase is particularly prevalent in women, with the age-adjusted prevalence of the metabolic syndrome increasing 24% in women and only 2% in men between the years 1988 and 1999 [10]. Obesity is a critical element of the "metabolic syndrome," also referred to as "insulin resistance syndrome." This entity combines insulin resistance, whether in the form of glucose intolerance or frank type 2 diabetes with a variety of factors. These factors include coronary heart disease (CHD), central or truncal obesity, hypertension, and dyslipidemia [11]. A model of the insulin resistance syndrome and its components is shown in Figure 1.3.

From a global perspective, the increasing incidence of the metabolic syndrome is due to changing dietary patterns, the trend toward obesity, and sedentary lifestyle. Interaction with other risk factors for diabetes has resulted in a changing pattern of public health and disease status. Figure 1.4 demonstrates how these interactions

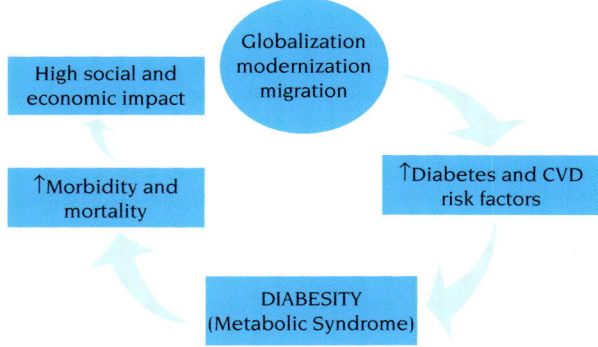

Figure 1.4. The metabolic syndrome.

Presence of classic symptoms
(fatigue, thirst, polyuria) and:

Fasting plasma glucose   ≥ 126 mg/dL

Random plasma glucose   ≥ 200 mg/dL

Type 2 diabetes affects about
18 million Americans

Figure 1.5. Diabetes: diagnostic criteria.

lead to development of the metabolic syndrome and the impact on public health. In the past, nomenclature often referred to diabetes as juvenile-onset or adult-onset. Since the metabolic syndrome and obesity can also affect children and adolescents, the incidence of type 2 diabetes is accelerating in these populations as well. In one large U.S. metropolitan area, 33% of new cases of diabetes in adolescents were type 2, representing a ten-fold increase between 1982 and 1994 [12]. Just as in the adult population, the primary risk factor appears to be obesity [13]. Therefore, insulin deficient or type 1 diabetes versus insulin resistant or type 2 diabetes are better descriptors for these diseases.

As the medical understanding of diabetes improves, the diagnostic criteria have become more focused and better defined. Eighteen million Americans are classified as having type 2 diabetes mellitus determined by elevated plasma glucose levels and classic symptoms such as fatigue, polydipsia, polyphagia, and polyuria. Current definitions include an elevated fasting plasma glucose level greater than 126 milligrams per deciliter (mg/dL), or a random plasma glucose in excess of 200 mg/dL. These criteria are summarized in Figure 1.5.

An additional 41 million Americans are currently classified as pre-diabetic. These patients have a fasting plasma glucose level between 100 and 125 mg/dL, or an impaired glucose tolerance test. These individuals are at increased risk for atherosclerosis and eventual conversion to type 2 diabetes. Figure 1.6 shows the current diagnostic criteria for pre-diabetes.

PRE-DIABETES: THE HIDDEN EPIDEMIC

Currently, patients diagnosed with diabetes represent only the tip of the diabetic epidemic iceberg. Studies show that patients with impaired glucose tolerance (the

Impaired fasting glucose (IFG)

Fasting glucose 100–125 mg/dL

Impaired glucose tolerance (IGT)

2 h glucose in glucose tolerance test: 140–199 mg/dl

Pre-diabetes affects about 41 million Americans. They are at risk of accelerated atherosclerosis and type 2 diabetes.

Figure 1.6. Prediabetes: diagnostic criteria.

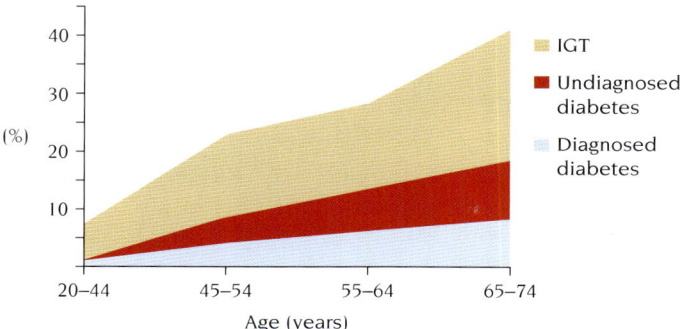

Figure 1.7. Prevalence of undiagnosed and diagnosed diabetes and impaired glucose tolerance (IGT) in a US population (20–74 year of age). (Source: Adapted from Harris ML. *Diabetes Care*. 1993;16:642–652.)

incidence of which is associated with advancing age) represent the largest group of potential diabetic patients. This represents an undiagnosed patient subgroup that far exceeds the number of diagnosed and undiagnosed persons with diabetes in the United States today (Fig. 1.7) [14].

Risk factors for type 2 diabetes are well recognized and include such uncontrollable issues as age, family history, and ethnicity. However, factors such as truncal obesity and dyslipidemia may be the result of physical inactivity and sedentary lifestyle (Fig. 1.8).

Prevention or delay of type 2 diabetes mellitus is of key concern when the population of persons with pre-diabetes is considered. Over a ten year period, 33% of patients with impaired glucose tolerance will progress to frank type 2 diabetes without intervention. Indeed, it is estimated that diabetes is undiagnosed in 30% to 50% of people with the disease and more than 50% of persons with newly diagnosed diabetes will have diabetic complications at the time of their diagnosis as a result of delayed detection. Obviously, delaying or reducing the conversion rate of people with pre-diabetes to type 2 diabetes would eliminate much of the end organ damage, and would reduce the great health care expense associated with treating these

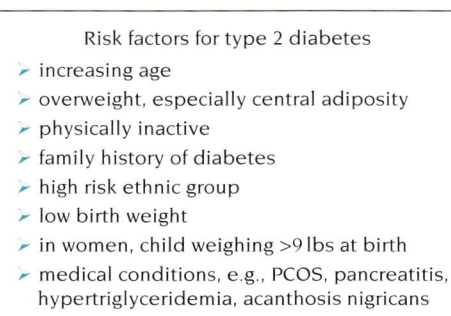

Figure 1.8. Risk factors for type 2 diabetes.

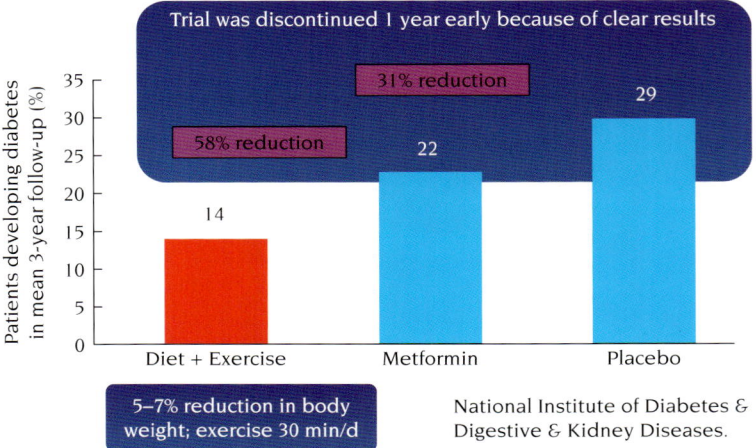

Figure 1.9. Diabetes Prevention Program preliminary results.

complications. The Diabetes Prevention Program (DPP) study looked at the role of the oral hypoglycemic agent metformin, as well as diet and exercise, in preventing progression to type 2 diabetes in patients with pre-diabetes. In the study, patients were divided into three groups. One was a control group. The second received metformin. The third group was treated with diet and exercise alone. While metformin was accompanied by a 31% reduction in the rate of development of disease, the diet and exercise group attained a 58% reduction. This decreased the rate of conversion to type 2 diabetes from 29% to 14% over a 3-year period [15]. This study confirms the fact that by addressing controllable risk factors, the rate of progression can be modified. The results of the DPP trial are summarized in Figure 1.9.

CONSEQUENCES OF DIABETES: COMPLICATIONS AND COSTS

Treatment of complications due to diabetes is a growing source of health care expenditures. While ophthalmologists focus on the retinal and ophthalmic complications of diabetes and their treatment costs, it is important to note that these represent only a fraction of the overall cost of uncontrolled diabetes. Chronic complications of diabetes include accelerated atherosclerosis and its associated macrovascular disease processes of CHD, stroke, and peripheral vascular disease. These are responsible for the majority of diabetes-associated morbidity and mortality. Peripheral and autonomic neuropathy, renal impairment and failure, and diabetic retinopathy are associated with the microvascular complications of diabetes. As an example, Haffner and colleagues compared the 7-year incidence of myocardial infarction (MI) in diabetic and nondiabetic subjects with and without prior CHD (Fig. 1.10). Their data suggest that diabetic patients without a previous MI have a higher risk of MI than nondiabetic patients who have had a previous history of MI. Persons with diabetes have a nearly seven-fold increase in heart disease compared to nondiabetic patients [16]. CHD is the number one cause of death in the

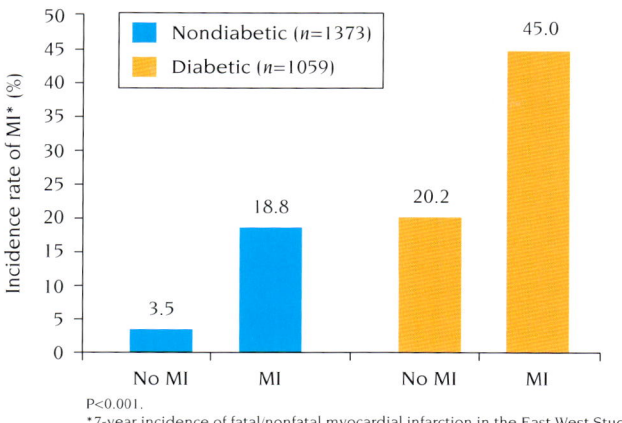

P<0.001.
*7-year incidence of fatal/nonfatal myocardial infarction in the East West Study.

Figure 1.10. Type 2 diabetes and coronary heart disease. (Source: Haffner SM et al. *N Engl J Med*. 1998;339:229–234.)

developed world, and accounts for over 500,000 deaths per year in the United States alone [17]. It is clear that the emerging diabetic epidemic facing the developing nations of the world will significantly change rates of CHD and associated mortality in coming years.

In the United States alone, the cost of treating uncomplicated diabetes is over 6 billion dollars per year. Acute complications of diabetes, such as emergent hypoglycemia or hyperglycemia, raise that cost significantly. The chronic complications of diabetes, as mentioned above, totaled over 44.1 billion dollars in 1997. That represented 10,071 dollars per each diabetic patient in the United States [18]. The total cost related to diabetic complications in the United States is estimated to be at least 100 billion dollars per year. Figure 1.11 shows that eye care expenditures are only a fraction of the total cost of treating diabetic complications in the United States.

Numerous studies have shown that the key to decreasing diabetic complications lies with strict glucose control. The Diabetes Control and Complications Trial (DCCT) has shown the benefits of intensive blood glucose control in patients with type 1 diabetes [19]. Intensive glucose control reduced the risk of developing

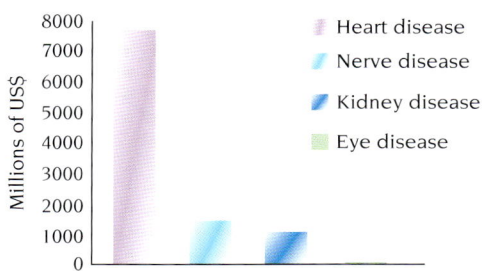

Figure 1.11. Cost of treating complications of diabetes. (Source: American Diabetes Association. *Diabetes Care*. 1998;21:296–309.)

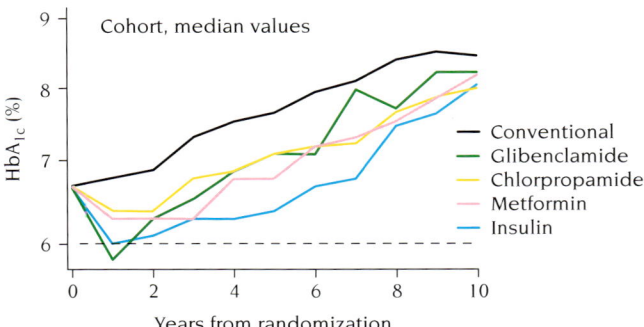

Figure 1.12. United Kingdom Prospective Diabetes Study: loss of long-term glycemic control. (Source: UKPDS. *Lancet*. 1998;352:837–853.)

retinopathy by 54%. Neuropathy was reduced by 60% and albuminuria by 54%, respectively. With regards to type 2 diabetes mellitus, the United Kingdom Prospective Diabetes Study (UKPDS) was a randomized clinical trial involving 3867 newly diagnosed patients with type 2 diabetes [20]. After 3 months of diet treatment alone, patients with a mean of two fasting plasma glucose concentrations of 6.1 to 15.0 mmol/L were randomly assigned to either an intensive glycemic control group or a conventional control group. This study showed a 21% reduction in risk for progression of diabetic retinopathy over a 12-year period in the intensive group. In addition, there was a 29% reduction in the need for retinal photocoagulation in the intensive group compared to the conventional group. Overall, there was a 37% reduction in the risk of an adverse microvascular complication with intensive control that was less strict than current guidelines. The UKPDS study also demonstrated that glycemic control appears to diminish with time (Fig. 1.12). Clearly, the best indicator of glycemic control continues to be hemoglobin A1C (HgbA1C). Skyler and associates have demonstrated that HgbA1C levels correlate in a direct relationship with the relative risk of diabetic microvascular complications (Fig. 1.13) [21]. Strict glucose control, weight

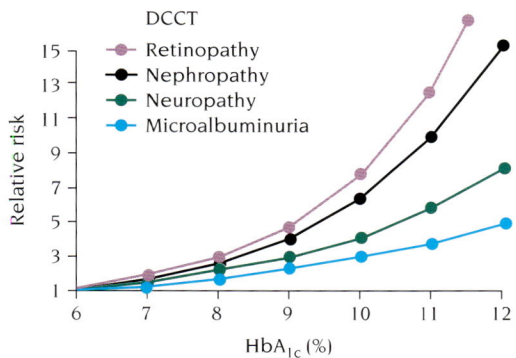

Figure 1.13. Relationship of HbA1c to risk of microvascular complications. (Source: Skyler. *Endocrinol Metab Clin*. 1996;25:243–254, with permission.)

control, and exercise, remain the essential elements to prevent the complications of diabetic disease.

CONCLUSION

Diabetes should be considered in the same context as AIDS—a global epidemic that is at least partially preventable—a chronic disease with quantifiable economic costs, and incalculable human costs whose effects span national boundaries and socioeconomic groups. As such, education and public policy initiatives play a critical role including screening programs and risk factor management directed at glycemic and blood pressure control, identification and control of hyperlipidemia, and cessation of smoking.

REFERENCES

1. World Health Organization, World Diabetes Day 2005, November 11, 2005.
2. Meyer JJ, Wung C, Shukla D. Diabetic retinopathy in Asia: the current trends and future challenges of managing this disease in China and India. *Cataract and Refractive Surgery Today.* 2005;Oct:64–68.
3. King H, Aubert RE, Herman WH. Global burden of diabetes, 1995–2025: prevalence, numerical estimates, and projections. *Diabetes Care.* 1995;21:1414–1431.
4. Mokdad AH, Ford ES, Bowman BA, et al. Diabetes trends in the U.S.: 1990–1998. *Diabetes Care.* 2000;23:1278–1283.
5. National Institute of Diabetes and Digestive and Kidney Diseases. National diabetes statistics fact sheet: general information and national estimates on diabetes in the United States. NIH Publication No. 04–3892. Bethesda, MD: US Department of Health and Human Services, National Institutes of Health; 2004.
6. National Institute of Diabetes and Digestive and Kidney Diseases. Diabetes in African Americans. NIH Publication No. 02–3266. Bethesda, MD: US Department of Health and Human Services, National Institutes of Health; 2002.
7. Centers for Disease Control and Prevention. Prevalence of overweight and obesity in the United States, 1999–2004. *JAMA.* 2006;295(13):1549–1555.
8. Bloomgarden ZT. Obesity and diabetes. *Diabetes Care.* 2000;23(10):1584–1590.
9. Colditz GA, Willett WC, Rotnitzky A, Manson JE. Weight gain as a risk factor for clinical diabetes mellitus in women. *Ann Intern Med.* 1995;122:481–486.
10. Ford ES, Giles WH, Mokdad AH. Increasing prevalence of the metabolic syndrome among U.S. adults. *Diabetes Care.* 2004;27:2444–2449.
11. Groop L, Orho-Melander M. The dysmetabolic syndrome. *J Intern Med.* 2001;250(2): 105–120.
12. Rosenbloom A. Increasing incidence of type 2 diabetes in children and adolescents. *Pediatr Drugs.* 2002;4:209–211.
13. Laron Z. Type 2 diabetes in childhood—a global perspective. *J Pediatr Endocrinol Metab.* 2002;15:459–469.
14. Harris MI. Undiagnosed NIDDM: clinical and public health issues. *Diabetes Care.* 1993;16:642–652.
15. Orchard TJ, Temprosa M, Goldberg R, et al. The effect of metformin and intensive lifestyle intervention on the metabolic syndrome: the Diabetes Prevention Program randomized trial. *Ann Intern Med.* 2005;142(8):611–619.

16. Haffner SM, Lehto S. Mortality from coronary heart disease in subjects with type 2 diabetes and in nondiabetic subjects with and without prior myocardial infarction. *N Engl J Med*. 1998;339:229–234.
17. Centers for Disease Control and Prevention. Mortality from coronary heart disease and acute myocardial infarction—United States, 1998. *MMWR Morb Mortal Wkly Rep*. 2001;50:90–93.
18. American Diabetes Association. Economic consequences of diabetes mellitus in the U.S. in 1997. *Diabetes Care*. 1998;21:296–309.
19. Diabetes Control and Complications Trial Research Group. The effect of intensive treatment of diabetes on the development and progression of long-term complications in insulin-dependent diabetes mellitus. *N Engl J Med*. 1993;329:977–986.
20. UK Prospective Diabetes Study Group. Intensive blood-glucose control with sulphony-lureas or insulin compared with conventional treatment and risk of complications in patients with type 2 diabetes. UKPDS 33. *Lancet*. 1998;352:837–853.
21. Skyler JS. Diabetic complications: the importance of glucose control. *Endocrinol Metab Clin*. 1996;25:243–254.

2

Classification of Diabetic Retinopathy

CHARLES P. WILKINSON, MD

CORE MESSAGES

- The prevalence of vision loss due to diabetic retinopathy can be expected to increase with growing numbers of patients with diabetes unless there is more effective screening of these patients.
- There is a need for improved communication between eye care professionals and physicians managing patients with diabetes.
- Development of a simplified classification system for diabetic retinopathy should lead to improved communication and improved patient outcomes.
- A 5-stage disease severity scale regarding diabetic retinopathy is proposed. This ranges from "no retinopathy" to "proliferative diabetic retinopathy."
- A 3-stage severity scale regarding edema of the central macula is proposed, and this is based upon the location and extent of the retinal thickening.

Diabetes mellitus is a significant public health issue. The World Health Organization (WHO) has estimated that there are approximately 150 million people with this disorder and that this number could double by the year 2025 [1]. In the U.S., diabetes affects over 18.2 million people (6.3% of the total population), and 800,000 new cases of type 2 diabetes are diagnosed each year [2]. As a frequent complication of diabetes, diabetic retinopathy can be expected to remain a significant cause of visual disability in an increasing number of patients.

In the U.S., diabetic retinopathy is the leading cause of blindness among adults aged 20 to 74 years of age; it is estimated that more than 10,000 individuals become legally blind from diabetic macular edema (DME) and/or proliferative diabetic retinopathy (PDR) each year [2]. The duration of diabetes is a strong risk factor for the development of retinopathy, as is the severity of the hypergly-cemia. Hypertension is an additional risk factor, and optimal control of serum glucose and systemic blood pressure is of utmost importance in the management of patients with diabetes [3]. The natural history of diabetic retinopathy is pro-gressive, and nearly all patients with type 1 and over 60% of patients with type 2 diabetes develop some degree of retinopathy over the course of 20 years [4]. The epidemiology of this disorder is discussed in detail in Chapter 5.

Visual morbidity and blindness can be combated effectively if treatment of retinopathy is instituted in a timely fashion. Landmark clinical trials, the Diabetic Retinopathy Study (DRS) and the Early Treatment Diabetic Retinopathy Study (ETDRS), demonstrated that effective treatment for retinopathy could reduce vision loss by 90% [4,5]. These studies underscored the critical need to have regu-lar eye examinations so that patients are identified reliably at the time when laser photocoagulation is most effective. Timely detection and treatment of diabetic retinopathy could result in major reductions in health expenditures—savings that are quite cost-effective compared with other health care interventions [6].

The disparity between the availability of effective treatment and the continued increase in the number of patients with symptomatic diabetic retinopathy implies that there are barriers to optimal management of diabetic patients. Part of the problem lies in diabetic individuals not being aware of their need to have dilated eye evaluations. In addition, many individuals lack health insurance, sufficient funds, or a means of reaching a physician. Several studies have documented that many patients with diabetes do not receive regular dilated eye examinations, with most reporting that no more than 50% of individuals with diabetes receive an annual dilated eye examination [4]. An additional negative factor is the lack of coordination between the systemic care of patients with diabetes and their eye care. Frequently, there does not appear to be a systematic approach for feedback and communication between the primary care physician (who might be a diabe-tologist/endocrinologist, family physician, or internist), and the ophthalmologist or eye care provider. Thus, patients may not be referred or reminded to keep their appointment with their ophthalmologist, even when there have been significant findings on past eye examinations. Physicians managing patients with diabetes fre-quently do not understand the retinopathy scales, and results of eye examinations are commonly not reported to them.

An additional issue is the lack of patient access to appropriate care. On a global basis, the WHO reported that many patients were not receiving appropriate care because of a lack of public and professional awareness as well as an absence of treatment facilities [1]. In several developing countries, optimal care is inaccessible to the majority of the population [1].

This need to provide a framework for improved communication between and among nurses, primary care physicians, internists, endocrinologists, ophthalmolo-gists, and other eye care providers is the key reason to develop a simplified clas-sification system that can be employed on an international scale. A standard set of definitions of severity of diabetic retinopathy and macular edema is critical for communication among colleagues, and improved communication should lead to better patient care.

THE ETDRS AND ADDITIONAL CLASSIFICATIONS
OF DIABETIC RETINOPATHY

The ETDRS grading scale is based upon the modified Airlie House classification of diabetic retinopathy [5]. This scheme is based on seven standard 30-degree photographic fields that provide sufficient depth of field, adequate area, and magnification to provide an accurate representation of the status of the retina. A standard set of definitions and a standard set of photographs of various lesions describing the severity of retinopathy is employed (Table 2.1). The ETDRS grading scale continues to be applied widely in research settings, publications, and in meetings of retina subspecialty groups, for it has demonstrated satisfactory reproducibility and

Table 2.1. Abbreviated Summary of the Early Treatment Diabetic Retinopathy Study Scale of Diabetic Retinopathy Severity for Individual Eyes [5,7].

Level	Severity	Definition
10	No retinopathy	Diabetic retinopathy absent
20	Very mild NPDR	Microaneurysms only
35	Mild NPDR	Hard exudates, soft exudates, and/or mild retinal hemorrhages
43	Moderate NPDR	43A Retinal hemorrhages moderate ($>$ photograph 1) in four quadrants or severe ($\geq$ photograph 2A) in one quadrant 43B Mild IRMA ($<$ photograph 8A) in one to three quadrants
47	Moderate NPDR	47A Both level 43 characteristics 47B Mild IRMA in four quadrants 47C Severe retinal hemorrhages in two to three quadrants 47D Venous beading in one quadrant
53A-D	Severe NPDR	53A $\geq$ 2 level 47 characteristics 53B Severe retinal hemorrhages in four quadrants 53C Moderate to severe IRMA ($\geq$ photograph 8A) in at least one quadrant 53D Venous beading in at least two quadrants
53E	Very severe NPDR	$\geq$2 level 53A-D characteristics
61	Mild PDR	NVE $<$ 0.5 disc areas in one or more quadrants
65	Moderate PDR	65A NVE $\geq$ 0.5 disc area in one or more quadrants 65B NVD $<$ photograph 10A ($<$0.24–0.33 disc area)
71,75	High risk PDR	NVD $\geq$ photograph 10A, or NVD $<$ photograph 10A or NVE $\geq$ 0.5 disc area plus VH or PRH, or VH or PRK obscuring $\geq$ 1 disc area
81, 85	Advanced PDR	Fundus partially or completed obscured by VH, new vessels ungradeable in at least one field, or retina detached at the center of the macula

The scale grades the following abnormalities: hemorrhages (HE), microaneurysms (MA), hard exudates (HE), soft exudates (SE), intraretinal microvascular abnormalities (IRMA), venous beading (VB), new vessels < 1 disc diameter (DD) from the disc (NVD), new vessels elsewhere (NVE), vitreous hemorrhages (VH), preretinal hemorrhage (PRH), fibrous proliferation on the optic nerve head (FPD), and fibrous proliferation elsewhere (FPE).

validity. Although it is recognized as the gold standard for grading the severity of diabetic retinopathy in clinical trials, its use in everyday clinical practice has not proven to be easy or practical. The grading system has more levels than may be necessary for clinical care, and the specific definitions of the levels are detailed, require comparison with standard photographs, and are difficult to remember and apply in a clinical setting. Several unpublished contemporary surveys have documented that the vast majority of physicians managing patients with diabetes do not employ the full ETDRS severity scale, because it is too complex for application in the clinical practices of retinal specialists, comprehensive ophthalmologists, endocrinologists, and primary care physicians [7].

In several countries, simplified classifications have been developed in an effort to improve both the screening of patients with diabetes and communication among caregivers. In 1993, a simplified diabetic retinopathy severity scale was developed as part of "The Initiative for the Prevention of Diabetic Eye Disease," sponsored by the German Society of Ophthalmology (Anselm Kampik, personal communication, 2003). Another similar severity scale has been used in Japan since 1983 [8]. The organizers of a recent massive screening campaign for diabetic retinopathy in 15 Latin American and the Caribbean countries developed a customized simplified classification based on another version of the ETDRS severity scale [9], and yet another system has been employed in Australia [10]. Because each of these grading systems is unique, it is very difficult to compare data from studies using these various classification schemes.

PROPOSED INTERNATIONAL CLASSIFICATION

Despite the development of the ETDRS and additional classifications in several countries, there remained a genuine need for a single standardized practical clinical disease severity scale that could be employed around the world to facilitate communication across groups of practitioners. The severity of retinopathy may lead to different treatment strategies and recommendations in different regions because practice patterns and health care delivery systems for patients with diabetes mellitus differ around the world. Nevertheless, an optimal clinical classification system should be useful for a broad range of caregivers with varying skills and diagnostic equipment, ranging from retinal specialists with contemporary equipment to trained physician assistants using only direct ophthalmoscopes.

In September 2001, the American Academy of Ophthalmology (AAO) launched a consensus development project with the goal of developing a new clinical severity scale for diabetic retinopathy [7]. The published report [7] reviews the deliberations that led to the establishment of the scale and presents a final document upon which consensus had been achieved. The development process was sponsored by the AAO, and the AAO Board of Trustees formally approved the final classification scales in February 2003.

At the time of the initiation of this project, it was agreed that the clinical disease severity scale should be evidence-based, employing data from important clinical studies such as the ETDRS and the Wisconsin Epidemiologic Study of Diabetic

Retinopathy (WESDR) [11,12]. The severity scale was intended primarily for comprehensive ophthalmologists and primary care physicians, because these individuals evaluate most patients with diabetes. Retinal specialists were considered to be familiar with the ETDRS classification system and expected to continue using either that or their personal customized modifications.

It was hoped that "most easily visible" lesions might serve as appropriate indicators of the likelihood of progression to severe forms of retinopathy. Unfortunately, this was not the case. Prior to the large meeting, data from the ETDRS and the WESDR were re-evaluated in an effort to document the association between specific lesions and the severity of diabetic retinopathy (Ronald Klein, MD, MPH, personal communication, 2002). In evaluations performed on the ETDRS data, intraretinal microvascular anomalies (IRMA) and venous beading (VB) were very predictive of the risk of developing proliferative retinopathy, but the presence of hard exudates or soft exudates was not very predictive. The most visible signs of retinopathy, hemorrhages/microaneurysms (H/MA), did not reliably predict the risk of progression to proliferative retinopathy. WESDR data demonstrated a lack of concordance of these lesions with the presence of IRMA and VB. For right eyes with IRMA present, 41% of patients with type 1 diabetes and 42% of patients with type 2 diabetes did not have H/MA ≥ standard photograph #1 in one or more fields. For right eyes with VB present, 29% of patients with type 1 diabetes and 31% with type 2 diabetes did not have H/MA ≥ standard photograph #1 in one or more fields. The sensitivity of using H/MA greater than standard photograph #1 in one or more fields for detecting the presence of IRMA or VB was about 60%, and the specificity about 97%. Therefore, it became clear that it would be necessary to identify the specific lesions of IRMA and VB, and not rely on H/MA alone, in order to differentiate moderate from severe nonproliferative diabetic retinopathy (NPDR).

Members of the Global Diabetic Retinopathy Project Group included retina specialists, comprehensive ophthalmologists, endocrinologists, and epidemiologists [7]. A modified nominal group technique or modified Delphi technique was utilized to evaluate the level of consensus regarding this initial clinical classification [13]. A 9-point rating scale was used, with 1 being strong disagreement and 9 being strong agreement. The results were aggregated mathematically to summarize the group results. To determine agreement and disagreement, a binomial distribution was applied. Depending on the number of participants, agreement was defined to exist if more than 80% rated within a 3-point range of 1–3, 4–6, and 7–9. Disagreement was defined as a 20% rate in the 7–9 range, and at least another 20% rate in the 1–3 range. Otherwise, agreement was rated as "equivocal" or "partial" (with many participants in the 4–6 range).

The most debated items in the discussions regarding the classification scheme included: (1) addition of a level of "no apparent retinopathy"; (2) determination of the extent of neovascularization required for a classification of "proliferative retinopathy"; (3) establishment of the lowest ETDRS level indicating "severe NPDR"; and (4) development of a grading scheme for DME. The results of the final ratings regarding the first three of these are presented in Figure 2.1. There was significant disagreement for including "no apparent retinopathy" and "minimal NPDR" in a single level (Fig. 2.1A). However, there was 100% agreement regarding the

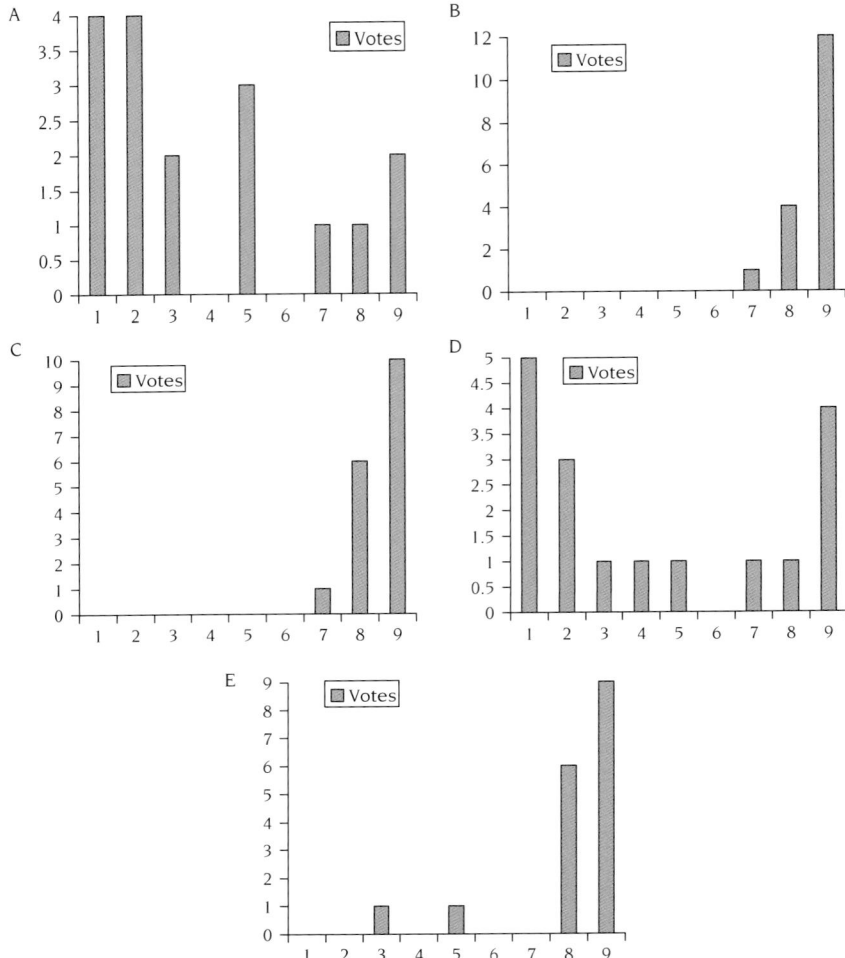

Figure 2.1. Participant votes for portions of the Diabetic Retinopathy Disease Severity Scale Employing the modified Delphi approach. Numbers 1–3 indicate levels of disagreement. Numbers 7–9 indicate levels of agreement. There were 17 voters. (A) Votes for including "No Retinopathy" and "Mild Retinopathy" as a single level. (B) Votes for including "No Retinopathy" as a single level. (C) Votes for any proliferation to be graded as "proliferative diabetic retinopathy." (D) Votes for including ETDRS level 47 in "Severe Retinopathy" Level. (E) Votes for *not* including ETDRS level 47 in "Severe Retinopathy" level.

desirability of including a single level for "no retinopathy" (Fig. 2.1B). There was also 100% agreement regarding a level for "PDR" that included all eyes with any neovascularization (Fig. 2.1C). However, a decision concerning whether or not to include ETDRS level 47 in the "severe NPDR" level was more controversial, and this ETDRS level was ultimately placed as the highest level in the "moderate NPDR" group (Figs. 2.1D and 2.1E). Regarding DME, there was significant agreement at all levels. High agreement was noted for levels of DME categorized as "apparently present" or "apparently absent" and for DME involving the fovea being designated in a separate level (assuming that examiner training and equipment allowed the location of edema to be documented). A minor degree of disagreement was noted in two subcategories of "apparently present" DME that did not involve the fovea. This was due primarily to the reality of the difficulties involved in assigning precise levels for stages that were admittedly difficult to specify.

The diabetic retinopathy disease severity levels are listed in Table 2.2 [7]. This consists of five scales with increasing severity of retinopathy. The first level is "no apparent retinopathy," and the absence of diabetic retinopathy is documented as a distinct first level. This designation of "no apparent retinopathy" was considered to be important in the care of patients with diabetes. Patients in particular may feel differently if they believe that they have no detectable signs of retinopathy than if definite retinopathy is detected. Although an examiner might miss one or two microaneurysms, if such a lesion is definitely detected, this indicates that retinopathy has begun, and this observation may make a difference to patients and their primary care physicians or endocrinologists.

The second level, "mild NPDR," includes ETDRS level 20 (microaneurysms only). The risk of significant progression over several years is very low in both this and the first group.

The third level, "moderate NPDR," includes eyes with ETDRS levels 35–47, and the risk of progression increases significantly by level 47, which is the reason that there was debate about placing level 47 in this third group (Fig. 2.1D).

The fourth level, "severe NPDR" (ETDRS stages 53 and higher), carries with it the most ominous prognosis for relatively rapid progression to PDR. The lower threshold for entry into this category was the presence of lesions consistent with the "4:2:1 rule" (Figs. 2.2–2.4). Continuing evaluations of ETDRS data have

Table 2.2. International Clinical Diabetic Retinopathy Disease Severity Scale [7]

Proposed Disease Severity Level	Findings Observable upon Dilated Ophthalmoscopy
No Apparent Retinopathy	No abnormalities
Mild Non-Proliferative Diabetic Retinopathy	• Microaneurysms only
Moderate Non-Proliferative Diabetic Retinopathy	• More than just microaneurysms but less than Severe NPDR
Severe Non-Proliferative Diabetic Retinopathy	Any of the following: • More than 20 intraretinal hemorrhages in each of 4 quadrants • Definite venous beading in 2+ quadrants • Prominent IRMA in 1+ quadrant And *no* signs of proliferative retinopathy
Proliferative Diabetic Retinopathy	One or more of the following: • Neovascularization • Vitreous/preretinal hemorrhage

demonstrated that severe NPDR can be identified reliably by the presence and severity of three retinopathy lesions. These include: four retinal quadrants containing extensive retinal hemorrhages (approximately 20 per quadrant) (Fig. 2.2), two quadrants containing definite significant VB (Fig. 2.3), or any single quadrant containing definite IRMA (Fig. 2.4). The workshop panel agreed that the 4:2:1 rule should remain the basis of classifying an eye as having "severe NPDR." Based on ETDRS data, 17% of eyes with this severity of retinopathy will develop ETDRS high-risk proliferative disease (HRPDR) within 1 year, and this rate increases to 44% within 3 years. The 1-year and 3-year rates for eyes with this severity of retinopathy developing any degree of PDR are 50% and 71%, respectively.

The fifth level, "PDR," includes all eyes with definite neovascularization. There was no attempt to subdivide this level as a function of ETDRS "high-risk characteristics," because significant rates of progression are expected to occur in all of these cases.

The DME Disease Severity Scale is listed in Table 2.3 [7]. The initial and most important designation is to separate the eyes with apparent DME from those with no apparent thickening or lipid in the macula. It was recognized that significant variation in examiner education and available equipment could make this grading relatively difficult, because many examiners would be employing direct ophthalmoscopy and, therefore, would not have the stereopsis necessary for a definitive diagnosis of retinal thickening in many cases. Thus, a two-tiered system was recommended. The initial decision is with regard to the presence or absence of apparent retinal thickening or lipid in the posterior pole. The ability to make the second level decision regarding thickening location will depend upon the ability of the examiner to document details related to the apparent DME. This may depend upon the equipment available to the examiner. These additional levels of DME are

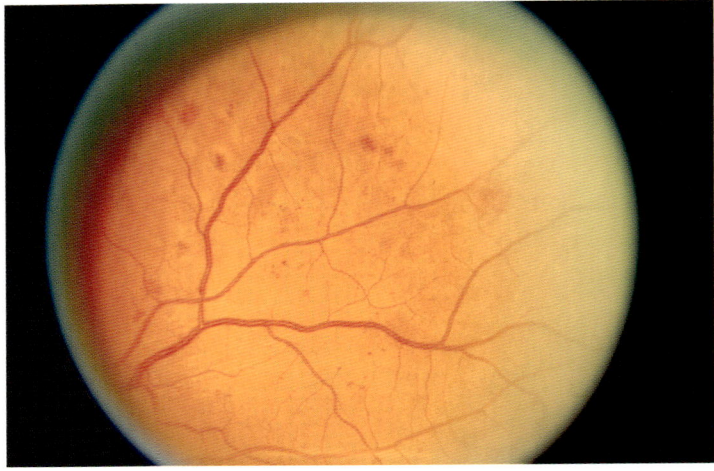

Figure 2.2. Early Treatment Diabetic Retinopathy Study standard photograph 2A. Hemorrhages and/or microaneurysms equaling or exceeding this severity in 4 quadrants indicates "Severe NPDR." (Source: Reprinted with permission from the Fundus Reading Center, Dept of Ophthalmology and Visual Sciences, University of Wisconsin, Madison, Wisconsin.)

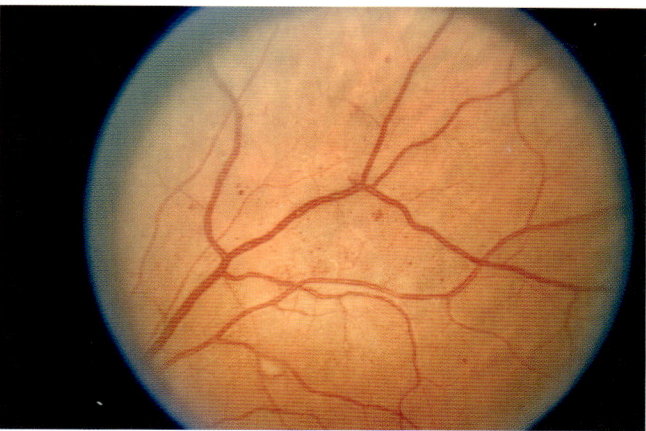

Figure 2.3. Early Treatment Diabetic Retinopathy Study standard photograph 6A. Venous beading equaling or exceeding this severity in 2 or more quadrants indicates "Severe NPDR." (Source: Reprinted with permission from the Fundus Reading Center, Dept of Ophthalmology and Visual Sciences, University of Wisconsin, Madison, Wisconsin.)

based on the distance of retinal thickening and/or lipid from the fovea. Eyes with obvious foveal involvement by edema or lipid are categorized as "severe DME." Eyes with edema and/or lipid relatively distant from the macula are graded as "mild DME." Although the term "moderate DME" was employed to identify cases in which retinal thickening and/or lipid are close to (or "threatening") the fovea, the specific distance from the fovea was deliberately not specified.

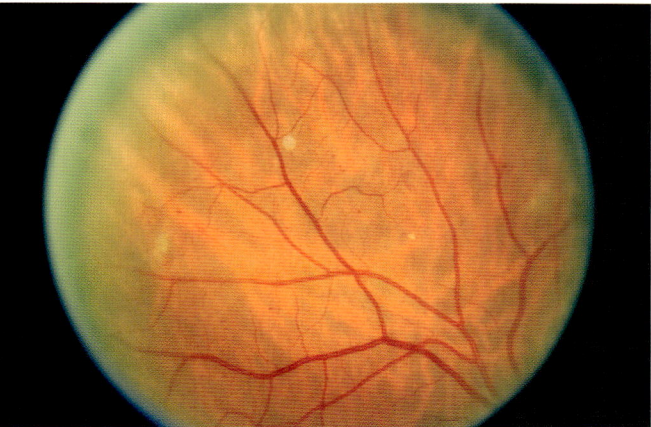

Figure 2.4. Early Treatment Diabetic Retinopathy Study standard photograph 8A. Intraretinal microvascular abnormalities equaling or exceeding this severity in one or more quadrants indicates "Severe NPDR." (Source: Reprinted with permission from the Fundus Reading Center, Dept of Ophthalmology and Visual Sciences, University of Wisconsin, Madison, Wisconsin.)

Table 2.3. International Clinical Diabetic Macular Edema Disease Severity Scale [7]

Proposed Disease Severity Level	Findings Observable Upon Dilated Ophthalmoscopy
Diabetic Macular Edema Apparently Absent	No apparent retinal thickening or hard exudates in posterior pole
Diabetic Macular Edema Apparently Present	Some apparent retinal thickening or hard exudates in posterior pole

If diabetic macular edema is present, it can be categorized as follows:

Proposed Disease Severity Level	Findings Observable Upon Dilated Ophthalmoscopy*
Diabetic Macular Edema Present	☐ Mild Diabetic Macular Edema
	Some retinal thickening or hard exudates in posterior pole but distant from the center of the macula
	☐ Moderate Diabetic Macular Edema
	Retinal thickening or hard exudates approaching the center of the macula but not involving the center
	☐ Severe Diabetic Macular Edema
	Retinal thickening or hard exudates involving the center of the macula

* Hard exudates are a sign of current or previous macular edema. Diabetic macular edema is defined as retinal thickening, and this requires a 3-dimensional assessment that is best performed by a dilated examination using slit-lamp biomicroscopy and/or stereo fundus photography.

CONCLUSIONS

The need to provide a framework for improved communication between the physicians' assistant, the primary care physician, endocrinologist, ophthalmologist, and other eye care providers was the major impetus to develop simplified clinical disease severity scales that could be employed internationally. This international clinical classification system is based on an evidence-based approach, particularly the findings of the ETDRS and the WESDR. Assessing these risks in various clinical settings can lead to appropriate clinical recommendations for follow-up or treatment.

The proposed clinical disease severity scale is intended to be a practical and valid method of grading severity of diabetic retinopathy and DME. It is recognized that examiner skills and equipment will vary widely around the world. Nevertheless, this system should allow observers to recognize and categorize levels of retinopathy and most DME. The identification of specific severity levels should result in more appropriate and consistent referrals to treatment centers. This system is not intended as a guide for treatment of diabetic retinopathy and DME. Although effective therapy for eyes with designated stages of NPDR, PDR, and DME was demonstrated in the DRS and ETDRS, the severity of these disorders may lead to somewhat different treatment and follow-up recommendations in different regions of the world, because specific practice patterns and health care delivery systems differ from country to country.

Although this staging system is intended primarily for comprehensive ophthalmologists and others with acquired skills necessary for evaluating the retina, it is hoped that this system will also allow better communication regarding retinopathy severity among all physicians and physician extenders caring for patients with diabetes. This improved communication should lead to more effective and consistent follow-up and better patient outcomes.

Implementation of this system will rely on its dissemination to ophthalmologists and other eye care providers, and it is also important that endocrinologists, diabetologists, and primary care physicians and physicians' assistants who care for patients with diabetes become familiar with these scales. Different localities and different structures for care will vary in approaches to implementation of care and will use different care providers and care delivery processes in managing patients with diabetes.

This scheme remains to be validated in appropriate studies. Hopefully, there will be processes to pilot test this system in a variety of local settings and to reevaluate its feasibility and utility in a variety of routine clinical environments around the world. As experience with the system is acquired, the reliability of the scales should be reevaluated. The classification scheme can be refined to maintain its currency as new developments occur in the management of diabetic retinopathy and DME.

ACKNOWLEDGMENTS

The author would like to thank the members of the Global Diabetic Retinopathy Project Group [7], and particularly Flora Lum, MD, for all of their efforts in developing the diabetic retinopathy disease severity scale.

REFERENCES

1. King, H, Aubert, RE, Herman, WH. Global burden of diabetes, 1995–2025: prevalence, numerical estimates, and projections. *Diabetes Care.* 1998;1998:1414–1431.
2. Fong DS, Aiello LP, Ferris FL, et al. Diabetic retinopathy. *Diabetes Care.* 2004; 27:2340–2553.
3. UK Prospective Diabetes Study (UKPDS) Group. Risks of progression of retinopathy and vision loss related to tight blood pressure control in type 2 diabetes mellitus. *Arch Ophthalmol.* 2004;122:1631–1640.
4. American Academy of Ophthalmology. *Diabetic Retinopathy Preferred Practice Pattern.* San Francisco: American Academy of Ophthalmology; 2008.
5. Diabetic Retinopathy Study Research Group. A modification of the Airlie House classification of diabetic retinopathy. Report 7. *Invest Ophthalmol Vis Sci.* 1981;21:210–226.
6. Javitt JC, Aiello LP, Bassi LP, et al. Detecting and treating retinopathy in patients with type I diabetes. Savings associated with improved implementation of current guidelines. *Ophthalmology.* 1991;98:1565–1573.

7. Wilkinson CP, Ferris FL III, Klein RE, et al. Proposed international clinical diabetic retinopathy and diabetic macular edema disease severity scales. *Ophthalmology.* 2003;110:1677–1682.

8. Fukuda M. Clinical arrangement of classification of diabetic retinopathy. *Tohoku J Exp Med.* 1983;141(Suppl):331–335.

9. Verdaguer TJ.Screening para retinopatia en latin America. *Rev Soc Brasil Retina Vitreo.* 2001;4:14–15.

10. National Health and Medical Research Council. *Clinical Practice Guidelines: Management of Diabetic Retinopathy.* Canberra: NHMRC; 1997.

11. Klein RE, Klein BE, Moss SE, et al. The Wisconsin Epidemiologic Study of Diabetic Retinopathy. IX. Four-year incidence and progression of diabetic retinopathy when age at diagnosis is less than 30 years. *Arch Ophthalmol.* 1989;107:237–243.

12. Klein RE, Klein BE, Moss SE, et al. The Wisconsin Epidemiologic Study of Diabetic Retinopathy. X. Four-year incidence and progression of diabetic retinopathy when age at diagnosis is 30 years or more. *Arch Ophthalmol.* 1989;107:244–249.

13. Shekelle PG, Kahan JP, Bernstein SJ, et al. The reproducibility of a method to identify the overuse and underuse of medical procedures. *N Engl J Med.* 1998;338:1888–1895.

3

Histopathology of Diabetic Retinopathy

MATTHEW GUESS, MD,
AND SANDER R. DUBOVY, MD

CORE MESSAGES

- The mechanisms that lead to the histopathologic changes in diabetes mellitus are complex and likely secondary to metabolic dysregulation including chronic hyperglycemia.
- Nonproliferative diabetic retinopathy (NPDR) describes intraretinal microvascular changes including basement membrane thickening, pericyte loss, microaneurysm formation, venous caliber abnormalities and intraretinal microvascular abnormalities (IRMAs).
- The vascular changes may lead to macular edema, hard exudate formation, cotton wool spots (microinfarctions), and intraretinal hemorrhages.
- Proliferative diabetic retinopathy (PDR) describes growth of new blood vessels at the optic nerve head, neovascularization of the disc (NVD) or on the surface of the retina, neovascularization elsewhere (NVE) that may lead to hemorrhage, vitreous traction, macular distortion, and retinal detachment.
- Other histopathologic changes in diabetes mellitus include cataract formation, recurrent corneal erosions, basement membrane thickening of the choroid and pigmented ciliary epithelium, rubeosis iridis and lacy vacuolization of the iris.

Chronic hyperglycemia appears to be the most important factor in promoting the microvascular changes in diabetic retinopathy, which include basement membrane thickening, pericyte loss, capillary closure, and neovascularization. Diabetic retinopathy can be grouped into two categories: nonproliferative and proliferative. Nonproliferative diabetic retinopathy (NPDR) involves intraretinal changes that may include microaneurysm formation, hemorrhage, cotton wool spots, exudates, microvascular abnormalities, venous caliber abnormalities, and macular edema. Proliferative diabetic retinopathy (PDR) describes both intraretinal pathology as well as neovascular changes that extend beyond the internal limiting membrane of the retina and may extend along the surface of the disc and retina or may be elevated by partial posterior vitreous detachment. Proliferative disease may lead to retinal detachment, preretinal hemorrhage, and neovascular glaucoma. The cornea, ciliary body, crystalline lens, and retinal glia may also be affected in patients with diabetes mellitus. In this chapter, the ocular histopathological changes of diabetes mellitus will be reviewed.

MECHANISM OF DIABETIC RETINOPATHY

The mechanisms that lead to the histopathologic changes in diabetes mellitus are complex and are likely secondary to dysregulation of a number of metabolic pathways. These include the polyol pathway, the formation of advanced glycosylation end products (AGEs), the pathological activation of protein kinase C (PKC), and increased oxidative stress by free radicals [1].

The polyol pathway, which becomes activated with high glucose levels, may lead to early changes in the retinal vasculature including loss of vascular pericytes and thickening of the basement membrane [2]. High intracellular levels of glucose may saturate the normal pathway and shunt the remaining glucose into the aldose reductase pathway. Aldose reductase reduces glucose to sorbitol and uses nicotinamide adenine dinucleotide phosphate (NADPH) as a cofactor. Sorbitol is then oxidized to fructose via sorbitol dehydrogenase with NAD(+) used as a cofactor. The overproduction of NADPH and increase in the NADH/NAD ratio is thought to alter enzyme activities and contribute to the formation of reactive metabolites that may lead to cellular dysfunction and damage [3]. Subsequent cellular dysfunction may cause pericyte loss [4–8] and basement membrane thickening [7,9]. While the use of an aldose reductase inhibitor has been proposed to reduce the formation of sorbitol and slow the progression of, or even prevent, diabetic retinopathy, studies have demonstrated mixed results. Aldose reductase inhibitors have been shown to prevent thickening of basement membrane in the retinal vessels in galactosemic and diabetic rats [10], while no benefit was shown in preventing or slowing retinopathy in a randomized clinical trial of sorbinil (aldose reductase inhibitor) in type 1 diabetic patients [7].

AGEs form as a result of the nonenzymatic glycation of intracellular and extracellular proteins and lipids. AGE formation is directly related to the amount and duration of hyperglycemia. Mild increases in glucose concentration have been shown to produce large increases in AGE accumulation [11]. AGEs alter the function of basement membrane matrix components including type IV collagen and laminin. AGEs interact with type IV collagen and inhibit the lateral association of these molecules into a network-like structure. Effects on laminin include decreased binding to type IV collagen and decreased self-assembly [12]. Alterations to the matrix components are thought to account for the thickening in the basement membranes of tissues seen in diabetic patients. AGEs alter the cellular function by binding to the receptors for advanced glycosylation end products (RAGEs) [13,14].

Ligand binding of AGE-specific receptors on endothelial cells increases coagulation factors (factors IX and X) [14], decreases anticoagulation factors (thrombomodulin) [14], and induces vasoconstrictive factors (endothelin-1) [15], which may lead to vasoconstriction and thrombosis in the setting of AGEs. AGEs may also alter DNA and the nuclear proteins of cells by nonenzymatic modification with resultant altered gene expression [16]. AGEs increase the extraluminal accumulation of plasma proteins including low density lipoproteins by chemically binding to reactive AGE precursors of matrix proteins [17,18]. These alterations caused by AGEs have been proposed to be responsible for the pathological changes seen in diabetic retinopathy [19].

Aminoguanidine, an AGE formation inhibitor, has been tested in animal models to evaluate the role of AGEs in the formation of diabetic retinopathy. Treatment with aminoguanidine for 26 weeks in diabetic rats prevented endothelial cell proliferation and reduced pericyte dropout when compared with controls. After 75 weeks, treated rats had an 80% reduction in the number of acellular capillaries and had no microaneurysm formation [20]. In addition, blockage of RAGEs has been shown to inhibit the AGE-induced impairment of endothelial barrier function and reverse the early vascular hyperpermeability seen in diabetic rats [21].

Free radical production is increased in states of hyperglycemia through oxidative phosphorylation and glucose autoxidation [22]. Reactive oxygen species are thought to contribute to some of the manifestations of diabetic retinopathy. [23–26].

PKC and diacylglycerol (DAG) are intracellular signaling molecules responsible for vascular functions including permeability, vasodilator release, endothelial activation, and growth factor signaling. PKC and DAG activation is increased in animal models with diabetes [27] and activated PKC may lead to vascular damage, increased growth factor expression and signaling, which has been proposed to account for the pathological changes seen in diabetic retinopathy [28–30].

The proposed pathways described above lead to alterations in gene expression and protein function, which may then manifest as cellular dysfunction with the resultant vascular changes seen in diabetes. While the relative roles of the different pathways is not clear, it is likely that the combined or interactive effects of all of these pathways may be responsible for the changes seen in diabetic retinopathy.

Nonproliferative Diabetic Retinopathy. NPDR describes intraretinal microvascular changes, which include basement membrane thickening, pericyte loss, microaneurysm formation, venous caliber abnormalities, and intraretinal microvascular abnormalities (IRMAs). The vascular changes may lead to macular edema, hard exudate formation, cotton-wool spots (soft exudates), and intraretinal hemorrhages. In the Early Treatment Diabetic Retinopathy Study (ETDRS), NPDR has been categorized as mild, moderate, severe, and very severe. Mild NPDR is defined as the presence of one microaneurysm, but hemorrhages and microaneurysms are less than ETDRS standard photograph 2A in all four retinal quadrants. There is no evidence of moderate, severe, or very severe disease. Moderate NPDR is defined as the presence of hemorrhages and/or microaneurysms greater than those pictured in ETDRS standard photograph 2A in at least one field but less than four retinal quadrants. Cotton-wool spots, venous beading, and IRMAs are present to a mild degree. Severe NPDR is present when there is hemorrhage/microaneurysms greater than standard photo 2A in four quadrants or venous caliber abnormalities in two or more quadrants or IRMAs greater than standard photo 8A in at least one quadrant. Very severe NPDR is present when eyes have two or more lesions of severe NPDR, but no neovascularization [31].

Early Histological Changes. The earliest changes in the retinal vasculature include pericyte loss and basement membrane thickening in the retinal microcirculation (Fig. 3.1) which occur before any clinical evidence of disease is present. The capillaries in the retina are composed of a lumen surrounded by a layer of endothelial cells with a basement membrane and a surrounding layer of intramural pericytes enclosed within the basement membrane. In the microcirculation of the retina, there are approximately equal numbers of endothelial cells and pericytes present in the capillary wall [32]. Pericyte loss and basement membrane thickening are two early histopathological changes that occur in the microcirculation of the retina in diabetic retinopathy.

Pericyte Loss. Pericytes are contractile cells that are responsible for blood flow regulation and have been shown in culture to contract in response to various stimulants [33–36]. In addition, pericytes appear to be necessary for the maintenance

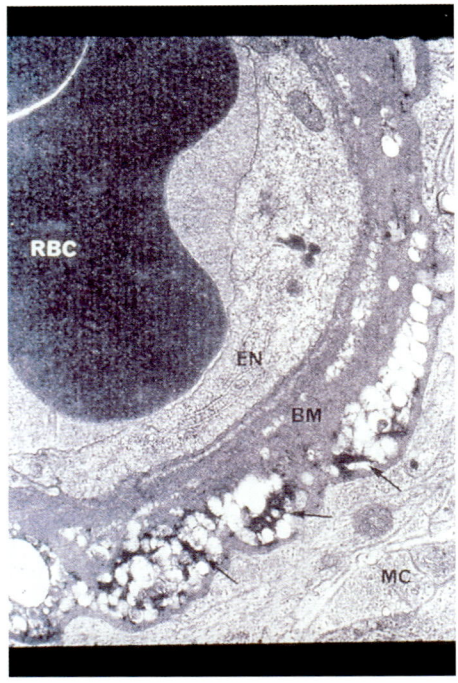

Figure 3.1. Electron micrograph demonstrating thickening of the basement membrane of the blood vessel wall. (Source: Courtesy W. Richard Green, MD.)

of normal growth and repair of the endothelial cells in the retinal vascular system [37]. Selective loss of intramural pericytes with a decreased ratio of intramural pericytes to endothelial cells occurs in the capillaries of the retina in patients with diabetic retinopathy [32,38–42]. Loss of pericytes leaves empty dropout spaces in the capillary wall that are referred to as pericyte "ghosts." Pericyte loss is only detectable by histological examination, and cannot be seen clinically.

Basement Membrane Thickening. Basement membrane is composed primarily of type IV collagen. Thickening of the vascular basement membrane is seen early in the course of patients with diabetes mellitus. Experimental studies in rats [43] and dogs [44] have shown that a high galactose diet can induce basement membrane thickening with striated collagen deposition. Clinical evidence has shown that basement membrane thickening is directly related to hyperglycemia and can be reversed with good diabetic control [45]. Increased synthesis of basement membrane with decreased turnover appears to be the cause of the thickening [46]. Decreased proteoglycan content is present in association with the thickening, which reduces the electrical charge barrier function and increases the membrane permeability [46,47]. The increase in membrane permeability may lead to the increased vascular permeability and the extravasation of intravascular fluid seen in diabetic retinopathy.

Microaneurysms. An early clinical manifestation of diabetic retinopathy is microaneurysm formation. Microaneurysms are dilations of the capillaries, terminal arterioles, or small venules caused by proliferation and outpouching of the capillary endothelium in areas of intramural pericyte loss [38,48]. These microaneurysms are located most often on the venous side, range in size from 25 to 100 microns in diameter, and are found in the posterior fundus, especially temporal to the macula [49]. Clinically, they appear as tiny red dots in the retina. The color is initially red because the wall of the microaneurysm is transparent and the red blood cells give the aneurysm a red hue. Over time, the wall of the microaneurysm thickens, becomes less transparent and may appear orange to yellow-white in color [50]. They may increase and decrease in number over time [51] secondary to the development of new aneurysms and the obliteration of some of the aneurysms by endothelial proliferation.

Microaneurysms are often difficult to identify through the ophthalmoscope and may be visualized best using fluorescein angiography. There are two types of aneurysms: saccular and fusiform (Fig. 3.2A and B). Saccular aneurysms involve the dilation of all sides of the vessel wall and fusiform aneurysms involve dilation of only one side of the vessel wall. An increase in the number of these microaneurysms in the retina is associated with progression of retinopathy [52–54]. When the number of microaneurysms in an eye exceeds 10, fluorescein angiography usually shows capillary abnormalities including dilation, nonperfusion, and leakage from capillaries or microaneurysms [55]. The microaneurysms occur adjacent to acellular capillaries and a proposed shunt theory suggests that the loss of pericytes leads to dilation of the capillaries and preemption of blood flow with secondary atrophy and obliteration of adjacent capillaries [56]. Other theories suggest that

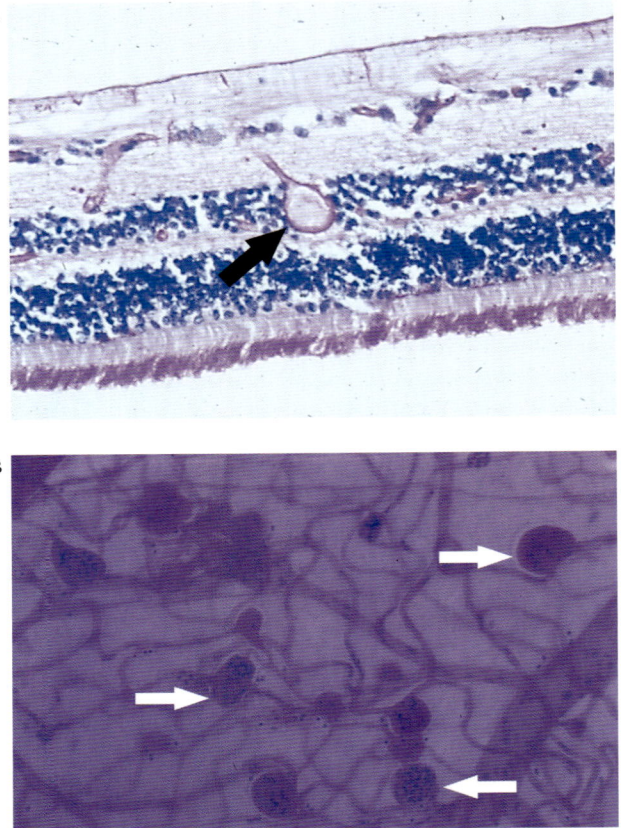

Figure 3.2. (A) A capillary microaneurysm is present that is dilated with a thinned wall (arrow) (Source: Courtesy W. Richard Green, MD.) (B) Capillary microaneurysms are present as saccular dilatations in the trypsin digest preparation. (Source: Courtesy W. Richard Green, MD.)

microaneurysm formation is a result of the net effects of pericyte loss and vascular endothelial growth factor (VEGF)-induced endothelial proliferation. Obstruction and occlusion of retinal vessels may occur secondary to the proliferation of endothelium into the lumen [57,58] with resultant ischemia of the adjacent retina.

Intraretinal microvascular abnormalities. IRMAs (Fig. 3.3) refer to shunt vessels and neovascularization within the neural retina located in areas of dilated capillaries and retinal nonperfusion [59,60] that may be associated with leakage, hard exudates, and hemorrhage [61]. IRMAs is a nonspecific term that was given to avoid the controversy of whether new tortuous, hypercellular retinal vessels in areas of occluded capillaries and nonperfused retina represent either retinal neovascularization, aberrant forms of aneurysms, or preexisting vessels that became dilated "shunts" in areas of nonperfusion [61,62]. Histologically, IRMAs have been described as thin-walled dilated vessels in the inner retina composed of endothelium with a thickened basement membrane and a decreased number of surrounding pericytes [63].

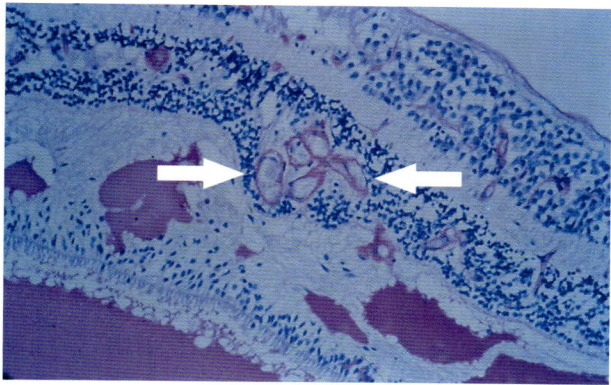

Figure 3.3. Intraretinal microvascular abnormalities: An area of intraretinal neovascularization with proliferation of blood vessels (arrows). (Source: Courtesy W. Richard Green, MD.)

Macular Edema. Macular edema develops secondary to microaneurysm formation, breakdown of the blood-retinal barrier, increased vascular permeability and leakage of fluid and exudate. It is the principal mechanism of vision loss in patients with NPDR. In the ETDRS, macular edema is defined as retinal thickening from accumulation of fluid within one disc diameter of the macula [64,65]. Macular edema is defined as clinically significant macular edema (CSME) if any of the following three features are present: (1) thickening of the retina at or within 500 microns of the center of the macula; (2) hard exudates at or within 500 microns of the center of the macula, if associated with thickening of the adjacent retina; or (3) a zone or zones of retinal thickening 1 disc area or larger, any part of which is within 1 disc diameter of the center of the macula [66] (Fig. 3.4A).

The incidence of macular edema over a 10-year period has been estimated at 20.1% of patients with type 1 diabetes, 25.4% of patients with type 2 diabetes who require insulin, and 13.9% of patients with type 2 diabetes who do not require insulin [67]. The fluid is composed of water, protein, and lipid material and often collects in the outer plexiform layer of the parafoveal region because more distension can occur in this area of the retina due to the anatomical configuration (Fig. 3.4B) [49]. The water and protein component of the exudates is absorbed by blood vessels and the retinal pigment epithelium, which leads to deposition of lipid-rich material in the outer plexiform layer [49] seen clinically as hard exudates. Hard exudates appear as well-defined yellowish-white intraretinal deposits at the border of edematous and nonedematous areas of the retina [68]. They typically form in clusters and may form a circinate pattern adjacent to groups of microaneurysms. A macular star pattern develops when these hard exudates form in a circinate pattern around the fovea. The exudates are composed of extracellular lipid-rich deposits consisting primarily of polyunsaturated fats [49]. In the ETDRS, it was determined that elevated serum lipid levels were associated with an increased risk of retinal hard exudate in persons with diabetic retinopathy [69]. Chronic macular edema may progress to macular retinoschisis and partial or complete macular hole formation [70].

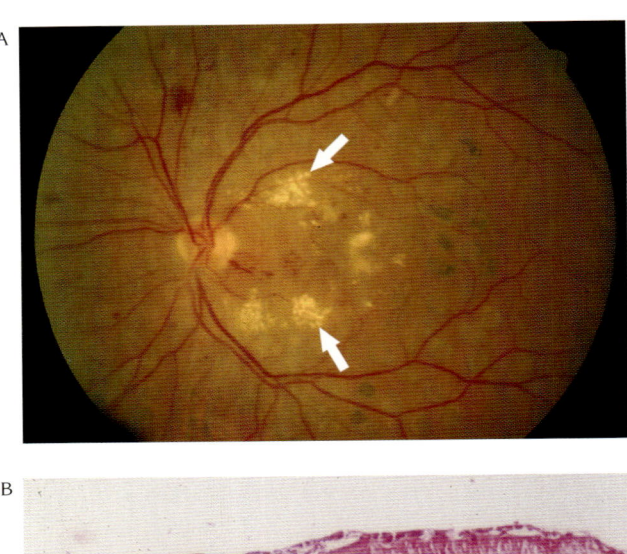

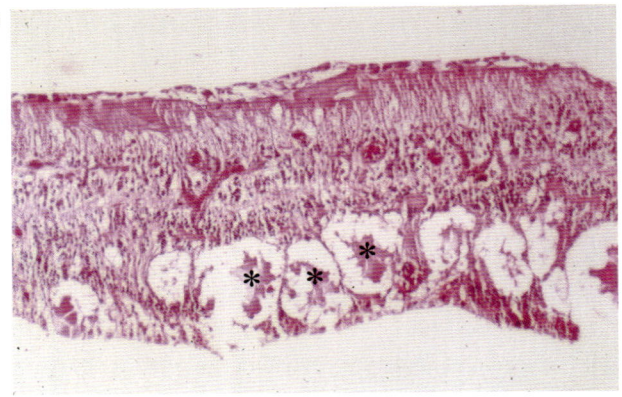

Figure 3.4. (A) Yellow material (hard exudates) is present within the posterior pole (arrows). (B) Proteinaceous material is present in the outer plexiform layer corresponding to that seen grossly (asterisk).

Intraretinal Hemorrhages. Intraretinal hemorrhages are an early sign of NPDR and are the result of ruptured microaneurysms, leaking capillaries, and IRMAs. The two types of hemorrhages that may be seen are dot-blot hemorrhages and flame-shaped hemorrhages (Fig. 3.5A–C). Dot-blot hemorrhages occur in the inner plexiform, inner nuclear, and outer plexiform layer and appear round because the cellular architecture in these areas runs perpendicular to the retinal surface. Flame-shaped hemorrhages occur in the nerve fiber layer and appear in this configuration because the nerve fiber layer runs parallel to the surface of the retina. The red blood cells may break through the internal limiting membrane and form preretinal or intravitreal hemorrhages [71,72].

Cotton-wool Spots (Soft Exudates). Cotton-wool spots are microinfarctions of the nerve fiber layer that appear clinically as gray and semiopaque lesions with poorly circumscribed, feathery edges (Fig. 3.6A). They frequently have striations running parallel to the nerve fiber layer and occur around blood vessels. The lesions were

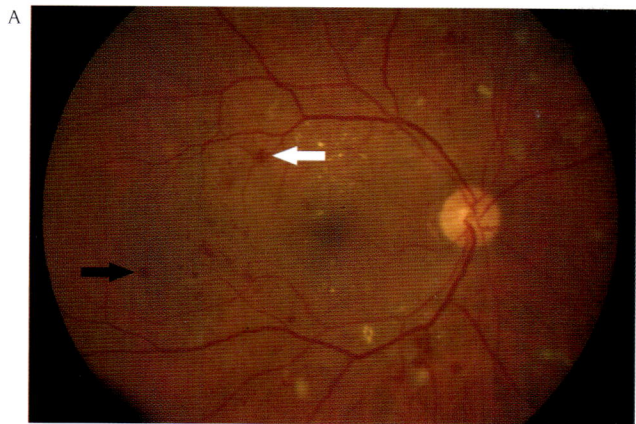

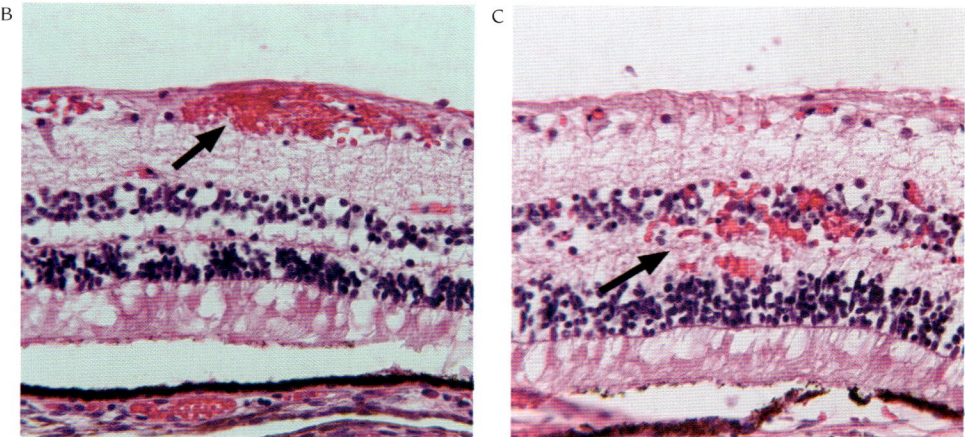

Figure 3.5. (A) Retinal hemorrhage. Fundus photograph demonstrates a flame-shaped hemorrhage (white arrow) and a dot-blot hemorrhage (black arrow). (B) The retinal hemorrhage is present in the nerve fiber layer which appears clinically as a flame-shaped hemorrhage. (C) Retinal hemorrhage is present in the outer plexiform and surrounding nuclear layers corresponding to a dot-blot hemorrhage seen clinically.

first observed microscopically as cellular appearing bodies with a "psuedonucleus" in the nerve fiber layer and given the name cytoid bodies [73–77]. They represent swollen nerve endings in the areas of ischemia. The swollen nerve endings are caused by the accumulation of cytoplasmic debris due to the interruption of axoplasmic flow [78] (Fig. 3.6B). Cotton-wool spots are not specific to diabetic retinopathy and can occur in a variety of disease processes, including systemic hypertension, retinal vein occlusions, and acquired immunodeficiency syndrome (AIDS) [79,80].

Venous Caliber Abnormalities. Venous caliber abnormalities in patients with diabetic retinopathy include venous dilation, venous beading, and venous loop formation. Venous dilation is a functional change in response to hyperglycemia and can

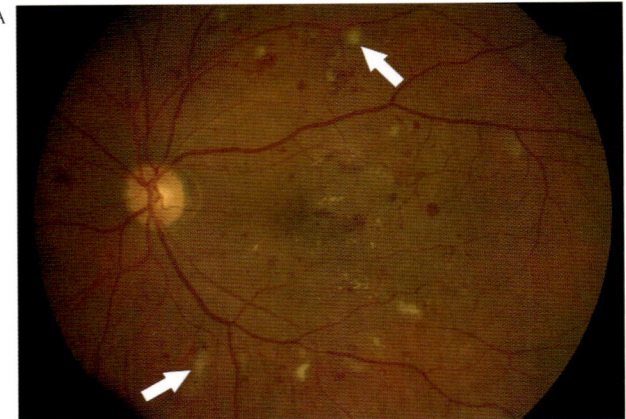

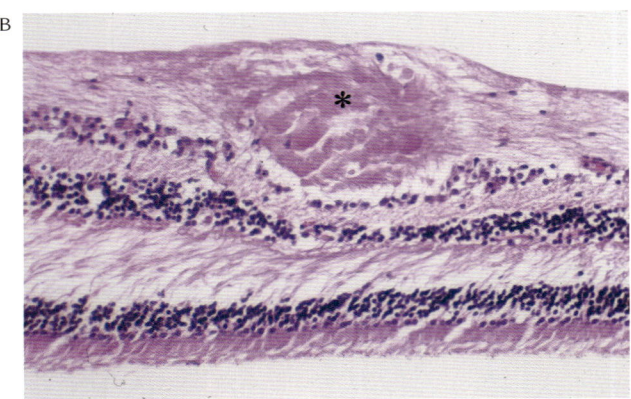

Figure 3.6. (A) Cotton wool spots are present throughout the fundus (arrows). (B) Micro-infarction of the nerve fiber layer is present with swelling, thickening, and cytoid body formation (asterisk).

be reversed by a return to normoglycemia [81]. In the hyperglycemic state, retinal blood flow is increased and oxygen autoregulation decreases. Increasing impairment of autoregulation correlates with increasing severity of diabetic retinopathy [82,83], which may explain venous dilation. Venous loops almost always form adjacent to large areas of capillary nonperfusion and may form secondary to focal vitreous contraction [84]. Venous beading describes focal dilation of the venous retinal vessel, is a sign of severe NPDR, and may occur in the setting of capillary closure and IRMAs.

Proliferative Diabetic Retinopathy. PDR occurs superimposed on nonproliferative retinal changes and is defined clinically as the presence of vitreous or preretinal hemorrhage, neovascularization of the disc (NVD) and/or neovascularization elsewhere (NVE). As defined by the diabetic retinopathy study (DRS) and ETDRS, NVD is new vessel or fibrous proliferation on or within one disc area of the optic nerve head (Fig. 3.7). NVE is defined as new vessel growth on the retina in locations greater than one disc area from the optic nerve head [31] (Fig. 3.8).

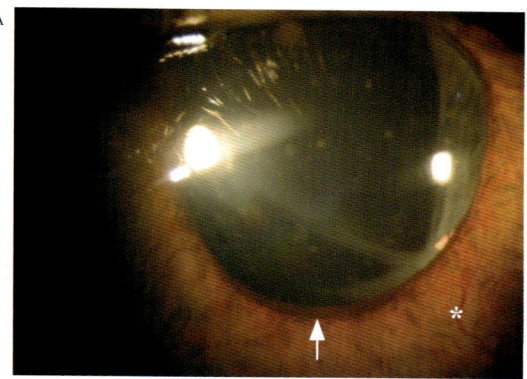

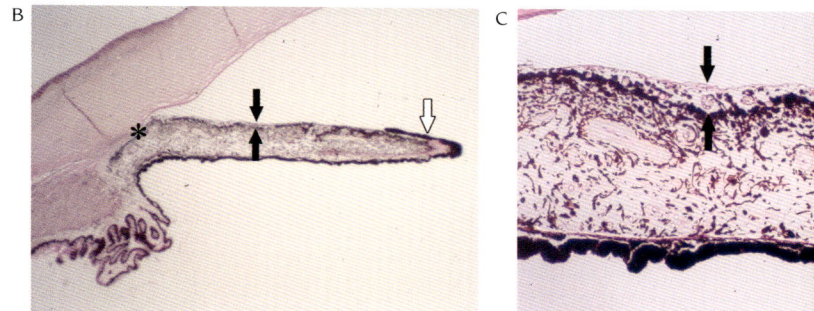

Figure 3.7. (A) Rubeosis iridis: slit lamp photograph discloses proliferation of blood vessels on the surface of the retina (asterisk) and ectropion uveae (arrow). (B) Proliferation of blood vessels on the surface of the iris (black arrows), with adherence between the peripheral iris and cornea (angle closure, asterisk), contraction of the neovascular tissue with resultant rotation of the iris pigment epithelium anteriorly (ectropion uveae, white arrow). (C) High power of the neovascular proliferation on the surface of the iris (arrows).

Proliferative retinopathy may occur in up to 50% of patients with type 1 diabetes [85] and 10% of patients with type 2 diabetes [86] who have had the disease for at least 15 years. The new vessels are seen most frequently in the posterior fundus, within 45 degrees of the optic disc [87,88], grow into the vitreous cavity perpendicular to the retina and have been shown to arise from the superficial veins and venules in the retinal vasculature [89]. The new vessels may grow in a carriage wheel configuration with new vessels forming a network and radiating peripherally to an encircling vessel. New vessels may also grow in irregular networks or grow across the retina for several disc diameters without forming networks. The rate of growth of these new vessels is variable with some patches of vessels showing no change over many months while the growth of other vessels may occur over a period of weeks. New vessels follow a pattern of proliferation and partial to complete regression [87,90]. Vessel regression in a carriage pattern of vessels begins with a decrease in the caliber and number of blood vessels in the center of the network, which is followed by replacement with fibrous tissue. The vessels in the periphery of the network tend to narrow while at the same time may increase in

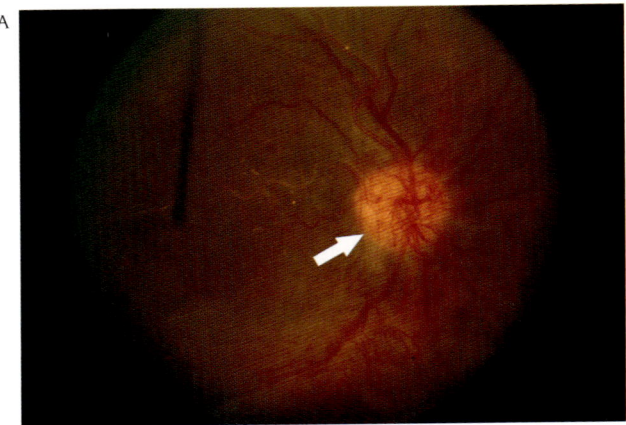

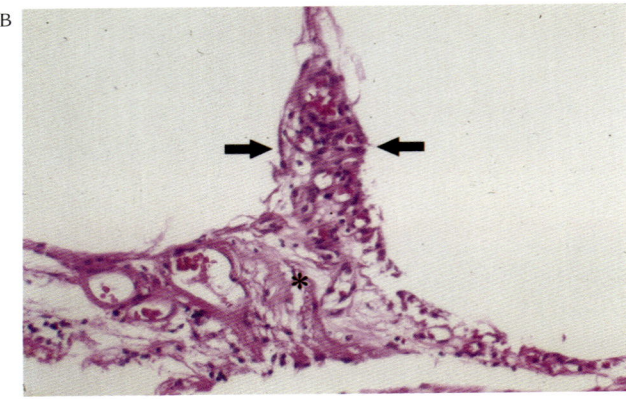

Figure 3.8. (A) Neovascularization of the disc: Proliferation of new blood vessels on the surface of the optic nerve (arrow). (B) Proliferation of immature blood vessels (between arrows) arising from the surface of the optic nerve head (asterisk).

length. New vessels may emanate from regressing vessels and vessel growth may be at different stages in different areas of the eye. Vessel sheathing may occur, which represents thickening of the vessel wall [91].

The risk of developing PDR is greatest in patients with severe NPDR. The features of severe NPDR may not be present when preretinal neovascularization is recognized because of the transient nature of the retinal lesions. Cotton-wool spots may disappear in 6 to 12 months and after extensive capillary closure, blot hemorrhages, and IRMAs may disappear. This clinical picture is called a featureless retina.

The cause for the vascular proliferation in diabetic retinopathy appears to be ischemia of the inner retinal layers secondary to closure of segments of the retinal capillary system [62,92–95] with subsequent production of vessel stimulating growth factors by the ischemic retina [93,95–97]. One vessel stimulating growth factor currently being studied is VEGF. VEGF is a group of proteins that initiates angiogenesis and increases permeability at blood–tissue barriers. VEGF is produced by the retina, choroid, and retinal pigment epithelium [98] and levels of VEGF are greatly increased in the aqueous and vitreous fluid of persons with diabetic retinopathy [99].

Vessel proliferation into the vitreous cavity first occurs with proliferating endothelium in the absence of accompanying intramural pericytes. Fibrosis, composed of fibrocytes and glial cells [100,101] later forms around the newly formed vessels. The new blood vessels have a propensity to rupture and cause vitreous hemorrhage, because of their delicate structure [102,103], lack of surrounding support [102] and traction placed on these vessels by surrounding fibrous tissue [90]. If the hemorrhage occurs in the subhyaloid space (between the vitreous and the retina) it may assume a boat shape with a rounded bottom and horizontal fluid level. Hemorrhage into the vitreous may remain localized or diffuse throughout the vitreous cavity. Scarring with shrinkage of the surrounding fibrotic tissue may occur and place traction on the vitreous and retina. This traction may cause a partial posterior vitreous detachment, which normally begins near the posterior pole in the region of the superotemporal vessels, temporal to the macula, and above and below the optic disc [87]. In addition, traction may lead to cystic degeneration of the retina and retinoschisis. Contraction of the fibrovascular tissue may also cause distortion of the macula, displacement of the macula, or macular holes by putting tangential traction on the retina and pulling it toward the area of fibrosis. A retinal detachment can result if the vitreous traction occurs in the area of new vessel formation and the retina is pulled with the new vessels and fibrotic material in a direction perpendicular to, and away from, the retinal pigment epithelium [50]. If contraction does not occur, new vessels can grow and regress without causing any visual disturbances to the patient [91]. With complete vitreous detachment from all areas of the retina, PDR may enter the burned-out, or involutional stage, which is characterized by vascular attenuation, optic nerve pallor, pigmentary dispersion, and replacement of neovascularization by avascular glial cells [104].

Other Diabetic Ocular Changes. The crystalline lens of diabetics may undergo cataractous changes. It has been demonstrated that there is an accumulation of sorbitol in diabetic lenses and may lead to an osmotic swelling of the lens and subsequent cataract formation [105]. In addition, sorbitol accumulation may damage the lens epithelium. Transient myopia in diabetics during periods of hyperglycemia is thought to be secondary to the osmotic swelling of the lens [106].

Corneal sensitivity and corneal epithelium adherence may be reduced in the setting of diabetes mellitus. Recurrent corneal erosions often develop in persons with diabetes. This may be due to a reduced adhesion of the epithelium to the basement membrane [107] secondary to decreased penetration of anchoring fibrils from the corneal epithelial basement membrane into the corneal stroma [108–110].

Involvement of the choriocapillaris may occur in diabetes. Basement membrane material of the choroidal vessels may thicken and may obliterate the lumen of vessels in the choriocapillaris [111]. The basement membrane of the pigmented ciliary epithelium may also become diffusely thickened [112] (Fig. 3.9).

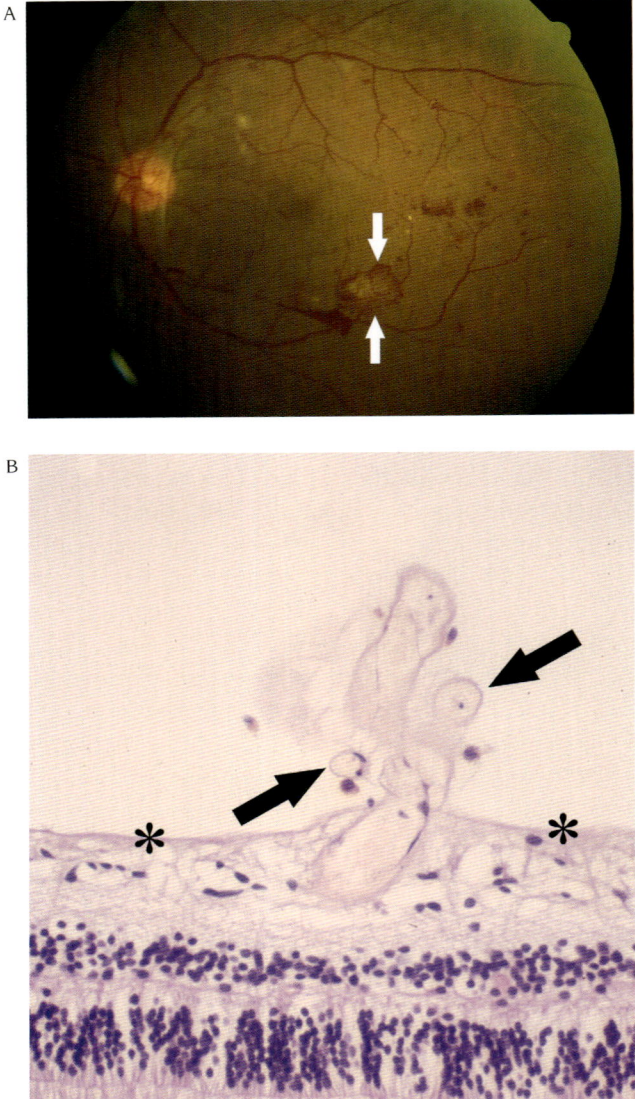

Figure 3.9. (A) Neovascularization elsewhere (NVE): Proliferation of blood vessels on the surface of the retina (arrow). (B) Proliferation of blood vessels through the internal limiting membrane (asterisks) onto the surface of the retina (arrows).

Neovascularization may occur along the anterior border of the iris in diabetics and is referred to as rubeosis iridis (Fig. 3.10A). The new vessel growth is thought to be initiated by vascular growth factors from the ischemic retina and these new vessels may arise from anywhere along the anterior iris border. Iris neovascularization is associated with significant retinal ischemia [113]. Neovascularization that involves the anterior chamber angle may cause a secondary open-angle glaucoma when the neovascular tissue blocks the outflow of aqueous through the trabecular meshwork and may progress to a closed-angle glaucoma caused by the formation of peripheral anterior synechiae. In addition, the neovascular tissue may cause the pupillary border of the iris to turn anteriorly and develop an ectropion uveae configuration (Fig. 3.10B and C). This is due to shrinkage of the neovascular membrane with traction placed on the iris pigment epithelium and subsequent pulling of the epithelium around the pupillary border [114]. Lacy

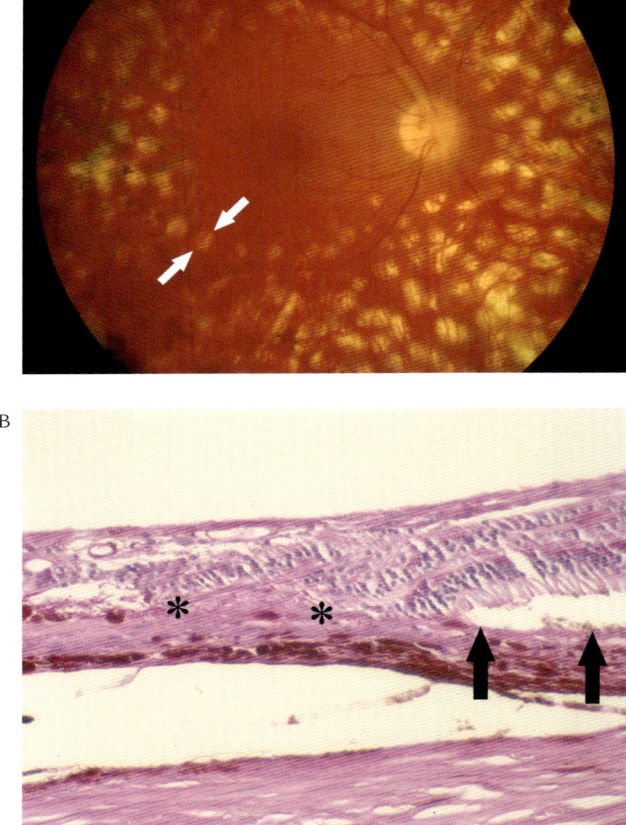

Figure 3.10. (A) Panretinal photocoagulation scars: gray white spots secondary to argon laser photocoagulation (arrow). (B) Intact outer retina (arrows) adjacent to an area of laser photocoagulation demonstrating loss of the inner choroid, retinal pigment epithelium, and scarring and gliosis of the outer neural retina (asterisk).

vacuolization, which is glycogen-containing vacuoles within the iris pigment epithelium, may occur in diabetic eyes. It is highly characteristic of diabetes mellitus although it may be seen in glycogen storage diseases [115–117]. If the vacuoles are manipulated during anterior chamber surgery, iris pigment epithelium may be released into the posterior chamber (so-called Schwarz-wasser or black water), and may be seen as pigment flowing through the pupil into the anterior chamber.

Macroglial and neuronal cells are also altered in diabetic retinopathy. Macroglial cells include astrocytes and Muller cells. These cells are responsible for integrating neuronal and vascular activity of the retina. Glial fibrillary acidic protein (GFAP) production is decreased in the astrocytes [118,119] and increased in the Muller cells [120] of patients with diabetes mellitus. These changes indicate that the macroglial cells, responsible for maintaining the blood-retinal barriers, have disrupted activity in diabetes. Neuronal cells, which include photoreceptors, bipolar, amacrine, and ganglion cells, are directly affected in diabetes. Retinal ganglion cells and inner nuclear layer cells degenerate by apoptosis early in the course of diabetes mellitus [121]. Color vision and contrast sensitivity are reduced in diabetics [122] and there is a reduction in the oscillatory potential of the electroretinogram (ERG) [123] sometimes before the onset of visible microvascular lesions [124].

TREATMENT

Treatment for macular edema and PDR includes the use of laser photocoagulation. The laser light is absorbed by the retinal pigment epithelium leading to coagulation of the retinal pigment epithelium, choriocapillaris, and outer segments of the photoreceptors (Fig. 3.11). The amount of coagulation is dependent on the amount of laser energy delivered. Endothelial cells in the retinal vessels have been shown to absorb the laser, which causes proliferation of these cells [125,126]. A

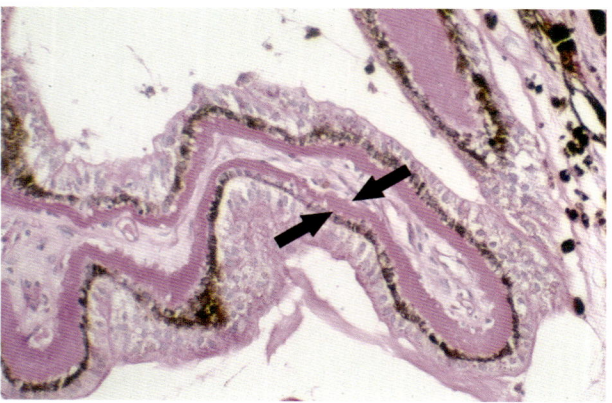

Figure 3.11. Basement membrane thickening of the pigmented ciliary epithelium (arrows).

chorioretinal scar develops, depending on the amount of laser delivered, and the scar is typically composed of retinal pigment epithelium hyperplasia and gliosis. Theories that explain the efficacy of photocoagulation for macular edema include: endothelial proliferation and occlusion of leaking microaneurysms, increased oxygen perfusion from the vitreous through the thinned retina in areas of lasering, with constriction of previously dilated blood vessels and reduction in hydrostatic pressure [127]. Theories that explain the efficacy of photocoagulation for PDR include decreased oxygen demand of the retina by destruction of the retinal pigment epithelium and outer segments of photoreceptors in areas of ischemic retina, destruction of VEGF-producing areas of the ischemic retina and retinal pigment epithelium [128], and production of angiogenesis inhibitors by cells in the chorioretinal scar [129].

CONCLUSION

In conclusion, the histopathologic changes in diabetic retinopathy are the result of retinal microvascular dysfunction in the setting of systemic hyperglycemia. Histological findings that occur before the disease is apparent clinically include pericyte dropout and thickening of the vascular basement membrane. The earliest clinical finding is microaneurysm formation, which is a preproliferative change. Other preproliferative changes include macular edema, cotton-wool spots (soft exudates), hard exudates, intraretinal hemorrhages, IRMAs, and venous caliber abnormalities (venous beading and dilation). Proliferative changes occur superimposed on the preproliferative changes and include vascular and fibrous tissue proliferation in the preretinal space, onto the vitreous framework and into the vitreous cavity. Numerous pathways and mechanisms have been proposed to explain the pathologic changes seen in diabetes mellitus. It is likely that the morphologic changes are the result of an interaction of numerous pathways leading to altered gene expression and protein function in the setting of systemic hyperglycemia. Understanding the pathophysiologic mechanisms of diabetic retinopathy allows the clinician to better identify and treat the vision-threatening changes encountered in patients. The information also provides researchers with potential new targets for therapy as attempts are made to decrease the morbidity from this sight-threatening disease.

REFERENCES

1. Frank RN. Diabetic retinopathy *N Engl J Med*. 2004;350(1):48–58. (PMID 14702427).
2. Lorenzi M. The polyol pathway as a mechanism for diabetic retinopathy: attractive, elusive and resilient. *Exp Diabetes Res*. 2007;2007:61038. (PMID 18224243).
3. Williamson JR, Chang K, Frangos M, et al. Hyperglycemic pseudohypoxia and diabetic complications. *Diabetes*. 1993;42: 801–813.
4. Mizutani M, Kern TS, Lorenzi M. Accelerated death of retinal microvascular cells in human and experimental diabetic retinopathy. *J Clin Inves*. 1996;97:2883–2890.

5. Kern TS, Engerman RL. Distribution of aldose reductase in ocular tissue. *Exp Eye Res.* 1981;33:175–182.
6. Tilton RG, Hoffmann PL, Kilo C, Williamson JR. Pericyte degeneration and basement membrane thickening in skeletal muscle capillaries of human diabetics. *Diabetes.* 1981;30:326–334.
7. Sorbinil Retinopathy Trail Research Group. A randomized trial of sorbinil, an aldose reductase inhibitor, in diabetic retinopathy. *Arch Ophthalmol.* 1990;108:1234–1244.
8. Buzney SM, Frank RN, Varma SD, et al. Aldose reductase in retinal mural cells. *Invest Ophthal Visual Sci.* 1977;16:392–396.
9. Kinoshita JH. Aldose reductase in the diabetic eye. XLIII Edward Jackson memorial lecture. *Am J Ophthal.* 1986;102:685–692.
10. Frank RN. Etiologic mechanisms in diabetic retinopathy. In: Ryan SJ, Schachat AP, eds. *Retina,* Vol. 2, Medical Retina. St. Louis: Mosby; 2001:1259–1294.
11. Tanaka S, Aviga G, Brodsky B, Eikenberry EF. Glycation induces expansion of the molecular packing of collagen. *J Mol Biol.* 1988;203:495–505.
12. Charonis AS, Reger LA, Dege JE, et al. Laminin alterations after in vitro nonenzymatic glucosylation. *Diabetes.* 1990;39:807–814.
13. Vlassara H, Brownlee M, Cerami A. High-affinity receptor-mediated uptake and degradation of glucose-modified proteins: a potential mechanism for the removal of senescent macromolecules. *Proc Natl Acad Sci USA.* 1985;82:5588–5592.
14. Esposito C, Gerlach H, Brett J, et al. Endothelial receptor-mediated binding of glucose modified albumin is associated with increased monolayer permeablility and modulation of cell surface coagulant properties. *J Exp Med.* 1989;170:1387–1407.
15. Schiekofer S, Balletshofer B, Andrassy M, Bierhaus A, Nawroth PP. Endothelial Dysfunction in diabetes mellitus. *Semin Thromb Hemost.* 2000;26(5):503–511.
16. Bucala R, Model P, Russel M, Cerami A. Modification of DNA by glucose-6-phosphate induces DNA rearrangements in an *E. coli* plasmid. *Proc Natl Acad Sci USA.* 1985;82:8439–8442.
17. Brownlee M, Vlassara H, Cerami A. Nonenzymatic glycosylation products on collagen covalently trap low-density lipoproteins. *Diabetes.* 1985;34:938–941.
18. Sensi M, Tanzi P, Bruno MR, Mancuso M, Andriani D. Human glomerular basement membrane: altered binding characteristics following in vitro non-enzymatic glycosylation. *Ann NY Acad Sci.* 1986;488:549–552.
19. Brownlee M. Glycation products and the pathogenesis of diabetic complications. *Diabetes Care.* 1992;15:1835–1842.
20. Hammes H-P, Martin S, Federlin K, et al. Aminoguanidine treatment inhibits the development of experimental diabetic retinopathy. *Proc Natl Acad Sci USA.* 1991;88:11555–11558.
21. Wautier JL, Zoukourian C, Chappey O, et al. Receptor-mediated endothelial cell dysfunction in diabetic vasculopathy. *J Clin Invest.* 1996;97:238–243.
22. Nishikawa T, Edelstein D, Du XL, et al. Normalizing mitochondrial superoxide production blocks three pathways of hyperglycemic damage. *Nature.* 2000;404:787–790.
23. Suzuki S, Hinokio Y, Komatu K, et al. Oxidative damage to mitochondrial DNA and its relationship to diabetic complications. *Diabetes Res Clin Pract.* 1999;45:161–168.
24. Giugliano D, Ceriello A, Paolisso G. Oxidative stress and diabetic vascular complications. *Diabetes Care.* 1996;19:257–267.
25. Baynes JW. Role of oxidative stress in development of complications in diabetes. *Diabetes.* 1991;40:405–412.

26. Anderson HR, Stitt AW, Gardiner TA, Archer DB. Diabetic retinopathy: morphometric analysis of basement membrane thickening of capillaries in different retinal layers within arterial and venous environments. *Brit J Ophthal*. 1995;79:1120–1123.
27. Ishi H, Koya D, King GL. Protein kinase C activation and its role in the development of vascular complications in diabetes mellitus. *J Mol Med*. 1998;76:21–31.
28. Nagpala PG, Malik AB, Vuong PT, Lum H. Protein kinase C B1 overexpression augments phorbol ester-induced increase in endothelial permeability. *J Cell Physiol*. 1996;166:249–255.
29. Williams B, Gallagher B, Patel H, Orme C. Glucose-induced protein kinase C activation regulates vascular permeability factor mRNA expression and peptide production by human vascular smooth muscle cells in vitro. *Diabetes*. 1997;46:1497–1503.
30. Aiello LP, Bursell SE, Clermont A, et al. Vascular endothelial growth factor-induced retinal permeability is mediated by protein kinase C in vivo and suppressed by an orally effective B-isoform-selective inhibitor. *Diabetes*. 1997;43:1473–1480.
31. Early Treatment Diabetic Retinopathy Study Research Group. ETDRS Report no. 12: Fundus photographic risk factors for progression of diabetic retinopathy. *Ophthalmology*. 1991;98:823–833. (PMID: 2062515).
32. Kuwabara T, Cogan DG. Retinal vascular patterns VI. Mural cells of the retinal capillaries. *Arch Ophthalmol*. 1963;69:492–502.
33. Kelley C, D'Amore P, Hechtman HB, Shepro D. Microvascular pericyte contractility in vitro: comparison with other cells of the vascular wall. *J Cell Biol*. 1987;104:483–490.
34. Chakravarthy U, Gardiner TA, Anderson P, Archer DB, Timble ER. The effects of endothelin 1 on the retinal microvascular pericyte. *Microvasc Res*. 1992;43:241–254.
35. Das A, Frank RN, Weber ML, Kennedy A, Reidy CA, Mancini MA. ATP causes retinal pericytes to contract in vitro. *Exp Eye Res*. 1988;46:349–362.
36. DiLorenzo AL, Sotolongo LB, Kennedy A, Frank RN. Effects of endothelin-1 and elevated glucose levels on contraction of retinal microvascular pericytes in vitro. *Invest Ophthalmol Vis Sci*. 1990;31(suppl):194.
37. Hammes HP, Lin J, Renner O, et al. Pericytes and the pathogenesis of diabetic retinopathy. *Diabetes*. 2002;51:3107–3112.
38. Cogan DG, Toussaint D, Kuwabara T. Retinal vascular patterns. IV. Diabetic retinopathy. *Arch Ophthalmol*. 1961;66:366–378.
39. Addison DF, Garner A, Ashton N. Degeneration of intramural pericytes in diabetic retinopathy. *BMJ*. 1970;1:264–266.
40. Yanoff M. Diabetic retinopathy. *N Engl J Med*. 1966;274:1344–1349.
41. Levene R, Horton G, Gorn R. Flat-mount studies of human retinal vessels. *Am J Ophthalmol*. 1966;61:283–289.
42. Speiser P, Gittelsohn AM, Patz A. Studies on diabetic retinopathy: III. Influence of diabetes on intramural pericytes. *Arch Ophthalmol*. 1968;80:332–337.
43. Frank RN, Keirn RJ, Kennedy A, Frank KW. Galactose-induced retinal capillary basement membrane thickening: prevention by sorbinil. *Invest Ophthalmol Vis Sci*. 1983;24:1519–1524.
44. Engerman RL, Kern TS. Experimental galactosemia produces diabetic-like retinopathy. *Diabetes*. 1984;33:97–100.
45. Sosenko JM, Miettinen OS, Williamson JR, Gabbay KH. Muscle capillary basement membrane thickess (CBMT) in relation to level of glycemia in type I diabetes. *Clin Res*. 1982;30:530a.

46. Abrahamson DR. Recent studies on the structure and pathology of basement membranes. *J Pathol.* 1986;149:257–278.
47. Sterberg M, Cohen-Forterre L, Peyroux J. Connective tissue in diabetes mellitus: biochemical alterations of the intercellular matrix with special reference to proteoglycans, collagens and basement membranes. *Diabetes Metab.* 1985;11:27–50.
48. Toussaint D, Dustin P. Electron microscopy of normal and diabetic retinal capillaries. *Arch Ophthalmol.* 1963;70:140–152.
49. Green WR. Retina. In: Spencer W, ed. *Ophthalmic Pathology.* Philadelphia: W.B. Saunders; 1996:1124–1128.
50. Davis MD. Diabetic retinopathy: a clinical overview. *Diabetes Care.* 1992;15: 1844–1874.
51. Bresnick GH, Segal P, Mattson D. Fluorescein angiographic and clinicopathologic findings. In: Little HL, Jack RL, Patz A, Forsham PH, eds. *Diabetic Retinopathy.* New York: Thieme-Stratton; 1983:37–71.
52. Klein R, Meuer SM, Moss SE, Klein BEK. Retinal microaneurysm counts to the 4-year progression of diabetic retinopathy. *Arch Ophthalmol.* 1989;107:1780–1785.
53. Klein R, Meuer SM, Moss SE, Klein BEK. Retinal microaneurysm counts and 10-year progression of diabetic retinopathy. *Arch Ophthalmol.* 1995;113:1386–1391.
54. Kohner EM, Sleightholm M, The Kroc Collaborative Study Group. Does microaneurysm count reflect severity of early diabetic retinopathy? *Ophthalmology.* 1986;93:586–589.
55. The Diabetes Control and Complications Trial Research Group. Color photography versus fluorescein angiography in the detection of diabetic retinopathy in the diabetes control and complications trial. *Arch Ophthalmol.* 1987;105:1344–1351.
56. Cogan DG, Kuwabara T. Capillary shunts in the pathogenesis of diabetic retinopathy. *Diabetes.* 1963;12:293–300.
57. Tolentino MJ, McLeod DS, Taomoto M, Otsuji T, Adamis AP, Lutty GA. Pathologic features of vascular endotheial growth factor-induced retinopathy in the nonhuman primate. *Am J Ophthalmol.* 2002;133:373–385.
58. Hofman P, van Blijswijk BC, Gaillard PJ, Vrensen GF, Schlingemann RO. Endotheial cell hypertrophy induced by vascular endotheial growth factor in the retina: new insights into the pathogenesis of capillary nonperfusion. *Arch Ophthalmol.* 2001;199:861–866.
59. Muraoka K, Shimizu K. Intraretinal neovascularization in diabetic retinopathy. *Ophthalmology.* 1984;91:1440–1446.
60. Davis MD, Myers FL, Engerman RL, et al. Clinical observations concerning the pathogenesis of diabetic retinopathy. In: Goldberg MF, Fine SL, eds. *Symposium on the Treatment of Diabetic Retinopathy (Public Health Service publication no.1890).* Washington, DC: US Government Printing Office; 1969:47–53.
61. Engerman RL. Pathogenesis of diabetic retinopathy. *Diabetes.* 1989;38:1203–1206.
62. Davis MD, Norton EWD, Myers FL. The Airlie classification of diabetic retinopathy. In: Goldberg MF, Fine SL, eds. *Symposium on the Treatment of Diabetic Retinopathy (Public Health Service publication no.1890).* Washington, DC: US Government Printing Office; 1969:47–53.
63. Imesch PD, Bindley CD, Wallow IHL. Clinicopathological correlation of intraretinal microvascular abnormalities. *Retina.* 1997;17:321–329.
64. Ferris FL III, Patz A. Macular edema: a complication of diabetic retinopathy. *Surv Ophthalmol.* 1984;28(suppl):452–461.
65. Patz A, Schatz H, Berkow JW, Gittelsohn AM, Ticho U. Macular edema-an overlooked complication of diabetic retinopathy. *Trans Am Acad Ophthalmol Otolaryngol.* 1977;77:34–42.

66. Early Treatment Diabetic Retinopathy Study Research Group. Photocoagulation for diabetic macular edema, ETDRS report no 1. *Arch Ophthalmol.* 1985;103:1796–1806.
67. Klein R, Klein BE, Moss SE, Cruickshanks KJ. The Wisconsin Epidemiologic Study of Diabetic Retinopathy. XV. The long-term incidence of macular edema. *Ophthalmology.* 1995;102:7–16.
68. Chew EY, Ferris FL III. Nonproliferative diabetic retinopathy. In: Ryan SJ, Schachat AP, eds. *Retina*, Vol. 2, Medical Retina. St. Louis: Mosby; 2001:1295–1308.
69. Chew EY, Klein ML, Ferris FL 3rd, et al. Association of elevated serum lipid levels with retinal hard exudates in diabetic retinopathy, early treatment diabetic retinopathy study (ETDRS) Report 22. *Arch Ophthalmol.* 1996;114:1079–1084.
70. Apple DJ, Rabb M. Fundus. In: *Ocular Pathology: Clinical Applications and Self Assessment.* St. Louis: Mosby; 1998:374–382.
71. Forrester JV, Grierson I, Lee WR. The pathology of vitreous hemorrhage. II. ultrastructure. *Arch Ophthalmol.* 1979;97:2368–2374.
72. Forrester V, Lee WR, Williamson J. The pathology of vitreous hemorrhage. I. gross and histological appearances. *Arch Ophthalmol.* 1978;96:703–710.
73. Ashton N. Pathological and ultrastructural aspect of the cotton-wool spots. *Proc R Soc Med.* 1969;62:1271–1276.
74. Ashton N. Pathophysiology of retinal cotton-wool spots. *Br Med Bull.* 1970;26: 143–150.
75. Ashton N, Harry J. The pathology of cotton-wool spots and cytoid bodies in hypertensive retinopathy and other diseases. *Trans Ophthalmol Soc UK.* 1963;83: 91–114.
76. Dollery CT. Circulatory, clinical and pathological aspects of the cotton-wool spot. *Proc R Soc Med.* 1969;62:1267–1269.
77. Ferry AP. Retinal cotton-wool spots and cytoid bodies. *Mt Sinai J Med.* 1972;39: 604–609.
78. McLeod D, Marshall J, Kohner EM, et al. The role of axoplasmic transport in the pathogenesis of cotton-wool spots. *Br J Ophthalmol.* 1977;61:177–191.
79. Brown GC, Brown MM, Hiller T, et al. Cotton-wool spots. *Retina.* 1985;5:206–214.
80. Mansour AM, Jampol LM, Logani S, et al. Cotton-wool spots in acquired immunodeficiency syndrome compared with diabetes mellitus, systemic hypertension, and central retinal vein occlusion. *Arch Ophthalmol.* 1988;106:1074–1077.
81. Laren HW. Diabetic retinopathy. *Acta Ophthalmol.* 1960;60(Suppl):1–89.
82. Grunwald JE, Riva CE, Brucker AJ, Sinclair SH, Petrig BL. Altered retinal vascular response to 100% oxygen breathing in diabetes mellitus. *Ophthalmology.* 1984;91:1447–1452.
83. Ernest JT, Goldstick TK, Engerman RL. Hyperglycemia impairs retinal oxygen autoregulation in normal and diabetic dogs. *Invest Ophthalmol Vis Sci.* 1983;24: 985–989.
84. Hersh PS, Green WR, Thoms JJV. Tractional venous loops in diabetic retinopathy. *Am J Ophthalmol.* 1981;92:661–671.
85. Klein R, Klein BEK, Moss SE, et al. The Wisconsin Epidemiologic Study of Diabetic Retinopathy. II. Prevalence and risk of diabetic retinopathy when age at diagnosis is less than 30 years. *Arch Ophthalmol.* 1984;102:520–526.
86. Klein R, Klein BEK, Moss SE, et al. The Wisconsin Epidemiologic Study of Diabetic Retinopathy. III. Prevalence and risk of diabetic retinopathy when age at diagnosis is 30 or more years. *Arch Ophthalmol.* 1984;102:527–532.
87. Davis M. Vitreous contraction in proliferative diabetic retinopathy. *Arch Ophthalmol.* 1965;74:741–751.

88. Dobree JH. Proliferative diabetic retinopathy: evolution of the retinal lesions. *Br J Ophthalmol.* 1964;48:637–649.

89. Garner A. Histopathology of diabetic retinopathy in man. *Eye.* 1993;7:250–253.

90. Davis MD. Natural Course of diabetic retinopathy. In: Kimua SJ, Caygill WM, eds. *Vascular Complications of Diabetes Mellitus.* St. Louis: Mosby Co; 1967:139–167.

91. Davis MD, Blodi BA. Etiologic proliferative diabetic retinopathy. In: Ryan SJ, Schachat AP, eds. *Retina,* Vol. 2, Medical Retina. St. Louis: Mosby; 2001:1309–1349.

92. Ashton N. Pathogenesis of diabetic retinopathy. In: Little H, Jack R, Patz A, and Forsham P, eds. *Diabetic Retinopathy.* New York: Thieme-Stratton; 1983:85–106.

93. Michelson I. The mode of development of the vascular system of the retina, with some observations on its significance for certain retinal diseases. *Trans Ophthalmol Soc UK.* 1948;68:137–180.

94. Shimizu K, Kobayashi Y, Muraoka K. Midperipheral fundus involvement in diabetic retinopathy. *Ophthalmology.* 1981;88:601–612.

95. Wise G. Retinal neovascularization. *Trans Am Ophthalmol Soc.* 1956;54:729–826.

96. Machemer R, Buettner H, Norton E, Parel J. Vitrectomy: a pars plana approach. *Trans Am Acad Ophthalmol Otolaryngol.* 1971;75:813–820.

97. Patz A. Clinical and experimental studies on retinal neovascularization. *Am J Ophthalmol.* 1982;94:715–743.

98. Kim I, Ryan AM, Rohan R, et al. Constitutive expression of VEGF, VEGFR-1, and VEGFR-2 in normal eyes. *Invest Ophthalmol Vis Sci.* 1999;40:2115–2121. [Erratum, *Invest Ophthalmol Vis Sci.* 2000;41:368.]

99. Aiello LP, Avery RL, Arrigg PG, et al. Vascular endothelial growth factor in ocular fluid of patients with diabetic retinopathy and other retinal disorders. *N Engl J Med.* 1994;331:1480–1487.

100. Kampik A, Kenyon K, Michels R, Green WR, de la Cruz Z. Epiretinal and vitreous membranes: comparative study of 56 cases. *Arch Ophthalmol.* 1981;99:1445–1454.

101. Nork T, Wallow I, Sramek S, Anderson G. Mueller's cell involvement in proliferative diabetic retinopathy. *Arch Ophthalmol.* 1987;105:1424–1429.

102. Wallow IHL, Geldner PS. Endothelial fenestrae in proliferative diabetic retinopathy. *Invest Ophthalmol Vis Sci.* 1980;19:1176–1183.

103. Taniguchi Y. Ultrastructure of newly formed blood vessels in diabetic retinopathy. *Jpn Ophthalmol.* 1976;20:19–31.

104. Ramsay WJ, Ramsay RC, Purple RL, Knobloch WH. Involutional diabetic retinopathy. *Am J Ophthalmol.* 1977;84:851–858.

105. Kinoshita JH. Mechanisms initiating cataract formation, proctor lecture. *Invest Ophthalmol.* 1974;13:713–724.

106. Brown C, Burman D. Transient cataracts in a diabetic child with hyperosmolar coma. *Br J Ophthalmol.* 1973;57:429.

107. Harry J, Mission G. *Clinical Ophthalmic Pathology: Principles of Diseases of the Eye and Associated Structure.* London: Butterworth-Heinemann; 2001:282–287.

108. Azar DT, Suprr-Michaud SJ, Tisdale AS, Gipson IK. Decreased penetration of anchoring fibrils into the diabetic stroma. *Arch Ophthalmol.* 1989;107:1520–1523.

109. Keoleian GM, Pach JM, Hodge DO. Structural and functional studies of the corneal endothelium in diabetes mellitus. *Am J Ophthalmol.* 1992;113:64–70.

110. Shetlar DJ, Bourne WM, Campbell RJ. Morphologic evaluation of descemet's membrane and corneal endothelium in diabetes mellitus. *Ophthalmology.* 1989;96:247–250.

111. Hidayat AA, Fine BS. Diabetic choroidopathy light and electron microscopic observations of seven cases. *Ophthalmology.* 1985;92:512–522.

112. Fisher RF. Factors which influence the thickness of basement membrane in diabetes: evidence of humoral control. *Trans Ophthalmol Soc UK*. 1979;99:10–21.

113. Wendel RT, Patel AC, Kelly NE, et al. Vitreous surgery for macular holes [see comment]. *Ophthalmology*. 1993;100:1671–1676.

114. John T, Sassani JW, Eagle RC Jr. The myofibroblastic component of rubeosis iridis. *Ophthalmology*. 1983;90:721–728.

115. Merritt JC, Risco JM, Pantell JP. Bilateral macular infarction in SS disease. *J Pediatr Ophthalmol Strabismus*. 1982;19:275.

116. Fine B, Berkow J, Helfgott J. Diabetic lacy vacuolation of iris pigment epithelium: a case report. *Am J Ophthalmol*. 1970;69:197–201.

117. Smith M, Glickman P. Diabetic vacuolation of the iris pigment epithelium. *Am J Ophthalmol*. 1975;79:875–877.

118. Barber AJ, Antonetti DA, Gardner TW. Altered expression of retinal occluding and glial fibrillary acidic protein in experimental diabetes. *Invest Ophthalmol Vis Sci*. 2000;41:3561–3568.

119. Rungger-Brandle E, Dosso AA, Leuenberger PM. Glial reactivity, an early feature of diabetic retinopathy. *Invest Ophthalmol Vis Sci*. 2000;41:1971–1980.

120. Lieth E, Barber AJ, Xu B, et al. Glial reactivity and impaired glutamate metabolism in short-term experimental diabetic retinopathy. *Diabetes*. 1998;47:815–820.

121. Barber AJ, Lieth E, Khin SA, et al. Neural apoptosis in the retina during experimental and human diabetes: early onset and effect of insulin. *J Clin Invest*. 1998;102:783–791.

122. Daley ML, Watzke RC, Riddle MC. Early loss of blue-sensitive color vision in patients with type I diabetes. *Diabetes Care*. 1987;10:777–781.

123. Simonsen SE. ERG in juvenile diabetics: a prognostic study. In: Goldberg M, Fine SL, eds. *Symposium on the Treatment of Diabetic Retinopathy*. Arlington, VA: US Department of Health, Education and Welfare; 1969:681–689.

124. Parisi V, Uccioli L. Visual electrophysiological responses in persons with type I diabetes. *Diabetes Metab Res Rev*. 2001;17:12–18.

125. Marshall J, Clover G, Rothery S. Some new findings on retinal irradiation by krypton and argon lasers. *Doc Ophthalmol Proc Ser*. 1984;36:21–37.

126. Clover GM. The effects of argon and krypton photocoagulation on the retina: implications for the inner and outer blood retinal barriers. In: Gitter KA, Shatz H, Yannuzzi LA, McDonald HR, eds. *Laser Photocoagulation of Retinal Disease*. (From International Laser Symposium of the Macula). San Francisco: Pacific Medical Press; 1988:11–78.

127. Gottfredsdottir MS, Stefansson E, Jonasson F, Gislason I. Retinal vasoconstriction after laser treatment for diabetic macular edema. *Am J Ophthalmol*. 1993;115:64–67.

128. Adamis AP, Shima DT, Yeo K-T, et al. Synthesis and secretion of vascular permeability factor/vascular endothelial growth factor by human retinal pigment epithelial cells. *Biochem biophys Res Commun*. 1993;193:631–638.

129. Glaser BM, Campochiaro PA, Davis JL Jr, et al. Retinal pigment epithelial cells release an inhibitor of neovascularization. *Arch Ophthalmol*. 1985;103:1870–1875.

4

Pathogenesis of Diabetic Retinopathy

THOMAS W. GARDNER, MD, MS,
AND LLOYD PAUL AIELLO, MD, PhD

CORE MESSAGES

- Diabetes impacts all retinal cell types, with changes beginning before the onset of clinically evident disease. Therefore, diabetic retinopathy is not merely a "microvascular disease."
- Vision impairment in persons with diabetes results from altered function of retinal neurons.
- Both ocular and systemic factors contribute to the pathogenesis of diabetic retinopathy and must be considered in evaluating and treating patients with diabetic macular edema.

This chapter reviews the clinical and cellular changes involved in the development and progression of diabetic retinopathy. The ocular and systemic factors that influence retinopathy and, in particular, its vision-threatening aspects are emphasized. The roles of these factors in the treatment of diabetic retinopathy are discussed in this chapter and in Chapter 20, "Future Therapies."

RETINAL ANATOMY AND PHYSIOLOGY

*T*he retina ("network") consists of five fundamental types of cellular elements: neurons, glial cells, microglia, blood vessels, and pigment epithelium (Fig. 4.1). Intact connections and communications between these cells are required for normal vision.

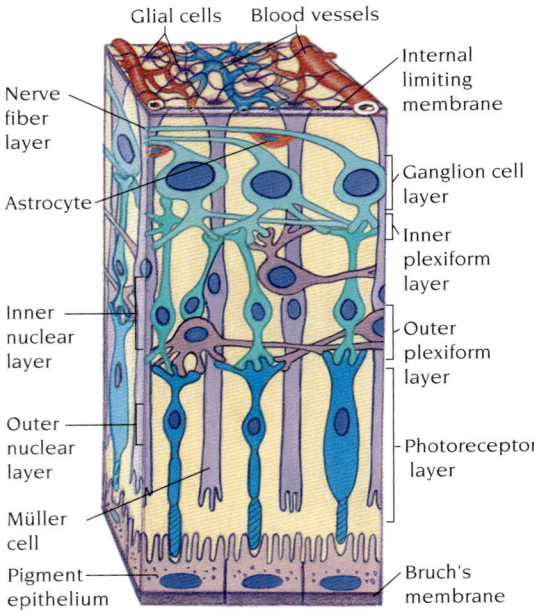

Figure 4.1. Anatomy of normal retina.

Neurons. The neurons and glial cells of the retina comprise more than 95% of the retinal mass, but they are transparent to visible light, so their structure and function are not readily apparent on clinical examination. As demonstrated in Figure 4.1, the retina is primarily a neural tissue, and retinal neurons, the cells that define vision, include photoreceptors, amacrine, bipolar, horizontal, and ganglion cells (reviewed in [1] and http://webvision.med.utah.edu). Electrical inputs from the first four types of neurons converge on the ganglia, and the ganglion cells' electrical output is conducted to the brain via axons of the nerve fiber layer and optic nerve. The high degree of convergence and integration of retinal signals is evident in the 10:1 ratio of photoreceptors (≈130 million) to ganglion cells (≈1.2 million) per human eye. Therefore, disruption of any of the neuronal layers interferes with vision, but redundancy of the neuronal architecture allows for many cells to die or malfunction before visual function is impaired. For example, at least 50% of ganglion cells in an area are lost before a clinically detectable visual defect is apparent in patients with glaucoma, and an eye can retain 20/20 acuity with less than 10% of cone photoreceptors.

Glial Cells. The glial ("glue") cells of the retina—Müller cells and astrocytes—serve as support cells for the neurons and blood vessels [2]. They regulate extracellular ion concentrations necessary for generating action potentials, metabolize neurotransmitters such as glutamate, and transport substrates for retinal metabolism (glucose, lipids, and amino acids) from blood vessels to neurons. Their role in glutamate handling is particularly important because excess glutamate in response to retinal ischemia or diabetes is toxic to neurons and may contribute to neuronal cell death [3].

In addition to their effects on neurons, astrocytes guide fetal vascular development from the optic nerve to the peripheral retina and influence the function and integrity of mature vessels [4]. Vascular endothelial growth factor (VEGF) is a major cytokine involved in this process and is produced by astrocytes and Müller cells. Astrocytes also signal blood vessels to acquire barrier properties to form the blood–retina barrier [5] and influence the development of tight junctions in retinal endothelial cells [6], and regulate the function of retinal synapses [7] and, therefore, visual function [8]. However, many details of the means by which glial cells control normal retinal function remain uncertain.

Microglial Cells. Microglia are bone marrow-derived macrophages that reside in the retina and sense the retinal metabolic environment. They respond to a variety of stimuli, such as retinal detachment, infection or trauma (including laser photocoagulation) by proliferating, migrating, and releasing inflammatory cytokines, such as interleukin-1, VEGF, and tumor necrosis factor-α [9,10]. Retinal injury increases the migration of bone marrow-derived immune cells into the retina and their differentiation into microglia cells [11]. In the short term, these responses may represent a beneficial response to the injury, but prolonged activation results in chronic inflammation and cellular damage.

Blood Vessels. The retinal vascular circuit consists of conduits into and out of the retina (Fig. 4.2A) [12]. The microcirculation includes precapillary arterioles, capillaries, and postcapillary venules. Arterioles possess smooth muscle cells, which allow the arterioles to change their radius and dynamically regulate local delivery of blood to the retina. Precapillary arterioles are the primary resistance vessels, whereas venules have a high density of receptors for vasoactive agents, such as histamine. Venules are primarily passive conducting tubes, which drain blood out of the retina. Capillaries and venules are the primary sites of fluid diffusion into the retina under normal conditions, and this diffusion increases in pathologic conditions such as diabetes [13].

Autoregulation is a general feature of blood vessels of the central nervous system by which the organ maintains appropriate blood flow despite changes in systemic arterial pressure [12]. Retinal arterial vessels have smooth muscle cells, while capillaries, arterioles, and venules possess pericytes, which function as modified smooth muscle cells. These features allow the retinal circulation to autoregulate in response to systemic and local metabolic demands (Fig. 4.2B). Blood vessels also autoregulate in response to the partial pressure of the oxygen (pO_2) and carbon dioxide (pCO_2). Therefore, vessels constrict in response to hyperoxemia and dilate in response to hypercapnea.

Retinal arteriolar narrowing in patients with hypertension is an ophthalmoscopic sign of autoregulatory responses to maintain normal intravascular (hydrostatic)

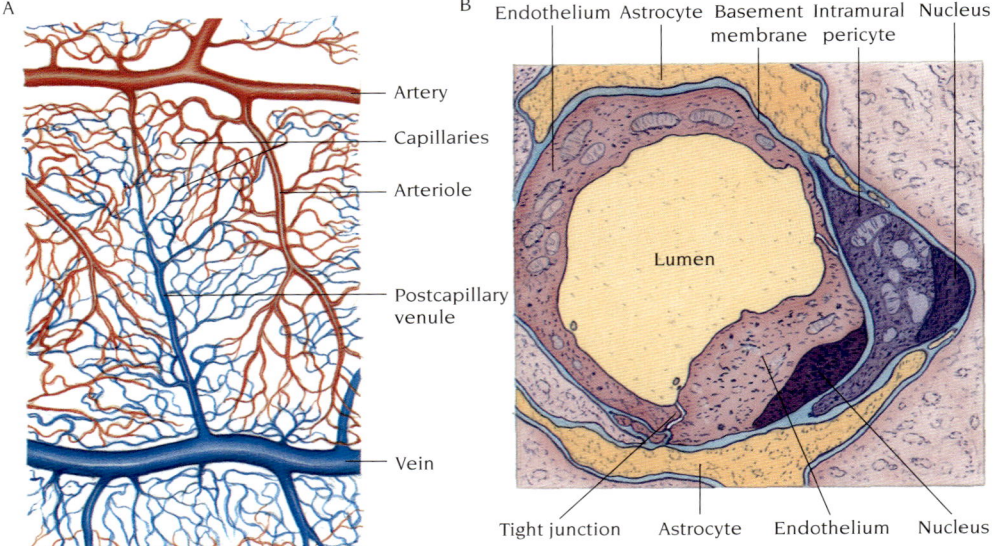

Figure 4.2. Retinal microcirculation. (A) Broad capillary-free zone is present around artery (red), and much narrower zone is seen about vein (blue). (B) Human retinal capillary shows endothelium with tight junctional complexes between adjacent cells, intramural pericyte, and basement membrane material with cavities.

pressure across the vascular wall and volume flow through the retina. When autoregulatory mechanisms and the blood–retina barrier are overwhelmed in hypertension, blood, serous fluid, and lipid exudates accumulate in the macula, and the optic disc may swell. Thus, the features of hypertensive retinopathy can be understood in light of these pathophysiologic processes [14].

Under normal conditions, retinal blood flow balances nutrient delivery and waste removal with retinal metabolism. Diabetes, a systemic malfunction of carbohydrate, lipid, and protein metabolism, leads to vascular and tissue damage in organs such as the retina. Thus, diabetic retinopathy is fundamentally a disorder of retinal and systemic metabolism that damages the retinal tissue elements and associated vessels; that is, a neurovascular degeneration or sensory neuropathy.

PRECLINICAL RETINOPATHY

In patients with type 1 diabetes in whom the duration of diabetes is well known, the interval between diagnosis and development of any retinopathy (microaneurysms) in half the patients is 7 years [15]. In patients with type 2 diabetes, it is more difficult to determine this interval between the development of diabetes and the development of retinopathy because it is believed that 4 to 7 years generally elapse between the onset of non-insulin dependent diabetes and its diagnosis [16]. There is now ample evidence that functional and anatomic changes occur before the onset of vascular lesions in both types of diabetes, as discussed below and shown in Table 4.1. This phase corresponds to Stage 0 in the International Diabetic Retinopathy classification [17].

Diabetic patients with clinically normal-appearing retinas generally lack specific visual symptoms. Nevertheless, sensitive testing methods have demonstrated subtle defects in neurosensory retinal function, including decreased blue-yellow color perception and contrast sensitivity [18,19]. In addition, the oscillatory amplitudes on the b-wave of electroretinogram (ERG) may be reduced. Mulifocal ERG and short-wavelength, and white-on-white perimetry testing reveal regional depression of retinal function in diabetic patients before the onset of vascular lesions [20,21]. These tests indicate dysfunction of the inner retina, especially bipolar, amacrine, and ganglion cell neurons. Nerve fiber layer defects may also be detected by red-free photography or scanning laser ophthalmoscopy in diabetic patients with minimal or no vascular lesions [22,23]. More than 45 years ago, Bloodworth [24] and Wolter [25] showed that diabetes damages retinal ganglion cells in regions remote from vascular pathology. Together, these findings provide strong evidence that retinal function may be altered prior to the onset of vascular lesions and that diabetic retinopathy is not strictly a vascular disease [19,26,27].

Experimental studies have demonstrated increased neural cell injury within 1 month of diabetes [28], long before the onset of typical vascular lesions. This accelerated cell death results in loss of the ganglion cell and inner plexiform layers, with retinal thinning. Recent studies reveal loss of cholinergic and dopaminergic amacrine cells [29], remodeling of dendrites [30], and reduction of essential proteins of synapses [31] as early neurodegenerative changes in diabetic retinopathy. Together, these subtle cellular changes may contribute to reduced oscillatory potentials in the ERG [32]. Optic nerve axon size also decreases [33] as part of the degenerative response of neural tissue to the metabolic stress of diabetes. The cause of these degenerative processes is highly complex but may include loss of neurotrophins (insulin, brain-derived neurotrophic factor), excess nutrients (glucose, amino

Table 4.1. Preclinical Retinopathy

Symptoms	Clinical Signs	Abnormal Test Results	Histopathology	Cellular Events
Usually none	Normal-appearing retina	Color perception: decreased blue-yellow sensation activation (deuteranomaly)	Neural cell apoptosis Microglial cell activation	Decreased vascular tight junctions
		ERG: decreased oscillatory potential amplitudes		Vascular basement membrane thickening
		Visual field defects	Nerve fiber layer loss	
		Vitreous fluorometry: increased blood–retina barrier permeability	Glial cell dysfunction: increased glutamate	

acids, and lipids), inflammation, and excitotoxicity. Müller cells and astrocytes control glutamate metabolism, so glutamate accumulation in the extracellular fluid between neurons and glia implies that glial cells are defective, and the clear-ance of retinal glutatmate is impaired in experimental diabetes [34,35]. Glutamate is a well-recognized cause of neuronal cell death in cerebral ischemia (glutamate excitotoxicity) [36].

Vascular changes that begin shortly after the onset of insulin-deficient diabetes include delayed leukocyte migration in the perifoveal capillaries [37], increased blood–retina barrier permeability [38], and increased retinal blood flow com-pared to nondiabetic control subjects [39]. Studies in diabetic animals have shown increased blood–retina barrier permeability and alterations in retinal blood flow within 1 to 3 months [40,41]. These findings suggest that vascular autoregulation is impaired before clinically evident vascular lesions appear [42]. Thus, humans and rodents exhibit similar cellular alterations in the preclinical phases of diabetic retinopathy.

Further evidence for early pathophysiologic abnormalities in the preclinical phase arises from studies in experimentally diabetic dogs. Engerman and Kern [43] showed that the intensive control of diabetes in dogs for the first 2.5 years deter-mined the subsequent development of vascular lesions, whether or not the animals were subsequently treated with high or low doses of insulin to achieve tight or poor metabolic control, respectively. Thus, while this early phase of diabetic retinopathy appears to be innocuous from a clinical standpoint, numerous cellular and meta-bolic processes are active that lead to the development of clinically evident nonpro-liferative diabetic retinopathy (NPDR). Indeed, a recent demonstration that retinal flavoprotein fluorescence increases in diabetic patients before the onset of visible retinopathy is strong evidence for early onset of metabolic dysregulation [44].

While it is reassuring that patients with diabetes may have no visible retinopathy, the absence of microaneurysms or hemorrhages should not lead to complacency on the part of patients or physicians. In fact, aggressive control of the metabolic and systemic cardiovascular risk factors known to exacerbate retinopathy onset and progression provides an ideal opportunity to prevent vision-threatening changes. Patients who have not developed retinopathy should have a treatment strategy designed to optimize the chance to maintain vision. These patients with healthy appearing retinas and good vision represent the greatest therapeutic opportunity, particularly in light of the emerging diabetes epidemic.

NONPROLIFERATIVE DIABETIC RETINOPATHY

NPDR is defined and staged by ophthalmoscopic features such as vascular lesions, including microaneurysms, intraretinal hemorrhages, and vasodilation. Table 4.2 summarizes the manifestations of NPDR.

Implicit in these classification terms is the concept of a primary vascular disor-der. The definitions (nonproliferative and proliferative) are useful clinically because they permit evaluation of ophthalmoscopically visible ocular risk factors for mod-erate and severe visual loss. The specific sequence of cellular events that lead to the features of NPDR remain uncertain because they occur below the resolution

Table 4.2. Nonproliferative Diabetic Retinopathy

Symptoms	Clinical Signs	Abnormal Test Results	Histopathology	Cellular Events
None, blurred vision, or glare	Retinal vasodilation Microaneurysms Cotton-wool spots	Intravenous fluorescein angiography: vascular leakage and occlusion ERG: depressed oscillatory amplitudes	Microaneurysms, intraretinal hemorrhages in nerve fiber layer and outer plexiform layer	Increased VEGF expression by neurons and glial cells
	Intraretinal hemorrhages	Increased retinal blood flow	Cytoid bodies, nerve fiber layer swelling	Vascular cell apoptosis
	IRMAs, Venous beading Retinal depression sign	Visual field defects	Neuronal loss and degeneration, lipid exudates and extracellular edema in outer plexiform layer; nerve fiber layer atrophy Glial cell occlusion of capillaries	Glial cell activation and macrophage infiltration

of any currently available clinical imaging tools. The sum of experimental and clinical studies strongly suggests that all retinal cells are affected in the preclinical stage of diabetic retinopathy (DR), and certainly by the time of development of NPDR, but there is no empirical evidence that retinopathy results from a specific or isolated vascular cell defect or biochemical pathway [45].

Capillary closure in the peripheral retina may lead to shunting of retinal blood flow into the posterior pole, where it increases the propensity for developing diabetic macular edema (DME) [46]. Capillary closure is a characteristic element of progressive NPDR, but it is unclear whether formed vascular elements—erythrocytes, leukocytes, or platelets—initiate vascular occlusion. Experimental studies demonstrate that transient leukocyte adherence to endothelial cells increases in diabetes [47], and this change may be part of a retina-wide chronic inflammatory process. Histopathologic studies have shown that glial cells migrate through the vessel wall and occlude vascular lumens in patients with diabetic retinopathy [48]. Whether this is a primary event related to glial cell proliferation or secondary to intraluminal capillary plugging is not known. Basement membrane thickening is a characteristic histopathologic feature of diabetic retinopathy and may contribute to capillary closure, but its cause is also unknown.

It has long been held that pericytes are among the first retinal cells to die in diabetes. Although pericytes and endothelial cells clearly undergo programmed cell death (apoptosis) [49], it is unproven whether pericytes are uniquely susceptible to diabetes. The original light microscopic study [50] of trypsin digest preparations in which the neural retina is removed to reveal the vascular network did not indicate the anatomic regions from which the images were taken, gave no statistical analysis of pericyte dropout or other morphologic lesions, and did not determine whether pericyte loss occurred in areas without microaneurysms. Another study [51] questioned whether pericytes are lost first or preferentially in diabetic retinopathy. Therefore, while pericytes undoubtedly change in diabetic retinopathy, they do not appear to be the earliest cellular defects, and the specific functional consequences are still unclear.

Cotton-wool spots have been considered to represent focal infarcts of the nerve fiber layer due to local microvascular occlusion [52]. However, cotton wool spots have also been described in diabetic persons without clinical or fluorescein angiographic evidence of vascular occlusion [53] and may resolve without detectable nerve fiber layer loss. Hence, it is likely that the loss of axonal transparency that appears as retinal whitening results from impaired axonal metabolism and axonal transport, particularly in patients with poorly controlled diabetes [54].

Some young patients (<45 years old) exhibit focal depressions in the macular reflex, the "retinal depression sign" (Fig. 4.3A and 4.3B) [55]. This sign results

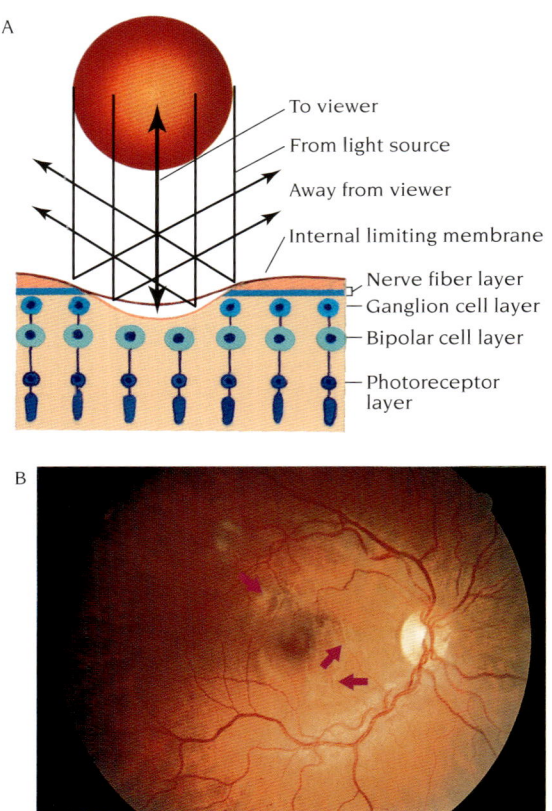

Figure 4.3. (A) Focal retinal depressions reflect light away from observer, so area appears relatively darker than normal regions. (B) Fundus photograph of retinal depression.

from small retinal depressions that reflect light away from the observer so that the macula appears slightly darker than the surrounding retina. The feature is best observed by slit-lamp biomicroscopy and is also noted on fundus photographs, particularly with red-free filters. It is more easily recognized in young patients who have a bright foveal reflex than in older persons. The thinning may result from macular ischemia and/or nonischemic neuroretinal degeneration (apoptosis). This finding may contribute to paracentral scotomas and may be confused with epiretinal membranes or macular edema.

The biochemical and cellular events that initiate vascular lesions in diabetic retinopathy are complex and uncertain in humans. Most of the available information is derived from studies in animals with experimental diabetes induced by streptozotocin or alloxan, or from vascular cell culture experiments. While it is clear that intensive treatment of diabetes in humans or animals significantly delays the onset and progression of retinopathy [56], it is not known whether the development of retinopathy represents a direct effect of insulin deficiency or insulin resistance, a consequence of hyperglycemia, or another metabolic derangement associated with diabetes, such as hyperlipidemia. The metabolic pathways that have been associated with diabetic retinopathy include activation of the polyol pathway, nonenzymatic glycosylation, and activation of the ß isoform of protein kinase C (PKC-ß) [57,58].

Increased glucose metabolism via the polyol pathway [59], first suggested as a cause of cataracts in diabetes, has also been considered to account for diabetic retinopathy and peripheral neuropathy. The hypothesis suggests that increased glucose metabolism via this pathway results in the accumulation of sorbitol, reduction of myo-inositol, and/or reduction in activity of sodium-potassium-ATPase, which may account for vascular dysfunction. Aldose reductase is a key enzyme in the polyol pathway. However, specific vascular functional or neuronal abnormalities, such as barrier breakdown or capillary closure, have not been fully explained by this hypothesis. Studies of aldose reductase inhibitors in diabetic dogs [60] and rats [61] have shown conflicting results. Several clinical trials of aldose reductase inhibitors (sorbinil, tolrestat) have failed to show a benefit on slowing human retinopathy progression [62]. After three decades of aldose reductase clinical trials, aldose reductase inhibitors have not yet proven to be a useful treatment for diabetic retinopathy.

Another theory for the development of diabetic retinopathy involves vascular damage by advanced glycosylation end products (AGEs). According to the concept of nonenzymatic glycosylation [63], sugar molecules bond covalently to reactive molecules and cause alterations in the functions of proteins, nucleic acids, and cells, such as macrophages. This reaction gives rise to the glycohemoglobin (hemoglobin A_{1c}) test, which measures integrated glucose levels over 3 months. Nonenzymatic glycosylation has been proposed to account for cross-linking of long-lived proteins such as collagens, which are found in vascular basement membranes and vitreous. Collagen cross-linking may reduce the turnover of collagen and allow for basement membrane thickening or may contribute to vitreous collagen contraction. Advanced glycation end products increase in Müller cells in experimental diabetes, and a soluble AGE receptor that blocks its activation, decreases neuronal cell death [64]. However, to date no clinical trials have shown that this mechanism can be safely inhibited as an efficacious treatment for diabetes complications. Thus, in spite of a likely role, there is no experimental evidence that demonstrates that excess glucose alone is necessary or sufficient to cause retinopathy or other complications in diabetes.

Another metabolic mechanism involves a specific molecule in signal transduction cascades. Protein kinase C adds phosphate groups to serine or threonine residues of cytoplasmic proteins (Fig. 4.4). Activation of PKC-ß has been observed in retinas of diabetic rats in response to vascular endothelial growth factor/ vascular permeability factor (VEGF/VPF) [57,58]. This enzyme also phosphorylates other proteins in the signal transduction cascade of VEGF and histamine, and is associated with alterations in retinal blood flow and blood–retina barrier breakdown [65]. An oral agent that inhibits PKC-ß activity (ruboxistaurin, Eli Lilly Co) reduces retinal and renal vascular dysfunction in experimental diabetes [66]. Ruboxistaurin reduced the risk of vision loss in persons with DME and visual acuity [67–69], although it did not alter the risk of developing neovascularization in patients with severe NPDR [70]. VEGF is produced by nonvascular retinal cells, including ganglion cells, Müller cells, and astrocytes [71], indicating that increased vascular permeability may be the consequence of vasoactive compounds originating in the neural retina acting secondarily on the microvasculature. This observation is further evidence that diabetic retinopathy may not be a primary vascular disease [19,26,27].

Diabetes is fundamentally a defect in insulin action, due to insulin deficiency (type 1) or insulin resistance (type 2). Patients with poorly controlled type 1 diabetes or who are overweight are also insulin resistant [72] and type 2 patients

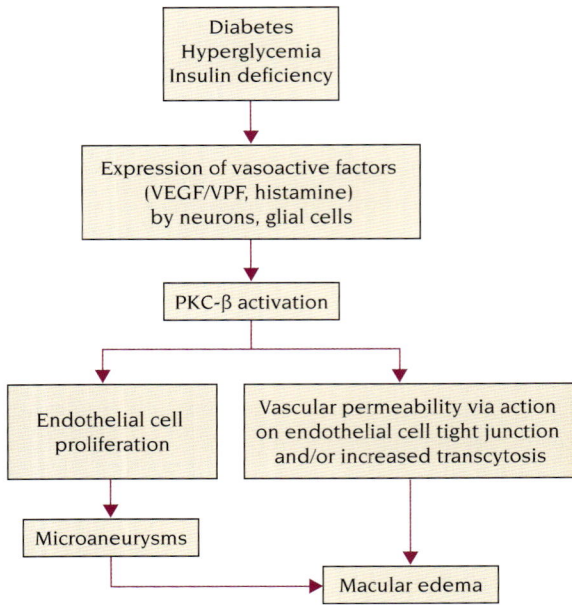

Figure 4.4. Possible mechanism for development of nonproliferative diabetic retinopathy.

become insulin deficient when their pancreatic ß-cells fail. Recent studies now show that impaired insulin action also occurs in the retinas of experimentally diabetic animals [73,74], indicating that diabetes itself directly impacts the retina. It is not certain how this change impacts the retina but it is likely to impair normal anabolic processes required for vision [45].

DIABETIC MACULAR EDEMA

The physiologic factors that govern the development of DME are similar to those involved in tissue edema elsewhere in the body, and understanding the pathophysiology of DME allows construction of a set of risk factors and treatment principles for DME.

Starling's law of the capillary states that edema formation in tissues from fluid flux across the capillary wall is related to the hydrostatic pressure gradient (blood pressure minus tissue pressure) less the oncotic pressure that draws water into the vessels. This relationship has recently been shown to also operate in the retina for DME [75]. That is, increased intravascular hydrostatic pressure from hypertension or intravascular fluid overload drives fluid across the vascular wall (Fig. 4.5) and

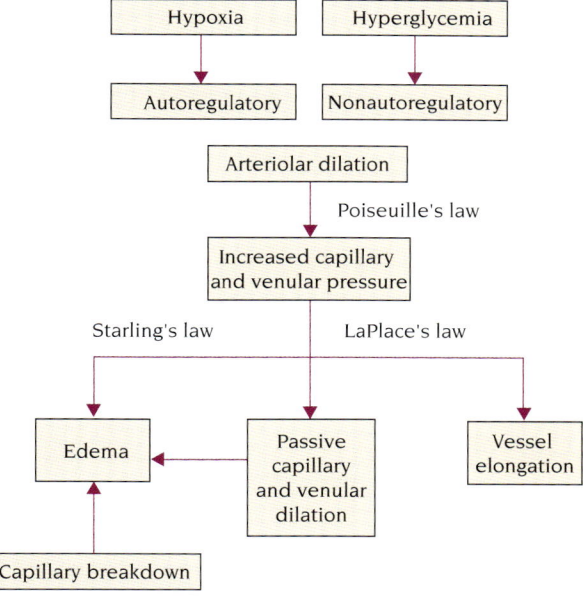

Figure 4.5. Relationship of altered vascular physiology to development of macular edema. Capillary occlusion with resulting nonperfusion has been confirmed as capillary dropout. Resulting retinal hypoxia produces autoregulatory arteriolar vasodilation with reduced pressure in arterioles and increase in capillary and venular hydrostatic pressure. Vessels dilate and increased capillary hydrostatic pressure leads to edema development, according to Starling's law. (Source: Redrawn from Kristinsson JK, Gottfredsdottir MS, Stefansson E: Retinal vessel dilatation and elongation precedes diabetic macular edema. *Br J Ophthalmol.* 1997;81:274–278, with permission from the BMJ Publishing Group.)

leads to increased fluid accumulation in the macula. The oncotic force that pulls water from tissue into capillaries is determined by the plasma albumin concentration, so when albumin levels decrease below 3.0 mg/dL, the oncotic pull is sufficiently diminished to contribute to tissue edema.

Patients with diabetes frequently have impaired Starling's equilibria. As shown in Table 4.3, the clinical risk factors for DME include increased intravascular volume due to hypertension, fluid overload (congestive heart failure and renal failure) and hypoalbuminemia from diabetic nephropathy.

Venous tortuosity and dilation are frequently noted in patients with progressive retinopathy. The physiologic basis of this feature owes to autoregulatory vasodilation of arterioles that causes intravascular pressure in the arterioles to decrease and that in the venules to increase, according to Poiseuille's Law. The increased hydrostatic pressure also leads to greater blood vessel length and tortuosity, per LaPlace's Law. Serial observations in patients with diabetes have shown that retinal vascular diameter and length increase prior to the onset of DME and improve following macular photocoagulation for DME [76] and after panretinal photocoagulation for proliferative diabetic retinopathy (PDR) [46].

In addition to altered autoregulation of vascular flow, the intrinsic integrity of the blood–retina barrier is also impaired. Studies with vitreous fluorometry in humans show that breakdown of the inner blood–retina barrier (formed by tight junctions between endothelial cells) predominates over changes in the outer barrier (tight junctions between retinal pigment epithelial cells) in early DME [77]. The outer barrier breaks down in patients with chronic DME. The proteins that comprise the tight junctions between vascular endothelial cells are reduced in early experimental diabetes, and this may account for increased vascular permeability [78]. As such, the hemodynamic abnormalities in the retina are analogous to those that occur in the kidney in early diabetes; that is, increased renal blood flow and increased glomerular permeability, with resultant albuminuria [79].

Other factors may also aggravate the overall severity of retinopathy. For example, hyperlipidemia has been associated with an increased risk of hard exudates and macular edema [80–82], and anemia is associated with worsening of retinopathy in general [83]. Anemia may impair oxygen delivery to the retina. In addition, erythropoietin may serve as a trophic factor for retinal cells [84] and its deficiency

Table 4.3. Mechanisms of Diabetic Macular Edema

Poor metabolic control
Increased hydrostatic pressure
Hypertension
Intravascular fluid overload (congestive heart failure, renal failure)
Decreased colloid oncotic pressure
Hypoalbuminemia
Hyperlipidemia
Anemia

might aggravate retinal cell death. Conversely, excessive intraocular erythropoietin levels may contribute to the development of DME and PDR [85,86].

Together, these risk factors give rise to principles of DME treatment, including improving metabolic control, blood pressure, fluid overload, anemia, and hyperlipidemia, as shown in Table 4.4.

Microaneurysms are the most characteristic ophthalmoscopic features of diabetic retinopathy. They occur throughout the posterior pole and are often first noted temporal to the macula. Their importance lies in their association with the retinopathy severity and as sources for leakage of fluid and lipid transudates. Histologically, they are outpouchings of the capillaries, with focal endothelial cell proliferation and pericyte loss, often adjacent to areas of nonperfusion. The factors that contribute to microaneurysm formation likely include structural features (loss of supporting pericytes and astrocytes), hemodynamic alterations (increased capillary intramural pressure), and local production of vasoproliferative factors, such as VEGF. Like cotton wool spots, retinal thickening, and hemorrhages, microaneurysms can wax and wane through the course of retinopathy [87].

Understanding the pathophysiology of DME allows construction of a set of systemic risk factors, such as poor diabetes control, systemic arterial hypertension, hyperlipidemia, and hypoalbuminemia.

PROLIFERATIVE DIABETIC RETINOPATHY

PDR, characterized by neovascularization of the optic disc, retina, and/or iris, may be an aberrant attempt to alleviate hypoxia in eyes with severe capillary closure or other retinal ischemia. However, despite the appearance of nonperfused retinal vessels in patients with PDR, retinal hypoxia has not been documented directly in patients [88]. Table 4.5 outlines the features of PDR. The new vessels grow perpendicular to the plane of the retina into the scaffolding provided by the vitreous cortex, typically from venules at the junction of perfused and nonperfused retina (Fig. 4.6). In contrast to normal retinal vessels, which are ensheathed by intact astrocytes, neovascularization is associated with reactive glial cells [89], which do

Table 4.4. Clinical Risk Factors for Diabetic Macular Edema and Retinopathy

Poor metabolic control
Hypertension (>130/80 mm Hg)
Intravascular fluid overload
Congestive heart failure
Renal failure
Hypoalbuminemia
Anemia—Erythropoietin effects on retina
Hyperlipidemia

not allow endothelial cell tight junctions to form completely, with resultant hyper-fluorescence noted on fluorescein angiography.

PDR, like wound healing in other tissues, first involves angiogenesis (neovascularization), followed by macrophage infiltration, remodeling of the vessels, with subsequent fibrosis, and eventual replacement of the vascular tissues by collagen.

Table 4.5. Proliferative Diabetic Retinopathy

Symptoms	Clinical Signs	Abnormal Test Results	Histopathology	Cellular Events
None, reduced vision, nyctalopia or floaters	Retinal signs: neovascularization of optic disc, retina and/or iris, retinal vasodilation beading, and IRMAs	Intravenous fluorescein angiography: severe capillary closure and hyperfluorescence of neovascularization with leakage	Glial cell proliferation and epiretinal membranes	Vitreous collagen cross-linking
			Endothelial cell proliferation	Endothelial cell mitosis
			Intraretinal hemorrhage	Glial cell proliferation
			Cystoid macular edema	Occluded capillaries
	Vitreous signs: vitreous cells, contraction, and opacification of posterior hyaloid face, partial posterior vitreous detachment with epiretinal membranes, and traction retinal detachment	Dark adaptation: impaired Ultrasonography: partial posterior vitreous detachment with vitreoretinal adhesions; retinal detachment	Neuronal loss, retinal detachment	

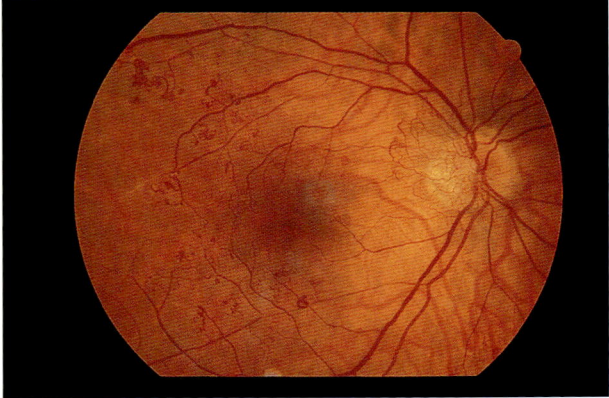

Figure 4.6. Growth of neovascularization at margin of perfused and nonperfused retina.

The natural history of untreated PDR includes fibrosis of the neovascularization, inducing traction on the retina. Subsequent contraction may induce preretinal hemorrhage, vitreous hemorrhage, and traction retinal detachment. Panretinal photocoagulation alters the healing response by reducing the neovascular proliferation, and inducing quiescence.

The cellular events that lead to neovascularization may include retinal hypoxia, elaboration of factors that stimulate endothelial cell proliferation, macrophages and vitreous contraction (Fig. 4.7) [90]. Numerous factors have been implicated in the pathogenesis of retinal neovascularization, including erythropoietin, growth hormone, insulin-like growth factor 1 (IGF-1), basic fibroblast growth factor (bFGF), and VEGF (reviewed in [88]). Together, these "growth factors," cytokines, and cells comprise an inflammatory response. As noted above, VEGF is produced by cells in the neurosensory retina and acts by specific endothelial cell surface receptors to induce neovascularization. VEGF levels are increased in the vitreous of eyes with neovascularization and diminish after panretinal photocoagulation [91]. Inhibition of VEGF action by antisense oligonucleotides that inhibit VEGF messenger RNA or by antibodies that bind the protein before it can activate its receptors reduces neovascularization [92]. After panretinal photocoagulation or intravitreal bevacizumab injection, VEGF levels diminish and those of connective tissue growth factor (CTGF) increase, changing the wound healing response from angiogenesis to fibrosis [93].

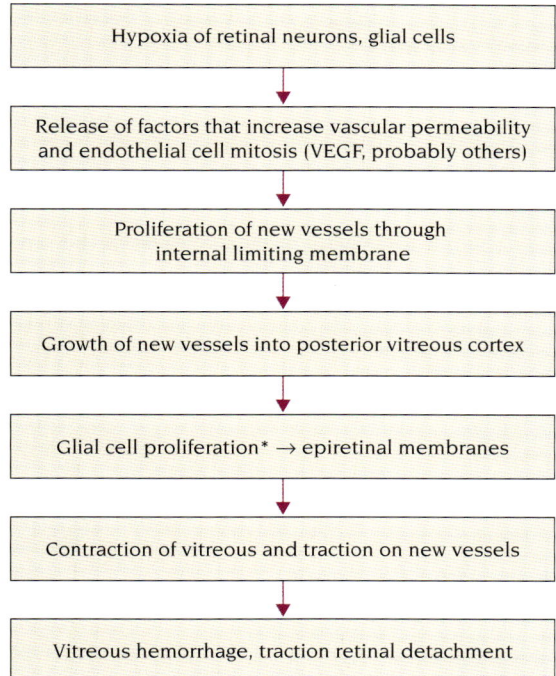

Figure 4.7. Mechanisms of proliferative diabetic retinopathy. *Point at which glial cell proliferation begins is not known, and may occur at same point as endothelial cell proliferation.

VEGF production is not unique to diabetic retinopathy, and is also increased in retinopathy of prematurity and other ocular neovascular processes, as well as in physiologic conditions (menstruation and wound healing) and in pathologic vascularization (tumors) throughout the body. The control of retinal angiogenesis is complex, and the molecular puzzle is still being unraveled [94]. Vitreous collagen crosslinking via nonenzymatic glycosylation may contribute to vitreous contraction.

WHY DO PERSONS WITH RETINOPATHY LOSE VISION?

Most ophthalmologists relate vision loss in persons with diabetic retinopathy to vascular changes seen in eyes with DME and PDR. However, studies detailed in this chapter indicate that multiple insults may contribute to visual loss. These changes may be categorized into abnormalities of the media and neurosensory system, with the latter subdivided into vascular and neural alterations, as shown in Table 4.6. A systematic approach to analysis of vision impairment in diabetes provides the best opportunity to maximize visual recovery by restoring optical, vascular, neural, and structural abnormalities. However, overlapping cellular mechanisms contribute to macular edema and other lesions because the vascular and neural elements of the retina are integrally linked. With the exception of media opacities, the final common pathway of vision loss in all cases includes neural dysfunction [95].

The mechanisms by which persons with diabetes lose sight underlie efforts to preserve vision. Clearly, it is beneficial to minimize retinal vascular leakage by laser photocoagulation, steroids or similar means. However, these therapies do not fully protect neuronal and glial cell function. Future treatments based on improved understanding of the complex biology of the retina that support the integrity of the whole retina may provide the best opportunity for persons with diabetes to maintain their vision.

Table 4.6. Mechanisms of Visual Loss in Diabetes Iterations in Ocular Media

Cornea: epithelial erosions

Lens: transient swelling associated with poor metabolic control; cataract

Vitreous: vitreous hemorrhage

Alterations in Neurosensory System

Retina:

    Vascular: macular edema or ischemia

    Neural: neuronal degeneration as direct effect of diabetes or secondary to vascular occlusion: macular heterotopia; traction or rhegmatogenous retinal detachment

Optic nerve:

    Vascular: diabetic papillopathy; nonarteritic anterior ischemic optic neuropathy

    Neural: axonal degeneration secondary to diabetes or to vascular lesions

CONCLUSIONS

Many steps in the pathogenesis of diabetic retinopathy are under intensive investigation. Diabetic retinopathy involves both vascular and neural elements of the retina from the early stages of diabetes through the development of PDR. Improved means of preventing visual loss in diabetes depend on a better understanding of the underlying mechanisms and the altered relationships between the neural retina and blood vessels.

REFERENCES

1. Masland RH. The fundamental plan of the retina. *Nat Neurosci*. 2001;4:877–886.
2. Stone J, Dreher Z. Relationship between astrocytes, ganglion cells and vasculature of the retina. *J Comp Neurol*. 1987;255:35–49.
3. Lieth E, LaNoue KF, Antonetti DA, Ratz M, Penn State Retina Research Group. Diabetes reduces glutamate oxidation and glutamine synthesis in the retina. *Exp Eye Res*. 2000;70:723–730.
4. Zhang Y, Stone J. Role of astrocytes in the control of developing retinal vessels. *Invest Ophthalmol Vis Sci*. 1997;38:1653–1666.
5. Janzer RC, Raff MC. Astrocytes induce blood-brain barrier properties in endothelial cells. *Nature*. 1987;325:253–257.
6. Gardner TW, Lieth E, Khin SA, et al. Astrocytes increase barrier properties and ZO-1 expression in retinal vascular endothelial cells. *Invest Ophthalmol Vis Sci*. 1997;38:2423–2427.
7. Newman EA. Glial modulation of synaptic transmission in the retina. *Glia*. 2004;47:268–274.
8. Newman EA. New roles for astrocytes: regulation of synaptic transmission. *Trends Neurosci*. 2003;26:536–542.
9. Schuetz E, Thanos S. Microglia-targeted pharmacotherapy in retinal neurodegenerative diseases. *Curr Drug Targets*. 2004;5:619–627.
10. Lee JE, Liang KJ, Fariss RN, Wong WT. Ex vivo dynamic imaging of retinal microglia using time-lapse confocal microscopy. *Invest Ophthalmol Vis Sci*. 2008;49:4169–4176.
11. Kaneko H, Nishiguchi KM, Nakamura M, Kachi S, Terasaki H. Characteristics of bone marrow-derived microglia in the normal and injured retina. *Invest Ophthalmol Vis Sci*. 2008;49:4162–4168.
12. Wise GN, Dollery CT, Henkind P. *The Retinal Circulation*. New York: Harper & Row; 1971:34–54.
13. Barber AJ, Antonetti DA. Mapping the blood vessels with paracellular permeability in the retinas of diabetic rats. *Invest Ophthalmol Vis Sci*. 2003;44:5410–5416.
14. Wong TY, Mitchell P. Current concepts: hypertensive retinopathy. *N Engl J Med*. 2004;351:2310–2317.
15. Klein R, Klein BE. *Vision Disorders in Diabetes*. Bethesda: NIH Publication 95–1468. 1995:311–338.
16. Harris MI, Klein R, Welborn TA, Knuiman MW. Onset of NIDDM occurs at least 4–7 yr before clinical diagnosis. *Diabetes Care*. 1992;15:815–819.
17. Wilkinson CP, Ferris FL, 3rd, Klein RE, et al. Proposed international clinical diabetic retinopathy and diabetic macular edema disease severity scales. *Ophthalmology*. 2003;110:1677–1682.

18. Sokol S, Moskowitz A, Skarf B. Contrast sensitivity in diabetics with and without background retinopathy. *Arch Ophthalmol.* 1985;103:51–54.

19. Ghirlanda G, Di Leo MA, Caputo S, Cercone S, Greco AV. From functional to microvascular abnormalities in early diabetic retinopathy. *Diabetes Metab Rev.* 1997;13:15–35.

20. Han Y, Bearse MA, Jr, Schneck ME, Barez S, Jacobsen CH, Adams AJ. Multifocal electroretinogram delays predict sites of subsequent diabetic retinopathy. *Invest Ophthalmol Vis Sci.* 2004;45:948–954.

21. Han Y, Adams AJ, Bearse MA, Jr, Schneck ME. Multifocal electroretinogram and short-wavelength automated perimetry measures in diabetic eyes with little or no retinopathy. *Arch Ophthalmol.* 2004;122:1809–1815.

22. Chihara E, Matsuoka T, Ogura Y, Matsumura M. Retinal nerve fiber layer defect as an early manifestation of diabetic retinopathy. *Ophthalmology.* 1993;100:1147–1151.

23. Takahashi H, Goto T, Shoji T, Tanito M, Park M, Chihara E. Diabetes-associated retinal nerve fiber damage evaluated with scanning laser polarimetry. *Am J Ophthalmol.* 2006;142:88–94.

24. Bloodworth JMB. Diabetic retinopathy. *Diabetes.* 1962;2:1–22.

25. Wolter JR. Diabetic retinopathy. *Am J Ophthalmol.* 1961;51:1123–1139.

26. Bresnick GH. Diabetic retinopathy viewed as a neurosensory disorder. *Arch Ophthalmol.* 1986;104:989–990.

27. Gardner TW, Antonetti DA, Barber AJ, LaNoue KF, Levison SW. Diabetic retinopathy: more than meets the eye. *Surv Ophthalmol.* 2002;47(Suppl 2):S253–S262.

28. Barber AJ, Lieth E, Khin SA, Antonetti DA, Buchanan AG, Gardner TW. Neural apoptosis in the retina during experimental and human diabetes. Early onset and effect of insulin. *J Clin Invest.* 1998;102:783–791.

29. Gastinger MJ, Singh RS, Barber AJ. Loss of cholinergic and dopaminergic amacrine cells in streptozotocin-diabetic rat and Ins2Akita-diabetic mouse retinas. *Invest Ophthalmol Vis Sci.* 2006;47:3143–3150.

30. Gastinger MJ, Kunselman AR, Conboy EE, Bronson SK, Barber AJ. Dendrite remodeling and other abnormalities in the retinal ganglion cells of Ins2 Akita diabetic mice. *Invest Ophthalmol Vis Sci.* 2008;49:2635–2642.

31. vanGuilder HD, Brucklacher AR, Conboy EE, Bronson SK, Barber AJ. Diabetes downregulates presynaptic proteins and reduces basal synapsin 1 phosphorylation in rat retina. *Eur J Neurosci.* 2008;28:1–11.

32. Hancock HA, Kraft TW. Oscillatory potential analysis and ERGs of normal and diabetic rats. *Invest Ophthalmol Vis Sci.* 2004;45:1002–1008.

33. Scott TM, Foote J, Peat B, Galway G. Vascular and neural changes in the rat optic nerve following induction of diabetes with streptozotocin. *J Anat.* 1986;144:145–152.

34. Lieth E, Barber AJ, Xu B, et al. Glial reactivity and impaired glutamate metabolism in short-term experimental diabetic retinopathy. *Diabetes.* 1998;47:815–820.

35. Mizutani M, Gerhardinger C, Lorenzi M. Müller cell changes in human diabetic retinopathy. *Diabetes.* 1998;47:445–449.

36. Lipton SA, Rosenberg PA. Excitatory amino acids as a final common pathway for neurologic disorders. *N Engl J Med.* 1994;330:613–622.

37. Sander B, Larsen M, Engler C, Lund-Andersen H, Parving HH. Early changes in diabetic retinopathy: capillary loss and blood-retina barrier permeability in relation to metabolic control. *Acta Ophthalmologica.* 1994;72:553–559.

38. Krogsaa B, Lund-Andersen H, Mehlsen J, Sestoft L. Blood-retinal barrier permeability versus diabetes duration and retinal morphology in insulin dependent diabetic patients. *Acta Ophthalmol (Copenh).* 1987;65:686–692.

39. Grunwald JE, DuPont J, Riva CE. Retinal haemodynamics in patients with early diabetes mellitus. *Br J Ophthalmol.* 1996;80:327–331.

40. Enea NA, Hollis TM, Kern JA, Gardner TW. Histamine H1 receptors mediate increased blood-retinal barrier permeability in experimental diabetes. *Arch Ophthalmol.* 1989;107:270–274.

41. Bursell SE, Clermont AC, Oren B, King GL. The in vivo effect of endothelins on retinal circulation in nondiabetic and diabetic rats. *Invest Ophthalmol Vis Sci.* 1995;36:596–607.

42. Tiedeman JS, Kirk SE, Srinivas S, Beach JM. Retinal oxygen consumption during hyperglycemia in patients with diabetes without retinopathy. *Ophthalmology.* 1998;105:31–36.

43. Engerman RL, Kern TS. Progression of incipient diabetic retinopathy during good glycemic control. *Diabetes.* 1987;36:808–812.

44. Field MG, Elner VM, Puro DG, et al. Rapid, noninvasive detection of diabetes-induced retinal metabolic stress. *Arch Ophthalmol.* 2008;126:934–938.

45. Antonetti DA, Barber AJ, Bronson SK, et al. Diabetic retinopathy: seeing beyond glucose-induced microvascular disease. *Diabetes.* 2006;55:2401–2411.

46. Grunwald JE, Brucker AJ, Petrig BL, Riva CE. Retinal blood flow regulation and the clinical response to panretinal photocoagulation in proliferative diabetic retinopathy. *Ophthalmology.* 1989;96:1518–1522.

47. Joussen AM, Murata T, Tsujikawa A, Kirchhof B, Bursell SE, Adamis AP. Leukocyte-mediated endothelial cell injury and death in the diabetic retina. *Am J Pathol.* 2001;158:147–152.

48. Bek T. Glial cell involvement in vascular occlusion of diabetic retinopathy. *Acta Ophthalmol Scand.* 1997;75:239–243.

49. Mizutani M, Kern TS, Lorenzi M. Accelerated death of retinal microvascular cells in human and experimental diabetic retinopathy. *J Clin Invest.* 1996;97:2883–2890.

50. Cogan DG, Toussaint D, Kuwabara T. Retinal vascular patterns. IV. Diabetic retinopathy. *Arch Ophthalmol.* 1961;66:366–378.

51. de Oliveira F. Pericytes in diabetic retinopathy. *Br J Ophthalmol.* 1966;50:134–143.

52. Yanoff M, Fine BS. *Ocular Pathology. A Text and Atlas.* Hagerstown: Harper & Row; 1975:397.

53. Roy MS, Rick ME, Higgins KE, Mc Culloch JC. Retinal cotton-wool spots: an early finding in diabetic retinopathy? *Br J Ophthalmol.* 1986;70:772–778.

54. McLeod D. Why cotton wool spots should not be regarded as retinal nerve fibre layer infarcts. *Br J Ophthalmol.* 2005;89:229–237.

55. Gardner TW, Miller ML, Cunningham D, Blankenship GW. The retinal depression sign in diabetic retinopathy. *Graefe's Arch Clin Exp Ophthalmol.* 1995;233:617–620.

56. Diabetes Control and Complications Trial Research Group. The effect of intensive treatment of diabetes on the development and progression of long-term complications in insulin-dependent diabetes mellitus. *N Engl J Med.* 1993;329:977–986.

57. Koya D, King GL. Protein Kinase-C activation and the development of diabetic complications. *Diabetes.* 1998;47:859–866.

58. Aiello LP, Bursell SE, Clermont A, et al. Vascular endothelial growth factor-induced retinal permeability is mediated by protein kinase C in vivo and suppressed by an orally effective beta-isoform-selective inhibitor. *Diabetes.* 1997;46:1473–1480.

59. Greene DA, Lattimer SA, Sima AAF. Sorbitol, phosphoinositides, and sodium-potassium-ATPase in the pathogenesis of diabetic complications. *N Engl J Med.* 1987;316:599–606.

60. Engerman RL, Kern TS. Aldose reductase inhibition fails to prevent retinopathy in diabetic and galactosemic dogs. [comment]. *Diabetes*. 1993;42:820–825.

61. McCaleb ML, McKean ML, Hohman TC, Laver N, Robison WG, Jr. Intervention with the aldose reductase inhibitor, tolrestat, in renal and retinal lesions of streptozotocin-diabetic rats. *Diabetologia*. 1991;34:695–701.

62. Anonymous. A randomized trial of sorbinil, an aldose reductase inhibitor, in diabetic retinopathy. Sorbinil Retinopathy Trial Research Group. *Arch Ophthalmol*. 1990;108:1234–1244.

63. Brownlee M. Glycation and diabetic complications [Lilly Lecture 1993]. *Diabetes*. 1993;43:836–841.

64. Barile GR, Pachydaki SI, Tari SR, et al. The RAGE axis in early diabetic retinopathy. *Invest Ophthalmol Vis Sci*. 2005;46:2916–2924.

65. Clermont AC, Aiello LP, Mori F, Aiello LM, Bursell SE. Vascular endothelial growth factor and severity of nonproliferative diabetic retinopathy mediate retinal hemodynamics in vivo: a potential role for vascular endothelial growth factor in the progression of nonproliferative diabetic retinopathy. *Am J Ophthalmol*. 1997;124:433–446.

66. Ishii H, Jirousek MR, Koya D, et al. Amelioration of vascular dysfunctions in diabetic rats by an oral PKC beta inhibitor. *Science*. 1996;272:728–731.

67. Aiello LP, Davis MD, Girach A, et al. Effect of ruboxistaurin on visual loss in patients with diabetic retinopathy. *Ophthalmology*. 2006;113:2221–2230.

68. Anonymous. Effect of ruboxistaurin in patients with diabetic macular edema: thirty-month results of the randomized PKC-DMES clinical trial. *Arch Ophthalmol*. 2007;125:318–324.

69. Davis MD, Sheetz MJ, Aiello LP, et al. Effect of ruboxistaurin on the visual acuity decline associated with long-standing diabetic macular edema. *Invest Ophthalmol Vis Sci*. 2009;50:1–4.

70. PKC-DRS Group. The effect of ruboxistaurin on visual loss in patients with moderately severe to very severe nonproliferative diabetic retinopathy. Initial results of the protein kinase Cbeta inhibitor diabetic retinopathy study (PKC-DRS) multicenter randomized clinical trial. *Diabetes*. 2005;54:2188–2197.

71. Lutty GA, McLeod DS, Merges C, Diggs A, Plouét J. Localization of vascular endothelial growth factor in human retina and choroid. *Arch Ophthalmol*. 1996;114:971–977.

72. Greenbaum CJ. Insulin resistance in type 1 diabetes. *Diabetes Metab Res Rev*. 2002;18:192–200.

73. Kondo T, Kahn CR. Altered insulin signaling in retinal tissue in diabetic states. *J Biol Chem*. 2004;279:37997–38006.

74. Reiter CEN, Wu X, Sandirasegarane L, et al. Diabetes reduces basal retinal insulin receptor signaling: reversal with systemic and local insulin. *Diabetes*. 2006;55:1148–1156.

75. Kristinsson JK, Gottfredsdottir MS, Stefansson E. Retinal vessel dilatation and elongation precedes diabetic macular oedema. *Br J Ophthalmol*. 1997;81:274–278.

76. Gottfredsdottir MS, Stefansson E, Jonasson F, Gislason I. Retinal vasoconstriction after laser treatment for diabetic macular edema. *Am J Ophthalmol*. 1993;115:64–67.

77. Larsen M, Dalgaard P, Lund-Andersen H. Differential spectrofluorometry in the human vitreous: blood-retina barrier permeability to fluorescein and fluorescein glucuronide. *Graefes Arch Clin Exp Ophthalmol*. 1991;229:350–357.

78. Antonetti DA, Barber AJ, Khin S, et al. Vascular permeability in experimental diabetes is associated with reduced endothelial occludin content: vascular endothelial growth factor decreases occludin in retinal endothelial cells. *Diabetes*. 1998;47:1953–1959.

79. Gardner TW, Lieth E, Antonetti DA, Barber AJ, Khin SA. A novel hypothesis on the molecular mechanisms of retinal vascular permeability in diabetes. In: Friedman EA, L'Esperance FA, eds. *The DiabeticRenal-Retinal Syndrome*. Dordrecht, Netherlands: Kluwer Publishers; 1998:169–179.

80. Gordon B, Chang S, Kavanagh M, et al. The effects of lipid lowering on diabetic retinopathy. *Am J Ophthalmol*. 1991;112:385–391.

81. Chew EY, Klein ML, Ferris FL, 3rd, et al. Association of elevated serum lipid levels with retinal hard exudate in diabetic retinopathy. Early Treatment Diabetic Retinopathy Study (ETDRS) Report 22. *Arch Ophthalmol*. 1996;114:1079–1084.

82. Miljanovic B, Glynn RJ, Nathan DM, Manson JE, Schaumberg DA. A prospective study of serum lipids and risk of diabetic macular edema in type 1 diabetes. *Diabetes*. 2004;53:2883–2892.

83. Sinclair SH, DelVecchio C, Levin A. Treatment of anemia in the diabetic patient with retinopathy and kidney disease. *Am J Ophthalmol*. 2003;135:740–743.

84. Becerra SP, Amaral J. Erythropoietin—an endogenous retinal survival factor. *N Engl J Med*. 2002;347:1968–1970.

85. Hernandez C, Fonollosa A, Garcia-Ramirez M, et al. Erythropoietin is expressed in the human retina and it is highly elevated in the vitreous fluid of patients with diabetic macular edema. *Diabetes Care*. 2006;29:2028–2033.

86. Katsura Y, Okano T, Matsuno K, et al. Erythropoietin is highly elevated in vitreous fluid of patients with proliferative diabetic retinopathy. *Diabetes Care*. 2005;28:2252–2254.

87. Bresnick GH, Segal P, Mattson D. *Fluorescein Angiographic and Clinicopathologic Findings*. New York: Thieme-Stratton; 1983:37–71.

88. Gariano RF, Gardner TW. Retinal angiogenesis in development and disease. *Nature*. 2005;438:960–966.

89. Ohira A, de Juan EJ. Characterization of glial involvement in proliferative diabetic retinopathy. *Ophthalmologica*. 1990;201:187–195.

90. Casey R, Li WW. Factors controlling ocular angiogenesis. *Am J Ophthalmol*. 1997;124:521–529.

91. Aiello LP, Avery RL, Arrigg PG, et al. Vascular endothelial growth factor in ocular fluid of patients with diabetic retinopathy and other retinal disorders. *N Engl J Med*. 1994;331:1480–1487.

92. Aiello LP. Vascular endothelial growth factor. 20th-century mechanisms, 21st-century therapies. *Invest Ophthalmol Vis Sci*. 1997;38:1647–1652.

93. Kuiper EJ, Van Nieuwenhoven FA, de Smet MD, et al. The angio-fibrotic switch of VEGF and CTGF in proliferative diabetic retinopathy. *PLoS ONE*. 2008;3:e2675.

94. Grant MB, Afzal A, Spoerri P, Pan H, Shaw LC, Mames RN. The role of growth factors in the pathogenesis of diabetic retinopathy. *Expert Opin Investig Drugs*. 2004;13:1275–1293.

95. Lieth E, Gardner TW, Barber AJ, Antonetti DA, Penn State Retina Research Group. Retinal neurodegeneration: early pathology in diabetes. *Clin Experiment Ophthalmol*. 2000;28:3–8.

5

Epidemiology and Risk Factors of Diabetic Retinopathy

TIEN Y. WONG, MD, PhD,
RONALD KLEIN, MD, MPH,
AND BARBARA E.K. KLEIN, MD, MPH

CORE MESSAGES

- Diabetic retinopathy is the leading cause of blindness among persons aged 20 to 64 years in the United States.
- In adult type 2 diabetic persons 40 years and older, 40% have retinopathy, and about 8% have vision-threatening disease (pre-proliferative retinopathy, proliferative retinopathy or macular edema).
- Incidence rates for new retinopathy signs vary from 5% to 10% per year, and are associated primarily with diabetes duration and glycemic control.
- Hyperglycemia, hypertension, and hyperlipidemia are independent risk factors for the presence, development, and progression of diabetic retinopathy. These factors should be monitored and controlled rigorously in the diabetic patient to prevent visual loss.
- Comprehensive, regular dilated eye examinations are important for early detection of potentially vision-threatening retinopathy.

Diabetes mellitus is a leading cause of morbidity and mortality in the United States [1]. Diabetic retinopathy is the most common specific complication of diabetes and is the leading cause of blindness among persons aged 20 to 64 years [2].

Epidemiological studies and clinical trials over the past 25 years have provided data on the prevalence, incidence, and natural history of retinopathy and its associated risk factors [3–5]. Although these findings have been used to develop guidelines for patient care around the world [2,6], considerable morbidity associated with diabetic retinopathy remains. The purpose of this chapter is to review the epidemiology and risk factors of diabetic retinopathy, and their relationship to systemic morbidity and mortality.

EPIDEMIOLOGY

Prevalence of Diabetic Retinopathy in the United States. There have been several epidemiological studies on the prevalence of diabetic retinopathy in the United States (U.S.). One of the largest, the Wisconsin Epidemiologic Study of Diabetic Retinopathy (WESDR), assessed both the prevalence and long-term incidence of retinopathy in a population-based cohort of white persons with diabetes residing in an 11-county area in Wisconsin in the 1980s and 1990s [7–9]. The WESDR used stereoscopic fundus photographs of seven standard fields to detect and grade retinopathy based on a modification of the Early Treatment Diabetic Retinopathy Study (ETDRS) protocol. Two groups of individuals were examined: persons diagnosed with diabetes before 30 years of age on insulin treatment (the younger-onset group) and those diagnosed after the age of 30 years (the older-onset group).

In the younger onset group, 71% had retinopathy (defined as microaneurysms only, or retinal hemorrhages or cotton wool spots in the absence of microaneurysms), 23% had proliferative retinopathy and 6% had clinically significant macular edema (CSME) (Fig. 5.1) [8,10]. The likelihood of retinopathy was strongly related to duration of diabetes, and the prevalence ranged from 2% among participants with less than 2 years of diabetes to 98% in those with 15 years or more of disease [8]. The prevalence of proliferative retinopathy ranged from 4% among participants with 10 years of diabetes to 56% in those with 20 or more years of disease [8].

In the older-onset group, retinopathy affected 39% of those who were not on insulin treatment and 70% of those on insulin treatment. Among older-onset participants not on insulin treatment, 3% had proliferative disease and 4% had CSME, but among those on insulin treatment, 14% had proliferative retinopathy and 11% had CSME [9,10]. As in the younger onset group, the prevalence of retinopathy was strongly related to duration of disease, and ranged from about 20% among participants with less than 2 years of diabetes to more than 60% in those with 15 years or more of diabetes.

Other studies conducted within the U.S. have reported on the prevalence of diabetic retinopathy in different populations and settings [11–21]. Variations in study design, population characteristics, definitions of diabetes, and in the ascertainment of retinopathy, however, make it difficult to compare rates directly across these studies. A recent pooled study examined the prevalence of retinopathy among people 40 years and older from eight population-based studies, including the WESDR [22]. The studies included in this meta-analysis used standardized methods to grade retinopathy from fundus photographs and estimated an overall prevalence of retinopathy of about 40% and a prevalence of sight-threatening disease (either pre-proliferative retinopathy, proliferative retinopathy, or macular edema) of about 8%. Thus, based on these estimates, approximately 4 million individuals with diabetes 40 years of age or older in the U.S. have retinopathy, with 900,000 having sight-threatening retinopathy.

Prevalence of Diabetic Retinopathy in Other Countries. There are fewer population-based data on the prevalence of retinopathy outside of the U.S. [23–33]. In general,

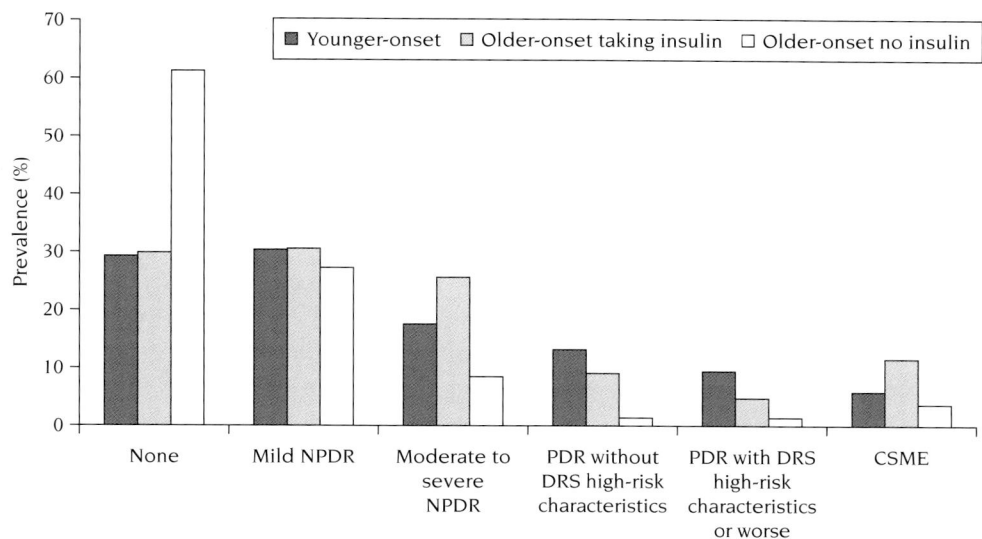

Figure 5.1. Prevalence and Severity of Retinopathy and Macular Edema at the Baseline Examination, the Wisconsin Epidemiologic Study of Diabetic Retinopathy, 1980–1982. (Source: Modified from Klein R, Klein BEK, Moss SE, et al: The Wisconsin Epidemiologic Study of Diabetic Retinopathy, IX: Four-year incidence and progression of diabetic retinopathy when age at diagnosis is less than 30 years. *Arch Ophthalmol.* 1989;107:237–243; and Klein R, Klein BEK, Moss SE, et al. The Wisconsin Epidemiologic Study of Diabetic Retinopathy, X: Four-year incidence and progression of diabetic retinopathy when age at diagnosis is 30 years or more. *Arch Ophthalmol.* 1989;107:244–249. Copyrighted © 1989 with permission from American Medical Association. All rights reserved.)

however, these studies show a similar pattern in both the prevalence and risk factors of diabetic retinopathy. There have been a number of epidemiological studies in England and Europe [23,27–30]. A population-based survey of diabetic patients in Melton Mowbray, England, evaluated the prevalence of retinopathy in insulin-treated [29] and non-insulin treated patients [30]. For insulin-treated patients, the prevalence of any retinopathy was 41%. For non-insulin treated patients, the prevalence of retinopathy was 52%. Data from western Scotland showed the prevalence of any diabetic retinopathy to be 26.7% and that of serious retinopathy (defined as maculopathy, pre-proliferative, or proliferative retinopathy) to be about 10% [31]. Studies from Danish populations have shown an overall prevalence of retinopathy of 77% in men and 74% in women with type 1 diabetes [32]. Variations in the prevalence of retinopathy may be due in part to differences in population selection and in methods for assessing retinopathy.

In Australia, three large population-based studies assessed diabetic retinopathy from a standardized grading of fundus photographs. The Melbourne Visual Impairment Project reported a retinopathy prevalence of 29.1% among persons aged 40 years or older with self-reported diabetes.[24] The prevalence of untreated, vision-threatening retinopathy in this population was 2.8%. The Blue Mountains Eye Study, west of Sydney, found a similar retinopathy prevalence of 32.4% among older persons aged 49 years and above with known or newly diagnosed diabetes [26], with signs of proliferative disease in 1.6% and macular edema in 5.5%. Among persons with newly diagnosed diabetes (i.e., undetected diabetes), retinopathy was present in about 16%. The Australian Diabetes Obesity and Lifestyle (AusDiab) study examined 11,247 adults aged 25 years or older from 42 randomly selected urban and rural communities [33]. Overall, 25% of participants with known diabetes were found to have retinopathy, including 2% with proliferative retinopathy. As in other studies, the prevalence of retinopathy was strongly related to the duration of diabetes, with a prevalence of 9.2% among those with duration less than 5 years, 23% for durations between 5 and 9 years, 33% for durations between 10 and 19 years, and 57% for those with duration of 20 or more years. In fact, after accounting for duration of diabetes, the prevalence findings from these three Australian studies were relatively similar.

In many Asian countries, the prevalence of diabetes has increased substantially over the past few decades [34–38]. In Singapore, for example, serial population surveys in 1975, 1985, and 1992 showed increasing prevalence rates of diabetes of 2%, 4.7%, and 8.6%, respectively, in the population between the ages of 15 and 69 years [37,38]. However, there remains limited information on the epidemiology of retinopathy among Asians. The Aravind Eye Disease Survey in southern India reported a retinopathy prevalence of 27% in a population aged 50 years or older with self-reported diabetes [39], similar to the 22% prevalence reported from another population-based study in an urban population in Hyderabad, India [40]. These rates are similar to those reported in the U.S. and elsewhere.

Incidence and Progression of Diabetic Retinopathy. There are few long-term data on the incidence and natural history of diabetic retinopathy. In the WESDR, the 4-year incidence of retinopathy in the entire cohort was 40% [41,42]. The 4-year incidence and progression rates of diabetic retinopathy in the WESDR are presented in Figure 5.2. The younger-onset group using insulin had the highest 4-year incidence, rate of progression, and rate of progression to proliferative retinopathy, while the older-onset group not using insulin had the lowest rates.

In the WESDR, the 10-year incidence of new retinopathy was 76% in the younger-onset group, 69% in the older-onset group on insulin and 53% in the non-insulin treated older-onset group [43]. The 10-year incidence of macular edema was 20% in the younger-onset group, 25% in the older-onset group on insulin and 14% in the older-onset group not on insulin (Fig. 5.3) [44]. WESDR also reported on the progression of retinopathy in diabetic persons with retinopathy at baseline. The 10-year progression to proliferative retinopathy was 30% in the younger-onset group, 24% in the older-onset group on insulin, and 10% in the older-onset group not on insulin [43]. Based on the WESDR data, it is estimated that each year, of the 10 million Americans with known diabetes mellitus, 96,000 will develop proliferative retinopathy, and 121,000 will develop macular edema.

There are few other long-term population-based incidence data using objective measures to detect retinopathy to compare with these findings [45–52]. In the United Kingdom Prospective Diabetes Study (UKPDS), a multicenter randomized clinical trial of the effects of targeted levels of glycemia on complications of diabetes, the 6-year incidence of retinopathy was 41% in the 1216 patients with

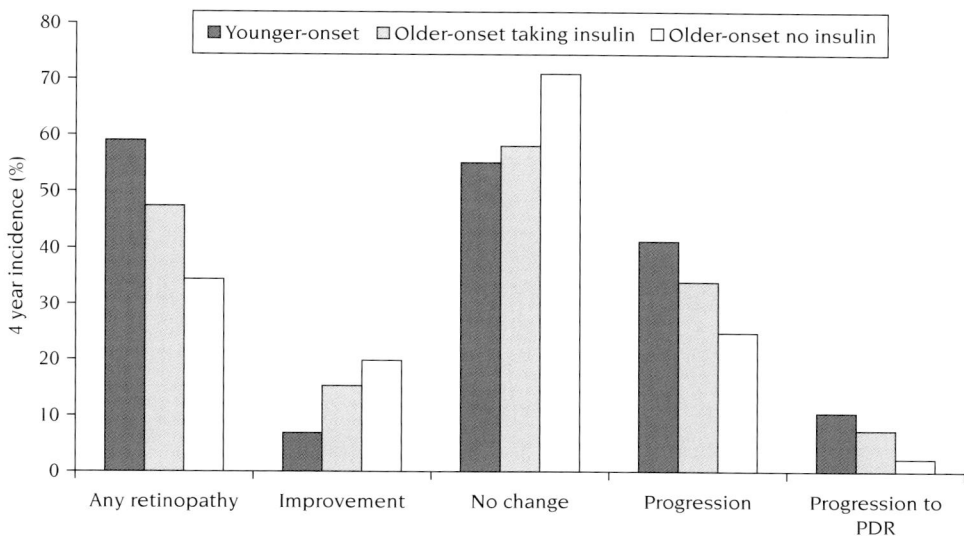

Figure 5.2. Four-Year Incidences of Any Retinopathy, Improvement or Progression of Retinopathy, and Progression to proliferative diabetic retinopathy in Wisconsin Epidemiologic Study Diabetic Retinopathy, 1980–1986. (Source: Modified from Klein R, Klein BEK, Moss SE, et al. The Wisconsin Epidemiologic Study of Diabetic Retinopathy, IX: Four-year incidence and progression of diabetic retinopathy when age at diagnosis is less than 30 years. *Arch Ophthalmol.* 1989;107:237–243; and Klein R, Klein BEK, Moss SE, et al. The Wisconsin Epidemiologic Study of Diabetic Retinopathy, X: Four-year incidence and progression of diabetic retinopathy when age at diagnosis is 30 years or more. *Arch Ophthalmol.* 1989;107:244–249. Copyrighted © 1989 with permission from American Medical Association. All rights reserved.)

newly diagnosed type 2 diabetes without retinopathy at baseline [51]. In the United Kingdom Prospective Diabetes Study (UKPDS), a multicenter randomized clinical trial of the effects of targeted levels of glycemia on complications of diabetes, the 6-year incidence of retinopathy was 41% in the 1,216 patients with newly diagnosed type 2 diabetes without retinopathy at baseline [51]. Of those with retinopathy at baseline, 30% progressed by two or more steps on the ETDRS scale over the 6- year period. As with WESDR, the incidence and progression of retinopathy was dependent on the level of hyperglycemia. Of those with retinopathy at baseline, 30% progressed by two or more steps on the ETDRS scale over the 6-year period. The Liverpool Diabetic Eye Study assessed a cohort of patients registered with general practices within the Liverpool Health Authority to investigate the yearly and cumulative incidence of any retinopathy in persons with type 2 diabetes [52]. The annual incidence of sight-threatening retinopathy in diabetic persons without retinopathy at baseline was 0.3% in the first year, rising to 1.8% in the fifth year, suggesting that the incidence of retinopathy, like the prevalence, increases with duration of diabetes [52].

Time Trends in the Epidemiology of Diabetic Retinopathy. There have been some suggestions that over the past 25 years, better recognition and management of retinopathy risk factors based on evidence from the Diabetes Control and

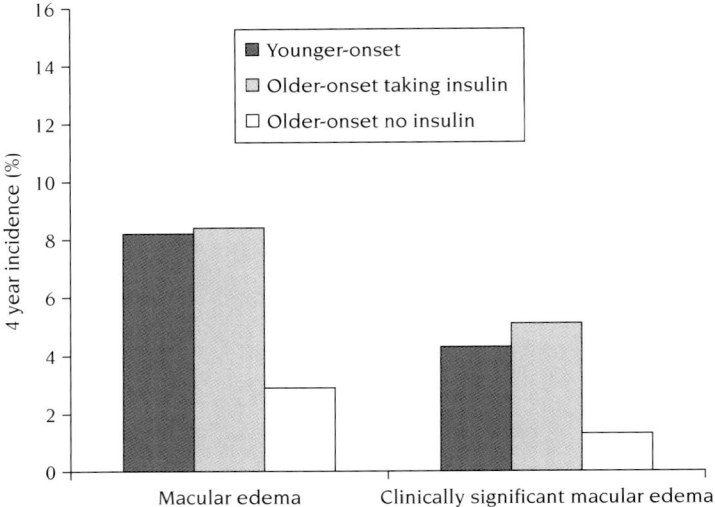

Figure 5.3. Four-Year Incidences of Macular Edema and clinically significant macular edema, by Diabetes Group, Wisconsin Epidomiologic Study of Diabetic Retinopathy, 1980–1986. (Source: Reprinted from Klein R, Moss SE, Klein BEK, et al. The Wisconsin Epidemiologic Study of Diabetic Retinopathy, XI: The incidence of macular edema. *Ophthalmology.* 1989;96:1501–1510. Copyright © 1989 with permission from *American Academy of Ophthalmology.* All rights reserved.)

Complications Trial (DCCT) and UKPDS and the institution of structured retinopathy screening programs have led to a decline in both the prevalence and incidence of moderate to severe microvascular diabetic complications.

Studies conducted in contemporary populations have suggested this to be the case, although differences in study design, population characteristics, and definitions of diabetes and retinopathy between earlier and newer studies make it difficult to draw definitive conclusions. For example, data from both the UKPDS [51] and the Liverpool Diabetic Eye Study [52] show lower incidence rates for retinopathy, particularly sight-threatening retinopathy, than was reported previously in the WESDR and studies in the early 1980s [53]. A recent study assessed the age at which retinopathy was first diagnosed in a sample of patients with type 1 diabetes and showed that the median diabetes duration until the first occurrence of retinopathy was 16.6 years [54], which is longer than reported in previous studies. Data from Sweden indicated that the prevalence of retinopathy appeared to be decreasing in the past decade [46]. The meta-analysis review showed that estimates of retinopathy prevalence was about 10% to 20% lower in the 7 later studies as compared to WESDR [22].

These data provide supporting evidence that improvements in diabetes management and improved levels of metabolic and blood pressure control may have had a positive impact in reducing the prevalence and incidence of retinopathy.

Retinopathy in Non-Diabetic Persons. There is increasing recognition that typical lesions of early retinopathy (retinal microaneuryms, hemorrhages and cotton wool spots) are also commonly seen in persons without clinically diagnosed diabetes [55]. Studies using fundus photographs to evaluate retinopathy have reported prevalence rates of up to 14% in some populations [56–59]. Prospective data from the Beaver Dam and Blue Mountains Eye Studies show that these retinopathy signs developed in 6% to 10% of nondiabetic persons over a 5-year period [59,60].

The risk factors associated with retinopathy signs in nondiabetic persons remain unclear. Various studies show that these retinopathy signs may be related to impaired glucose tolerance [61–63], components related to the metabolic syndrome [64] and hypertension [65–67]. However, population-based studies in nondiabetic adult patients show that while hypertension is strongly associated with prevalence of retinal hemorrhages and microaneurysms [55,56,58], higher blood pressure is not associated with the incidence of these retinopathy signs [47,60].

Few studies have investigated if these retinopathy signs are preclinical markers of diabetes. In the Atherosclerosis Risk in Communities (ARIC) study, retinopathy signs in nondiabetic persons were not significantly associated with the subsequent incidence of diabetes, except among individuals with a positive family history of diabetes [68]. This suggests that in persons with underlying predisposition to diabetes, retinopathy signs may be markers of underlying abnormalities in glucose metabolism or microvascular disease.

DEMOGRAPHIC VARIATIONS

Age. In type 1 diabetes, the prevalence and severity of diabetic retinopathy appear to increase with age. In the WESDR, diabetic retinopathy was infrequent in persons younger than 13 years of age, irrespective of the duration of the disease [9]. The 4-year incidence and progression of retinopathy also increased with age, rising steadily until 15 to 19 years of age, after which there was a gradual decline [41]. Because none of the participants younger than 13 years of age at baseline developed proliferative retinopathy at the 4-year follow-up. These data are supported by similar observations in other cohorts with type 1 diabetes [69,70]. It has therefore been recommended that retinopathy screening may not be necessary in young children with type 1 diabetes [71].

Among persons with older-onset type 2 diabetes, the risk of retinopathy may decrease with age. In the older-onset group taking insulin in WESDR, the 4-year incidence of retinopathy and progression of retinopathy was lower in older compared to younger persons [42]. For those not taking insulin, the 4-year rate of progression to proliferative retinopathy decreased with increasing age. In fact, few participants 75 years or older developed proliferative retinopathy over the 10 years of follow-up in WESDR [43].

These findings are supported by data from other population-based studies [44,45]. In a study of people with type 2 diabetes in Rochester, Minnesota, a lower incidence of retinopathy with increasing age in diabetic people older than 60 years of age was found [12]. It is possible that older persons have less severe retinopathy. Alternatively, these findings may indicate selective mortality, that is, older persons with severe retinopathy are more likely to die and are not followed-up.

Gender. Epidemiological studies have not shown a consistent pattern of gender variation in either prevalence or incidence of retinopathy. In the WESDR, younger-onset men were more likely to have proliferative retinopathy than younger women [8], but there were no significant differences in the incidence or progression of diabetic retinopathy between younger-onset men and women [41,43]. In older-onset diabetes participants in the WESDR, there were no significant differences by gender in either the prevalence or incidence of retinopathy [9,42,43].

Race/Ethnicity. There is a substantial body of evidence that the prevalence of diabetes and diabetic retinopathy varies among racial/ethnic groups [13,16,17,19–22].

Studies comparing rates of retinopathy between African Americans and whites have consistently shown a higher prevalence of diabetic retinopathy in African Americans. Three population-based studies, the National Health and Nutrition Examination Survey III (NHANES III) [17], the ARIC study [20], and the Cardiovascular Health Study [21], showed that retinopathy was more prevalent in African Americans with type 2 diabetes than in whites. In the NHANES III, the higher prevalence of retinopathy in African Americans compared to whites disappeared after controlling for retinopathy risk factors, such as glycemic and blood pressure levels [17]. Likewise, in the ARIC study, the higher prevalence of retinopathy in African Americans (28%) than whites (17%) was largely explained by black–white differences in glycemic control, duration of diabetes, and blood pressure [20]. Thus, the higher prevalence of retinopathy in African Americans with type 2 diabetes is partly due to poorer metabolic and blood pressure control in this racial group, and reinforces the need to achieve tight glycemic and blood pressure control in African Americans.

Similar to African Americans, Hispanics have been reported to have higher prevalence of both diabetes and diabetic retinopathy [22]. However, the higher prevalence in Hispanics is not entirely explained by higher frequency of retinopathy risk factors in this racial group. Haffner and colleagues showed that even in multivariate analysis controlling for glycemia and other risk factors, retinopathy in Hispanics living in San Antonio was 2.4 times higher than non-Hispanic whites in the WESDR [13]. Similarly, in the NHANES III, retinopathy was significantly more frequent among adult Hispanics than non-Hispanic whites with type 2 diabetes, despite controlling for duration of diabetes, glycosylated hemoglobin level, blood pressure, and type of antihyperglycemic medication used [17]. Varma et al. recently found Mexican Americans living in Los Angeles to have a higher prevalence of proliferative retinopathy and macular edema than whites living in Beaver Dam, Wisconsin [72].

Native American groups, such as the Pima Indians, have long been known to have a higher prevalence of type 2 diabetes and to have more advanced retinopathy for a given duration of diabetes as compared to whites [73,74]. It has been suggested that Native American groups may have been exposed to longer periods of more severe hyperglycemia at a younger age than whites with type 2 diabetes. In addition, even among different Native American groups, the prevalence and severity of retinopathy appears to vary [75–77], possibly related to different levels or impact of retinopathy risk factors or genetic differences.

Few studies have examined the prevalence of retinopathy in Asian Americans [78,79]. Retinopathy in second generation Japanese American males (Nisei), 12%, was significantly lower than that reported in the diabetes clinic in Tokyo (49% among patients with an onset of diabetes from 20 to 59 years of age and 47% among those with an onset after 59 years of age) and in whites reported in the WESDR (36%) [9,80]. One of the few studies to directly compare rates of retinopathy among different racial/ethnic groups in the U.S. was the Multi-Ethnic Study of Atherosclerosis, which examined the prevalence of diabetic retinopathy among whites, African Americans, Hispanics and Chinese Americans aged 45 years and older [81]. This study showed that the prevalence of retinopathy was similar between African Americans (37%) and Hispanics (37%) and was lower in whites (25%) and Chinese Americans (26%).

In summary, there is substantial variation in the rates of diabetic retinopathy among racial/ethnic groups, but the underlying reasons for these differences are complex, and likely to reflect a combination of variations in health care access, genetic susceptibility and other risk factors for retinopathy, such as duration of diabetes, levels of glycemia, and blood pressure. Nonetheless, it is worth noting that in many studies, controlling for these known risk factors had only a minor effect on the higher retinopathy prevalence among racial/ethnic groups, suggesting that other unmeasured possible risk factors (genetic or otherwise) may account for these variations.

RISK FACTORS

Duration of Diabetes. The strongest predictor for the prevalence of retinopathy in persons with type 1 and type 2 diabetes is the duration of diabetes. In the younger-onset group in the WESDR, the prevalence of any retinopathy was 8% among participants with diabetes duration of 3 years, 25% for 5 years, 60% for 10 years, and 80% for 15 years [8]. The prevalence of proliferative retinopathy was 0% for those with diabetes duration of 3 years, increasing to 25% for 15 years.

In general, the higher prevalence of retinopathy at presentation in type 2 diabetes as compared to type 1 diabetes is a reflection of the longer duration of diabetes before diagnosis in patients with type 2 diabetes. Extrapolating data of retinopathy prevalence for different durations of diabetes from older-onset participants in the WESDR and from a study in Australia, Harris et al. estimated that the onset of detectable retinopathy occurred approximately 4 to 7 years before diagnosis of type 2 diabetes [82].

The incidence of retinopathy also increases with increasing duration of diabetes [41–43,83]. The 4-year incidence of proliferative retinopathy in the WESDR younger-onset group increased from 0% among participants with diabetes duration of 5 years to 28% for those with diabetes duration of 13 to 14 years. After 15 years of diabetes, the incidence of proliferative retinopathy remained stable. In the older-onset WESDR group, 2% of those with diabetes for less than 5 years and 5% of those with diabetes for 15 or more years who were not taking insulin at baseline developed signs of proliferative disease at the 4-year follow-up [58].

Other epidemiological and clinical studies have corroborated the WESDR findings. For example, a Swedish study of type 1 diabetic persons showed an increase in prevalence of retinopathy from 4% in patients with duration of diabetes less than 2 years to 32% among those with duration of diabetes between 10 and 12 years [84].

Hyperglycemia. One of the most important predictive factors for diabetic retinopathy is the level of glycemic control [8,9,12,14,15,20,27,28,30,33,85–94]. The WESDR showed that both the younger-onset and older-onset patients with diabetes who had no retinopathy had significantly lower mean glycosylated hemoglobin values than those patients with retinopathy [93]. Patients with higher glycosylated hemoglobin values were shown to have a higher risk of retinopathy, such that those with mean HbA1c levels over 12% were 3.2 times more likely to have retinopathy after 4 years than subjects with HbA1c levels under 12% [93].

Two landmark multicentered clinical trials, the DCCT [3,90,95,96] and the UKPDS [4,5], assessed the relationship between glycemic control and vascular complications of diabetes (Table 5.1).

The DCCT randomized patients with type 1 diabetes to strict glycemic control (intensive group) or conventional treatment. Over a 6.5 year period, intensive glycemic control reduced the incidence of retinopathy by 76% and progression from early to advanced retinopathy by 54% [3]. For each 10% decrease in HbA1c (e.g., from 9.0% to 8.1% or from 8.0% to 7.2%) there was a 39% decrease in risk of retinopathy. In the DCCT, tight glycemic control was associated with an early worsening in retinopathy in the first year of treatment in the intensive control [90], consistent with observations in other studies [97]. However, after 18 months, the early worsening in retinopathy reversed and the overall beneficial effect of intensive treatment increased with time. It is unclear whether a slower correction of hyperglycemia in poorly controlled diabetic patients may reduce the risk of early worsening.

The DCCT addressed three important clinical questions regarding diabetic retinopathy. First, it examined whether there is a threshold glycosylated hemoglobin level (suggested to be around 8%) above which the risk of retinopathy increased markedly [98]. The DCCT study could not demonstrate any definite threshold level. This was supported by the EURODIAB prospective complications study that showed no glycemic threshold for incident retinopathy in 764 patients with type 1 diabetes followed for an average of 7 years [99]. Second, the DCCT examined whether intensive glycemic control is more beneficial when started earlier in the course of type 1 diabetes [96]. The study found that in the intensive therapy group, the progression of retinopathy was lower among patients with retinopathy for less than 2.5 years (7%) compared to those with more than 2.5 years (20%). This supports the concept that beginning intensive treatment earlier in the course of diabetes, prior to the onset of diabetic retinopathy, may have added benefit. Third, the DCCT, via the Epidemiology of Diabetes Interventions and Complications (EDIC) study, an observational follow-up study of the DCCT cohort, addressed the issue of

Table 5.1. Summary of Findings from the Diabetes Control and Complications Trial (DCCT) and the United Kingdom Prospective Diabetes Study (UKPDS) in Relation to Glycemic Control and Risk of Retinopathy [3,4]

	DCCT	UKPDS
Inclusion criteria	Type 1 diabetes patients who were C-peptide deficient, 13 to 39 years of age, in general good health	Type 2 diabetes patients who had mean fasting plasma glucose of 6.1 to 15.0 mmol/L, after three months of diet treatment
Number of subjects	1441	3867
Treatment group	Intensive therapy consisted of administration of insulin three or more times daily by injections or an external pump, with adjustment of dosage under the direction of an expert team, taking into account self-monitoring of blood glucose performed four times per day, dietary intake, and anticipated exercise	Intensive therapy aimed at achieving fasting plasma glucose of 6.0 mmol/L using various pharmacological agents
Control group	Conventional therapy consisted of one or two daily injections of insulin, daily self-monitoring of urine or blood glucose, and education about exercise and diet, with no adjustment of insulin dosage on a daily basis	Conventional treatment initially involve diet control, with addition of pharmacological therapy when symptoms developed, or if fasting plasma glucose exceeded 15.0 mmol/L
Retinopathy outcome measures	Development of new retinopathy (primary prevention) and progression from early to advanced retinopathy (secondary intervention)	Development of any microvascular complications (retinopathy requiring laser photocoagulation, vitreous hemorrhage and renal failure)
Mean follow-up	6.5 years	12 years
Mean HbA1c difference	1.9% difference between intensive (9.1%) and conventional (7.2%) group	0.9% difference between intensive (7.0%) and conventional (7.9%) group
Main findings	Intensive therapy reduced the incidence of retinopathy by 76% and progression from early to advanced retinopathy by 54%	Intensive therapy reduced the risk of retinopathy progression by 21% and reduction in need for laser photocoagulation by 29%

whether the beneficial effects of intensive therapy persisted in the long term [100]. The EDIC study demonstrated that, 4 years after the end of the DCCT, the reduction in retinopathy progression persisted in the original intensive therapy group, despite a convergence in HbA1c values between the original intensive therapy and original conventional therapy group.

From the results of the DCCT, it was estimated that intensive therapy would result in a "gain of 920,000 years of sight, 691,000 years free from end-stage renal disease, 678,000 years free from lower extremity amputation, and 611,000 years of life at an additional cost of $4.0 billion over the lifetime" of the 120,000 persons with type 1 diabetes in the U.S. who meet DCCT eligibility criteria [3]. The incremental cost per year of life gained was $28,661, and, when adjusted for quality of life, intensive therapy costs $19,987 per quality of life year gained, similar to cost effectiveness of other medical interventions for chronic diseases in the U.S.

In the UKPDS, intensive therapy reduced the risk of retinopathy progression by 21% and reduced the need for laser photocoagulation by 29% as compared to conventional treatment [4,101]. A 1% reduction in mean HbA1c level was associated with a reduction in the risk of any microvascular complications by 37%. Intensive treatment, however, did not appear to have a significant impact on the risk for macrovascular events [5]. In the UKPDS, a 6-year sub-study using detailed grading of retinal photographs showed that the development of retinopathy was strongly influenced by baseline glycemia and glycemic exposure over the follow-up period [51].

There is some suggestion that overall risk reductions associated with glycemic control is greater for type 1 patients in DCCT than in type 2 patients in the UKPDS. For example, in the DCCT, the 1.9% difference in HbA1c between the intensive (9.1%) and conventional group (7.2%, a 21% reduction in HbA1c) was associated with a 63% reduction in retinopathy progression [3]. However, in the UKPDS, the 0.9% difference in HbA1c between the intensive (7.0%) and conventional group (7.9%, an 11% reduction) was associated with only a 21% reduction in retinopathy progression [4].

Recent epidemiological studies have added further evidence to the clinical trial findings. For example, a population-based cohort study of 339 patients with type 1 diabetes in Denmark showed that elevated HbA1c ($p < 0.0001$) and longer diabetes duration ($p < 0.0001$) were independent factors for the 6-year risk of retinopathy [102]. In fact, among patients with high HbA1c (10% or higher), retinopathy risk increased rapidly within a few years of developing diabetes, but in patients with low HbA1c (less than 6%), retinopathy risk remained low during the first 8 years of diabetes.

In summary, there is strong epidemiological and clinical trials evidence that intensive metabolic therapy maintaining near-normal glycosylated hemoglobin levels has a substantial long-term beneficial effect on the development of diabetic retinopathy and that this effect has no threshold and persists long after the initiation of such therapy. However, it is worth emphasizing that retinopathy risk appears not greatly affected in the short term by tight glycemic control, and that there is a lag of about 1½ to 2½ years between metabolic control and measureable changes to the risk of retinopathy.

Hypertension. A common comorbid condition in patients with diabetes is hypertension. The WESDR found that 17% of patients with type 1 diabetes at baseline had hypertension, and a further 25% developed hypertension after 10 years [103].

Hypertension has long been hypothesized to be a risk factor for retinopathy in patients with diabetes. Several mechanisms have been postulated to support this hypothesis. Impairment of retinal vascular autoregulation in response to elevated blood pressure may play a role, based on observations that diabetic patients with hypertension appear to have an impaired ability to regulate retinal blood flow when compared with nondiabetic patients [104]. Hypertension may also result in endothelial damage in the retinal vasculature [105], and an increase in expression of vascular endothelial growth factor and its receptors in diabetic patients [106]. Population-based studies show that, in nondiabetic adult patients, hypertension is strongly associated with presence of retinal hemorrhages and microaneurysms [55,56,58].

However, epidemiological studies in diabetic patients have provided inconsistent evidence regarding the relationship between hypertension and retinopathy development or progression, which has been demonstrated in some studies [8–10,15,83] but not others [12,20,99,102,107]. In the WESDR, higher blood pressure was associated with an increased 14-year incidence of diabetic retinopathy in younger-onset type 1 diabetes [83], independent of other risk factors such as baseline retinopathy status, glycosylated hemoglobin, and duration of diabetes. However, in older onset type 2 diabetes, neither systolic nor diastolic blood pressure was related to the 10-year incidence and progression of retinopathy [107]. No relationship between blood pressure and incident retinopathy was demonstrated in two other prospective studies of type 1 diabetes; the EURODIAB Study [99] and a Danish study of children and adolescents [102]. Other studies document an association between diabetic retinopathy severity with systolic, but not diastolic, blood pressure [14,17,45]. Associations also seem to be weaker among elderly type 2 patients [21,26]. The variability of these results may be related to inherent limitations in study design, selection bias in clinic-based studies, selective mortality in older patients with type 2 diabetes, lack of statistical adjustment for use of anti-hypertensive medications, and measurement errors in the assessment and definition of blood pressure and hypertension.

Clinical trial data, however, have provided much clearer and stronger evidence of the role of hypertension in retinopathy development and progression. In the UKPDS, 1048 patients with hypertension were randomized to a regimen of tight control (aiming for blood pressure less than 150/85 mmHg with atenolol or captopril) and less tight control (less than 180/105 mmHg) [5]. The group with tight blood pressure control had a 37% reduction in the risk of microvascular disease, a 34% reduction in the rate of progression of retinopathy by two or more steps using the modified ETDRS severity scale, and a 47% reduction in the deterioration of visual acuity by three lines or more using the ETDRS charts (for example, a reduction in vision from 20/30 to 20/60 or worse on a Snellen chart). In the tight control group, atenolol and captopril were equally effective in reducing the risk of developing these microvascular complications, suggesting that blood pressure reduction was more important than the type of medication used to reduce it. The effects of blood pressure control were independent of those of glycemic control. After 6 years of follow-up in the UKPDS, subjects with baseline blood pressure in the highest third of the study population (systolic blood pressure ≥ 140 mmHg) were 2.8 times as likely to develop retinopathy as those in the lowest third (systolic blood pressure < 125 mmHg) [51]. There was no relation of systolic blood pressure with retinopathy progression [51] and no threshold systolic blood pressure was evident [108]. Based on the UKPDS data, each 10 mmHg reduction in systolic blood pressure could be expected to reduce the risk of retinopathy by 10% [51].

Two other clinical trials have provided further evidence that blood pressure control is useful in preventing retinopathy and other microvascular complications in type 2 diabetes. The Appropriate Blood Pressure Control in Diabetes (ABCD) trial, a randomized controlled clinical trial of intensive versus conventional blood pressure control, showed benefit of intensive control in normotensive but not hypertensive patients with type 2 diabetes [109]. The Steno-2 Study showed that in patients with type 2 diabetes and microalbuminuria, an intensive, multifactorial approach that targeted hyperglycemia, hypertension, and dyslipidemia, reduced the risk of retinopathy by 58% as compared to conventional treatment alone [110].

In conclusion, data from epidemiological studies and clinical trials support clinical guidelines to control elevated blood pressure in patients with type 2 diabetes to reduce visual loss from retinopathy, as well as morbidity and mortality from cardiovascular diseases.

Hyperlipidemia. There is increasing evidence that dyslipidemia is an important risk factor for retinopathy and macular edema. Epidemiological studies show an association of dyslipidemia with retinopathy [20,111–117], CSME [20], and possibly proliferative retinopathy [118]. In the WESDR, higher total serum cholesterol was associated with retinal hard exudates in both the younger- and the older-onset groups taking insulin but not in those with type 2 diabetes using oral hypoglycemic agents [119]. In the 2709 patients in the ETDRS in whom serum lipids were measured, higher levels of triglycerides, low-density lipoproteins, and very-low-density lipoproteins at baseline were associated with an increased risk of hard exudates and decreased visual acuity [120].

A recent large clinical trial has provided the initial evidence that lipid-lowering therapy may prevent visual loss from diabetic retinopathy. In the Fenofibrate Intervention and Event Lowering in Diabetes (FIELD) study, the effect of fenofibrate on vascular events was examined in 9795 participants with type 2 diabetes who were not taking statin therapy at study entry [121]. Patients had a total cholesterol concentration of 3.0 to 6.5 mmol/L and a total cholesterol/HDL-cholesterol ratio of 4.0 or more, or plasma triglyceride of 1.0 to 5.0 mmol/L. After 5 years, participants treated on fenofibrate were less likely to have retinopathy needing laser treatment (5.2% vs 3.6%, $p = 0.0003$). However, the severity of retinopathy, the indication of laser treatment, and the type of laser treatment (focal or pan-retinal) was not reported in the FIELD study. This study is supported by smaller clinical case series [122–124] that suggest lipid-lowering therapy with statins could be useful as an adjunct therapy to laser treatment. Thus, lipid lowering therapy may be beneficial for patients with diabetes and dyslipidemia not only for its effects on cardiovascular morbidity, but also for its possible effects on retinopathy.

Endogenous and Exogenous Insulin. Whether endogenous and exogenous insulin has an independent effect on risk of diabetic retinopathy is uncertain [125–128]. In the WESDR, persons with undetectable or low plasma C-peptide (a marker for low endogenous insulin) were more likely to have retinopathy and to have more severe retinopathy at baseline [126]. However, there was no relationship between baseline C-peptide level and the incidence or progression of retinopathy in persons with type 1 diabetes [127]. This contrasts somewhat to findings from the DCCT in which lower C-peptide levels were associated with an increased risk of retinopathy [128].

Exogenous insulin has been suggested as a possible cause of both macrovascular and microvascular disease, including retinopathy, in people with type 2 diabetes. However, in the WESDR, there was no association between the amount or type of exogenous insulin used and the presence, severity, incidence or progression of retinopathy in the older-onset group using insulin with high C-peptide levels (0.3 nM or greater) [126,127]. Thus, exogenous insulin is unlikely to be a significant independent risk factor for retinopathy incidence or progression in persons with diabetes.

Proteinuria and Nephropathy. Diabetic retinopathy is closely linked with nephropathy, as both frequently coexist in diabetic patients, and are thought to be microangiopathies reflecting common predisposing factors and pathogenic mechanisms [129]. Longer duration of diabetes, hyperglycemia and hypertension, for example, are well-established risk factors for both retinopathy and nephropathy.

Independent of duration of diabetes, blood pressure, and glycemic control, retinopathy is associated with preclinical morphological changes of diabetic nephropathy in normotensive diabetic patients prior to the development of nephropathy [130]. The presence of retinopathy is also a risk factor for the subsequent development of clinical nephropathy, estimated in one study to be 50% at 5 years, and 75% at 12 years [131]. At the same time, the presence of diabetic nephropathy is a risk factor for the development and progression of retinopathy [132,133]. In the WESDR, younger-onset diabetic persons with gross proteinuria at baseline were 2.3 times more likely to develop proliferative retinopathy over 4 years than those without gross proteinuria [133]. The presence of gross proteinuria at baseline was also associated with a 95% increased risk of developing macular edema among this group in the WESDR 14-year follow-up examination [83]. However, these associations reached only borderline significance when other retinopathy risk factors were controlled for, supporting the fact that similar processes may explain both microvascular complications. For older-onset diabetic patients taking insulin, the relationship was less consistent.

There are clinical case series of patients with renal failure having more severe macular edema that resolves after either peritoneal or hemodialysis [134,135], but no benefit was observed in a small uncontrolled prospective study of diabetic patients with renal failure [136]. There are no clinical trial data to show that interventions that prevent or slow diabetic nephropathy will reduce the incidence and progression of retinopathy.

Cigarette Smoking and Alcohol Consumption. Cigarette smoking is a known risk factor for atherosclerotic diseases while moderate alcohol consumption has been suggested to be cardioprotective [137,138]. However, most epidemiological studies, including the WESDR, have not found a consistent pattern of association between either smoking [12,15,77,139] or alcohol consumption [26,140] and risk of retinopathy.

Unexpectedly, in the UKPDS, cigarette smoking was suggested to be associated with a reduced incidence of retinopathy [59], while alcohol consumption was found to increase the risk of retinopathy in newly diagnosed men with type 2 diabetes [28]. In the WESDR, alcohol consumption was associated with a lower frequency of proliferative retinopathy in the younger-onset group [139]. However, there was no relationship between alcohol consumption at the 4-year examination and the incidence and progression of retinopathy in either the younger- or older-onset groups at the 10-year follow-up [140].

Obesity. The association between obesity and diabetic retinopathy has been investigated in several studies. Some [12,64,70,81,141–144] but not others [9,77,78,145,146], have documented a relationship between larger body mass index (BMI) and risk of retinopathy. In the WESDR, higher body mass was related to presence and severity of retinopathy only in the older-onset people not using insulin [144]. Those who were underweight at baseline (BMI < 20 kg/m² for both men and women) were three times more likely to develop retinopathy as those who were of normal weight (BMI of 20–27.7 kg/m² for men and 20–27.2 kg/m² for women). It has been suggested that this may reflect a "severe" phase of diabetes in underweight older-onset subjects, or that these underweight patients may be a subset of late-onset type 1 diabetes. Persons obese at baseline (BMI > 31.0 kg/m² for men and 32.1 kg/m² for women) were 34% (95% confidence intervals, 0.97, 1.86) more likely to have progression of retinopathy and 41% (95% confidence intervals, 0.76, 2.62) more likely to develop proliferative retinopathy than those who were of normal weight at baseline, although these associations were not statistically significant.

Exercise. Exercise and physical activity may have a positive effect in reducing the risk of diabetic complications, either directly (e.g., lowering blood glucose levels and increasing insulin sensitivity), or indirectly via improved cardiovascular function (e.g., increasing high density lipoprotein (HDL), lowering risk of hypertension). However, there is also the concern that physical activity may have potentially adverse effects on retinopathy in patients with more advanced disease (e.g., risk of vitreous hemorrhage in patients with proliferative retinopathy due to transiently elevated blood pressure).

However, the few epidemiologic data available have not shown a consistent relationship between physical exercise and diabetic retinopathy [147,148]. In the WESDR, women diagnosed with diabetes before 14 years of age who participated in team sports were less likely to have proliferative diabetic retinopathy than those who did not [147]. However, there was no association between physical activity or leisure-time energy expenditure and the presence and severity of diabetic retinopathy in men. In addition, in a more recent analysis of prospective WESDR data, there was no effect of exercise in preventing retinopathy in either men or women [148].

Pregnancy and Reproductive Measures. Diabetic retinopathy can progress rapidly during pregnancy [149,150], but this is thought to be usually a transient effect. Whether pregnancy is an independent risk factor for long-term incidence and progression of retinopathy is less clear. In the WESDR, when compared with nonpregnant diabetic women of similar age and duration of diabetes, pregnant women were more likely to develop retinopathy and have progression of retinopathy, when the groups were followed for a time interval about equal to the length of the pregnancy and when other risk factors were accounted for [150]. Similar findings have been reported in other studies [151,152]. In addition, progression of retinopathy was increased in pre-eclamptic diabetic women when compared to those without pre-eclampsia [153]. While the mechanisms underlying this exacerbation are unclear, retinal hemodynamics are altered by pregnancy [154,155] and progesterone may induce the production of vascular endothelial growth factor [156].

In pregnancy, the risk factors for retinopathy progression are similar to retinopathy risk factors in nonpregnant diabetic individuals, and include poorer glycemic control, longer duration of diabetes prior to pregnancy, and presence of concomitant hypertension [151,153,157]. The Diabetes in Early Pregnancy Study, a prospective study of 140 pregnant diabetic patients, showed that women with the poorest glycemic control at baseline, but with the greatest reduction in HbA1c during the first trimester, were at increased risk of retinopathy progression [151]. These findings underscore the importance of good metabolic and blood pressure control and close monitoring of retinopathy status in diabetic patients who are pregnant.

The higher risk of developing retinopathy after puberty may be related to sex hormones. In the WESDR, menarchal status at the baseline examination was related to the prevalence and severity of retinopathy [158]. However, increased estrogen occurring with puberty is unlikely to be an important risk factor, because use of oral contraceptives does not appear to increase the risk of retinopathy [159]. Similarly, use of hormone replacement therapy has not been found to increase the risk of diabetic retinopathy in the WESDR [160].

Inflammation. Chronic inflammation and dysfunction of the vascular endothelium have been proposed as possible pathogenic factors in type 2 diabetes development [161,162]. There is increasing evidence from animal models and human studies that chronic inflammation and glucose-induced arteriolar endothelial dysfunction are related to development, severity, and progression of diabetic retinopathy [163–165]. Studies have shown that inflammatory protein levels of cytokines, chemokines, and adhesion molecules are elevated in both the vitreous [166] and serum [167] of patients with diabetic retinopathy. Epidemiological studies have provided further support. In the Hoorn study and the EURODIAB Prospective Complications Study, systemic markers of inflammation and endothelial activation (e.g., C-reactive protein, soluble intercellular adhesion molecule-1, von Willebrand factor) were associated with retinopathy, independent of other risk factors [168,169]. However, whether anti-inflammatory treatment can delay the onset or progression of retinopathy is unclear. In the ETDRS, patients with mild-to-severe nonproliferative diabetic retinopathy (NPDR) or early proliferative diabetic retinopathy (PDR) were assigned randomly to either aspirin (650 mg per day) or placebo. Aspirin did not prevent the development of high-risk PDR and did not reduce the risk of visual loss, or increase the risk of vitreous hemorrhage [170].

MORBIDITY AND MORTALITY ASSOCIATED WITH RETINOPATHY

Diabetic retinopathy, reflecting systemic microvascular dysfunction, may be linked with cardiovascular diseases elsewhere in the body [55]. In the WESDR, participants with proliferative retinopathy had a higher risk of incident myocardial infarction, stroke, nephropathy, and lower leg amputation as compared to those with no or minimal retinopathy at baseline [171]. In younger-onset diabetics, after adjusting for age and sex, retinopathy severity was associated with all-cause and coronary heart disease mortality, and in older-onset persons with all-cause, coronary heart disease mortality, and stroke [172]. After controlling for systemic factors, only the associations with all-cause and stroke mortality in older-onset persons remained. In the ARIC study, the presence of retinopathy was associated with a four-fold risk of congestive heart failure among type 2 diabetic participants without previous coronary heart disease or hypertension, independent of standard risk factors [173].

Epidemiological studies in fact indicate that typical retinopathy signs predict systemic vascular diseases even in persons without diabetes [173]. In the ARIC study, retinopathy was associated with two- to four-fold risk of incident clinical stroke, independent of blood pressure, cigarette smoking, lipids, and other risk factors [66]. Among participants without stroke or transient ischemic attack, retinopathy was significantly related to magnetic resonance imaging (MRI)-defined cerebral white matter lesions, which are markers of subclinical small vessel cerebral disease [67].

These data suggest that the presence of retinopathy in both diabetic and non-diabetic patients may be an indicator for increased cardiovascular risk, and may, therefore, help identify individuals who should be under close scrutiny for systemic vascular diseases.

CONCLUSION

Prevention of diabetes, diabetic retinopathy, and other microvascular and macrovascular complications is an important goal in reducing the public health impact of diabetes. Clinical trials have demonstrated that, until approaches for primary prevention of diabetes itself become available, secondary prevention through risk factor reduction (e.g., controlling hyperglycemia and hypertension) can reduce the incidence and progression of retinopathy and visual loss. Because retinopathy may progress despite good glycemic and blood pressure control, it is important that early detection of retinopathy through comprehensive dilated eye examinations by appropriate eye care providers be performed.

SUMMARY FOR CLINICIANS

- Retinopathy is the most common specific complication of patients with diabetes.
- The risk of retinopathy is strongly associated with duration of diabetes. Between 60% and 90% of persons who have diabetes for 15 years or longer will have signs of retinopathy.
- Hyperglycemia is an important modifiable risk factor for the development and progression of retinopathy in both type 1 and type 2 diabetes. In the DCCT, a 1% reduction in HbA1c levels is associated with an approximately 30% reduction in risk of retinopathy in type 1 patients. In the UKPDS, a similar 1% reduction in HbA1c levels is associated with an approximately 20% reduction in the risk of retinopathy in type 2 patients.
- Hypertension is another important risk factor for retinopathy in type 2 patients. The UKPDS showed that a 10 mmHg reduction in systolic blood pressure is associated with a 10% reduction in the risk of retinopathy. Moreover, the beneficial effects of tight blood pressure control appear to additive and independent of tight glycemic control.
- Lipid-lowering therapy may be useful as an adjunct in the management of diabetic retinopathy. However, there have been no large randomized clinical trials that have shown efficacy of lipid-lowering therapy in reducing the risk of macular edema or progression of retinopathy.
- The presence of retinopathy in both diabetic and nondiabetic patients may be an indicator for increased cardiovascular risk.
- Comprehensive dilated eye examinations are important for early detection of sight-threatening retinopathy in patients with diabetes.

REFERENCES

1. Centers for Disease Control and Prevention. US Department of Health and Human Services. National Diabetes Fact Sheet: General information and national estimates on diabetes in the United States 2002. Atlanta, GA; 2003.
2. Fong DS, Aiello LP, Ferris FL, 3rd, Klein R. Diabetic retinopathy. *Diabetes Care.* 2004;10:2540–2553.
3. The Diabetes Control and Complications Trial Research Group. The effect of intensive treatment of diabetes on the development and progression of long-term complications in insulin-dependent diabetes mellitus. *N Engl J Med.* 1993;329(14):977–986.
4. UK Prospective Diabetes Study (UKPDS) Group. Intensive blood-glucose control with sulphonylureas or insulin compared with conventional treatment and risk of complications in patients with type 2 diabetes (UKPDS 33). *Lancet.* 1998;352(9131):837–853.
5. UK Prospective Diabetes Study Group. Tight blood pressure control and risk of macrovascular and microvascular complications in type 2 diabetes: UKPDS 38. *Br Med J.* 1998;317(7160):703–713.
6. McCarty CA, McKay R, Keeffe JE. Management of diabetic retinopathy by Australian ophthalmologists. Working Group on Evaluation of the NHMRC Retinopathy Guideline Distribution. National Health and Medical Research Council. *Clin Experiment Ophthalmol.* 2000;28(2):107–112.
7. Klein R, Klein BE, Moss SE, DeMets DL, Kaufman I, Voss PS. Prevalence of diabetes mellitus in southern Wisconsin. *Am J Epidemiol.* 1984;119(1):54–61.
8. Klein R, Klein BE, Moss SE, Davis MD, DeMets DL. The Wisconsin epidemiologic study of diabetic retinopathy. II. Prevalence and risk of diabetic retinopathy when age at diagnosis is less than 30 years. *Arch Ophthalmol.* 1984;102(4):520–526.

9. Klein R, Klein BE, Moss SE, Davis MD, DeMets DL. The Wisconsin epidemiologic study of diabetic retinopathy. III. Prevalence and risk of diabetic retinopathy when age at diagnosis is 30 or more years. *Arch Ophthalmol.* 1984;102(4):527–532.

10. Klein R, Klein BE, Moss SE, Davis MD, DeMets DL. The Wisconsin epidemiologic study of diabetic retinopathy. IV. Diabetic macular edema. *Ophthalmology.* 1984;91(12):1464–1474.

11. Kahn HA, Leibowitz HM, Ganley JP, et al. The Framingham Eye Study. I. Outline and major prevalence findings. *Am J Epidemiol.* 1977;106(1):17–32.

12. Ballard DJ, Melton LJ, 3rd, Dwyer MS, et al. Risk factors for diabetic retinopathy: a population-based study in Rochester, Minnesota. *Diabetes Care.* 1986;9(4):334–342.

13. Haffner SM, Fong D, Stern MP, et al. Diabetic retinopathy in Mexican Americans and non-Hispanic whites. *Diabetes.* 1988;37(7):878–884.

14. Hamman RF, Mayer EJ, Moo-Young GA, Hildebrandt W, Marshall JA, Baxter J. Prevalence and risk factors of diabetic retinopathy in non-Hispanic whites and Hispanics with NIDDM. San Luis Valley Diabetes Study. *Diabetes.* 1989;38(10):1231–1237.

15. Kostraba JN, Klein R, Dorman JS, et al. The epidemiology of diabetes complications study. IV. Correlates of diabetic background and proliferative retinopathy. *Am J Epidemiol.* 1991;133(4):381–391.

16. West SK, Klein R, Rodriguez J, et al. Diabetes and diabetic retinopathy in a Mexican-American population: Proyecto VER. *Diabetes Care.* 2001;24(7):1204–1209.

17. Harris MI, Klein R, Cowie CC, Rowland M, Byrd-Holt DD. Is the risk of diabetic retinopathy greater in non-Hispanic blacks and Mexican Americans than in non-Hispanic whites with type 2 diabetes? A U.S. population study. *Diabetes Care.* 1998;21(8):1230–1235.

18. Klein R, Klein BE, Moss SE, Linton KL. The Beaver Dam Eye Study. Retinopathy in adults with newly discovered and previously diagnosed diabetes mellitus. *Ophthalmology.* 1992;99(1):58–62.

19. Roy MS. Diabetic retinopathy in African Americans with type 1 diabetes: The New Jersey 725: I. Methodology, population, frequency of retinopathy, and visual impairment. *Arch Ophthalmol.* 2000;118(1):97–104.

20. Klein R, Sharrett AR, Klein BE, et al. The association of atherosclerosis, vascular risk factors, and retinopathy in adults with diabetes: the atherosclerosis risk in communities study. *Ophthalmology.* 2002;109(7):1225–1234.

21. Klein R, Marino EK, Kuller LH, et al. The relation of atherosclerotic cardiovascular disease to retinopathy in people with diabetes in the Cardiovascular Health Study. *Br J Ophthalmol.* 2002;86(1):84–90.

22. Kempen JH, O'Colmain BJ, Leske MC, et al. The prevalence of diabetic retinopathy among adults in the United States. *Arch Ophthalmol.* 2004;122(4):552–563.

23. Broadbent DM, Scott JA, Vora JP, Harding SP. Prevalence of diabetic eye disease in an inner city population: the Liverpool Diabetic Eye Study. *Eye.* 1999;13(Pt 2):160–165.

24. McKay R, McCarty CA, Taylor HR. Diabetic retinopathy in Victoria, Australia: the Visual Impairment Project. *Br J Ophthalmol.* 2000;84(8):865–870.

25. Leske MC, Wu SY, Hyman L, et al. Diabetic retinopathy in a black population: the Barbados Eye Study. *Ophthalmology.* 1999;106(10):1893–1899 [erratum appears in *Ophthalmology.* 2000 March;107(3):412].

26. Mitchell P, Smith W, Wang JJ, Attebo K. Prevalence of diabetic retinopathy in an older community. The Blue Mountains Eye Study. *Ophthalmology.* 1998;105(3):406–411.

27. Stolk RP, Vingerling JR, de Jong PT, et al. Retinopathy, glucose, and insulin in an elderly population. The Rotterdam Study. *Diabetes.* 1995;44(1):11–15.

28. van Leiden HA, Dekker JM, Moll AC, et al. Risk factors for incident retinopathy in a diabetic and nondiabetic population: the Hoorn study. *Arch Ophthalmol.* 2003;121(2):245–251.

29. McLeod BK, Thompson JR, Rosenthal AR. The prevalence of retinopathy in the insulin-requiring diabetic patients of an English country town. *Eye.* 1988;2(Pt 4): 424–430.

30. Sparrow JM, McLeod BK, Smith TD, Birch MK, Rosenthal AR. The prevalence of diabetic retinopathy and maculopathy and their risk factors in the non-insulin-treated diabetic patients of an English town. *Eye.* 1993;7(Pt 1):158–163.

31. Foulds WS, McCuish A, Barrie T, et al. Diabetic retinopathy in the West of Scotland: its detection and prevalence, and the cost-effectiveness of a proposed screening programme. *Health Bull.* 1983;41(6):318–326.

32. Sjolie AK. Ocular complications in insulin treated diabetes mellitus. An epidemiological study. *Acta Ophthalmol Suppl.* 1985;172:1–77.

33. Tapp RJ, Shaw JE, Harper CA, et al. The prevalence of and factors associated with diabetic retinopathy in the Australian population. *Diabetes Care.* 2003;26(6):1731–1737.

34. Zimmet P, Alberti KG, Shaw J. Global and societal implications of the diabetes epidemic. *Nature.* 2001;414(6865):782–787.

35. Pan XR, Yang WY, Li GW, Liu J. Prevalence of diabetes and its risk factors in China, 1994. National Diabetes Prevention and Control Cooperative Group. *Diabetes Care.* 1997;20(11):1664–1669.

36. Ramachandran A, Snehalatha C, Latha E, Vijay V, Viswanathan M. Rising prevalence of NIDDM in an urban population in India. *Diabetologia.* 1997;40(2):232–237.

37. Tan CE, Emmanuel SC, Tan BY, Jacob E. Prevalence of diabetes and ethnic differences in cardiovascular risk factors. The 1992 Singapore National Health Survey. *Diabetes Care.* 1999;22(2):241–247.

38. Cheah JS, Yeo PP, Thai AC, et al. Epidemiology of diabetes mellitus in Singapore: comparison with other ASEAN countries. *Ann Acad Med Singapore.* 1985;14(2):232–239.

39. Narendran V, John RK, Raghuram A, Ravindran RD, Nirmalan PK, Thulasiraj RD. Diabetic retinopathy among self reported diabetics in southern India: a population based assessment. *Br J Ophthalmol.* 2002;86(9):1014–1018.

40. Dandona L, Dandona R, Naduvilath TJ, McCarty CA, Rao GN. Population based assessment of diabetic retinopathy in an urban population in southern India. *Br J Ophthalmol.* 1999;83(8):937–940.

41. Klein R, Klein BE, Moss SE, Davis MD, DeMets DL. The Wisconsin Epidemiologic Study of Diabetic Retinopathy. IX. Four-year incidence and progression of diabetic retinopathy when age at diagnosis is less than 30 years. *Arch Ophthalmol.* 1989;107(2):237–243.

42. Klein R, Klein BE, Moss SE, Davis MD, DeMets DL. The Wisconsin Epidemiologic Study of Diabetic Retinopathy. X. Four-year incidence and progression of diabetic retinopathy when age at diagnosis is 30 years or more. *Arch Ophthalmol.* 1989;107(2):244–249.

43. Klein R, Klein BE, Moss SE, Cruickshanks KJ. The Wisconsin Epidemiologic Study of diabetic retinopathy. XIV. Ten-year incidence and progression of diabetic retinopathy. *Arch Ophthalmol.* 1994;112(9):1217–1228.

44. Klein R, Moss SE, Klein BE, Davis MD, DeMets DL. The Wisconsin epidemiologic study of diabetic retinopathy. XI. The incidence of macular edema. *Ophthalmology.* 1989;96(10):1501–1510.

45. Teuscher A, Schnell H, Wilson PW. Incidence of diabetic retinopathy and relationship to baseline plasma glucose and blood pressure. *Diabetes Care.* 1988;11(3):246–251.

46. Henricsson M, Nystrom L, Blohme G, et al. The incidence of retinopathy 10 years after diagnosis in young adult people with diabetes: results from the nationwide population-based Diabetes Incidence Study in Sweden (DISS). *Diabetes Care.* 2003;26(2):349–354.

47. Klein R, Palta M, Allen C, Shen G, Han DP, D'Alessio DJ. Incidence of retinopathy and associated risk factors from time of diagnosis of insulin-dependent diabetes. *Arch Ophthalmol.* 1997;115(3):351–356.

48. Tudor SM, Hamman RF, Baron A, Johnson DW, Shetterly SM. Incidence and progression of diabetic retinopathy in Hispanics and non-Hispanic whites with type 2 diabetes. San Luis Valley Diabetes Study, Colorado. *Diabetes Care.* 1998;21(1):53–61.

49. Porta M, Sjoelie AK, Chaturvedi N, et al. Risk factors for progression to proliferative diabetic retinopathy in the EURODIAB Prospective Complications Study. *Diabetologia.* 2001;44(12):2203–2209.

50. Nielsen NV. Diabetic retinopathy I. The course of retinopathy in insulin-treated diabetics. A one year epidemiological cohort study of diabetes mellitus. The Island of Falster, Denmark. *Acta Ophthalmol.* 1984;62(2):256–265.

51. Stratton IM, Kohner EM, Aldington SJ, et al. UKPDS 50: risk factors for incidence and progression of retinopathy in Type II diabetes over 6 years from diagnosis. *Diabetologia.* 2001;44(2):156–163.

52. Younis N, Broadbent DM, Vora JP, Harding SP, Liverpool Diabetic Eye S. Incidence of sight-threatening retinopathy in patients with type 2 diabetes in the Liverpool Diabetic Eye Study: a cohort study. *Lancet.* 2003;361(9353):195–200.

53. Mitchell P. The prevalence of diabetic retinopathy: a study of 1300 diabetics from Newcastle and the Hunter Valley. *Aust J Ophthalmol.* 1980;8(3):241–246.

54. Holl RW, Lang GE, Grabert M, Heinze E, Lang GK, Debatin KM. Diabetic retinopathy in pediatric patients with type-1 diabetes: effect of diabetes duration, prepubertal and pubertal onset of diabetes, and metabolic control. *J Pediatr.* 1998;132(5): 790–794.

55. Wong TY, Klein R, Klein BE, Tielsch JM, Hubbard L, Nieto FJ. Retinal microvascular abnormalities and their relationship with hypertension, cardiovascular disease, and mortality. *Surv Ophthalmol.* 2001;46(1):59–80.

56. Wong TY, Hubbard LD, Klein R, et al. Retinal microvascular abnormalities and blood pressure in older people: the Cardiovascular Health Study. *Br J Ophthalmol.* 2002;86(9):1007–1013.

57. Wong TY, Klein R, Sharrett AR, et al. The prevalence and risk factors of retinal microvascular abnormalities in older persons: The Cardiovascular Health Study. *Ophthalmology.* 2003;110(4):658–666.

58. Yu T, Mitchell P, Berry G, Li W, Wang JJ. Retinopathy in older persons without diabetes and its relationship to hypertension. *Arch Ophthalmol.* 1998;116(1):83–89.

59. Klein R, Klein BE, Moss SE. The relation of systemic hypertension to changes in the retinal vasculature: the Beaver Dam Eye Study. *Trans Am Ophthalmol Soc.* 1997;95:329–348; discussion 348–350.

60. Cugati S, Cikamatana L, Wang JJ, Kifley A, Liew G, Mitchell P. Five-year incidence and progression of vascular retinopathy in persons without diabetes: the Blue Mountains Eye Study. *Eye.* 2006;20(11):1239–1245.

61. Wong TY, Barr EL, Tapp RJ, et al. Retinopathy in persons with impaired glucose metabolism: the Australian Diabetes Obesity and Lifestyle (AusDiab) study. *Am J Ophthalmol.* 2005;140(6):1157–1159.

62. Rajala U, Laakso M, Qiao Q, Keinanen-Kiukaanniemi S. Prevalence of retinopathy in people with diabetes, impaired glucose tolerance, and normal glucose tolerance. *Diabetes Care*. 1998;21(10):1664–1669.
63. Singleton JR, Smith AG, Russell JW, Feldman EL. Microvascular complications of impaired glucose tolerance. *Diabetes*. 2003;52(12):2867–2873.
64. Wong TY, Duncan BB, Golden SH, et al. Associations between the metabolic syndrome and retinal microvascular signs: the Atherosclerosis Risk in Communities study. *Invest Ophthalmol Vis Sci*. 2004;45(9):2949–2954.
65. Wong TY, Mitchell P. Hypertensive retinopathy. *N Engl J Med*. 2004;351(22):2310–2317.
66. Wong TY, Klein R, Couper DJ, et al. Retinal microvascular abnormalities and incident stroke: the Atherosclerosis Risk in Communities Study. *Lancet*. 2001;358 (9288):1134–1140.
67. Wong TY, Klein R, Sharrett AR, et al. Cerebral white matter lesions, retinopathy, and incident clinical stroke. *JAMA*. 2002;288(1):67–74.
68. Wong TY, Mohamed Q, Klein R, Couper DJ. Do retinopathy signs in non-diabetic individuals predict the subsequent risk of diabetes? *Br J Ophthalmol*. 2006;90(3):301–303.
69. Fairchild JM, Hing SJ, Donaghue KC, et al. Prevalence and risk factors for retinopathy in adolescents with type 1 diabetes. *Med J Aust*. 1994;160(12):757–762.
70. Zhang L, Krzentowski G, Albert A, Lefebvre PJ. Risk of developing retinopathy in Diabetes Control and Complications Trial type 1 diabetic patients with good or poor metabolic control. *Diabetes Care*. 2001;24(7):1275–1279.
71. Maguire A, Chan A, Cusumano J, et al. The case for biennial retinopathy screening in children and adolescents. *Diabetes Care*. 2005;28(3):509–513.
72. Varma R, Torres M, Pena F, Klein R, Azen SP. Prevalence of diabetic retinopathy in adult Latinos: the Los Angeles Latino eye study. *Ophthalmology*. 2004;111(7):1298–1306.
73. Dorf A, Ballintine EJ, Bennett PH, Miller M. Retinopathy in Pima Indians. Relationships to glucose level, duration of diabetes, age at diagnosis of diabetes, and age at examination in a population with a high prevalence of diabetes mellitus. *Diabetes*. 1976;25(7):554–560.
74. Bennett PH, Rushforth NB, Miller M, LeCompte PM. Epidemiologic studies of diabetes in the Pima Indians. *Recent Prog Horm Res*. 1976;32:333–376.
75. Berinstein DM, Stahn RM, Welty TK, Leonardson GR, Herlihy JJ. The prevalence of diabetic retinopathy and associated risk factors among Sioux Indians. *Diabetes Care*. 1997;20(5):757–759.
76. Lee ET, Lee VS, Lu M, Russell D. Development of proliferative retinopathy in NIDDM. A follow-up study of American Indians in Oklahoma. *Diabetes*. 1992; 41(3):359–367.
77. Lee ET, Lee VS, Kingsley RM, et al. Diabetic retinopathy in Oklahoma Indians with NIDDM. Incidence and risk factors. *Diabetes Care*. 1992;15(11):1620–1627.
78. Dowse GK, Humphrey AR, Collins VR, et al. Prevalence and risk factors for diabetic retinopathy in the multiethnic population of Mauritius. *Am J Epidemiol*. 1998;147(5):448–457.
79. Collins VR, Dowse GK, Plehwe WE, et al. High prevalence of diabetic retinopathy and nephropathy in Polynesians of Western Samoa. *Diabetes Care*. 1995;18(8):1140–1149.
80. Fujimoto W, Fukuda, M. Natural history of diabetic retinopathy and its treatment in Japan. In: Baba S, Goto Y, Fukui I, eds. *Diabetes Mellitus in Asia. Excerpta Med*. 1976:225–231.

81. Wong TY, Klein R, Islam FM, et al. The Multi Ethnic Study of Atherosclerosis (MESA). Diabetic retinopathy in a Multi Ethnic Cohort in the United States. *Am J Ophthalmol.* 2006;141(3):446–455.

82. Harris MI, Klein R, Welborn TA, Knuiman MW. Onset of NIDDM occurs at least 4–7 yr before clinical diagnosis. *Diabetes Care.* 1992;15(7):815–819.

83. Klein R, Klein BE, Moss SE, Cruickshanks KJ. The Wisconsin Epidemiologic Study of Diabetic Retinopathy: XVII. The 14-year incidence and progression of diabetic retinopathy and associated risk factors in type 1 diabetes. *Ophthalmology.* 1998; 105(10):1801–1815.

84. Kernell A, Dedorsson I, Johansson B, et al. Prevalence of diabetic retinopathy in children and adolescents with IDDM. A population-based multicentre study. *Diabetologia.* 1997;40(3):307–310.

85. Krolewski AS, Warram JH, Rand LI, Christlieb AR, Busick EJ, Kahn CR. Risk of proliferative diabetic retinopathy in juvenile-onset type I diabetes: a 40-yr follow-up study. *Diabetes Care.* 1986;9(5):443–452.

86. Colwell JA. Effect of diabetic control on retinopathy. *Diabetes.* 1966;15(7):497–499.

87. Miki E, Fukuda M, Kuzuya T, Kosaka K, Nakao K. Relation of the course of retinopathy to control of diabetes, age, and therapeutic agents in diabetic Japanese patients. *Diabetes.* 1969;18(11):773–780.

88. Doft BH, Kingsley LA, Orchard TJ, Kuller L, Drash A, Becker D. The association between long-term diabetic control and early retinopathy. *Ophthalmology.* 1984;91(7):763–769.

89. Friberg TR, Rosenstock J, Sanborn G, Vaghefi A, Raskin P. The effect of long-term near normal glycemic control on mild diabetic retinopathy. *Ophthalmology.* 1985; 92(8):1051–1058.

90. The Kroc Collaborative Study Group. Blood glucose control and the evolution of diabetic retinopathy and albuminuria. A preliminary multicenter trial. The Kroc Collaborative Study Group. *N Engl J Med.* 1984;311(6):365–372.

91. Lauritzen T, Frost-Larsen K, Larsen HW, Deckert T. Effect of 1 year of near-normal blood glucose levels on retinopathy in insulin-dependent diabetics. *Lancet.* 1983;1(8318):200–204.

92. Klein R. The epidemiology of diabetic retinopathy: findings from the Wisconsin Epidemiologic Study of Diabetic Retinopathy. *Int Ophthalmol Clin.* 1987;27(4): 230–238.

93. Klein R, Klein BE, Moss SE, Davis MD, DeMets DL. Glycosylated hemoglobin predicts the incidence and progression of diabetic retinopathy. *JAMA.* 1988; 260(19):2864–2871.

94. Klein R, Klein BE, Moss SE, Cruickshanks KJ. Relationship of hyperglycemia to the long-term incidence and progression of diabetic retinopathy. *Arch Intern Med.* 1994;154(19):2169–2178.

95. The Diabetes Control and Complications Trial. The effect of intensive diabetes treatment on the progression of diabetic retinopathy in insulin-dependent diabetes mellitus. *Arch Ophthalmol.* 1995;113(1):36–51.

96. The Diabetes Control and Complications Trial Research Group. Progression of retinopathy with intensive versus conventional treatment in the Diabetes Control and Complications Trial. Diabetes Control and Complications Trial Research Group. *Ophthalmology.* 1995;102(4):647–661.

97. Dahl-Jorgensen K, Brinchmann-Hansen O, Hanssen KF, et al. Effect of near normoglycaemia for two years on progression of early diabetic retinopathy, nephropathy, and neuropathy: the Oslo study. *BMJ.* 1986;293(6556):1195–1199.

98. The Diabetes Control and Complications Trial. The absence of a glycemic threshold for the development of long-term complications: the perspective of the Diabetes Control and Complications Trial. *Diabetes*. 1996;45(10):1289–1298.

99. Chaturvedi N, Sjoelie AK, Porta M, et al. Markers of insulin resistance are strong risk factors for retinopathy incidence in type 1 diabetes. *Diabetes Care*. 2001;24(2): 284–289.

100. The Diabetes Control and Complications Trial. Epidemiology of Diabetes Interventions and Complications Research Group. Retinopathy and nephropathy in patients with type 1 diabetes four years after a trial of intensive therapy. *N Engl J Med*. 2000;342(6):381–389.

101. UK Prospective Diabetes Study (UKPDS) Group. Effect of intensive blood-glucose control with metformin on complications in overweight patients with type 2 diabetes (UKPDS 34). *Lancet*. 1998;352(9131):854–865. [erratum appears in *Lancet*. November 7, 1998;352(9139):1557].

102. Olsen BS, Sjolie A, Hougaard P, et al. A 6-year nationwide cohort study of glycaemic control in young people with type 1 diabetes. Risk markers for the development of retinopathy, nephropathy and neuropathy. Danish Study Group of Diabetes in Childhood. *J Diabetes Complicat*. 2000;14(6):295–300.

103. Klein R, Klein BE, Lee KE, Cruickshanks KJ, Moss SE. The incidence of hypertension in insulin-dependent diabetes. *Arch Intern Med*. 1996;156(6):622–627.

104. Rassam SM, Patel V, Kohner EM. The effect of experimental hypertension on retinal vascular autoregulation in humans: a mechanism for the progression of diabetic retinopathy. *Exp Physiol*. 1995;80(1):53–68.

105. Hsueh WA, Anderson PW. Hypertension, the endothelial cell, and the vascular complications of diabetes mellitus. *Hypertension*. 1992;20(2):253–263.

106. Suzuma I, Hata Y, Clermont A, et al. Cyclic stretch and hypertension induce retinal expression of vascular endothelial growth factor and vascular endothelial growth factor receptor-2: potential mechanisms for exacerbation of diabetic retinopathy by hypertension. *Diabetes*. 2001;50(2):444–454.

107. Klein R, Klein BE, Moss SE, Davis MD, DeMets DL. Is blood pressure a predictor of the incidence or progression of diabetic retinopathy? *Arch Intern Med*. 1989;149(11):2427–2432.

108. Adler AI, Stratton IM, Neil HA, et al. Association of systolic blood pressure with macrovascular and microvascular complications of type 2 diabetes (UKPDS 36): prospective observational study. *BMJ*. 2000;321(7258):412–419.

109. Schrier RW, Estacio RO, Esler A, Mehler P. Effects of aggressive blood pressure control in normotensive type 2 diabetic patients on albuminuria, retinopathy and strokes. *Kidney Int*. 2002;61(3):1086–1097.

110. Gaede P, Vedel P, Larsen N, Jensen GV, Parving HH, Pedersen O. Multifactorial intervention and cardiovascular disease in patients with type 2 diabetes. *N Engl J Med*. 2003;348(5):383–393.

111. Ferris FL, 3rd, Chew EY, Hoogwerf BJ. Serum lipids and diabetic retinopathy. Early Treatment Diabetic Retinopathy Study Research Group. *Diabetes Care*. 1996;19(11):1291–1293.

112. Lyons TJ, Jenkins AJ, Zheng D, et al. Diabetic retinopathy and serum lipoprotein subclasses in the DCCT/EDIC cohort. *Invest Ophthalmol Vis Sci*. 2004;45(3):910–918.

113. Chew EY. Diabetic retinopathy and lipid abnormalities. *Curr Opin Ophthalmol*. 1997;8(3):59–62.

114. Su DH, Yeo KT. Diabetic retinopathy and serum lipids. *Singapore Med J*. 2000;41(6):295–297.

115. Cusick M, Chew EY, Chan CC, Kruth HS, Murphy RP, Ferris FL, 3rd. Histopathology and regression of retinal hard exudates in diabetic retinopathy after reduction of elevated serum lipid levels. *Ophthalmology.* 2003;110(11):2126–2133.
116. Curtis TM, Scholfield CN. The role of lipids and protein kinase Cs in the pathogenesis of diabetic retinopathy. *Diabetes Metab Res Rev.* 2004;20(1):28–43.
117. Cohen RA, Hennekens CH, Christen WG, et al. Determinants of retinopathy progression in type 1 diabetes mellitus. *Am J Med.* 1999;107(1):45–51.
118. Nazimek-Siewniak B, Moczulski D, Grzeszczak W. Risk of macrovascular and microvascular complications in Type 2 diabetes: results of longitudinal study design. *J Diabet Complications.* 2002;16(4):271–276.
119. Klein BE, Moss SE, Klein R, Surawicz TS. The Wisconsin Epidemiologic Study of Diabetic Retinopathy. XIII. Relationship of serum cholesterol to retinopathy and hard exudate. *Ophthalmology.* 1991;98(8):1261–1265.
120. Chew EY, Klein ML, Ferris FL, 3rd, et al. Association of elevated serum lipid levels with retinal hard exudate in diabetic retinopathy. Early Treatment Diabetic Retinopathy Study (ETDRS) Report 22. *Arch Ophthalmol.* 1996;114(9):1079–1084.
121. Keech A, Simes RJ, Barter P, et al. Effects of long-term fenofibrate therapy on cardiovascular events in 9795 people with type 2 diabetes mellitus (the FIELD study): randomised controlled trial. *Lancet.* 2005;366(9500):1849–1861.
122. Gupta A, Gupta V, Thapar S, Bhansali A. Lipid-lowering drug atorvastatin as an adjunct in the management of diabetic macular edema. *Am J Ophthalmol.* 2004;137(4):675–682.
123. Sen K, Misra A, Kumar A, Pandey RM. Simvastatin retards progression of retinopathy in diabetic patients with hypercholesterolemia. *Diabetes Res Clin Pract.* 2002;56(1):1–11.
124. Gordon B, Chang S, Kavanagh M, et al. The effects of lipid lowering on diabetic retinopathy. *Am J Ophthalmol.* 1991;112(4):385–391.
125. Sjoberg S, Gunnarsson R, Gjotterberg M, Lefvert AK, Persson A, Ostman J. Residual insulin production, glycaemic control and prevalence of microvascular lesions and polyneuropathy in long-term type 1 (insulin-dependent) diabetes mellitus. *Diabetologia.* 1987;30(4):208–213.
126. Klein R, Moss SE, Klein BE, Davis MD, DeMets DL. Wisconsin Epidemiologic Study of Diabetic Retinopathy. XII. Relationship of C-peptide and diabetic retinopathy. *Diabetes.* 1990;39(11):1445–1450.
127. Klein R, Klein BE, Moss SE. The Wisconsin Epidemiologic Study of Diabetic Retinopathy. XVI. The relationship of C-peptide to the incidence and progression of diabetic retinopathy. *Diabetes.* 1995;44(7):796–801.
128. Steffes MW, Sibley S, Jackson M, Thomas W. Beta-cell function and the development of diabetes-related complications in the diabetes control and complications trial. *Diabetes Care.* 2003;26(3):832–836.
129. Root H, Pote WH, Frehner H. Triopathy of diabetes; sequence of neuropathy, retinopathy and nephropathy in one hundred fifty-five patients. *Arch Intern Med.* 1954;94(6):931–941.
130. Klein R, Zinman B, Gardiner R, et al. The relationship of diabetic retinopathy to preclinical diabetic glomerulopathy lesions in type 1 diabetic patients: the Renin-Angiotensin System Study. *Diabetes.* 2005;54(2):527–533.
131. Ballone E, Colagrande V, Di Nicola M, Di Mascio R, Di Mascio C, Capani F. Probabilistic approach to developing nephropathy in diabetic patients with retinopathy. *Stat Med.* 2003;22(24):3889–3897.

132. Cruickshanks KJ, Ritter LL, Klein R, Moss SE. The association of microalbumin-uria with diabetic retinopathy. The Wisconsin Epidemiologic Study of Diabetic Retinopathy. *Ophthalmology*. 1993;100(6):862–867.

133. Klein R, Moss SE, Klein BE. Is gross proteinuria a risk factor for the incidence of proliferative diabetic retinopathy? *Ophthalmology*. 1993;100(8):1140–1146.

134. Bresnick GH. Diabetic maculopathy. A critical review highlighting diffuse macular edema. *Ophthalmology*. 1983;90(11):1301–1317.

135. Perkovich BT, Meyers SM. Systemic factors affecting diabetic macular edema. *Am J Ophthalmol*. 1988;105(2):211–212.

136. Tokuyama T, Ikeda T, Sato K. Effects of haemodialysis on diabetic macular leakage. *Br J Ophthalmol*. 2000;84(12):1397–1400.

137. Freund KM, Belanger AJ, D'Agostino RB, Kannel WB. The health risks of smoking. The Framingham Study: 34 years of follow-up. *Ann Epidemiol*. 1993;3(4): 417–424.

138. Gaziano JM, Buring JE, Breslow JL, et al. Moderate alcohol intake, increased levels of high-density lipoprotein and its subfractions, and decreased risk of myocardial infarction. *N Engl J Med*. 1993;329(25):1829–1834.

139. Moss SE, Klein R, Klein BE. Cigarette smoking and ten-year progression of diabetic retinopathy. *Ophthalmology*. 1996;103(9):1438–1442.

140. Moss SE, Klein R, Klein BE. The association of alcohol consumption with the incidence and progression of diabetic retinopathy. *Ophthalmology*. 1994;101(12): 1962–1968.

141. Uckaya G, Ozata M, Bayraktar Z, Erten V, Bingol N, Ozdemir IC. Is leptin associated with diabetic retinopathy? *Diabetes Care*. 2000;23(3):371–376.

142. van Leiden HA, Dekker JM, Moll AC, et al. Blood pressure, lipids, and obesity are associated with retinopathy: the hoorn study. *Diabetes Care*. 2002;25(8):1320–1325.

143. De Block CE, De Leeuw IH, Van Gaal LF. Impact of overweight on chronic microvascular complications in type 1 diabetic patients. *Diabetes Care*. 2005;28(7): 1649–1655.

144. Klein R, Klein BE, Moss SE. Is obesity related to microvascular and macrovascular complications in diabetes? The Wisconsin Epidemiologic Study of Diabetic Retinopathy. *Arch Intern Med*. 1997;157(6):650–656.

145. Chaturvedi N, Fuller JH. Mortality risk by body weight and weight change in people with NIDDM. The WHO Multinational Study of Vascular Disease in Diabetes. *Diabetes Care*. 1995;18(6):766–774.

146. Nelson RG, Wolfe JA, Horton MB, Pettitt DJ, Bennett PH, Knowler WC. Proliferative retinopathy in NIDDM. Incidence and risk factors in Pima Indians. *Diabetes*. 1989;38(4):435–440.

147. Kriska AM, LaPorte RE, Patrick SL, Kuller LH, Orchard TJ. The association of physical activity and diabetic complications in individuals with insulin-dependent diabetes mellitus: the Epidemiology of Diabetes Complications Study—VII. *J Clin Epidemiol*. 1991;44(11):1207–1214.

148. Cruickshanks KJ, Moss SE, Klein R, Klein BE. Physical activity and proliferative retinopathy in people diagnosed with diabetes before age 30 yr. *Diabetes Care*. 1992;15(10):1267–1272.

149. Moloney JB, Drury MI. The effect of pregnancy on the natural course of diabetic retinopathy. *Am J Ophthalmol*. 1982;93(6):745–756.

150. Klein BE, Moss SE, Klein R. Effect of pregnancy on progression of diabetic retinopathy. *Diabetes Care*. 1990;13(1):34–40.

151. Chew EY, Mills JL, Metzger BE, et al. Metabolic control and progression of retinopathy. The Diabetes in Early Pregnancy Study. National Institute of Child Health
and Human Development Diabetes in Early Pregnancy Study. *Diabetes Care.*
1995;18(5):631–637.

152. Hemachandra A, Ellis D, Lloyd CE, Orchard TJ. The influence of pregnancy on
IDDM complications. *Diabetes Care.* 1995;18(7):950–954.

153. Lovestam-Adrian M, Agardh CD, Aberg A, Agardh E. Pre-eclampsia is a potent risk
factor for deterioration of retinopathy during pregnancy in Type 1 diabetic patients.
Diabetic Med. 1997;14(12):1059–1065.

154. Chen HC, Newsom RS, Patel V, Cassar J, Mather H, Kohner EM. Retinal blood
flow changes during pregnancy in women with diabetes. *Invest Ophthalmol Vis Sci.*
1994;35(8):3199–3208.

155. Schocket LS, Grunwald JE, Tsang AF, DuPont J. The effect of pregnancy on retinal hemodynamics in diabetic versus nondiabetic mothers. *Am J Ophthalmol.*
1999;128(4):477–484.

156. Sone H, Okuda Y, Kawakami Y, et al. Progesterone induces vascular endothelial growth
factor on retinal pigment epithelial cells in culture. *Life Sci.* 1996;59(1):21–25.

157. Rosenn B, Miodovnik M, Kranias G, et al. Progression of diabetic retinopathy in
pregnancy: association with hypertension in pregnancy. *Am J Obstet Gynecol.*
1992;166(4):1214–1218.

158. Klein BE, Moss SE, Klein R. Is menarche associated with diabetic retinopathy?
Diabetes Care. 1990;13(10):1034–1038.

159. Klein BE, Moss SE, Klein R. Oral contraceptives in women with diabetes. *Diabetes
Care.* 1990;13(8):895–898.

160. Klein BE, Klein R, Moss SE. Exogenous estrogen exposures and changes in diabetic
retinopathy. The Wisconsin Epidemiologic Study of Diabetic Retinopathy. *Diabetes
Care.* 1999;22(12):1984–1987.

161. Meigs JB, Hu FB, Rifai N, Manson JE. Biomarkers of endothelial dysfunction and
risk of type 2 diabetes mellitus. *JAMA.* 2004;291(16):1978–1986.

162. Pradhan AD, Manson JE, Rifai N, Buring JE, Ridker PM. C-reactive protein, interleukin 6, and risk of developing type 2 diabetes mellitus. *JAMA.*
2001;286(3):327–334.

163. Miyamoto K, Khosrof S, Bursell SE, et al. Prevention of leukostasis and vascular
leakage in streptozotocin-induced diabetic retinopathy via intercellular adhesion
molecule-1 inhibition. *Proc Natl Acad Sci USA.* 1999;96(19):10836–10841.

164. Izuora KE, Chase HP, Jackson WE, et al. Inflammatory markers and diabetic retinopathy in type 1 diabetes. *Diabetes Care.* 2005;28(3):714–715.

165. Joussen AM, Poulaki V, Le ML, et al. A central role for inflammation in the pathogenesis of diabetic retinopathy. *FASEB J.* 2004;18(12):1450–1452.

166. Mitamura Y, Takeuchi S, Yamamoto S, et al. Monocyte chemotactic protein-1 levels
in the vitreous of patients with proliferative vitreoretinopathy. *Jpn J Ophthalmol.*
2002;46(2):218–221.

167. Meleth AD, Agron E, Chan CC, et al. Serum inflammatory markers in diabetic retinopathy. *Invest Ophthalmol Vis Sci.* 2005;46(11):4295–4301.

168. van Hecke MV, Dekker JM, Nijpels G, et al. Inflammation and endothelial dysfunction are associated with retinopathy: the Hoorn Study. *Diabetologia.*
2005;48(7):1300–1306.

169. Schram MT, Chaturvedi N, Schalkwijk CG, Fuller JH, Stehouwer CD, Group
EPCS. Markers of inflammation are cross-sectionally associated with microvascular

complications and cardiovascular disease in type 1 diabetes—the EURODIAB Prospective Complications Study. *Diabetologia*. 2005;48(2):370–378.

170. Early Treatment Diabetic Retinopathy Study Research Group. Effects of aspirin treatment on diabetic retinopathy. ETDRS report number 8. Early Treatment Diabetic Retinopathy Study Research Group. *Ophthalmology*. 1991;98(5 Suppl):757–765.

171. Klein R, Klein BE, Moss SE. Epidemiology of proliferative diabetic retinopathy. *Diabetes Care*. 1992;15(12):1875–1891.

172. Klein R, Klein BE, Moss SE, Cruickshanks KJ. Association of ocular disease and mortality in a diabetic population. *Arch Ophthalmol*. 1999;117(11):1487–1495.

173. Wong TY, Rosamond W, Chang PP, et al. Retinopathy and risk of congestive heart failure. *JAMA*. 2005;293(1):63–69.

6

History of Evolving Treatments for Diabetic Retinopathy

GEORGE W. BLANKENSHIP, MD

CORE MESSAGES

- Creative concepts, research, clinical observations, and sharing information and ideas have resulted in successful treatments for diabetic retinopathy.
- Professor Meyer-Schwickerath introduced photocoagulation for developing and refining the use of light energy to treat retinal diseases in the late 1940s and 1950s.
- Dr. Robert Machemer is appropriately recognized as the father of vitreous surgery for developing the initial concepts, instruments, and procedures for pars plana vitreous surgery in the 1960s and 1970s.
- Collaborative clinical trials sponsored by the National Eye Institute defined the natural history, indications, techniques, and results of treatment for diabetic retinopathy.

The earliest known written record of diabetes was by the Hindu physician Susruta who described a condition of honey urine. Descriptions of diabetes also appear in early Egyptian records, and Greek physicians reported the melting away of flesh and limbs to urine. Other diabetic complications such as blindness undoubtedly occurred, but were probably rare because of the patients' relatively short life span following the development of diabetes.

Diabetic retinopathy was first described by von Jager in 1855 [1]. Initially, the fundus changes were thought to be the result of hypertension that often coexisted with diabetes, or an inflammatory response to elevated albumin and urea levels resulting in the descriptive term diabetic retinitis. Later, the specific relationship between diabetes and retinal vascular changes was recognized, but diabetic retinopathy remained a relatively uncommon complication.

CONTROL OF DIABETES AND RETINOPATHY

The discovery of insulin by Banting and Best [2] in 1921 revolutionized the treatment of diabetes and markedly extended the lives of people with this disease. The increased longevity provided more time for the development of late complications such as retinopathy. Loss of vision and blindness from diabetic retinopathy became an increasing problem without successful treatment.

The direct relationship of blood sugar levels and diabetic retinopathy was suspected but not proven or universally accepted. Some argued that diabetes had a primary effect on the basement membrane of blood vessels, independent of blood sugar [3], while others believed that tight control of blood glucose levels would inhibit the progression of the vascular changes. Only when instruments were developed, which patients could use to check their blood sugar repeatedly throughout the day, did intensive control of blood sugar level become feasible.

Later, the National Institutes of Health supported a large multicenter clinical trial, the Diabetes Control and Complication Trial (DCCT), which proved that good control of blood sugar was a very important factor in preventing and slowing the progression of retinopathy [4].

PHOTOCOAGULATION

The risk of losing vision from looking at the sun had been known for centuries, and solar retinal burns were observed after the development of the ophthalmoscope. The possibility of using light to treat retinal diseases gradually evolved from these observations. Following a solar eclipse on July 10, 1945, Meyer-Schwickerath (Fig. 6.1) in Hamburg-Eppendorf, Germany, became interested in the possible use of light energy to treat retinal diseases. He initially used focused sunlight (Fig. 6.2) but found this to be impractical, and tried other sources of light (Fig. 6.3) before refining the use of light produced by a high pressure xenon arc bulb (Fig. 6.4). His results of treating retinal tears and small suspected melanomas were first published in 1949 [5–7]. Moran-Sales had been doing similar research independently and he published his results shortly thereafter in 1950 [8].

The initial results of treating diabetic retinopathy lesions with photocoagulation were discouraging, but persistent efforts during the 1950s and 1960s by Wetzig (Fig. 6.5) [9,10], Amalric (Fig 6.6) [11,12], Okun (Fig 6.7) [13–15], Wessing [16], and numerous other ophthalmologists began to produce better visual and anatomical results than those reported for the natural course of the disease by Caird [17] and Beetham (Fig. 6.8) [18]. Various techniques of photocoagulation treatment of diabetic retinopathy were tried and advocated. Treatment strategies ranged from coagulating everything that was red (retinal hemorrhages and microaneurysms) to producing a line of coagulation along the sides of the major vessels to direct confluent treatment of neovascularization.

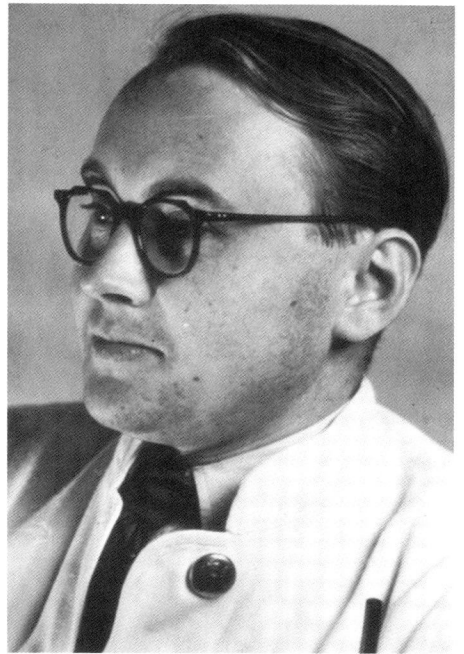

Figure 6.1. Meyer-Schwickerath in Hamburg, Germany, when initially developing photocoagulation. Professor Meyer-Schwickerath is universally recognized as the father of photocoagulation.

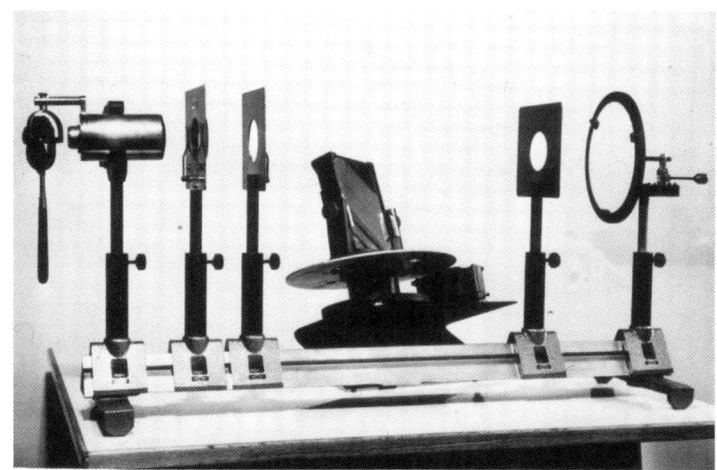

Figure 6.2. Meyer-Schwickerath's lens system for focusing sunlight for photocoagulation.

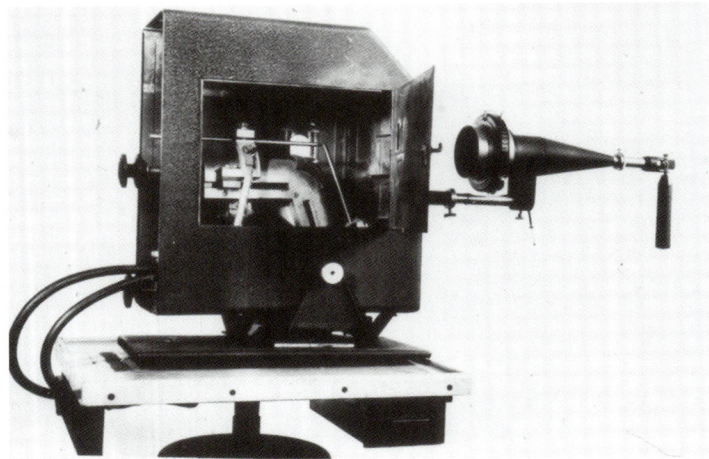

Figure 6.3. Meyer-Schwickerath's early photocoagulator using a carbon arc light source.

LASER PHOTOCOAGULATION

During this time, there was increasing interest and research to adapt wavelengths produced by newly invented lasers for photocoagulation. Campbell [19,20] and Zweng (Fig. 6.9) [21] independently used ruby laser wavelengths with limited success in the early 1960s. Beetham [22] and Aiello (Fig. 6.8) [23] had better results treating diabetic retinopathy with ruby laser photocoagulation a few years later, especially with widespread scatter panretinal photocoagulation (PRP).

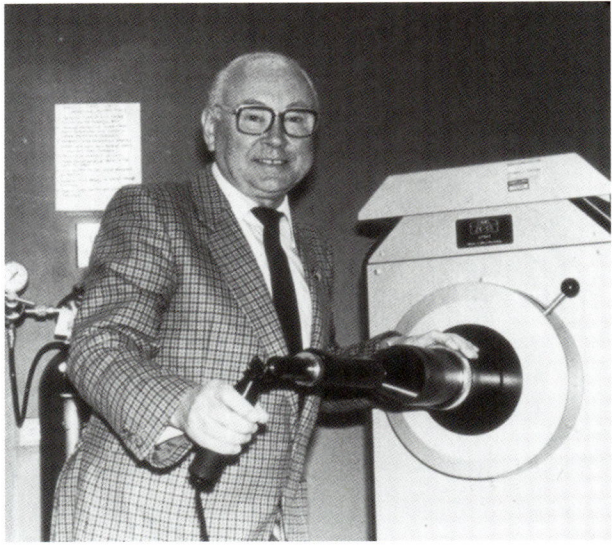

Figure 6.4. Meyer-Schwickerath with photocoagulator using a xenon light source.

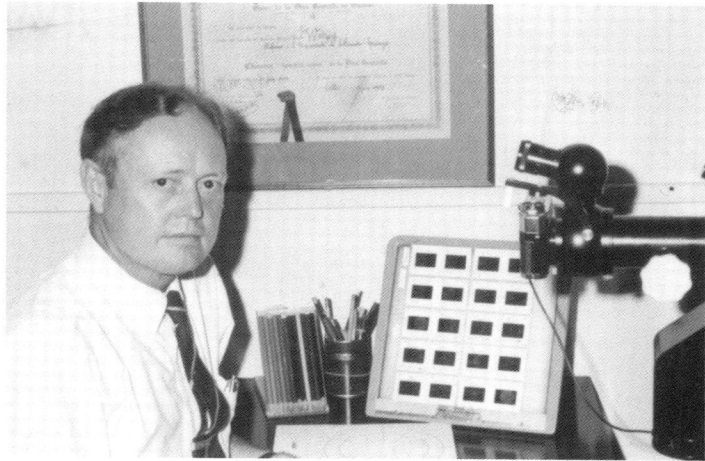

Figure 6.5. Paul Wetzig, M.D.

In the late 1960s, the potential value of laser wavelengths produced with argon gas was recognized. Independent research by L'Esperance (Fig. 6.10) and coworkers [24,25], and Little (Fig. 6.11) and Zweng [26,27] and their associates resulted in the adaptation of argon laser wavelengths with delivery systems for successful retinal photocoagulation.

The successful treatment of diabetic retinopathy with argon laser wavelengths was also reported by Patz (Fig. 6.12) [28]. When the argon laser was developed, it was hoped that the absorption of green wavelengths by hemoglobin would allow direct treatment of elevated neovascularization. Efforts to close neovascularization

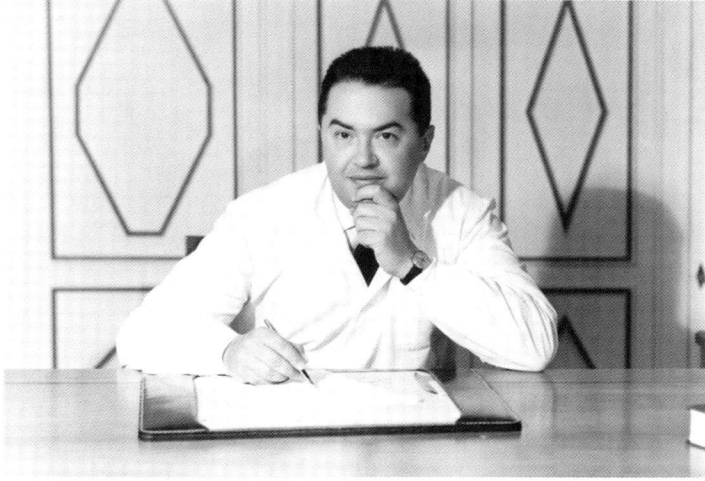

Figure 6.6. Professor Pierre Amalric.

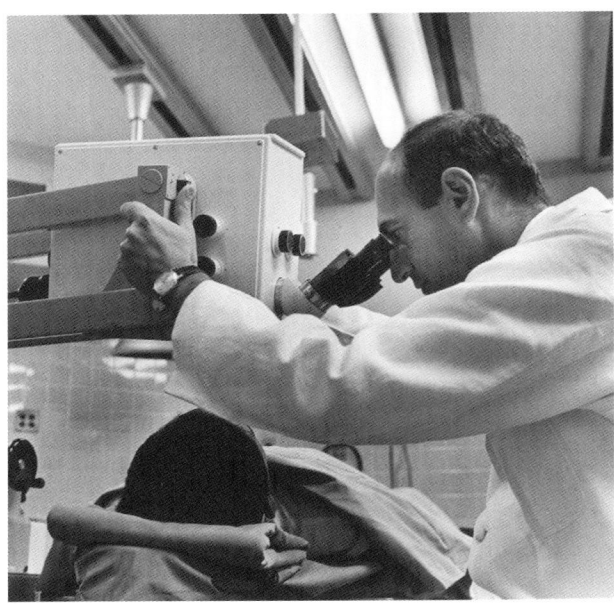

Figure 6.7. Edward Okun, M.D., Professor of Ophthalmology at Washington University School of Medicine and Director of Washington University Ophthalmology Department Retina Service using binocular xenon photocoagulation.

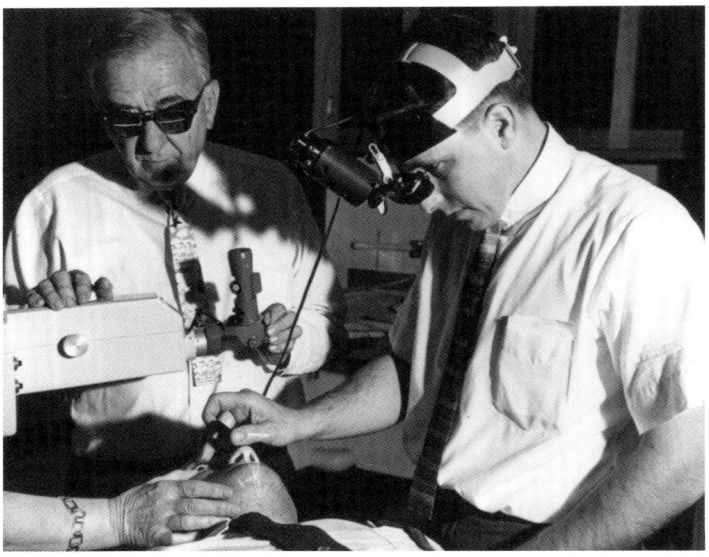

Figure 6.8. William Beetham, M.D., and Lloyd M. Aiello, M.D., Directors of Beetham Eye Unit of Joslin Diabetes Center, Boston, Massachusetts evaluating panretinal photocoagulation with a ruby laser.

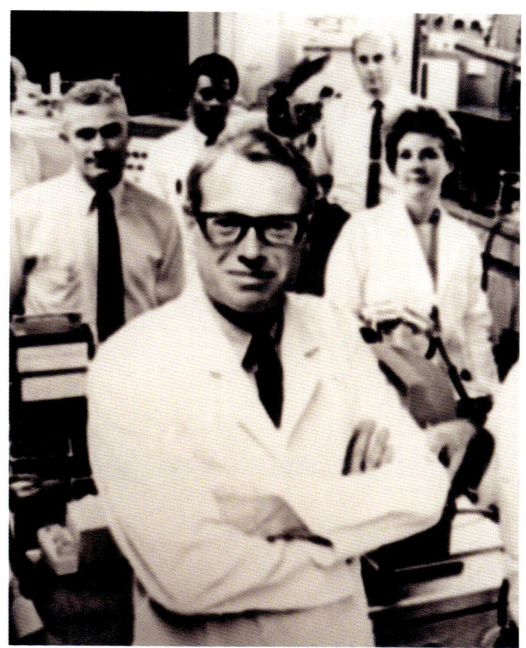

Figure 6.9. Christopher Zweng, M.D., adapting laser wavelengths for retinal photocoagulation.

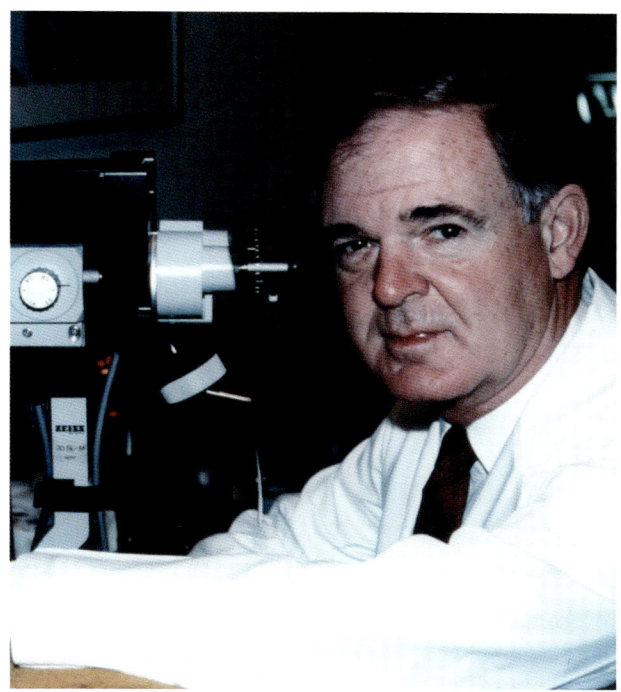

Figure 6.10. Francis L'Esperance, M.D., adapting laser wavelengths for retinal photocoagulation.

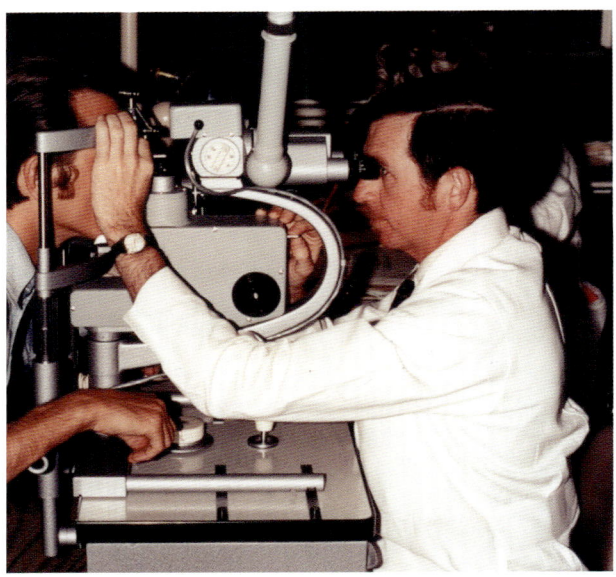

Figure 6.11. Hunter Little, M.D., adapting laser wavelengths for retinal photocoagulation.

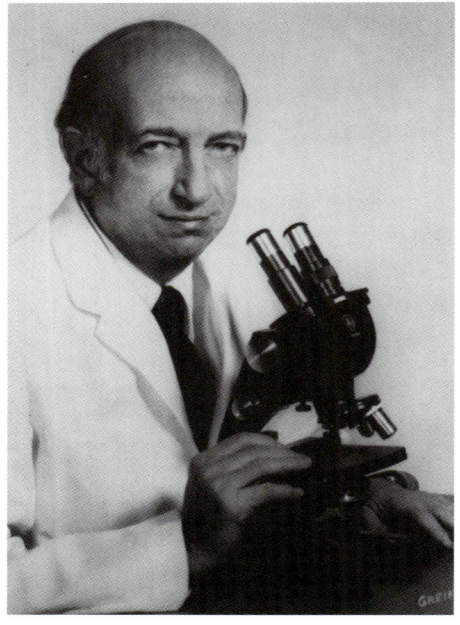

Figure 6.12. Arnall Patz, Professor and Chair of Johns Hopkins Department of Ophthalmology and Director of Wilmer Ophthalmological Institute evaluating histopathology of diabetic retinopathy.

by treating feeder arteriolar vessels of elevated neovascular fronds were usually unsuccessful, despite retreatments several times within a few days. This technique was abandoned because of its lack of efficacy and because it often produced vitreous hemorrhages. Unless the stimulus for neovascularization was reduced, the treated new vessels simply reopened and continued to proliferate.

The studies of Davis (Fig. 6.13) on the natural history of diabetic retinopathy [29,30] had documented that the neovascular component in some cases resolved spontaneously into a fibrotic scar before loss of vision occurred. Another important observation [13,16] was the apparent protection against developing diabetic retinopathy in eyes with extensive chorioretinal scarring and optic atrophy. This led to further attempts to induce regression of neovascularization to preserve vision by applying a standardized pattern of PRP that would spare the macula but reduce the stimulus for neovascular proliferation.

Fundus photography and fluorescein angiography provided valuable additional information on the vascular changes of diabetic retinopathy progressing from capillary damage, edema, nonperfusion and ischemia, and neovascular proliferation [31–37]. Specific identification of leakage sites for focal laser photocoagulation when treating macular edema [38–42], and areas of nonperfusion for PRP when treating neovascular proliferation became possible.

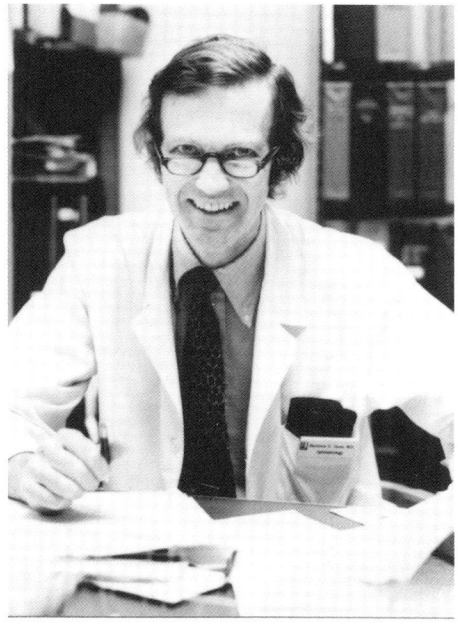

Figure 6.13. Matthew Davis, M.D., Professor and Chair of University of Wisconsin Ophthalmology Department, Director of Diabetic Retinopathy Study, Director of Diabetic Retinopathy Vitrectomy Study.

Regression of diabetic retinopathy and preservation of vision had also been observed following loss of pituitary function, and therapeutic roles of pituitary ablation were also being studied.

Various surgical and irradiation procedures were developed for pituitary ablation [43–46], but this form of therapy was abandoned with the development of photocoagulation, which was much simpler to perform, had fewer systemic side effects, and produced better results.

There was increasing awareness of the number of people developing diabetes and having loss of vision from diabetic retinopathy complications. In 1968, Drs. Stuart Fine and Morton Goldberg of the United States Public Health Service organized an international meeting on diabetic retinopathy and its treatment at the Airlie House Convention Center near Washington, DC (Fig. 6.14).

Although numerous scientific presentations were given on the natural history of diabetic retinopathy and its treatment with photocoagulation and pituitary gland suppression, the need for more and better data on the natural history and the indications, techniques, and results of photocoagulation collected in a standardized manner at multiple clinical centers was recognized.

The National Eye Institute (NEI), under the direction of Dr. Carl Kupfer, supplied the necessary funding for a series of very successful large collaborative clinical trials on the natural history and treatment of various stages of diabetic retinopathy. In addition, Dr. Frederick Ferris (Fig. 6.15), Director, Division of Epidemiology and Clinical Research, and Clinical Director of the NEI, provided equally important encouragement, advice, and leadership for these projects.

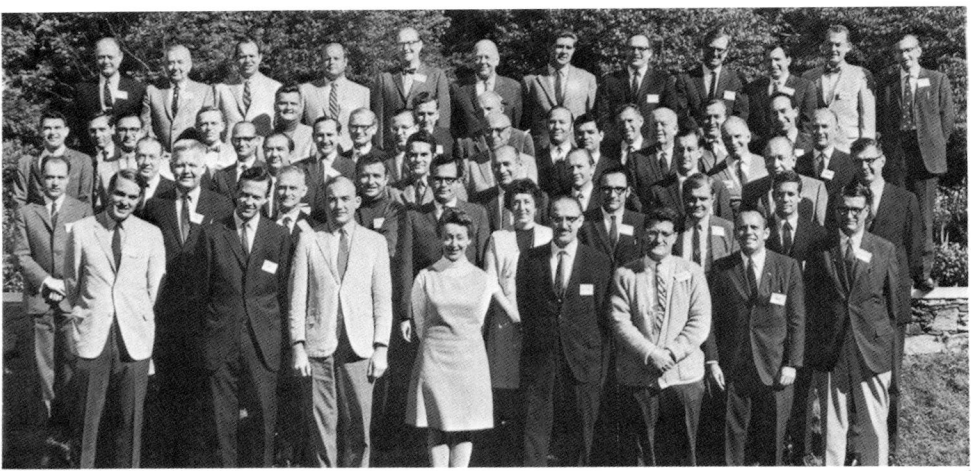

Row 1 (front): S. L. Fine, M. D. Davis, N. Oakley, E. Kohner, M. Balodimos, H. Spalter, J. Linfoot, T. Duane. Row 2: A. Wessing, R. Kjellberg, W. Sweet, N. Zervas, E. Finkelstein, E. Hallworth, L. Jagerman, E. W. D. Norton, H. Lester. Row 3: B. Ray, J. Hardy, A. Panisset, E. Okun. B. Straatsma, G. Cleasby, O. Pearson, J. W. McMeel. Row 4: F. Myers, M. Goldberg, H.-W. Larsen, R. Blach, T. R. Fraser, W. van Heuven, R. Feinberg, K. Gabbay, G. McDonald, J. Dobree, R. Schimek. Row 5: R. Packman, R. Bradley, P. Jahnke, F. Caird, P. Thornfeldt, C. Mortimer, G. Harris, K. Lundbaek, H. Keen. Row 6: P. Wetzig, W. Beetham, W. Peretz, J. Glaser, M. Rubin, J. Ferree, Sv. Simonsen, N. Roth, H. C. Zweng, L. Aiello, E. Greenberg, G. Joplin.

Figure 6.14. Participants of U.S. Public Health Service International Meeting on diabetic retinopathy organized by Dr. Stuart Fine and Dr. Morton Goldberg at the Airlie House Convention Center in 1968.

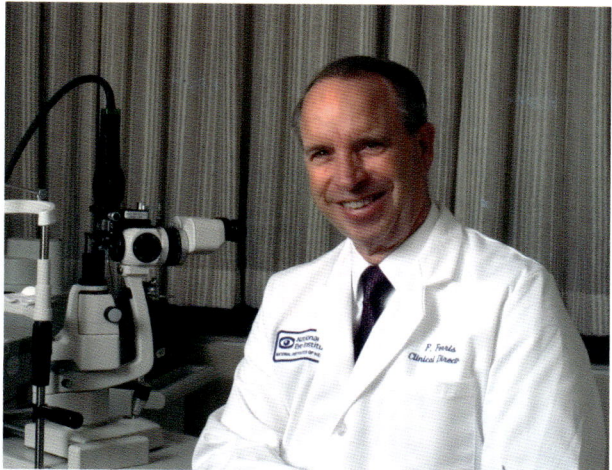

Figure 6.15. Frederick Ferris, M.D., Director of the National Eye Institute's Division of Epidemiology and Clinical Research, and Clinical Director of the National Eye Institute.

The first of these clinical trials, the Diabetic Retinopathy Study (DRS) [47], was directed by Dr. Matthew Davis. It documented the increased risk of blindness with progression of diabetic retinopathy, and the success of PRP produced with either xenon light or argon laser wavelengths in regressing diabetic retinopathy and preserving vision. The very successful DRS was followed by the Early Treatment Diabetic Retinopathy Study (ETDRS) [48] with Dr. Lloyd M. Aiello as Director. It documented the value of argon laser photocoagulation in treating macular edema and reducing loss of vision. Each of these important clinical trials, their major findings and impact on establishing the standards of care for diabetic retinopathy, are presented in much more detail elsewhere in this book.

Additional studies further evaluated laser treatment procedures and techniques for treating diabetic retinopathy [49–54].

VITREOUS SURGERY

Coincidental with the development of photocoagulation treatment of diabetic retinopathy, radical new concepts and revolutionary surgery for the management of diseases and disorders affecting the vitreous were being developed at the Bascom Palmer Eye Institute of the University of Miami School of Medicine in Florida. Dr. David Kasner (Fig. 6.16) had successfully restored vision in an eye with amyloidosis by removing a large portion of the opaque formed vitreous. He had achieved good results with similar aggressive techniques while teaching ophthalmology residents how to manage loss of vitreous during cataract surgery at the Miami Veterans Administration Hospital.

Dr. Robert Machemer (Fig. 6.17), also at the Bascom Palmer Eye Institute and the Miami Veterans Administration Hospital, was intrigued with Dr. Kasner's

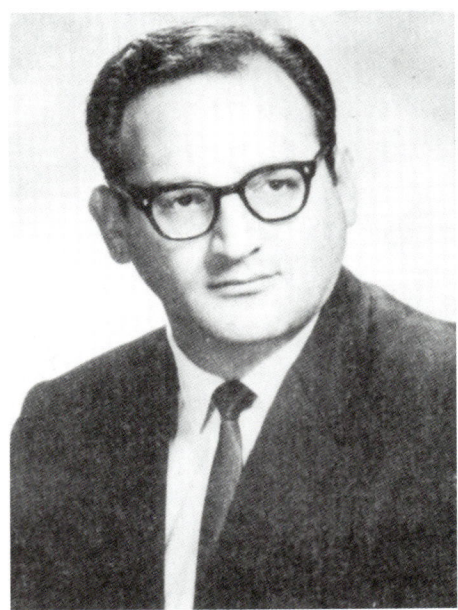

Figure 6.16. David Kasner, M.D., Clinical Faculty of Bascom Palmer Eye Institute of the University of Miami School of Medicine and Veterans Administrative Hospital of Miami, Florida.

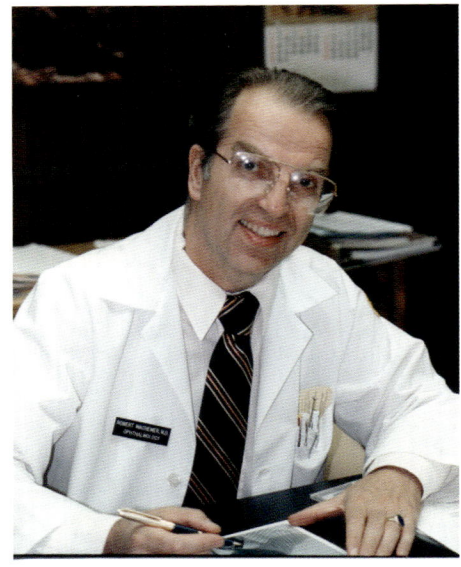

Figure 6.17. Robert Machemer, M.D., Professor of Ophthalmology at Bascom Palmer Eye Institute of the University of Miami, and Professor and Chair of Duke University's Ophthalmology Department and Director of Duke University's Eye Center. Dr. Machemer is universally recognized as the father of vitreous surgery.

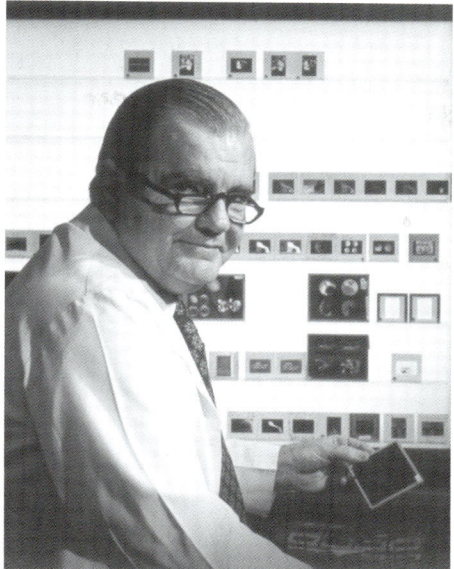

Figure 6.18. Edward W. D. Norton, M.D., Professor and Chair of University of Miami's Department of Ophthalmology and Director of the Bascom Palmer Eye Institute.

success, and began a research program to develop surgery to correct vitreous diseases and restore vision. With the support and encouragement of Dr. Edward W.D. Norton (Fig. 6.18), Chairman of the Bascom Palmer Eye Institute, Dr. Machemer worked with Dr. Helmut Buettner and Mr. Jean Marie Parel and their coworkers to develop microsurgical instruments (Fig. 6.19) and procedures with which the contents of the vitreous cavity could be safely removed through the pars plana while maintaining intraocular pressure and a formed globe [55,56].

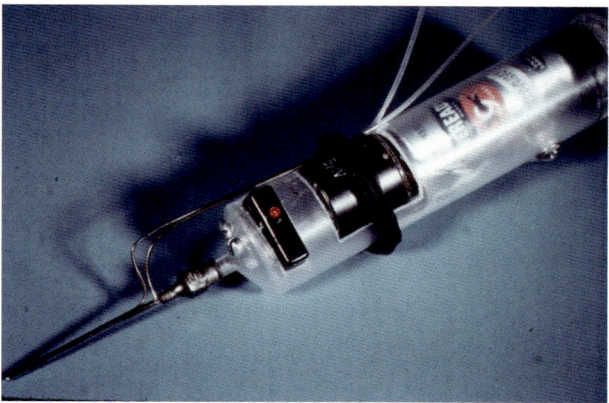

Figure 6.19. First prototype of pars plana vitrectomy instrument combining vitreous infusion, suction, and cutting by a rotating auger enclosed in the tip in a single instrument.

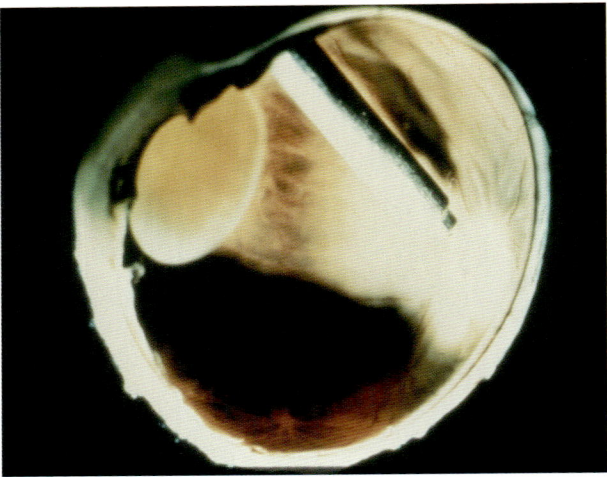

Figure 6.20. Vitreous infusion suction cutter (VISC) with surrounding fiber optics inserted through the pars plana into the vitreous cavity.

Dr. Machemer performed the first pars plana vitrectomy in 1970 and soon realized the potential value of removing not only opaque vitreous hemorrhages but also proliferative membranes, and repairing retinal detachments by releasing vitreous traction [57]. This new surgery provided a way to restore sight for people who had become blind from diabetic retinopathy.

At this early stage, the vitrectomy instruments evolved rapidly with a single hand-held instrument named the vitreous infusion suction cutter (VISC) (Fig. 6.20) providing vitreous infusion, suction, and cutting. The advantages of having a second instrument in the vitreous cavity for additional infusion, diathermy, tissue retraction, aspiration, etc. were soon recognized and bimanual surgical techniques and additional instruments were developed [58].

The initial vitrectomies were performed with just coaxial light from the operating microscope, but intraocular visualization was soon improved by the introduction of fiber-optic light sources into the vitreous cavity.

O'Malley [59,60] emphasized the value of decreasing the diameter of the instrument used in the eye by separating the functions and introducing the guillotine type cutter and 3-port system separating the suction-cutter from the infusion and the fiber-optic light source (Fig. 6.21). Aaberg [61–63], Charles (Fig. 6.22) [64,65], Douvas [66], Federman [67], Kloti [68,69], McCuen [70], Michels (Fig. 6.23) [71–79], Peyman [80], Tolentino [81,82], and many others [83–86] expanded and clarified the indications for vitrectomy and made important contributions to instrumentation and surgical techniques. Recently, the size of vitrectomy instruments has been further reduced to 25 gauge [87]; their use decreases postoperative morbidity and recovery time in selected cases.

Improvements in evaluating eyes with opaque media by ultrasound dramatically increased the success of pars plana vitreous surgery. Coleman and coworkers

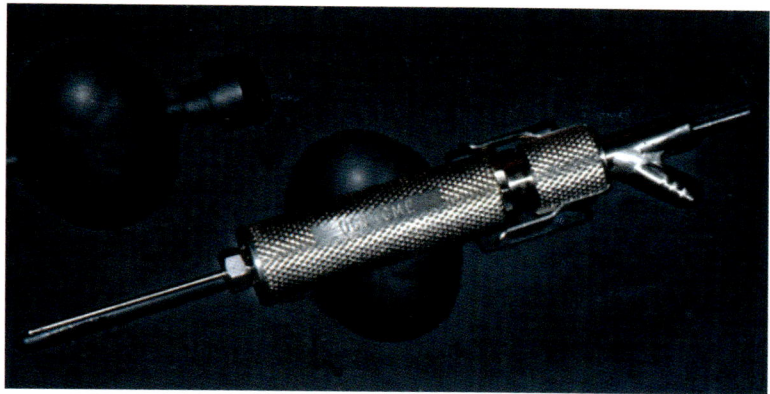

Figure 6.21. Early version of Ocutome vitrectomy instrument developed by O'Malley and Heintz, which utilized a back and forth guillotine cutting action of formed vitreous and proliferative tissue aspirated into the side of the instrument tip.

[88,89], and others, developed and refined ultrasound procedures to identify areas of vitreoretinal traction, and the presence, location, and extent of retinal detachments, better.

The use of pars plana vitreous surgery spread rapidly because of its potential to dramatically restore functioning vision for patients who had lost their sight most frequently from complications of diabetic retinopathy, and because of a philosophy of openly sharing experiences and ideas by Dr. Machemer and others involved with the development of pars plana vitreous surgery.

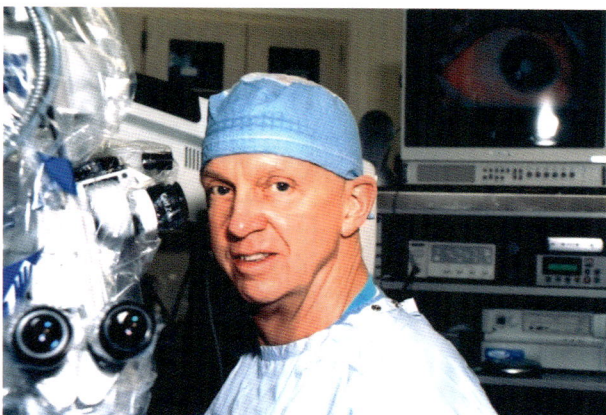

Figure 6.22. Steven T. Charles, M.D., Director of Charles Eye Institute of Memphis, Tennessee. Dr. Charles made many contributions to the development of vitreous surgical instruments and developed numerous creative procedures for vitreous surgery.

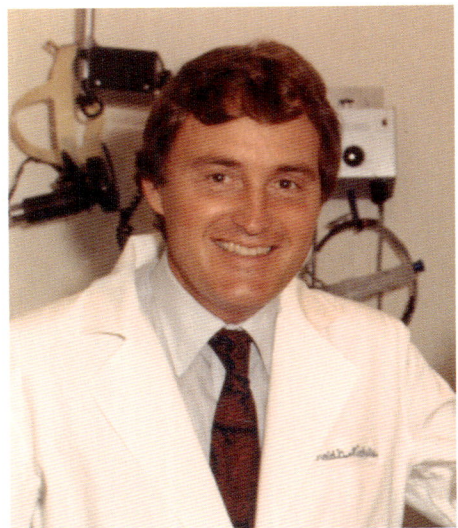

Figure 6.23. Ronald G. Michels, M.D., Professor of Ophthalmology at the Johns Hopkins University School of Medicine, former Director of Wilmer Ophthalmological Institute Vitreoretinal Surgery Service, and Co-Director of The Retina Center in Baltimore, Maryland. Dr. Michels made invaluable contributions to the development of pars plana vitreous surgery by developing new vitreous surgery procedures and publishing extensively on vitreous surgery.

Still, questions remained about when to recommend vitreous surgery for dense nonclearing vitreous hemorrhages, and for eyes with functioning vision but very extensive neovascular proliferation beyond what could reasonably be treated with photocoagulation. Once again, the NEI provided funding for a large multicenter clinical trial named the Diabetic Retinopathy Vitrectomy Study (DRVS) [90], with Dr. Matthew Davis as Director. The DRVS confirmed the benefits of pars plana vitrectomy in removing dense vitreous hemorrhages and extensive neovascularization caused by diabetic retinopathy.

CONCLUSION

The history of the treatment for diabetic retinopathy encompasses almost 60 years and continues to evolve with new innovations. It is composed of many important observations, creative new concepts, elaborate laboratory and clinical research projects, development and refinement of revolutionary instruments and procedures, sophisticated evaluations confirming the benefits of good control of blood sugar levels, and appropriate photocoagulation and vitreous surgery. A very large number of people have made important contributions to the current level of knowledge and treatment abilities, and the future is even more encouraging for additional discoveries that will further enhance the ability to preserve and regain vision for people with diabetes.

REFERENCES

1. von Jaeger E. Beitrage zur Pathologie des Auges. 2. Lieferung, S. 33, Tafel XII. Wien, K.K. Hof- and Staatsdruckerei; 1855.
2. Banting FG, Best CH. The internal secretion of the pancreas. *J Lab Clin Med.* 1922;7:251–266.
3. Hutton WL, Snyder WB, Vaiser A, Siperstein MD. Retinal microangiopathy without associated glucose intolerance. *Trans Amer Acad Ophthalmol Otolaryngol.* 1972;76:968–980.
4. Diabetes Control and Complications Trial Research Group. The effect of intensive treatment of diabetes on the development and progression of long-term complications in insulin dependent diabetes mellitus. *N Engl J Med.* 1993;329:977–986.
5. Meyer-Schwickerath G. *Verh Dtsch Ges Ophthalmol Heidelberg.* 1949;55:256.
6. Meyer-Schwickerath G. Licktkoagulation. *Buech Augenarzt.* 1959;33:1–96.
7. Meyer-Schwickerath G. *Light Coagulation.* Translated by SM Drance. St. Louis: CV Mosby Co; 1960:114.
8. Moran-Salas J. *Arch Soc Oftal Hispano-Am.* 1950;10:566–578.
9. Wetzig PC, Worlton JT. Treatment of diabetic retinopathy by light coagulation: a preliminary study. *Br J Ophthalmol.* 1963;47:539–541.
10. Wetzig PC, Jepson CN. Treatment of diabetic retinopathy by light coagulation. *Am J Ophthalmol.* 1966;62:459–465.
11. Amalric MP. Essai de traitement de la retinopathie diabetique exsudative. *Bulletin des Societes d'Ophtalmologie de France.* 1960;5–6:1–4.
12. Amalric P. Nouvelles considerations concernant l'evolution et le traitment de la retinopathie diabetique. *Ophthalmologica.* 1967;154:151–160.
13. Okun E, Cibis P. The role of photocoagulation in the treatment of proliferative diabetic retinopathy. *Arch Ophthalmol.* 1966;75:337–352.
14. Okun E. The effectiveness of photocoagulation in the therapy of proliferative diabetic retinopathy (PDR); (controlled study in 50 patients). *Trans Am Acad Ophthalmol Otolaryngol.* 1968;72:246–252.
15. Okun E, Johnston G, Boniuk I. *Management of Diabetic Retinopathy; a Stereoscopic Presentation.* St. Louis: The C.V. Mosby Co; 1971.
16. Wessing AK, Meyer-Schwickerath G. Results of photocoagulation in diabetic retinopathy. In: Goldberg MF, Fine SL, eds. *Symposium on the Treatment of Diabetic Retinopathy.* Airlie House, Warrenton, VA, September 29 to October 1, 1968. Washington, DC, US Government Printing Office (PHS Publ No 1980), 1969: 569–592.
17. Caird FI, Garrett CJ. Prognosis for vision in diabetic retinopathy. *Diabetes.* 1963;12: 389–397.
18. Beetham WP. Visual prognosis of proliferating diabetic retinopathy. *Br J Ophthalmol.* 1963;47:611–619.
19. Campbell CJ, Rittler MC, Koester CJ. The optical maser as a retinal coagulator: an evaluation. *Trans Am Acad Ophthalmol Otolaryngol.* 1963;67:58–67.
20. Campbell CJ, Koester CJ, Curtice V, et al. Clinical studies in laser photocoagulation. *Arch Ophthalmol.* 1965;74:57–65.
21. Zweng HC, Flocks M, Kapany NS, et al. Experimental laser photocoagulation. *Am J Ophthalmol.* 1964;58:353–362.
22. Beetham WP, Aiello LM, Balodimos MC, et al. Ruby laser photocoagulation of early diabetic neovascular retinopathy: preliminary results of a long-term controlled study. *Arch Ophthalmol.* 1970;83:261–272.

23. Aiello LM, Beetham WP, Balodimos MC, et al. Ruby laser photocoagulation in treatment of diabetic proliferating retinopathy: preliminary report. In: Goldberg MF, Fine SL, eds. *Symposium on the Treatment of Diabetic Retinopathy*. Airlie House, Warrenton, VA, September 29–October 1, 1968. Washington, DC, US Government Printing Office (PHS Publ No 1980), 1968:437–463.

24. L'Esperance FA. An ophthalmic argon laser photocoagulation system: design, construction, and laboratory investigations. *Trans Am Ophthalmol Soc*. 1968;66:827–904.

25. L'Esperance FA. Argon laser photocoagulation of diabetic retinal neovascularization: a five year appraisal. *Trans Am Acad Ophthalmol Otolaryngol*. 1973;77:OP6–OP24.

26. Little HL, Zweng HC, Peabody RR. Argon laser slit lamp retinal photocoagulation. *Trans Am Acad Ophthalmol Otolaryngol*. 1970;74:85–97.

27. Zweng HC, Little HL, Peabody RR. Further observations on argon laser photocoagulation of diabetic retinopathy. *Trans Am Acad Ophthalmol Otolaryngol*. 1972;76:990–1004.

28. Patz A, Maumanee AE, Ryan SJ. Argon laser photocoagulation: advantages and limitations. *Trans Am Acad Ophthalmol Otolaryngol*. 1971;75:569–579.

29. Davis MD. Natural course of diabetic retinopathy. In: Kimura SJ, Caygill WM, eds. *Vascular Complications of Diabetes Mellitus with Special Emphasis on Microangiopathy of the Eye*. St. Louis: C.V. Mosby; 1967:139–169, Chapter 10.

30. Davis MD. The natural course of diabetic retinopathy. *Trans Am Acad Ophthalmol Otolaryngol*. 1968;72:237–240.

31. Gass JDM. A fluoroscein angriographic study of macular dysfunction secondary to retinal vascular disease. IV Diabetic retinal angiopathy. *Arch Ophthalmol*. 1968;80:583–591.

32. Kohner EM, Dollery CT. Fluoroscein angiography of the fundus in diabetic retinopathy. *Br Med Bull*. 1970;26:166–170.

33. Bresnick GH, de Venecia G, Myers FL, et al. Retinal ischemia in diabetic retinopathy. *Arch Ophthalmol*. 1975;93:1300–1310.

34. Bresnick GH, Engerman R, Davis MD, et al. Patterns of ischemia in diabetic retinopathy. *Trans Am Acad Ophthalmol Otolaryngol*. 1976;81:OP694.

35. Kohner EM. The evolution and natural history of diabetic retinopathy. *Int Ophthalmol Clin*. 1978;18:1–16.

36. Patz A. Clinical and experimental studies on retinal neovascularization, Thirty-Ninth Edward Jackson Memorial Lecture. *Am J Ophthalmol*. 1982;94:715–743.

37. Shimizu K, Kobayashi Y, Muraoka K. Midperipheral fundus involvement in diabetic retinopathy. *Ophthalmology*. 1981;88:601–612.

38. Patz A, Schatz H, Ryan SJ, et al. Argon laser photocoagulation for treatment of advanced diabetic retinopathy. *Trans Am Acad Ophthalmol Otolaryngol*. 1972;76:984.

39. Patz A, Schatz H, Berkow JW, et al. Macular edema-an overlooked complication of diabetic retinopathy. *Trans Am Acad Ophthalmol Otolaryngol*. 1973;77:OP34–OP42.

40. Merin S, Yanko L, Ivry M. Treatment of diabetic maculopathy by argon-laser. *Br J Ophthalmol*. 1974;58:85–91.

41. Blankenship GW. Diabetic macular edema and argon laser photocoagulation: a prospective randomized study. *Ophthalmology*. 1979;86:69–75.

42. British Multicentre Study Group. Photocoagulation for diabetic maculopathy: a randomized controlled clinical trial using the xenon arc. *Diabetes*. 1983;32:1010–1016.

43. Luft R, et al. Hypophysectomy in man. Further experiences in severe diabetes mellitus. *Br Med J*. 1955;2:752–756.

44. Bradley RF, Rees SB. Surgical pituitary ablation for diabetic retinopathy. In: Goldberg MF, Fine SL, eds. *Symposium on the Treatment of Diabetic Retinopathy.* Airlie House, Warrenton, VA, September 29–October 1, 1968. Washington, DC, US Government Printing Office (PHS Publ No 1980), 1968:171–191.

45. Field RA, McMeel JW, Sweet WH, Schepens CL. Hypophyseal stalk section for angiopathic diabetic retinopathy. In: Goldberg MF, Fine SL, eds. *Symposium on the Treatment of Diabetic Retinopathy.* Airlie House, Warrenton, VA, September 29–October 1, 1968. Washington, DC, US Government Printing Office (PHS Publ No 1980), 1968:213–225.

46. Oakley NW, Joplin GF, Kohner EM, Fraser TR. The treatment of diabetic retinopathy by pituitary implantation of radioactive yttrium. In: Goldberg MF, Fine SL, eds. *Symposium on the Treatment of Diabetic Retinopathy.* Airlie House, Warrenton, VA, September 29–October 1, 1968. Washington, DC, US Government Printing Office (PHS Publ No 1980), 1968:317–329.

47. Diabetic Retinopathy Study Research Group. Preliminary report on effects of photocoagulation therapy. *Am J Ophthalmol.* 1976;81:383–396.

48. Early Treatment Diabetic Retinopathy Study Research Group. Photocoagulation for diabetic macular edema, Early Treatment Diabetic Retinopathy Study (ETDRS) Report No. 1. *Arch Ophthalmol.* 1985;103:1796–1806.

49. Doft BH, Blankenship GW. Single versus multiple treatment sessions of argon laser panretinal photocoagulation for proliferative diabetic retinopathy. *Ophthalmology.* 1982;89:772–779.

50. Blankenship GW, Machemer R. Long term diabetic vitrectomy results, report of 10 year follow-up. *Ophthalmology.* 1985;92:503–506.

51. Blankenship GW. Red krypton and blue-green argon panretinal laser photocoagulation for proliferative diabetic retinopathy: a laboratory and clinical comparison. *Trans Am Acad Ophth Soc.* 1986;84:967–1003.

52. Blankenship GW. A clinical comparison of central and peripheral argon laser panretinal photocoagulation for proliferative diabetic retinopathy. *Ophthalmology.* 1988;95:170–177.

53. Blankenship GW. Fifteen-year argon laser and xenon photocoagulation results of Bascom Palmer Eye Institute's patients participating in the Diabetic Retinopathy Study. *Ophthalmology.* 1991;98:125–128.

54. Wade EC, Blankenship GW. The effect of short versus long exposure times of argon laser photocoagulation on proliferative diabetic retinopathy. *Graefe's Arch Clin Exp Ophthalmol.* 1990;228:226–231.

55. Machemer R, Buettner H, Norton EWD, Parel JM. Vitrectomy: a pars plana approach. *Trans Am Acad Ophthalmol Otolaryngol.* 1971;75:813–820.

56. Machemer R, Parel JM, Buettner H. A new concept for vitreous surgery. 1. Instrumentation. *Am J Ophthalmol.* 1972;73:1–7.

57. Machemer R. Vitrectomy in diabetic retinopathy; removal of preretinal proliferations. *Trans Am Acad Ophthalmol Otolaryngol.* 1975;79:OP394–OP395.

58. Machemer R. A new concept for vitreous surgery. 7. Two instrument techniques in pars plana vitrectomy. *Arch Ophthalmol.* 1974;92:407–412.

59. O'Malley C, Heintz RM. Vitrectomy via the pars plana, a new instrument system. *Trans Pac Coast Otoophthalmol Soc.* 1972;50:121–137.

60. O'Malley C, Heintz RM. Vitrectomy with an alternative instrument system. *Ann Ophthalmol.* 1975;7:585–588.

61. Aaberg TM. Clinical results in vitrectomy for diabetic traction retinal detachment. *Am J Ophthalmol.* 1979;88:246–253.

62. Aaberg TM. Pars plana vitrectomy for diabetic traction retinal detachment. *Ophthalmology.* 1981;88:639–642.

63. Aaberg TM, Abrams GW. Changing indications and techniques for vitrectomy in management of complications of diabetic retinopathy. *Ophthalmology.* 1987;94:775–779.

64. Charles S. Endophotocoagulation. *Retina.* 1981;1:117–120.

65. Charles S. *Vitreous Microsurgery,* 2nd edn. Baltimore: Williams & Wilkins Co; 1987.

66. Douvas NG. Microsurgical roto-extractor instrument for vitrectomy. *Mod Probl Ophthalmol.* 1975;15:253–260.

67. Federman JL, Cook K, Bross R, et al. Intraocular microsurgery: I. New instrumentation (SITE). *Ophthalmic Surg.* 1976;7:82–87.

68. Kloti R. Vitrektomie I. Ein neues instrument fur die hintere vitrektomie. *Graefe's Arch Klin Ophthalmol.* 1973;187:161–170.

69. Kloti R. Indications for vitrectomy and results in 115 cases. In: McPherson A, ed. *New and Controversial Aspects of Vitreoretinal Surgery.* St. Louis: The CV Mosby Co.; 1977:237–244.

70. McCuen BW, Rinkoff JS. Silicone oil for progressive anterior ocular neovascularization after failed diabetic vitrectomy. *Arch Ophthalmol.* 1989;107:677–682.

71. Michels RG, Ryan SJ. Results and complications of 100 consecutive cases of pars plana vitrectomy. *Am J Ophthalmol.* 1975;80:24–29.

72. Michels RG. Vitrectomy for complications of diabetic retinopathy. *Arch Ophthalmol.* 1978;96:237–246.

73. Rice TA, Michels RG. Long-term anatomic and functional results of vitrectomy for diabetic retinopathy. *Am J Ophthalmol.* 1980;90:297–303.

74. Michels RG. *Vitreous Surgery.* St. Louis: The CV Mosby Co; 1981.

75. Thompson JT, Auer CL, de Bustros S, et al. Prognostic indicators of success and failure in vitrectomy for diabetic retinopathy. *Ophthalmology.* 1986;93:290–295.

76. Thompson JT, de Bustros S, Michels RG, et al. Results of vitrectomy for proliferative diabetic retinopathy. *Ophthalmology.* 1986;93:1571–1574.

77. Thompson JT, de Bustros S, Michels RG, Rice TA. Results and prognostic factors in vitrectomy for diabetic vitreous hemorrhage. *Arch Ophthalmol.* 1987;105:191–195.

78. de Bustros S, Thompson JT, Michels RG, Rice TA. Vitrectomy for progressive proliferative diabetic retinopathy. *Arch Ophthalmol.* 1987;105:196–199.

79. Thompson JT, de Bustros S, Michels RG, Rice TA. Results and prognostic factors in vitrectomy for diabetic traction retinal detachment of the macula. *Arch Ophthalmol.* 1987;105:497–502.

80. Peyman GA, Dodich NA. Experimental vitrectomy. Instrumentation and surgical technique. *Arch Ophthalmol.* 1971;86:548–551.

81. Tolentino FI, Banko A, Schepens CL, et al. Vitreous surgery. XII. New instrumentation for vitrectomy. *Arch Ophthalmol.* 1975;93:667–672.

82. Tolentino FI, Freeman HM, Tolentino FL. Closed vitrectomy in the management of diabetic traction retinal detachment. *Ophthalmology.* 1980;87:1078–1089.

83. Mandelcorn MS, Blankenship GW, Machemer R. Pars plana vitrectomy for the management of severe diabetic retinopathy. *Am J Ophthalmol.* 1976;81:561–570.

84. Blankenship GW, Machemer R. Pars plana vitrectomy for the management of severe diabetic retinopathy and analysis of results five years following surgery. *Ophthalmology.* 1978;85:553–559.

85. Blankenship GW. Stability of pars plana vitrectomy results for diabetic retinopathy complications, a comparison of five-year and six-month post-vitrectomy findings. *Arch Ophthalmol.* 1981;99:1009–1012.

86. Blankenship GW, Machemer R. Long term diabetic vitrectomy results, report of 10 year follow-up. *Ophthalmology.* 1985;92:503–506.
87. Fujii GY, de Juan E, Humayun MS, et al. A new 25 gauge instrument system for transconjunctival sutureless vitrectomy surgery. *Ophthalmology.* 2002;109:1807–1813.
88. Coleman DJ. Ultrasound in vitreous surgery. *Trans Am Acad Ophthalmol Otolaryngol.* 1972;76:467–479.
89. Coleman DJ, Franzen LA. Preoperative evaluation and prognostic value of ultrasonic display of vitreous hemorrhage. *Arch Ophthalmol.* 1974;92:375–381.
90. Diabetic Retinopathy Vitrectomy Study Research Group. Early vitrectomy for severe proliferative diabetic retinopathy in eyes with useful vision: results of a randomized trial. DRVS Report Number 3. *Ophthalmology.* 1988;95:1307–1320.

Photography, Angiography, and Ultrasonography in Diabetic Retinopathy

ANDREW LAM, MD,
NICHOLAS G. ANDERSON, MD,
CARL D. REGILLO, MD,
AND GARY C. BROWN, MD, MBA

CORE MESSAGES

- Fundus photography plays an important role in monitoring progression of diabetic retinopathy.
- Fundus photography is becoming a popular method of screening large populations for diabetic retinopathy.
- Fluorescein angiography is useful to identify areas of nonperfusion, increased vascular permeability, and neovascularization.
- Fluorescein angiography is useful to guide laser treatment of clinically significant macular edema.
- Ultrasound is useful when media opacity obscures visualization of the fundus and often helps determine appropriate timing of surgical intervention.

Fundus photography, fluorescein angiography, and ultrasonography are valuable tools in the management of diabetic retinopathy. These modalities enable clinicians to document pathology, monitor progression, and guide treatment of this increasingly prevalent disease. In this chapter, the indications and clinical utility of these tests in the management of diabetic retinopathy will be reviewed.

FUNDUS PHOTOGRAPHY

Background. In 1886, Jackman and Webster published the first report of a retinal photograph taken of a living human [1]. An albo-carbon light source provided illumination for their 2.5 min exposure. While the quality of this first image was limited, by the early 20th century, Fredrick Dimmer had produced photographs of sufficient quality to be incorporated into the first photographic atlas of

123

ophthalmology [2,3]. The first color fundus photographs appeared in 1929. Today, ophthalmologists are fortunate to have wide-angle fundus cameras, nonmydriatic cameras, and digital imaging at their disposal.

Clinical Indications. Fundus photography is an invaluable tool with which diabetic retinopathy can be followed up [4]. Photographs can be used to monitor progression of disease, particularly when following subtle changes in the posterior pole. The use of fundus photography to screen for diabetic retinopathy is also becoming more common [5,6].

It is critical to employ standardized photographic technique and parameters when using photographs to follow up any disease process. Accurate comparisons can only be made through photographs that reflect the same exposure and field of view. Color fundus photos can be taken in stereoscopic or nonstereoscopic mode and can be performed in the traditional seven stereoscopic 30° fields or wide angle 60° fields. Both 30° and 60° have advantages and disadvantages, but generally the seven stereoscopic 30° fields provide the most complete coverage.

As the prevalence of diabetes rises, the challenge of screening large patient populations for diabetic retinopathy also increases, particularly in underserved areas. Direct ophthalmoscopy, either by primary care physicians or ophthalmologists, has a sensitivity as low as 65% for the detection of sight-threatening disease [7]. Digital retinal photography has therefore become an important method of screening diabetic patients. Photos provide a permanent image of the retina that can be easily stored, enhanced, and transferred electronically for remote interpretation. Multiple studies have confirmed that digital photos can be an excellent screening tool when evaluated by a trained clinician [8–10]. Nonmydriatic cameras and automated screening systems to analyze digital retinal photographs have been used successfully in screening for diabetic retinopathy and will allow for more rapid evaluation of large patient populations in the future [11–13].

FLUORESCEIN ANGIOGRAPHY

Background. In 1955, MacClean and Maumenee first used intravenous fluorescein in humans to assist in diagnosing choroidal hemangiomas and choroidal melanomas [14]. In 1961, Novotny and Alvis described the current technique for retinal angiography [15].

Sodium fluorescein is a hydrocarbon that is 80% bound to albumin in the circulation. The unbound molecule diffuses freely through the choriocapillaris, Bruch's membrane, optic nerve, and sclera. However, it does not diffuse through the tight junctions of the retinal endothelial cells, the retinal pigment epithelium, or the larger choroidal vessels. A physiologic inner blood–retina barrier exists at the level of the retinal capillaries because of the tight junctions within these vessels. When there is a disruption of this inner blood–retina barrier, dye leakage occurs. The outer blood–retina barrier is formed by tight junctions between the retinal pigment epithelial cells and is also normally impermeable to fluorescein. Understanding these vascular barriers is critical to interpreting fluorescein angiograms.

Fluorescence occurs when light of a specific wavelength excites the electrons of a substance to a higher level of energy. When these electrons return to their original energy level, a longer wavelength is emitted. Sodium fluorescein is excited by blue light with wavelengths between 465 and 490 nm and fluoresces green-yellow light at wavelengths of 520 to 530 nm. The blue flash of the fundus camera excites both the 20% of fluorescein molecules that are unbound to albumin and any fluorescein that has leaked out of the vessels. A blue filter blocks all other light entering the eye. Reflected back into the camera is the green-yellow light emitted from the fluorescein molecules and reflected blue light. Another filter blocks the unwanted blue light and transmits the green-yellow light. "Autofluorescence" refers to areas of hyperfluorescence seen in preinjection fundus photographs when using the filters. It is produced by highly reflective structures such as optic disc drusen, astrocytic hamartomas, or exudates.

Image quality is dependent on technique, filters, film or digital processing equipment, ocular media, and patient cooperation. Intravenously administered fluorescein allows for high resolution images and standardized circulation times, although orally administered fluorescein is still occasionally used in limited clinical settings.

Although sodium fluorescein is generally safe, adverse reactions such as itching, nausea, or vomiting may occur. Severe anaphylactic reactions can rarely occur (1 in 200,000) [16,17]. All angiography facilities should have a clear protocol for managing such emergencies.

Clinical Indications. Fluorescein angiography plays an important role in the diagnosis and treatment of retinal and choroidal vascular pathology. It is particularly useful in identifying areas of nonperfusion, increased vascular permeability, and neovascularization. These characteristics make fluorescein angiography a valuable tool in managing the vascular complications commonly associated with diabetic retinopathy.

Nonproliferative Diabetic Retinopathy. The earliest detectable clinical change in diabetic retinopathy is the presence of microaneurysms (MAs). Histologic studies have demonstrated that the blood–retinal barrier is compromised within MAs because of loss of tight junction anchor proteins in the capillary endothelial cells. This breakdown results in leakage of fluid and retinal edema [18,19]. MAs therefore typically leak fluorescein and are easy to detect with angiography (Fig. 7.1). Angiography often shows more MAs than are seen either clinically or with color stereoscopic photographs. One study estimated that fluorescein angiogram could detect four times as many MAs than can be seen on fundus photos [20]. Other retinal vascular changes, such as altered caliber of vessels and focal areas of capillary nonperfusion, are also better seen angiographically than on clinical exam. Despite this high sensitivity in detecting the earliest changes in diabetic retinopathy, fluorescein angiography is not typically indicated for management at this early stage as the presence of these lesions is not in itself an indication for treatment [21].

As diabetic retinopathy progresses, intraretinal hemorrhages, cotton wool spots, and hard exudates may be seen. These lesions may produce blocking defects

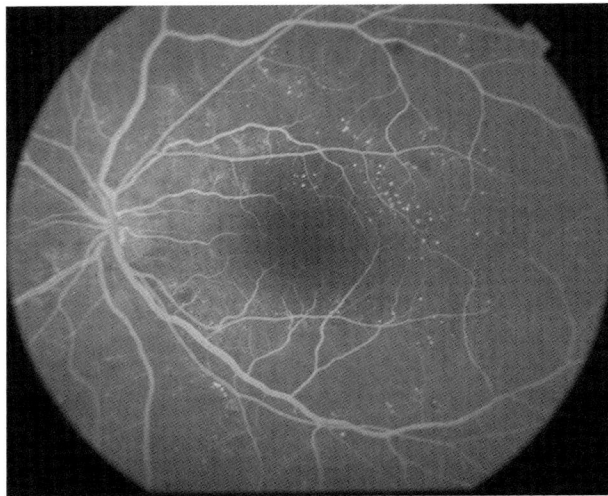

Figure 7.1. Early fluorescein angiogram demonstrates multiple microaneurysms scattered throughout the macula.

on fluorescein angiogram. Fluorescein angiography is usually not indicated for patients with moderate nonproliferative diabetic retinopathy (NPDR), unless the level of visual loss seems to surpass the degree of diabetic retinopathy seen clinically. In these cases, ischemic diabetic maculopathy that may be present can be identified angiographically (Fig. 7.2).

Severe NPDR is characterized by numerous hemorrhages and MAs in four quadrants, venous beading in two or more quadrants, or intraretinal microvascular abnormalities (IRMA) in at least one quadrant (Figs. 7.3 and 7.4). The risk of progression from severe NPDR to high risk proliferative diabetic retinopathy (PDR) is 15% within 1 year and 56% within 5 years. The risk of progression to PDR from very severe NPDR, defined by the presence of any two of the above features, is 45% within 1 year and 71% within 5 years [22]. Although fluorescein angiography well delineates the defining vascular abnormalities of severe NPDR, the presence of these features alone is not an indication for testing. At this advanced stage of NPDR, however, it may be helpful to follow disease progression with color fundus photographs [23].

Wide-angle fluorescein angiography can be directed to detect peripheral capillary nonperfusion, a feature that has been shown to be associated with progression of PDR (Fig. 7.5A and 7.5B). Investigators from Japan demonstrated that the peripheral retina was much more likely to undergo capillary nonperfusion than the posterior retina [24]. The same group later found a positive correlation between the initial site of capillary nonperfusion and progression of retinopathy. Progression was more rapid when nonperfused areas were, in ascending order: peripheral, midperipheral, central, and generalized [25].

Proliferative Diabetic Retinopathy. While fluorescein angiography is not typically necessary to make the diagnosis of PDR, the angiographic characteristics of

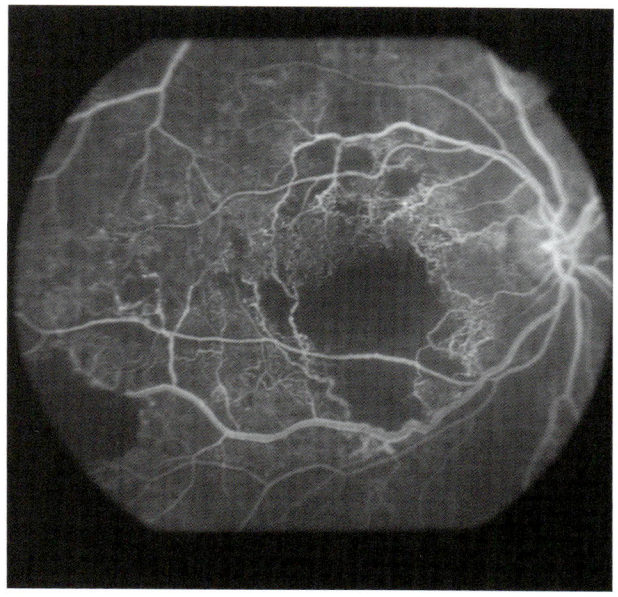

Figure 7.2. Fluorescein angiogram reveals extensive capillary nonperfusion within the macula.

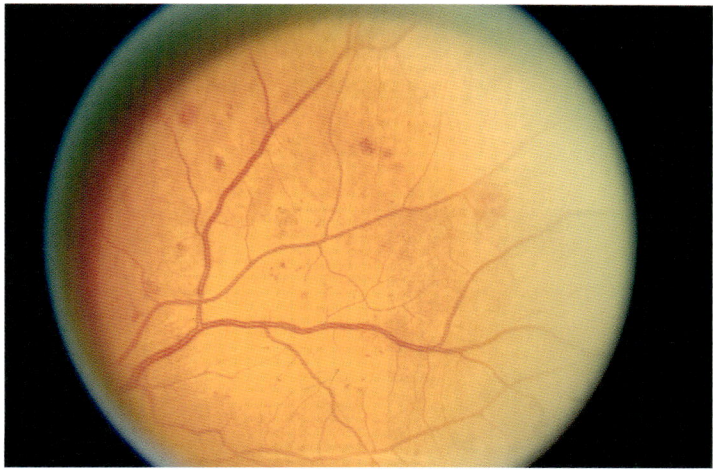

Figure 7.3. Color photograph of severe nonproliferative diabetic retinopathy with intraretinal microvascular abnormalities and extensive intraretinal hemorrhages. (Source: Courtesy of ETDRS.)

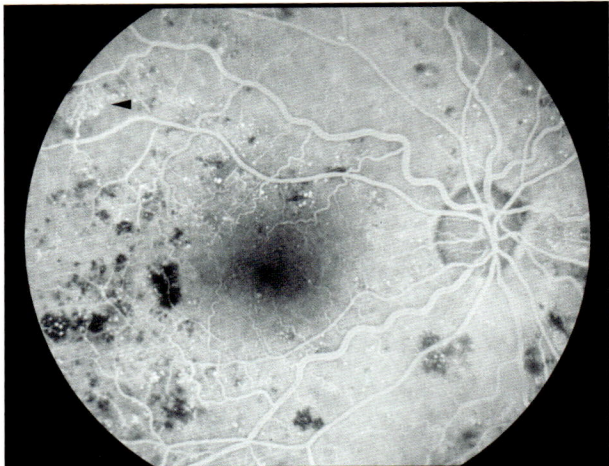

Figure 7.4. Fluorescein angiogram demonstrates characteristics of severe nonproliferative diabetic retinopathy including blocking defects from extensive intraretinal hemorrhages and intraretinal microvascular abnormalities (arrowhead), as well as diffuse microaneurysms.

neovascularization are accentuated on angiography. Fronds of neovascularization, often occurring at the junction of perfused and nonperfused retina, leak fluorescein dye abundantly (Fig. 7.6). They sometimes have a propensity to fill before the normal retinal arteries, suggesting a choroidal blood source for these vessels. After panretinal photocoagulation, a decrease in the leakage from the fronds is noted.

The decision to treat PDR with scatter photocoagulation is also typically based on clinical findings rather than fluorescein findings. The "high risk" characteristics for severe visual loss in PDR as defined by the Diabetic Retinopathy Study are based on clinical ophthalmic examination [26]. One study, however, has found

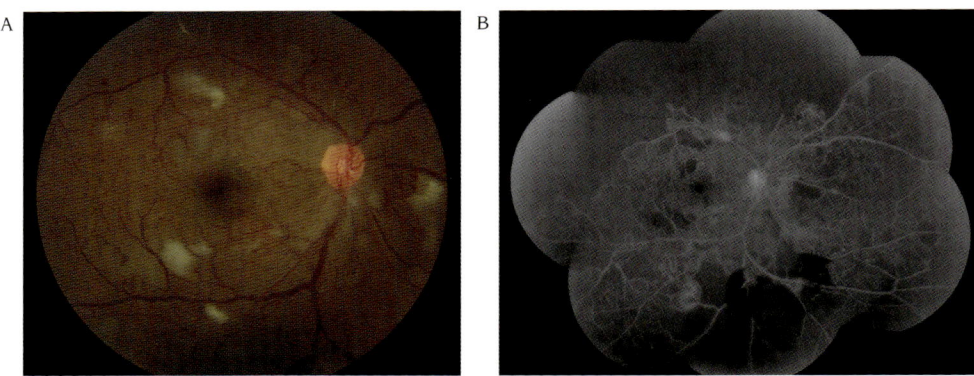

Figure 7.5. (A) Color photograph displaying numerous hemorrhages, microaneurysms, cotton wool spots, and intraretinal microvascular abnormalities. (B) Wide-angle fluorescein angiogram of the same patient reveals significant capillary nonperfusion centrally and in the periphery.

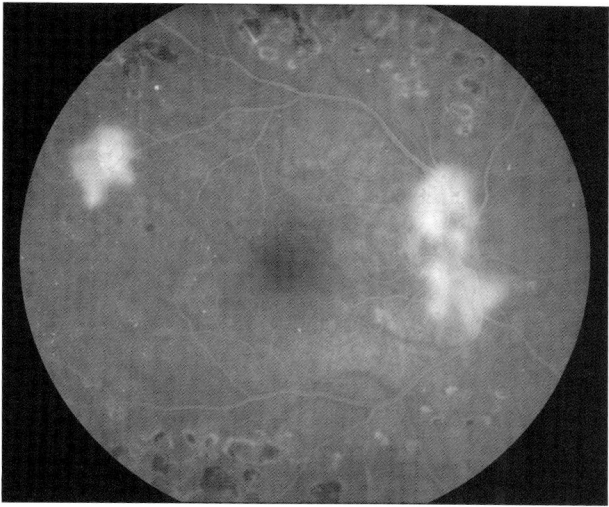

Figure 7.6. Pronounced fluorescein leakage from neovascularization of the disc (NVD) and neovascularization elsewhere (NVE) in proliferative diabetic retinopathy.

that peripheral angiography may be useful in identifying patients likely to develop anterior segment neovascularization [27].

Macular Edema. The most common indication for fluorescein angiography in diabetic retinopathy is in the management of macular edema. The incidence of macular edema in diabetic retinopathy is between 13.9% and 25.4% [28]. The Early Treatment Diabetic Retinopathy Study (ETDRS) defined edema characteristics that are associated with more pronounced treatment effect [29]:

1. Thickening of the retina at or within 500 microns of the center of the macula
2. Hard exudates at or within 500 microns of the center of the macula if associated with thickening of the adjacent retina
3. A zone or zones of retinal thickening one disc area or larger in size, any part of which is within one disc diameter of the center of the macula

Diabetic macular edema that meets any one of the above criteria is termed "clinically significant macular edema" (CSME). The incidence of CSME in diabetic retinopathy is between 9.2% and 17.6% [22]. It is important to note that the diagnosis of CSME is made on the basis of clinical exam rather than on fluorescein angiogram findings. Eyes with macular edema that is not clinically significant are usually not treated with laser photocoagulation and, therefore, are primarily followed by clinical examination.

In eyes with CSME, the fluorescein angiogram is useful in guiding focal or grid laser treatment [22,30,31]. Although some clinicians feel that fluorescein angiography is not necessary prior to laser treatment, a study found that preoperative imaging improves the accuracy and probably the effectiveness of laser treatment

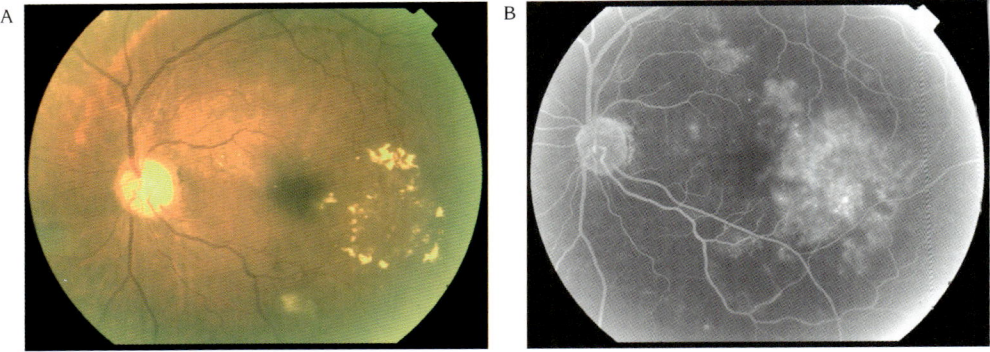

Figure 7.7. (A) Circinate lipid and thickening consistent with focal clinically significant macular edema. (B) Extensive fluorescein leakage is present in the area of macular edema seen clinically.

[32]. Focal diabetic maculopathy is characterized by areas of discrete leakage with sufficient macular perfusion (Fig. 7.7A and 7.7B). These areas can be treated with focal laser directed at individual lesions. Diffuse diabetic maculopathy, however, results from hyperpermeability of the entire perimacular capillary bed secondary to breakdown of the inner blood–retina barrier (Fig. 7.8A and 7.8B) [33]. Areas of diffuse leakage are typically treated with grid laser, although treatment outcome may be less favorable [34]. Fluorescein angiography is also helpful in guiding laser treatment by demonstrating the border of the foveal avascular zone. When considering retreatment, fluorescein angiogram is useful in identifying areas of persistent leakage, capillary nonperfusion, and previous laser treatment.

Angiography is also useful for evaluating macular edema in patients with some degree of diabetic retinopathy after cataract extraction, where differentiating diabetic CSME from post-cataract extraction cystoid macular edema (the Irvine-Gass Syndrome) may be difficult based on clinical exam alone. The leakage pattern in Irvine-Gass syndrome is typically "petalloid" in appearance as opposed to the

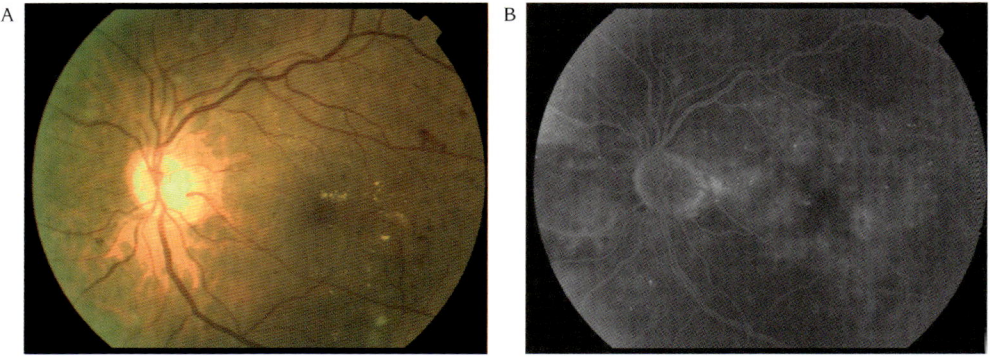

Figure 7.8. (A) Extensive hard exudates with associated clinically significant macular edema. (B) Fluorescein angiogram of the same patient demonstrates diffuse leakage in the macula.

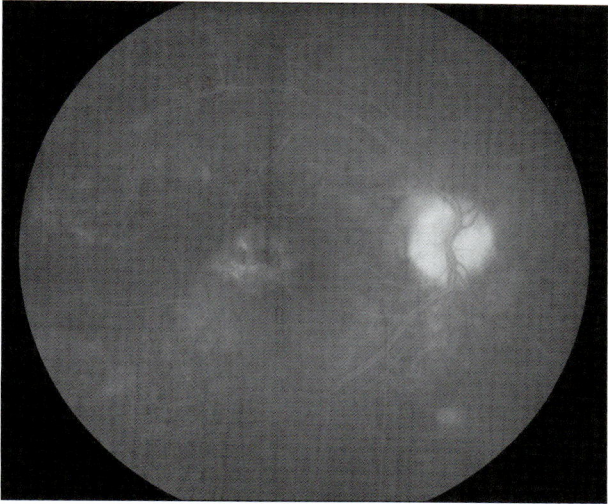

Figure 7.9. A "petalloid" pattern of leakage reflecting fluid accumulation in Henle's layer is seen angiographically in cystoid macular edema. Note that the disc is hyperfluorescent.

focal or diffuse leakage seen in diabetic macular edema (Fig. 7.9). Reports have also noted that the disc is more likely to hyperfluoresce in Irvine-Gass Syndrome and less likely in exacerbation of CSME [35]. Differentiating these two entities is important in guiding treatment. In some cases, however, both forms of leakage may be present.

FLUORESCEIN ANGIOSCOPY

In fluorescein angioscopy, indirect ophthalmoscopy rather than photography is used in conjunction with fluorescein injection to directly evaluate retinal vascular abnormalities. This technique may allow for better visualization of the fundus as compared to standard angiography in eyes with hazy media. Peripheral retinal lesions may also be better visualized with fluorescein angioscopy. In the operating room, angioscopy may be used if standard angiography equipment is not available. The main disadvantage of fluorescein angioscopy, however, is that no permanent record of the exam is created.

INDOCYANINE GREEN ANGIOGRAPHY

Indocyanine green (ICG) fluorescence angiography was first introduced in 1973 by Robert Flower and Bernard Hochheimer [36]. The technique did not become widely used, however, until the 1990s with the advent of sensitive infrared video imaging and high resolution digital equipment. The ICG molecule is 98% protein-bound and, unlike sodium fluorescein, does not extravasate from the fenestrated choriocapillaris. The excitation and emission wavelengths at the near-infrared region allow penetration to deeper fundus structures as well as through overlying hemorrhage. Owing to these characteristics, visualization of the choroidal circulation is better with ICG angiography as compared to fluorescein angiography.

While ICG is not commonly used in diabetic retinopathy, studies have suggested that ICG could be a complementary test to fluorescein angiography in NPDR. One study showed that NPDR exhibits lobular spotty ("salt and pepper") hyperfluorescence and hypofluorescence, diffuse late-phase hyperfluorescence in areas of retinal thickening and edema, and MAs not seen on fluorescein angiogram [37]. This suggests that the degree of diabetic retinopathy seen clinically and by fluorescein angiography may reveal only part of the pathology in the chorioretinal vasculature. ICG may better highlight these abnormalities. Currently, the clinical utility of this information is unclear.

ULTRASONOGRAPHY

Background. The use of ultrasonography in ophthalmology has become a critical tool to enable evaluation of intraocular pathology when ophthalmoscopic examination is limited by media opacity. Ultrasound waves have frequencies greater than 20 kHz. Ophthalmic ultrasonography utilizes frequencies in the range of 8–10 MHz. The sound wave is emitted from a probe that can be positioned on the globe or eyelid. The velocity of the emitted sound wave in the eye is dependent on the density of the medium through which it passes. When the sound wave strikes an interface of two media with different densities, part of the wave is reflected back to the probe where it is reacquired and the acoustic energy is converted to electrical energy that is depicted on an oscilloscope. B-scan ultrasound is a brightness-modulated display in which echoes are represented by pixels on the monitor that form a two-dimensional image, whereas A-scan ultrasound is a one dimensional representation of the amplitude of the reflected sound waves. The amplification of the signal may be increased or decreased by adjusting the gain setting on the instrument.

Clinical Indications. Ultrasound is most commonly indicated when media opacity, such as cataract or vitreous hemorrhage, prevents an adequate view of the fundus. In these cases, ultrasound can be used to monitor progression of posterior segment disease and assist in deciding when surgical intervention is appropriate. The major pathologic processes that should be differentiated include: vitreous hemorrhage, posterior vitreous detachment (PVD), fibrovascular proliferation, blood layered on the retina, and retinal detachment [38].

Vitreous hemorrhage is a common complication of diabetic retinopathy. Blood can be positioned in the subhyaloid space or within the vitreous gel itself. While vitreous hemorrhage usually results from primary disease in diabetic patients, the possibility of other causes, such as a retinal tear or detachment should be considered. Therefore, any patient who presents with a vitreous hemorrhage should be evaluated with ultrasonography if an adequate view of the retina is not sufficient to rule out these processes. On ultrasound, vitreous hemorrhage is usually represented by diffuse, mobile, minimally reflective opacities in the vitreous cavity

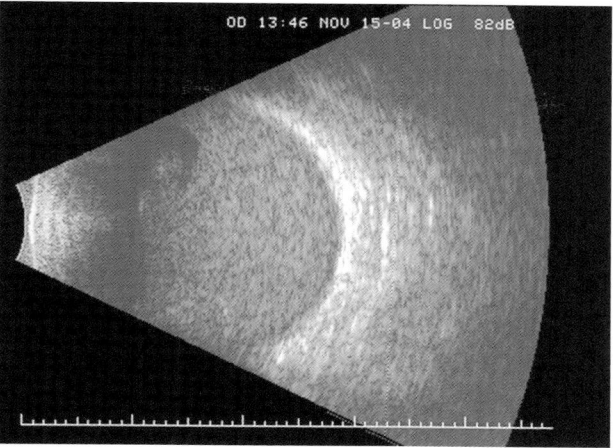

Figure 7.10. Vitreous hemorrhage is seen on ultrasound as a diffuse, minimally reflective opacity in the vitreous cavity.

(Fig. 7.10). Serial exams should be performed until the hemorrhage has sufficiently cleared to allow ophthalmoscopic evaluation.

Ultrasound is also useful in detecting fibrovascular membranes on the retinal surface [39,40]. Such membranes can cause fibrous contraction resulting in tangential traction or exaggerated adhesions between the vitreous and retina. Fibrovascular tissue can also cause splitting of the cortical vitreous (posterior vitreoschisis) that may simulate PVD on ultrasound [41,42].

Ultrasound plays an important role in managing tractional retinal detachment. These detachments are usually located in the peripapillary area or along the arcades. Common patterns of traction detachment include "tent-like" or "table-top." A tent-like detachment has a concave appearance and results from vitreoretinal adherence at a focal point Fig. 7.11). This elevation of the retina is immobile

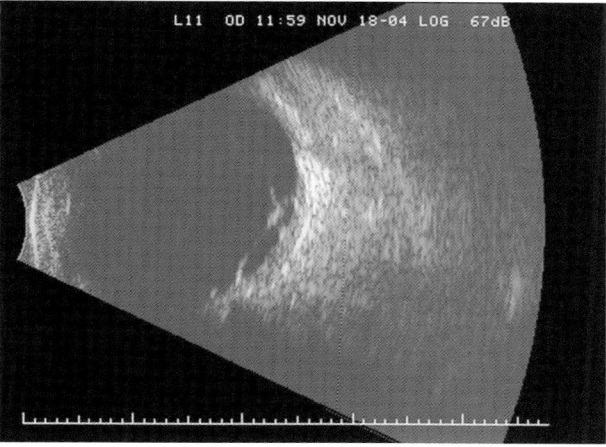

Figure 7.11. With ultrasonography, the posterior hyaloid is seen attaching to the retina at a focal point, resulting in a "tent-like" tractional retinal detachment.

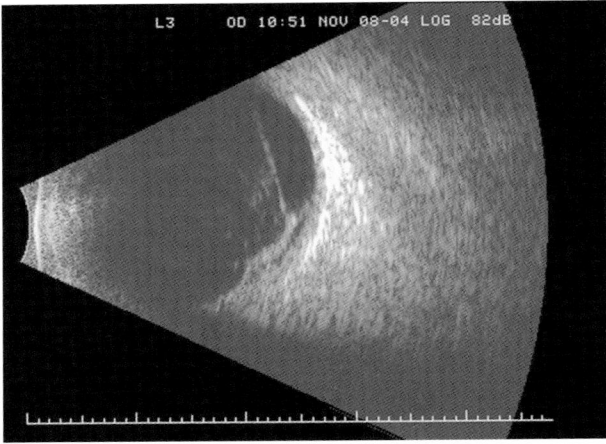

Figure 7.12. Ultrasonography reveals a broad vitreoretinal interface causing a "table-top" tractional retinal detachment.

on kinetic testing. In contrast, table-top detachments exhibit a broader area of vitreoretinal adherence. Ultrasonographically, the detachment is seen as a highly reflective membrane with an adherent posterior hyaloid (Fig. 7.12). The decision to intervene surgically is often based on the location and progression of the detachment as seen on ultrasound.

At times, it may be difficult to distinguish between vitreous hemorrhage, PVD, fibrovascular membrane, and retinal detachment on ultrasound. Furthermore, subretinal blood may simulate a shallow retinal detachment. Several modalities may be used to differentiate these entities. The A-scan spike is higher with a retinal detachment, often a 100% signal, as compared to vitreous detachment. Similarly, on B-Scan, the signal from a retinal detachment generally persists with lower gain settings. Furthermore, the reflectivity of a PVD will decrease in the periphery, whereas a retinal detachment will retain its high reflectivity in the periphery. A retinal detachment always remains attached at the optic nerve (Fig. 7.13). Therefore, a signal that does not insert on the nerve represents a PVD. Finally, kinetic B-scan can be helpful in discriminating between retina, vitreous, and blood.

CONCLUSIONS

Fundus photography has an important role in monitoring progression of diabetic retinopathy. It is also becoming a popular method of screening for diabetic retinopathy in the community setting. Fluorescein angiography is useful in identifying areas of nonperfusion, increased vascular permeability, and neovascularization. It has an essential role in guiding laser treatment of CSME. Ultrasound is useful when cataract or vitreous hemorrhage obscures visualization of the posterior segment. It is important for identifying fibrovascular proliferation, vitreous hemorrhage,

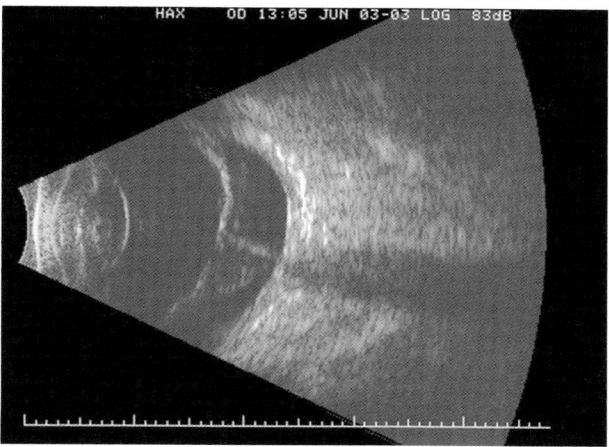

Figure 7.13. Ultrasound demonstrates a total retinal detachment inserting on the optic nerve.

and retinal detachments. Timing of surgical intervention frequently depends on findings from ultrasound examination.

REFERENCES

1. Jackman WT, Webster JD. On photographing the retina of the living human eye. *Philadelphia Photographer* 1886;23:275.
2. Dimmer F. *Der Augenspiegel und die Ophthalmoskopische Diagnostik.* Leipzig, Germany: F. Deuticke; 1921.
3. Dimmer F, Pillat A. *Atlas photographischer Bilder des Menschlichen Augenhintergrundes.* Leipzig, Germany: F. Deuticke; 1927.
4. Klein R, Klein BE, Neider MW, et al. Diabetic retinopathy as detected using ophthalmoscopy, a nonmydriatic camera and a standard fundus camera. *Ophthalmology.* 1985;92:485–491.
5. Moss SE, Klein R, Kessler SD, et al. Comparison between ophthalmoscopy and fundus photography in determining severity of diabetic retinopathy. *Ophthalmology.* 1985;92:62–67.
6. Gonzalez ME, Gonzalez C, Stern MP, et al. Concordance in diagnosis of diabetic retinopathy by fundus photography between retina specialists and standardized reading center. Mexico City Diabetes Study Retinopathy Group. *Arch Med Res.* 1995;26:127–130.
7. Harding SP, Broadbent DM, Neoh C, et al. Sensitivity and specificity of photography and direct ophthalmoscopy in screening for sight threatening eye disease: the Liverpool Diabetic Eye Study. *Br Med J.* 1995;331:1131–1135.
8. Newsom R, Moate B, Casswell T. Screening for diabetic retinopathy using digital colour photography and oral fluorescein angiography. *Eye.* 2000;14:579–582.
9. Agargh E, Cavallin-Sjoberg U. Peripheral retinal evaluation comparing fundus photography with fluorescein angiograms in patients with diabetes mellitus. *Retina.* 1998;18:420–423.
10. George LD, Halliwell M, Hill R, et al. A comparison of digital retinal images and 35 mm colour transparencies in detecting and grading diabetic retinopathy. *Diabet Med.* 1998;15:254–258.

11. Massin P, Erginay A, Mehidi B, et al. Evaluation of a new non-mydriatic digital camera for detection of diabetic retinopathy. *Diabetes UK*. 2003;20:635–641.

12. Hipwell JH, Strachan F, Olson JA, et al. Automated detection of microaneuryms in digital red-free photographs: a diabetic retinopathy screening tool. *Diabet Med*. 2000;17:588–594.

13. Sinthanayothin C, Boyce JF, Williamson TH. Automated detection of diabetic retinopathy on digital fundus images. *Diabet Med*. 2002;19:105–112.

14. MacClean AL, Maumenee AE. Hemangioma of the choroid. *Am J Ophthalmol*. 1959;57:171–176.

15. Novotny HR, Alvis DL. A method of photographing fluorescein in the human retina. *Circulation*. 1961;24:72–77.

16. Yannuzzi LA, Rohrer KT, Tindel LJ, et al. Fluorescein angiography complication survey. *Ophthalmology*. 1986;93:611–617.

17. Stein MR, Parker CW. Reactions following intravenous fluorescein. *Am J Ophthalmol*. 1971;72:861–868.

18. Antonetti DA, Barber AJ, Khin S, et al. Vascular permeability in experimental diabetes is associated with reduced endothelial occluding content: vascular endothelium growth factor decreases occluding in retinal endothelial cells. *Diabetes*. 1998;12:1953–1959.

19. Ishibashi T, Inomata H. Ultrastructure of retinal vessels in diabetic patients. *Br J Ophthalmol*. 1993;77:574–578.

20. Hellstedt T, Vesti E, Immonen I. Identification of individual microaneurysms: a comparison between fluorescein angiograms and red-free and colour photographs. *Graefes Arch Klin Exp Ophthalmol*. 1996;234(suppl 1):S13–S17.

21. Diabetes Control and Complications Trial Research Group. Color photography versus fluorescein angiography in the detection of diabetic retinopathy in the Diabetes Control and Complications Trial. *Arch Ophthalmol*. 1987;105:1344–1351.

22. Early Treatment Diabetic Retinopathy Study Research Group. Early photocoagulation for diabetic retinopathy. ETDRS report number 9. *Ophthalmology*. 1991;98:766–785.

23. Early Treatment Diabetic Retinopathy Study Research Group. Fundus photographic risk factors for progression of diabetic retinopathy. ETDRS report number 12. *Ophthalmology*. 1991;98:823–833.

24. Shimizu K, Kobayashi Y, Muraoka K. Mid-peripheral fundus involvement in diabetic retinopathy. *Ophthalmology*. 1981;88:601–612.

25. Niki, T, Muraoka K, Shimizu K. Distribution of capillary nonperfusion in early-stage diabetic retinopathy. *Ophthalmology*. 1984;91:1431–1439.

26. Diabetic Retinopathy Study Research Group. Four risk factors for severe visual loss in diabetic retinopathy. DRS Report 3. *Arch Ophthalmol*. 1979;97:654–655.

27. Terasaki H, Miyake Y, Mori M, et al. Fluorescein angiography of extreme peripheral retina and rubeosis iridis in proliferative diabetic retinopathy. *Retina*. 1999;19:302–308.

28. Klein R, Klein BE, Moss SE, et al. The Wisconsin Epidemiologic Study of Diabetic Retinopathy XV. The long term incidence of macular edema. *Ophthalmology*. 1995;102:7–16.

29. Early Treatment Diabetic Retinopathy Study Research Group. Photocoagulation for diabetic macular edema. ETDRS report number 4. *Int Ophthalmol Clin*. 1987;27:265–272.

30. Early Treatment Diabetic Retinopathy Study Research Group. Treatment techniques and clinical guidelines for photocoagulation of diabetic macular edema. ETDRS report number 2. *Ophthalmology*. 1987;94:761–774.

31. Early Treatment Diabetic Retinopathy Study Research Group. Techniques for scatter and focal photocoagulation treatment of diabetic retinopathy. ETDRS report number 3. *Int Ophthalmol Clin*. 1987;27:254–264.
32. Kylstra JA, Brown JC, Jaffe GJ, et al. The importance of fluorescein angiography in planning laser treatment of diabetic macular edema. *Ophthalmology*. 1999;106:2068–2073.
33. Bresnick GH. Diabetic maculopathy: a critical review highlighting diffuse macular edema. *Ophthalmology*. 1983;90:1301–1317.
34. Early Treatment Diabetic Retinopathy Study Research Group. Focal photocoagulation treatment of diabetic macular edema: relationship of treatment effect to fluorescein angiographic and other retinal characteristics at baseline. ETDRS report number 19. *Arch Ophthalmol*. 1995;113:1144–1155.
35. Dowler J, Sehmi K, Hykin P, et al. The natural history of macular edema after cataract surgery in diabetes. *Ophthalmology*. 1999;106:663–668.
36. Flower RW, Hochheimer BF. A clinical technique and apparatus for simultaneous angiography of the separate retinal and choroidal circulations. *Invest Ophthalmol*. 1973;12:248–261.
37. Weinberger D, Kramer M, Priel E, et al. Indocyanine green angiographic findings in nonproliferative diabetic retinopathy. *Am J Ophthalmol*. 1998;126:238–247.
38. DiBernardo CW, Schachat AP, Fekrat S. Ophthalmic Ultrasound: A Diagnostic Atlas. New York: Thieme; 1998; 1: 3–45.
39. Restori M, McLeod D. Ultrasound in previtrectomy assessment. *Trans Ophthalmol Soc UK*. 1977;97:232–234.
40. Arzabe CW, Akiba J, Jalkh AE, et al. Comparative study of vitreoretinal relationships using biomicroscopy and ultrasound. *Grafes Arch Klin Exp Ophthalmol*. 1991;229:66–68.
41. Chu TG, Lopez PF, Cano MR, et al. Posterior vitreoschisis. An echographic finding in proliferative diabetic retinopathy. *Ophthalmology*. 1996;103:315.
42. Schwartz SD, Alexander R, Hiscott P, et al. Recognition of vitreoschisis in proliferative diabetic retinopathy. A useful landmark in vitrectomy for diabetic traction retinal detachment. *Ophthalmology*. 1996;103:323.

8

Optical Coherence Tomography in the Management of Diabetic Retinopathy

ANDREW A. MOSHFEGHI, MD,
INGRID U. SCOTT, MD, MPH,
HARRY W. FLYNN, JR., MD,
AND CARMEN A. PULIAFITO, MD, MBA

CORE MESSAGES

- Optical coherence tomography (OCT) is a noninvasive test that evaluates diabetic retinopathy both quantitatively and qualitatively.
  - Time-domain (Stratus OCT)
  - Spectral-domain (Fourier domain OCT)
- Retinal thickness evaluation with OCT is often inversely correlated with visual acuity in patients with diabetic macular edema, although this association has been reported to be modest.
- OCT abnormalities due to diabetic retinopathy include the following:
  - Cystoid macular edema
  - Vitreoretinal traction and posterior hyaloid abnormalities
  - Subretinal fluid
- OCT is useful to monitor the clinical course as well as the response to treatment.
  - Laser photocoagulation
  - Intravitreal pharmacotherapies
    - Intravitreal steroids
    - Intravitreal vascular endothelial growth factor (VEGF) inhibitors
  - Vitreoretinal surgery
- Correlation of clinical examination, fluorescein angiography, and OCT findings can provide a comprehensive assessment and understanding of visual dysfunction in patients with diabetic retinopathy.

Optical coherence tomography (OCT) has emerged as an important diagnostic adjunct and management tool for ophthalmologists managing patients with diabetic retinopathy [1–4]. In addition to medical history, laboratory review, and clinical examination (stereoscopic slit-lamp biomicroscopy of the anterior and posterior segment), ancillary tests such as fundus photography, fluorescein angiography, and OCT has provided the ophthalmologist with a new appreciation for the dynamics of vision loss in eyes with a spectrum of diabetic retinopathy (Table 8.1) [4,5]. Although OCT was not available for the Diabetic Retinopathy Study (DRS) and the Early Treatment Diabetic Retinopathy Study (ETDRS) [6–10], virtually every new and ongoing clinical trial (e.g., Diabetic Retinopathy Clinical Research network, unpublished data) includes OCT as an important secondary outcome variable [11–22]. This chapter focuses on clinical examples that demonstrate the utility of OCT in the evaluation and management of patients with diabetic retinopathy and diabetic macular edema (DME) [23–30]. The following examples (Figs. 8.1–8.15) illustrate how both the qualitative evaluation and quantitative assessment provided by OCT aids in the diagnosis and management of various vitreoretinal abnormalities in eyes with diabetic retinopathy.

BACKGROUND

Although OCT has been commercially available since 1996, its popularity among ophthalmologists and retina specialists flourished with the introduction of the most recent version of the technology known as Stratus OCT, colloquially referred to as OCT-3 (Carl Zeiss Meditec, Dublin, CA) [11–23,31–33]. A detailed explanation of OCT technology, the various OCT image acquisition sequences, and an extended discussion of OCT image creation are beyond the scope of this chapter. A more comprehensive evaluation of the technology is reviewed in several excellent sources [34–37].

Briefly, the OCT unit utilizes a noncontact transpupillary infrared laser to illuminate the retina with multiple axial scans in a rapid fashion and a detector to capture the reflected light [34,37]. The basis for OCT is the Michelson interferometer that measures the phase difference between the reflected light from the retinal tissue as compared to an internal reference beam [34,37]. This difference is plotted as a false-color image of individual axial scans of the retina, with pixels of varying colors corresponding to areas of differential light reflectivity within the retina.

Table 8.1. Application of OCT in the Management of Diabetic Retinopathy

Evaluate Pathology	Retinal Thickness
	Cystoid Macular Edema
	Vitreoretinal Traction
	Subretinal Fluid
Monitor Response	Standard Laser Treatment
	Intravitreal Pharmacotherapies
	Vitreoretinal Surgery

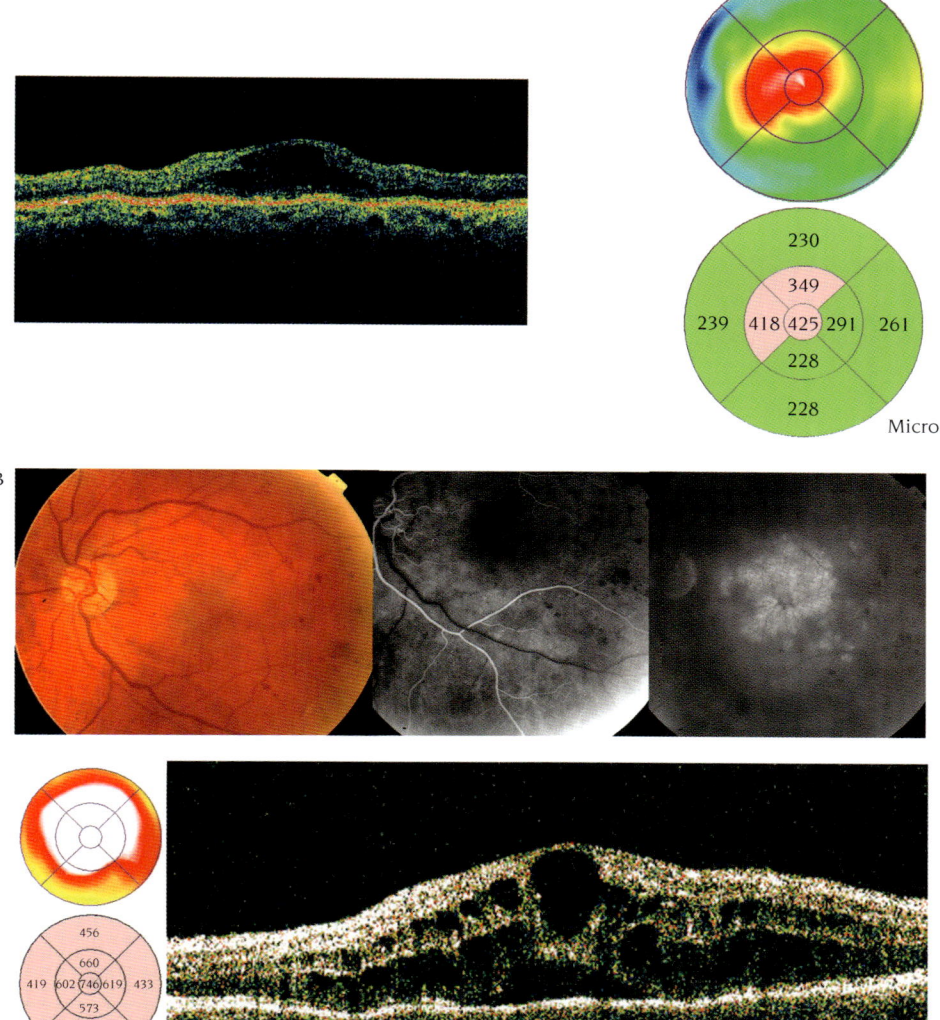

Figure 8.1. (A) This is a representative vertical radial line scan (left) and macular contour map (right) from a 54-year-old patient with nonproliferative diabetic retinopathy and diabetic macular edema. Marked intraretinal cystic thickening involving the foveal and parafoveal region is appreciated on the radial line scan. The macular thickness map demonstrates areas of increased retinal thickness using both a false-color map (right, top) and a numerically annotated topographical map (right, bottom). (B) The left eye color fundus photograph (top row, left) demonstrates severe nonproliferative diabetic retinopathy, microaneurysms and diffuse macular leakage on the fluorescein angiogram early (top row, middle) and late-phases (top row, right), and diffuse cystoid macular edema on the optical coherence tomography macular thickness map (bottom row, left) and radial line scan (bottom row, right) demonstrating inner and outer retinal cysts with a subfoveal fluid collection. Central foveal thickness measured 746 microns. Visual acuity was 20/80.

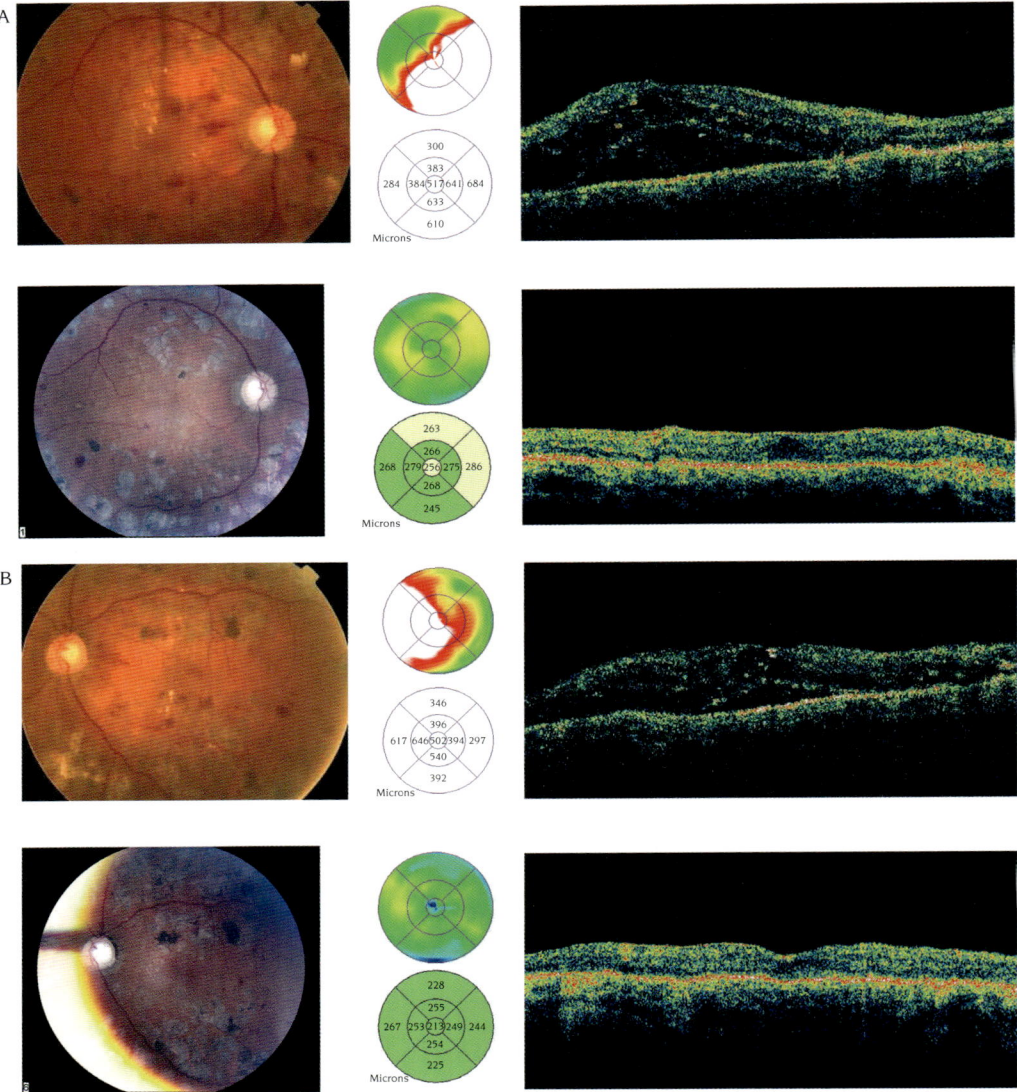

Figure 8.2. (A) The color fundus photograph at baseline (top row, left) demonstrates diffuse DME with exudates and evidence of prior focal/grid laser and peripheral cotton-wool spots. The OCT macular contour map helps delineate the extent of the massively swollen retina as depicted by the white color coding (top row, middle). Central foveal thickness measures 517 microns. The vertically oriented radial OCT scan demonstrates a faint surface membrane, scattered intraretinal hyperreflective foci consistent with hard exudates, and a subfoveal fluid collection (top row, left). This eye received panretinal laser photocoagulation (PRP) and six intravitreal triamcinolone acetonide injections over a 2.5-year period with VA benefit. After the sixth intravitreal triamcinolone acetonide injection, there was marked reduction in the macular edema as well as an overall less pronounced degree of diabetic retinopathy (bottom row, left). The macular contour map has flattened (bottom row, center) and the central foveal thickness measured 256 microns. No subfoveal fluid is seen on the vertically oriented radial OCT scan and although there is a blunted foveal depression with thin epiretinal membrane, marked reduction in CME resulted in improvement in VA from 20/100 to 20/25. (B) This same patient's left eye color fundus photograph (top row, left) is quite similar with a diffuse and sectoral DME

142

The OCT unit has image interpolation software that allows it to identify the inner and outer retinal boundaries. The inner retinal boundary is identified by the OCT unit as the interface between the typically low reflectance of the vitreous cavity with the high reflectance associated with the internal limiting membrane and nerve fiber layer. The outer retinal boundary is identified as the so-called highly-reflective external band, consisting of the retinal pigment epithelium (RPE), Bruch's membrane, and the choriocapillaris. The highly reflective external band is often incorrectly labeled the RPE, but this discrimination of the RPE from Bruch's membrane and the choriocapillaris is beyond the resolution capabilities of the current commercially available OCT technology. Once the inner and outer retinal boundaries are identified, a simple arithmetical calculation allows determination of the retinal thickness along the scan length. Several of these individual axial scans from various vantages can be combined to create an interpolated *en face* image of the macula, with an appearance much like a topographical map (Fig. 8.1A) with color coding or number labels indicating relative and absolute average retinal thicknesses for each region of the macula, respectively. Macular volume can be calculated in a similar manner [34,37].

RADIAL LINES SCAN

The most common scan type for the Stratus OCT is the radial lines scan (Fig. 8.1A). With the patient fixating, six consecutive 6 mm scans are obtained from various directions. All six scans have their center on the fovea. The scans are: inferior to superior (one vertical scan at 90°), inferotemporal to superonasal (two separate oblique scans, one at 60° and one at 30°), temporal to nasal (one horizontal scan at 0°), and superotemporal to inferonasal (two oblique scans, one at 330° and one at 300°) [37].

By the machine operator moving the fixation target, it is possible to evaluate extrafoveal regions with the radial lines scan. This is helpful, for example, when trying to characterize a traction retinal detachment along the temporal vascular arcades or when evaluating peripapillary traction. In the latter case, a radial line can be obtained by sweeping the scan horizontally from the temporal peripapillary retina, over the optic disc, and then to the nasal peripapillary retina. This type of scan helps determine the status of the posterior hyaloid in relation to the optic nerve and helps determine if abnormally firm vitreopapillary traction is present in

---

pattern with hard exudates and numerous dot and blot hemorrhages throughout the posterior pole. The macular thickness map shows a mirror image of the right eye, with a sector of massively thickened retina involving the foveal center. Central foveal thickness measured 502 microns. The vertically oriented radial OCT scan (top row, right) shows a faint surface membrane, microcystic retinal thickening, scattered highly reflective intraretinal foci consistent with hard exudates, and a shallow foveal detachment. This eye also received PRP and multiple intravitreal triamcinolone acetonide injections with interval and sustained benefit over a 2.5-year period. After the 6th intravitreal triamcinolone acetonide injection, the color fundus photograph shows marked reduction in macular edema (bottom row, left), the contour map has flattened and reveals a central foveal thickness of 213 microns (bottom row, center), and nearly normal appearing foveal contour is shown on the vertically oriented radial OCT scan (bottom row, right). As a result, the VA improved to 20/40.

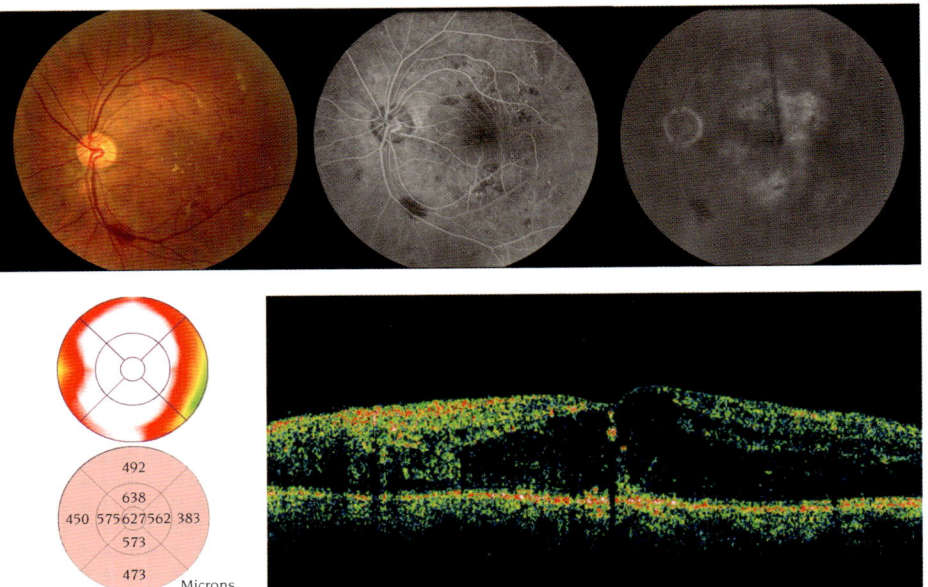

Figure 8.3. The color fundus photograph (top row, left) demonstrates severe nonproliferative diabetic retinopathy with multiple large blot retinal hemorrhages and numerous scattered microaneurysms and hard exudates throughout the posterior pole causing gross macular edema. The early- (top row, center) and late-phase (top row, right) fluorescein angiogram show a diffuse pattern of fluorescein leakage in a circinate arrangement about the foveal center. Enlargement of the foveal avascular zone is also appreciated. The optical coherence tomography (OCT) macular contour map (bottom row, left) depicts a broad zone of extensive macular thickening with a central foveal thickness measuring 627 microns and similar thickness levels noted in the adjacent subfields. The vertically oriented radial OCT scan (bottom row, right) shows an incomplete posterior vitreous detachment, massive outer retinal cystic elements and a peaked fovea. Small hyperreflective intraretinal foci with posterior optical shadowing are consistent with hard exudates. No foveal detachment is noted.

cases where the vision is more significantly compromised than can be explained by the clinical examination [37]. One shortcoming of OCT is the inability, at present, to evaluate the retinal periphery anterior to the equator. B-scan ultrasound remains the most useful adjunct to clinical examination for this region.

FAST MACULAR THICKNESS MAP

The fast scan is similar to the radial lines scan on the Stratus OCT, except that the scan speed is approximately twice that of the radial lines scan. This results in a lower resolution compared to the radial lines scan, but the fast scan is the one most often used in retinal thickness measurements because it is typically less prone to sampling artifacts than the slower scan [34,37]. It is also a good second-choice scan, when poor patient cooperation limits the acquisition of a normal resolution radial lines scan. Even patients with poor cooperation can generally be imaged

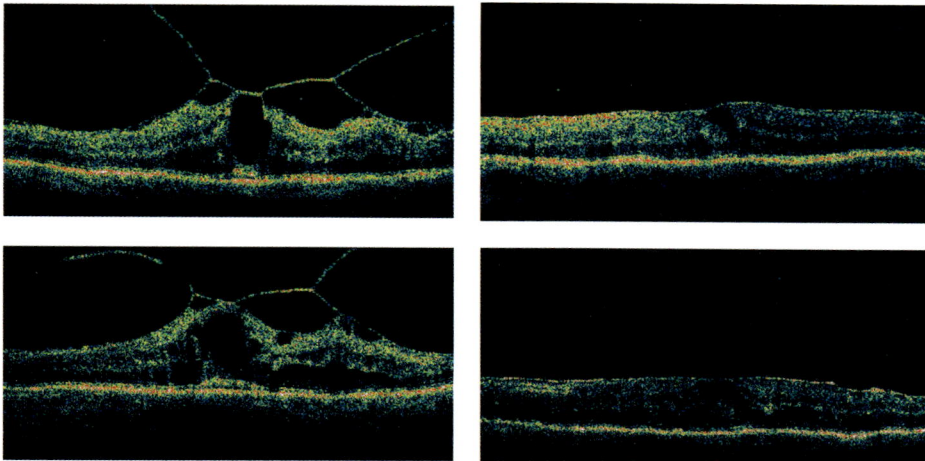

Figure 8.4. This is a 74-year-old man with type 2 diabetes mellitus and regressed proliferative diabetic retinopathy following pan retinal photocoagulation. Visual acuity at presentation was 20/200. He developed complex vitreomacular traction, epiretinal membrane, and cystoid macular edema as shown on the vertical (top row, left) and horizontal (bottom row, left) optical coherence tomography (OCT) scans. A shallow foveal detachment is also noted. After pars plana vitrectomy with membrane peeling, resolution of the vitreomacular traction, and residual epiretinal membrane and cystoid macular edema are noted on the vertical (top, right) and horizontal (bottom, right) OCT scans. Visual acuity improved to 20/60 postoperatively.

with the fast scan protocol because all six fast scans are obtained automatically in rapid sequence without interruption between scans, whereas each individual normal resolution radial lines scan is obtained by the OCT operator separately in sequence. Because the fast macular thickness map is easier to obtain, it is used as the primary scan by some practitioners. If the fast macular thickness map appears normal, no further scanning is performed. If the fast macular thickness map scans are abnormal, then additional higher resolution radial line scans are performed to better assess the pathology.

PERIPAPILLARY RETINAL NERVE FIBER LAYER (RNFL) ANALYSIS

Used most often as a glaucoma screening and monitoring tool, the peripapillary RNFL analysis quantifies the thickness of the peripapillary RNFL and compares a patient's thickness with a normative database [38,39]. A circular scan is obtained in the peripapillary region [37]. RNFL thickness is obtained via boundary analysis and arithmetic difference calculations; however, instead of measuring the inner and outer retinal boundaries, the inner and outer boundaries of the RNFL are identified. Significant deviations in RNFL thickness from the normative database indicate a greater risk for glaucomatous thinning of the peripapillary RNFL in each of the four peripapillary quadrants (inferior, superior, nasal, and temporal) [37–39].

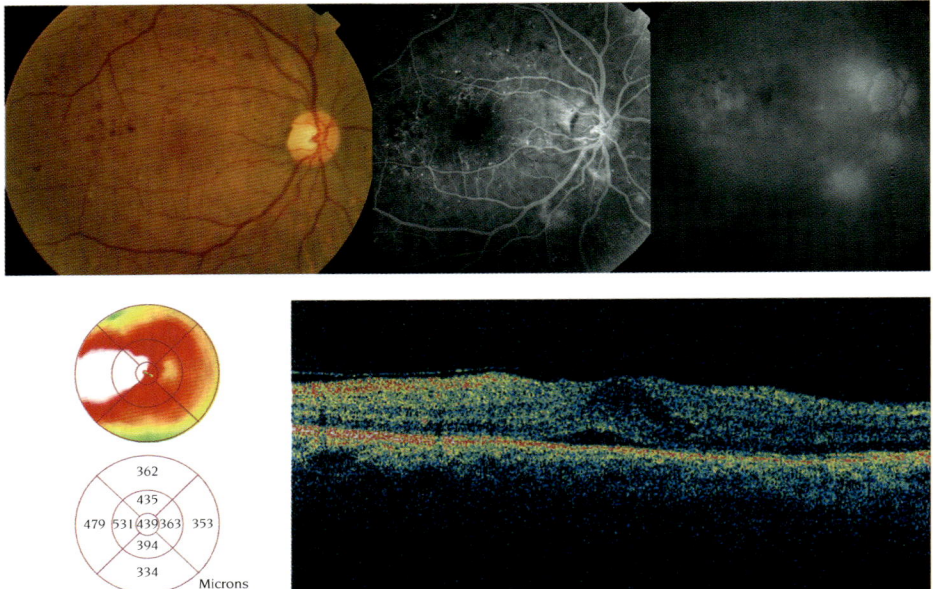

Figure 8.5. This is a 45 year-old man with type 2 diabetes mellitus and complaints of decreased visual acuity (VA) in the right and left eyes. VA measures 20/20. Compared to the left eye, the color fundus photograph of the right eye (top row, left) shows fewer blot retinal hemorrhages and microaneurysms. Similar to the left eye, the microaneurysms are temporally located. The mid-(top row, center) and late-phase (top row, right) fluorescein angiogram shows an enlarged foveal avascular zone, numerous microaneurysms, and a temporal pattern of diffuse leakage late in the study. Once again, the fluorescein leakage pattern corresponds well with the optical coherence tomography (OCT) macular contour map (bottom row, left) which reveals the greatest retinal thickening temporally. Despite good VA, the central foveal thickness measures 439 microns. The vertically oriented radial OCT scan (bottom row, right) reveals an incomplete posterior vitreous detachment over the macula, foveal cystic elements, and a foveal detachment.

NONPROLIFERATIVE DIABETIC RETINOPATHY (NPDR) AND DIABETIC MACULAR EDEMA (DME)

OCT's greatest utility in evaluating patients with nonproliferative diabetic retinopathy (NPDR) is the ability to detect and quantify the central retinal thickness in patients with clinically diagnosed DME [1,2,40–47]. In patients with mild NPDR and vision loss, OCT is often a good first diagnostic test if clinical exam and refractive changes do not account for vision loss (Figs. 8.1B–8.7) [40–42].

Structural macular derangements in patients with CSME include OCT patterns that demonstrate: (1) focal foveal and parafoveal intraretinal cystic thickening (Figs. 8.1B and 8.2); (2) diffuse intraretinal cystic thickening throughout the macular region (Fig. 8.3); (3) focal or broad vitreoretinal adhesions with resultant cystic retinal thickening and loss of the foveal contour consistent with a clinical diagnosis of taut posterior hyaloidal traction (Figs. 8.4 and 8.5) [1,2].

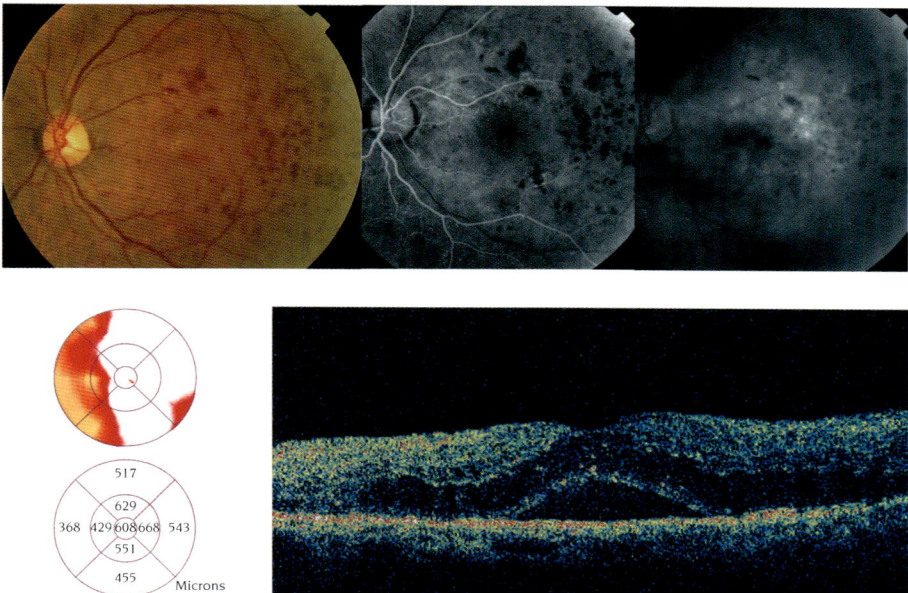

Figure 8.6. This is the left eye of the same patient in Figure 8.5. Visual acuity is 20/40. The color fundus photograph (top row, left) shows several areas of blot hemorrhages and numerous microaneurysms that are grouped temporal to the thickened fovea. The early- (top row, center) and late-phase (top row, right) fluorescein angiogram shows diffuse leakage on the temporal aspect of the macula and throughout the posterior pole. The optical coherence tomography (OCT) macular contour map (bottom row, left) matches the areas of leakage, showing the greatest retinal thickness in the temporal and superior macular regions. Central retinal thickness measures 608 microns. The vertically oriented radial OCT scan through the macula demonstrates incomplete posterior hyaloidal separation and a faint surface membrane with a blunted foveal depression, the presence of moderately sized cystic spaces in the outer retina, multiple highly-reflective foci in the fovea consistent with hard exudates, and a foveal detachment.

Historically, DME has been characterized as being focal or diffuse [48], but OCT has broadened our understanding of the relationship between DME and visual acuity. There is some controversy regarding the notion that OCT may serve as a proxy for visual acuity insofar as DME with significant central foveal thickening is associated with poor vision, while a nonedematous macula with a normal central retinal thickness is associated with good vision [49,50]. This somewhat simplified view does not take into consideration causes of vision loss other than macular swelling (e.g., foveal ischemia, epiretinal membrane, vitreomacular traction). It is true that not all visual loss in patients with diabetic retinopathy may be attributable to retinal thickening, cystoid macular edema, or subretinal fluid seen with OCT. Sometimes, occult concomitant retinal vascular disease is present that can confuse the clinical evaluation and OCT can be helpful in addition to clinical examination and fluorescein angiography. Commonly, macular ischemia may be present and appear as a relatively thin-appearing retina on OCT. Fluorescein angiography best characterizes macular ischemia by demonstrating enlargement of the capillary free zone (or foveal avascular zone), but can also demonstrate leakage

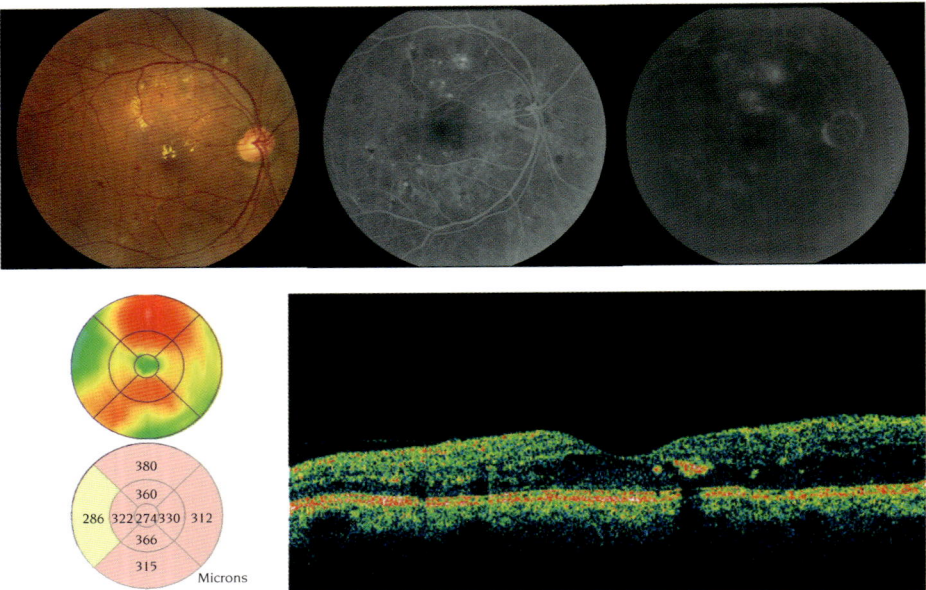

Figure 8.7. These images are from a 65-year-old man with type 2 diabetes mellitus and moderate to severe nonproliferative diabetic retinopathy. Visual acuity in the right eye is 20/25. The color fundus photograph (top row, left) shows several dot-blot hemorrhages and scattered hard exudates throughout the posterior pole. Although foveal exudates are present, questionable thickening is seen centrally. The mid- (top row, center) and late-phase (top row, right) fluorescein angiogram show leakage in an area superior to the fovea, although the foveal region is not affected by leakage. The optical coherence tomography (OCT) macular contour map (bottom row, left) mirrors the pattern of OCT leakage, ascribing the greatest thickening to the perifoveal region in the superior macula. The central 1-mm subfield foveal thickness measures just 274 microns, while more peripheral subfields show greater thickening, ranging from 360 to 380 microns. The vertically oriented radial OCT scan through the fovea demonstrates an incomplete posterior vitreous detachment, a relatively normal foveal contour with small cystic elements, and hyperreflective retinal foci consistent with foveal hard exudates. No subretinal fluid is appreciated in this case.

late in the study in patients with chronic macular ischemia. This synergy of diagnostic modalities is especially helpful when considering laser or pharmacologic treatment options for vision loss in diabetic retinopathy. Pharmacotherapies (e.g., triamcinolone acetonide, antivascular endothelial growth factor agents) typically improve vision, by reducing the vascular permeability that is causing CME. In the instance of thin/atrophic-appearing retina on OCT with nonperfusion (early) and leakage (late) in the angiogram, it would therefore not be anticipated that a pharmacologic agent would be effective at improving vision.

Spectral domain OCT (SD-OCT) is also able to quantify and qualitatively evaluate DME [51]. Although quantitative comparisons may be made between central retinal thickness measurements for the same patient imaged on the same SD-OCT unit, it appears that such comparisons cannot be made for a patient imaged on one visit with a time domain OCT unit and on another visit with an SD-OCT unit [51]. SD-OCT does provide spectacular views of macular anatomy in diabetic patients

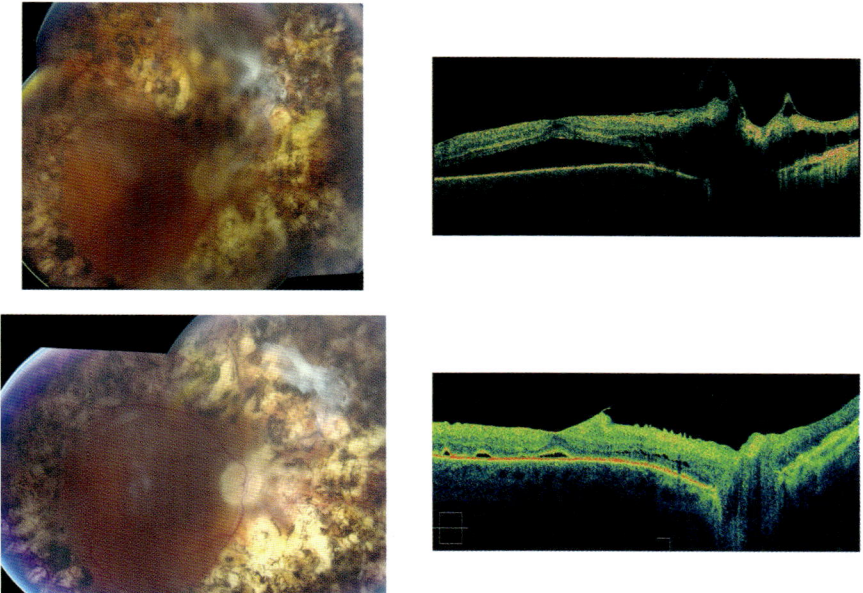

Figure 8.8. A 45-year-old man with proliferative diabetic retinopathy (PDR) presented with macular tractional retinal detachment (TRD) in his right eye. Preoperative montage color fundus photography revealing PDR with fibrous tuft on the optic disk with macular TRD (top row, left). Postoperative montage color fundus photography (bottom row, left) showing surgical release of fibrous epiretinal membranes and retinal reattachment. Preoperative SD-OCT revealing extensive subretinal fluid and intraretinal fluid below a tractional membrane (top row, right). The central subfield in the macula was 682 microns. Postoperative SD-OCT (bottom row, right) showing significant improvement in subretinal fluid, absence of the membrane, and retinal reattachment. The central subfield in the macula was 312 microns. (Source: Adapted from Kay et al, *Ophthalmic Surg Lasers Imaging* [61].)

and is particularly helpful in evaluating the vitreoretinal interface when planning the surgical approach to a patient with PDR and tractional retinal detachment of the macula (Figs. 8.8, 8.12, and 8.14).

TREATMENT MONITORING WITH OCT

OCT's qualitative and quantitative analytical capabilities make it a versatile tool not only for static evaluation of the patient, but also to monitor changes in the patient's condition from one visit to the next. One thing we have learned is that OCT is more sensitive than the ophthalmologist's clinical examination (even with stereoscopic contact lens biomicroscopy) at detecting macular edema [40–42,52]. Although some interoperator variability exists, overall, OCT has been found to be quite reproducible in its ability to detect and quantify DME [43–45,53].

For many, if not the majority, of cases of typical DME (patients without foveal ischemia, vitreomacular traction, foveal exudates (Fig. 8.7), or epiretinal membrane), CME with markedly increased central foveal thickness is the

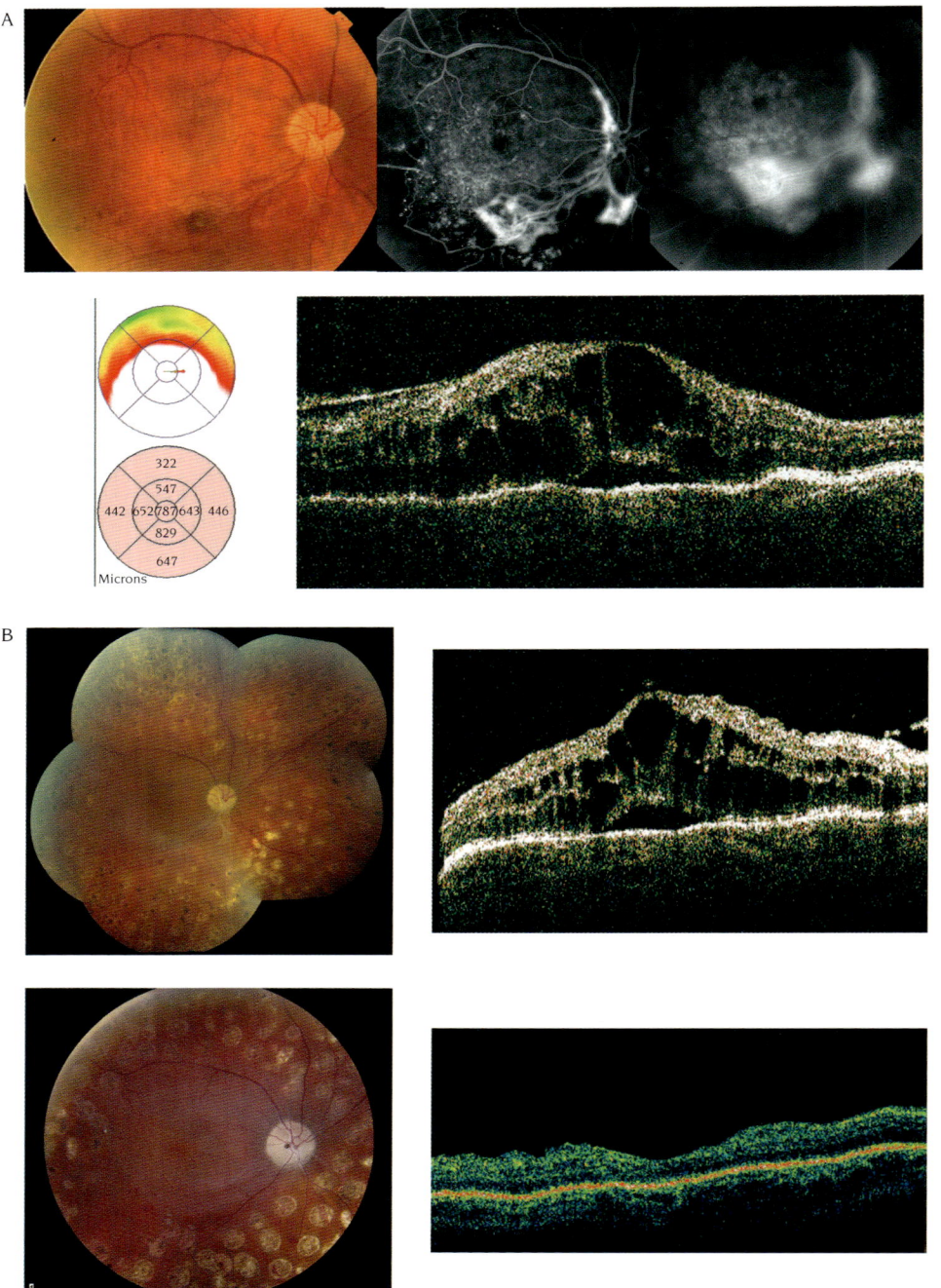

Figure 8.9. (A) Baseline studies from a 54-year-old non-insulin dependent diabetic man with complaints of progressively decreased vision in both eyes over the past 6 months. Fundus photograph (top row, left), early- (top row, middle) and late-phase (top row, right) fluorescein angiogram, OCT macular thickness map (bottom row, left) and radial line scan through the foveal center (bottom row, right) are shown for the right eye (Figure 8.9A). These demonstrate proliferative diabetic retinopathy with high risk features, diffuse macular leakage on the fluorescein

150

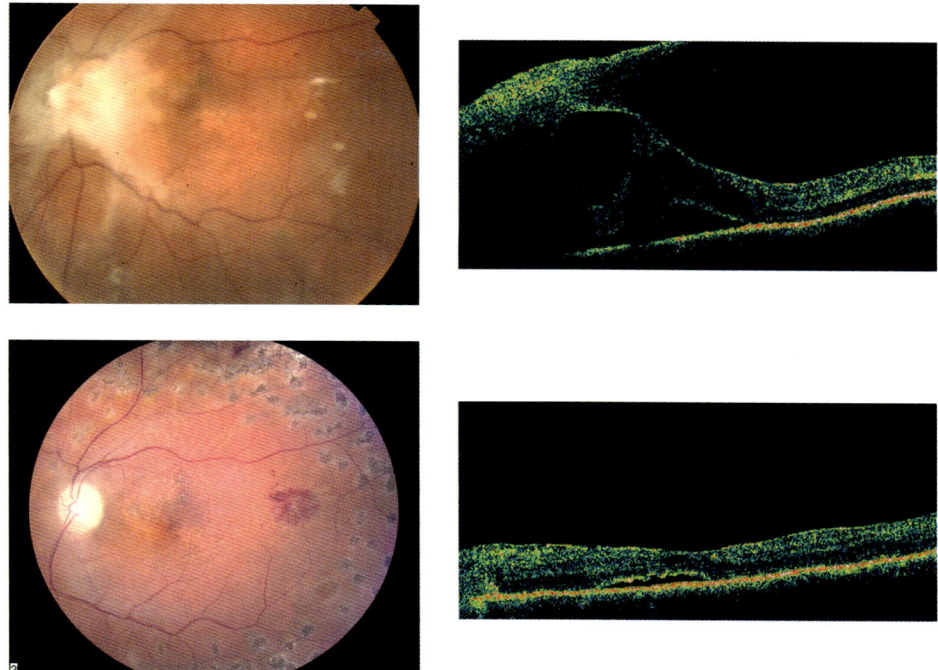

Figure 8.10. This is a 74-year-old man with type-2 diabetes mellitus and decreased visual acuity to the 20/200 level as a result of a macular tractional retinal detachment as shown in the presenting color fundus photograph (top row, left). The horizontal optical coherence tomography (OCT) scan of the left macula (top row, right) demonstrates a subfoveal fluid collection with overlying cystic retinal thickening, and insertion of the tractional membrane at the nasal aspect of the fovea (left of the scan). A relative normal appearing macular contour without cystoid macular edema is noted on the right half of this scan (temporal to the fovea). He underwent pars plana vitrectomy, membrane peeling, and endolaser and vision improved to 20/40 postoperatively. The postoperative color fundus photograph (bottom row, left) demonstrates absence of neovascular traction; however, the inferotemporal arcade remains slightly dystopic. Marked reduction in subfoveal fluid, intraretinal cytsts, and absence of tractional forces are noted on the postoperative horizontal OCT scan (bottom row, right).

---

angiogram and staining and leakage of the extraretinal fibrovascular neovascular membrane along the inferotemporal arcade, marked peripheral capillary nonperfusion, and diffuse cystoid macular edema on the OCT with a central foveal thickness of 787 microns. Visual acuity was 20/50. (B) Montage color fundus photograph of the right eye (top row, left) is shown six months after panretinal photocoagulation was performed on the patient in Figure 8.9A. The neovascular membrane along the inferotemporal arcade has involuted and, despite an intravitreal triamcinolone acetonide injection 4 months earlier, diffuse cystoid macular edema with a subfoveal fluid collection is noted on the radial line OCT scan (top row, right). Visual acuity was 20/70 and the central foveal thickness measured 840 microns. Subtly noted is an incomplete posterior vitreous detachment over the central macula, becoming more evident as a hyperreflective focus above the retina on the right side of the scan. Pars plana vitrectomy, membrane peeling, and endolaser was then performed. Six weeks postoperatively, color fundus photographs (bottom row, left) and OCT (bottom row, right) were obtained. These demonstrated resolution of both the traction and cystoid macular edema, with minimal irregularity to the inner foveal contour. Visual acuity improved to 20/50 and the central foveal thickness measured 225 microns.

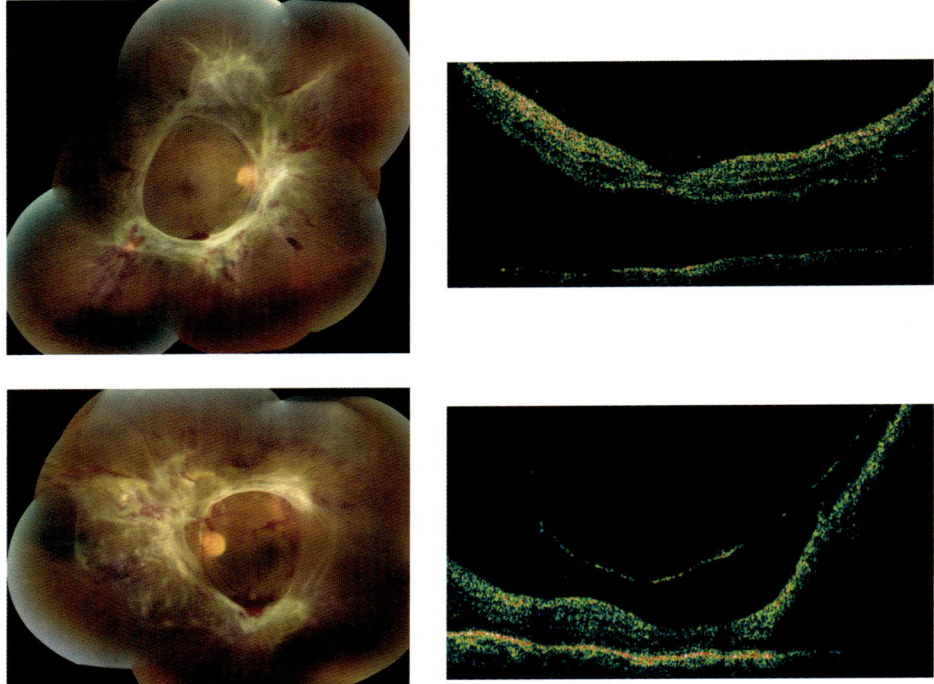

Figure 8.11. This is a 42-year-old type 1 diabetic man with bilateral "table-top" traction retinal detachments involving the macula due to advanced proliferative diabetic retinopathy as shown in the montage color fundus photographs of the right (top row, left) and left (bottom row, left) eye. The hyperreflective membrane shallowly separated from the inner retinal surface in both optical coherence tomography (OCT) scans represents the posterior hyaloid face. The oblique optical coherence tomography (OCT) scan (starting superonasal to the fovea and ending inferotemporal to the fovea) of the left macula (bottom row, right) shows the proximity of the subretinal fluid to the foveal center. Remarkably, visual acuity was 20/80 (right eye) and 20/60 (left eye).

usual presentation in patients with vision loss (Fig. 8.6). In these cases, changes in the central foveal thickness often do correlate with changes in visual acuity (Fig. 8.7) [54]. Patients generally appreciate improved vision (subjectively and objectively) associated with the rapid reduction in central foveal thickness following intraocular pharmacotherapy and, conversely, notice the rebound increase in their central foveal thickness (and worsening vision) after the anatomic effects of pharmacotherapy have subsided. Likely because of the multifactorial nature of vision fluctuation in diabetic eyes [40–47,55], the correlation between central retinal thickness and visual acuity is not always appreciated [49,50,56,61,62].

Nevertheless, OCT is a valuable tool to monitor treatment response. Following focal laser photocoagulation or intraocular pharmacotherapy, documented reduction in macular thickness confirms a positive anatomic response. In addition, maintenance of reduced macular thickness may help aid the clinician in deciding to withhold follow-up treatments. Recrudescence of macular edema and associated

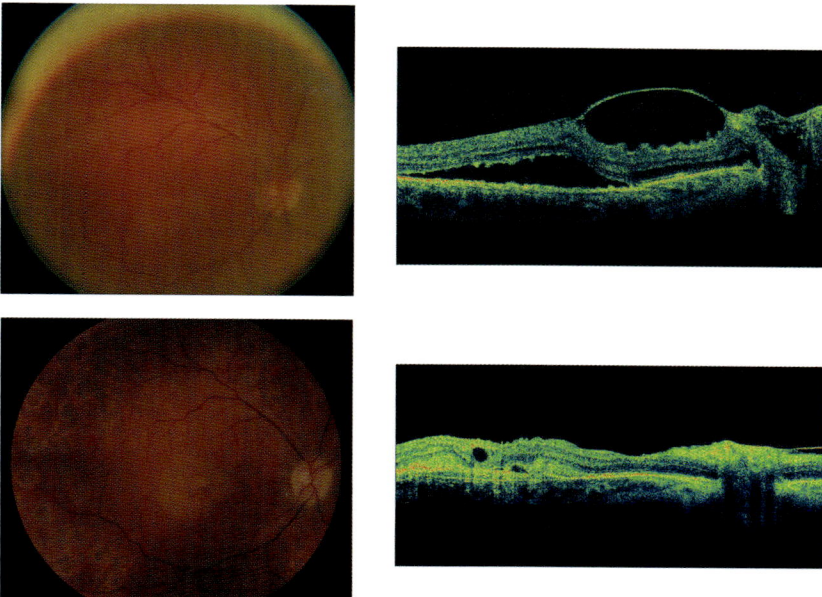

Figure 8.12. A 71-year-old man with proliferative diabetic retinopathy (PDR) presented with macular traction retinal detachment in his right eye. Preoperative color fundus photography demonstrates macular traction retinal detachment from PDR (top row, left). Postoperative color fundus photography (bottom row, left) demonstrates absence of epiretinal membranes and retinal reattachment. Preoperative spectral domain OCT (SD-OCT) (top row, right) reveals extensive subretinal fluid and epiretinal membranes. The central subfield in the macula was 476 microns. Postoperative SD-OCT (bottom row, right) depicts considerable resolution of this fluid, absence of the membrane, and retinal reattachment. The central subfield in the macula was 333 microns. (Source: Adapted from Kay et al., *Ophthalmic Surg Lasers Imaging* [61].)

increases in the central retinal thickness after a period of stability may indicate the need for additional therapy. Besides the valuable quantitative and qualitative information that the OCT provides on each patient longitudinally, the physician obviously integrates all available patient data to make informed and appropriate treatment decisions.

VITREORETINAL TRACTIONAL ABNORMALITIES AND DME

In the early 1990s, there was a recognition that diffuse DME was often associated with a taut and thickened posterior hyaloidal face that exerted tractional forces on the macula [57]. Without the benefit of OCT, it was recognized that a shallow foveal detachment was also present in these cases (Figs. 8.4, 8.5, and 8.7) [57]. Later evaluation of such patients with OCT documented the presence of both the posterior hyaloidal traction and the foveal detachment, although the latter was not always appreciated [58]. In these cases of posterior hyaloidal traction, OCT demonstrates resolution of the macular edema and foveal detachment after vitrectomy relieves the tangential traction exerted by the taut and thickened posterior hyaloid

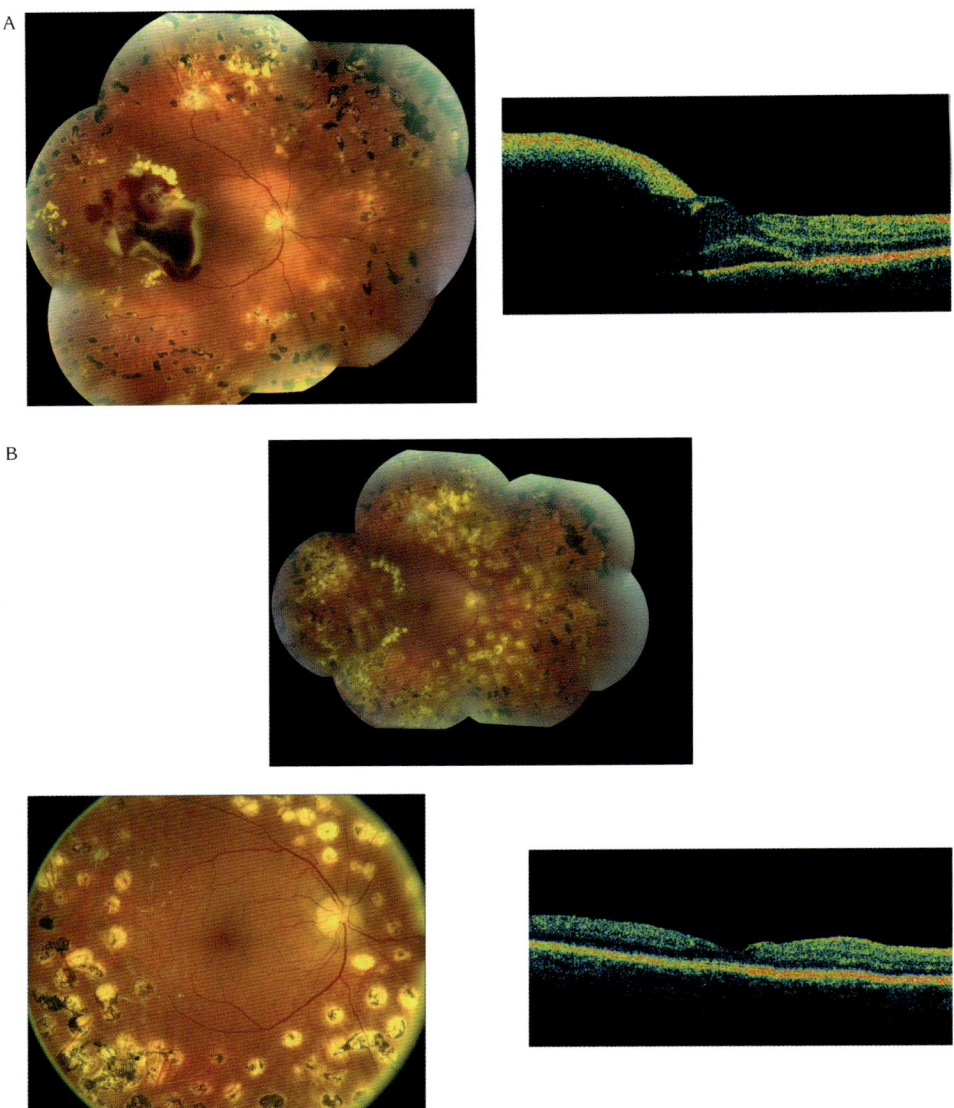

Figure 8.13. (A) This color fundus photograph montage (left) is from a 45-year-old man with proliferative diabetic retinopathy status post partial panretinal photocoagulation who developed a massive preretinal hemorrhage, splitting the fovea. Dehemoglobinized hemorrhage is appreciated on the nasal border of the hemorrhage and lipid exudates are seen temporally. Visual acuity is 20/80. The horizontal optical coherence tomography (OCT) scan (right) that sweeps horizontally from the papillomacular bundle through the fovea and then into the area of the hemorrhage (nasal to temporal) demonstrates progressively increasing microcystic retinal thickening, subfoveal fluid collection, and blocked reflections (red and yellow false color representation) due to the thick preretinal hemorrhage. (B) This is the same patient as Figure 8.13A. A color montage photograph of the right fundus (top) 1 month status post pars plana vitrectomy and endolaser demonstrates resolved pre-retinal hemorrhage, residual hard exudates in the temporal macula, and peripheral laser photocoagulation. Visual acuity is 20/30. A color fundus photograph focusing on the macula (bottom, left) 2 months later demonstrates continued resolution of the hard exudates. The corresponding horizontal OCT scan (sweeping from temporal to nasal) from the same day (bottom right) demonstrates a relatively normal foveal contour, free of cystoid macular edema.

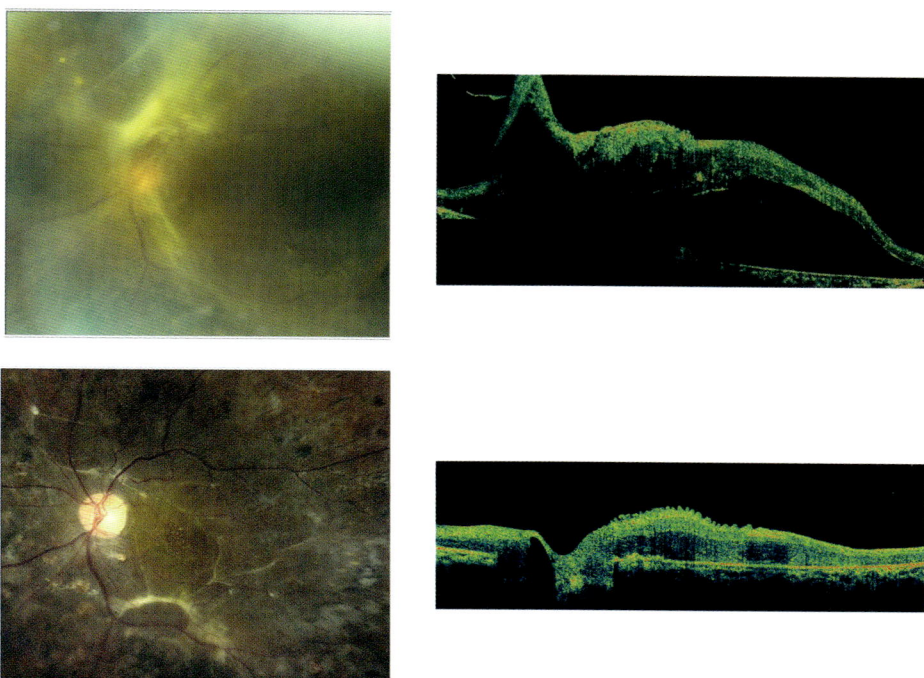

Figure 8.14. A 47-year-old man with proliferative diabetic retinopathy presented with macular tractional retinal detachment in his left eye. Preoperative color appearance showing extensive tractional fibrotic membranes and macular TRD (top, left). Preoperative spectral domain OCT (SD-OCT) revealing extensive subretinal fluid and epiretinal membrane (top, right). The central subfield retinal thickness in the macula was 1003 microns. Postoperative appearance showing removal of tractional epiretinal membrane and retinal reattachment (bottom, left). Postoperative SD-OCT showing resolution of this fluid, absence of the membrane, and retinal reattachment (bottom, right). The central subfield retinal thickness in the macula was 338 microns postoperatively. (Source: Adapted from Kay et al., *Ophthalmic Surg Lasers Imaging* [61].)

[58]. Pathologic vitreous adherence to the macula and posterior pole is now a well-recognized cause of vision loss in diabetics [57–60].

PROLIFERATIVE DIABETIC RETINOPATHY (PDR)

Proliferative diabetic retinopathy (PDR) is best evaluated with clinical examination, fluorescein angiography and, in cases with media opacity, B-scan ultrasonography. Extraretinal neovascularization and vitreous hemorrhage in PDR are traditionally evaluated and monitored with serial fundus photographs or echography before and after intervention (e.g., panretinal laser photocoagulation, pars plana vitrectomy). Left untreated, neovascular complexes often result in the development of complex tractional retinal detachment (Figs. 8.9–8.15). OCT can help determine macular involvement of the traction retinal detachment and further characterize the nature and extent of the traction [35–37]. In addition, vision loss

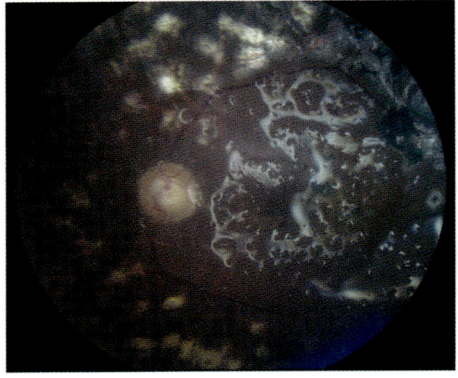 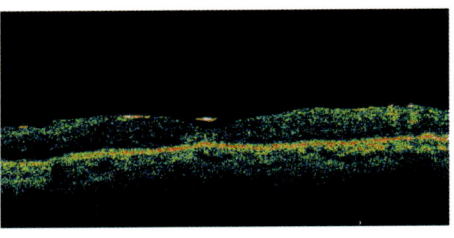

Figure 8.15. These images are of a 53-year-old diabetic man who underwent pars plana vitrectomy, membrane peeling, and silicone oil injection for management of proliferative diabetic retinopathy with traction retinal detachment. The color fundus photograph (top, left) demonstrates peripheral laser ablation and an attached macular with typical silicone oil light reflex (normal artifact in eyes with silicone oil). The optical coherence tomography (OCT) radial line scan demonstrates the ability of OCT to visualize the macula through silicone oil, revealing a relatively normal appearing macular contour that is free of vitreoretinal traction, cystoid macular edema, or subretinal fluid. Visual acuity is 20/400. The yellow hyper-reflective line anterior to the fovea is characteristically seen on OCT Scans of eyes harboring silicone oil.

following panretinal laser photocoagulation can be evaluated with OCT to determine whether a serous retinal detachment, new or exacerbated cystoid macular edema, or new preretinal hemorrhage (Fig. 8.13A) may be present and accounting for the vision fluctuation.

If surgical repair of a complex traction retinal detachment requires silicone oil, OCT is useful to assess for post-silicone oil visual acuity fluctuations. This information is often helpful when determining the proper time for silicone oil removal, because a macular cause for visual loss can be ruled out in most cases. Physicians should know that a normal artifact of OCT scans from eyes with silicone oil consists of a characteristic linear or crescentic hyperreflective focus just above the fovea, representing the posterior silicone oil/retina junction (Fig. 8.15).

SUMMARY

In conclusion, OCT has become an essential tool in the evaluation of patients with diabetic retinopathy. Along the wide spectrum of the disease, OCT has clinical utility, but its greatest application is in the diagnosis and management of patients with DME. Quantifying macular thickness and monitoring response to treatment are two features of this technology that make it so popular amongst vitreoretinal specialists. Its ability to assess vitreoretinal tractional abnormalities is also quite valuable, especially when these are unsuspected. More severe diabetic retinopathy that is associated with traction retinal detachment can be better characterized with OCT, insofar as subtle and progressive involvement of the macula can be ascertained.

OCT is continually being validated and it has been shown to be a reproducible technology. Virtually all new clinical trial protocols have included OCT outcomes—in addition to visual acuity—as one of their main outcome measures. Clinical examination, fundus photography, fluorescein angiography, and ultrasonography all remain important tools in the management of diabetic retinopathy. OCT has not, and likely will not, replace any of these useful diagnostic modalties, but instead it serves to enhance our understanding of this difficult disease in new ways. Technological advancements in OCT have incorporated image registration with an accompanying fundus photograph (ability to superimpose the scan on the fundus image), ultra-high-resolution image quality, entire macular capture at one sitting (compared to the individual radial line scans captured now), and three-dimensional topographical image rendering. All of these improvements are anticipated to improve the reliability and reproducibility of the technology as well as the longitudinal comparison of the patient over time. Enhanced understanding of the dynamics of the vitreomacular relationship is also anticipated.

REFERENCES

1. Hee MR, Puliafito CA, Wong C, et al. Quantitative assessment of macular edema with optical coherence tomography. *Arch Ophthalmol.* August 1995;113(8):1019–1029.
2. Hee MR, Puliafito CA, Duker JS, et al. Topography of diabetic macular edema with optical coherence tomography. *Ophthalmology.* February 1998;105(2):360–370.
3. Brancato R. Optical coherence tomography (OCT) in macular edema. *Doc Ophthalmol.* 1999;97(3–4):337–339.
4. Frank RN. Diabetic retinopathy. *N Engl J Med.* January 1, 2004;350(1):48–58.
5. Shah GK, Brown GC. Photography, angiography, and ultrasonography in diabetic retinopathy. In: Flynn HW Jr, Smiddy WE (Eds.), *Diabetes and Ocular Disease; Past, Present, and Future Therapies.* San Francisco: The Foundation of the American Academy of Ophthalmology; 2000:101–114.
6. Preliminary report on effects of photocoagulation therapy. The Diabetic Retinopathy Study Research Group. *Am J Ophthalmol.* April 1976;81(4):383–396.
7. Photocoagulation treatment of proliferative diabetic retinopathy: the second report of diabetic retinopathy study findings. *Ophthalmology.* January 1978;85(1):82–106.
8. Ferris FL 3rd, Podgor MJ, Davis MD. Macular edema in Diabetic Retinopathy Study patients. Diabetic Retinopathy Study Report Number 12. *Ophthalmology.* July 1987;94(7):754–760.
9. Photocoagulation for diabetic macular edema. Early Treatment Diabetic Retinopathy Study report number 1. Early Treatment Diabetic Retinopathy Study research group. *Arch Ophthalmol.* December 1985;103(12):1796–1806.
10. Kinyoun J, Barton F, Fisher M, Hubbard L, Aiello L, Ferris F 3rd. Detection of diabetic macular edema. Ophthalmoscopy versus photography—Early Treatment Diabetic Retinopathy Study Report Number 5. The ETDRS Research Group. *Ophthalmology.* June 1989;96(6):746–750; discussion 750–751.
11. Cunningham ET Jr, Adamis AP, Altaweel M, et al. A phase II randomized double-masked trial of pegaptanib, an anti-vascular endothelial growth factor aptamer, for diabetic macular edema. *Ophthalmology.* October 2005r;112(10):1747–1757.
12. Sutter FK, Simpson JM, Gillies MC. Intravitreal triamcinolone for diabetic macular edema that persists after laser treatment: three-month efficacy and safety results

of a prospective, randomized, double-masked, placebo-controlled clinical trial. *Ophthalmology*. November 2004;111(11):2044–2049.

13. Bonini-Filho MA, Jorge R, Barbosa JC, Calucci D, Cardillo JA, Costa RA. Intravitreal injection versus sub-Tenon's infusion of triamcinolone acetonide for refractory diabetic macular edema: a randomized clinical trial. *Invest Ophthalmol Vis Sci*. October 2005;46(10):3845–3849.

14. Cardillo JA, Melo LA Jr, Costa RA, et al. Comparison of intravitreal versus posterior sub-Tenon's capsule injection of triamcinolone acetonide for diffuse diabetic macular edema. *Ophthalmology*. September 2005;112(9):1557–1563.

15. Massin P, Audren F, Haouchine B, et al. Intravitreal triamcinolone acetonide for diabetic diffuse macular edema: preliminary results of a prospective controlled trial. *Ophthalmology*. February 2004;111(2):218–224; discussion 224–225.

16. Avitabile T, Longo A, Reibaldi A. Intravitreal triamcinolone compared with macular laser grid photocoagulation for the treatment of cystoid macular edema. *Am J Ophthalmol*. October 2005;140(4):695–702.

17. Parolini B, Panozzo G, Gusson E, et al. Diode laser, vitrectomy and intravitreal triamcinolone. A comparative study for the treatment of diffuse non tractional diabetic macular edema. *Semin Ophthalmol*. March–June 2004;19(1–2):1–12.

18. Patelli F, Fasolino G, Radice P, et al. Time course of changes in retinal thickness and visual acuity after intravitreal triamcinolone acetonide for diffuse diabetic macular edema with and without previous macular laser treatment. *Retina*. October–November 2005;25(7):840–845.

19. Yanyali A, Nohutcu AF, Horozoglu F, Celik E. Modified grid laser photocoagulation versus pars plana vitrectomy with internal limiting membrane removal in diabetic macular edema. *Am J Ophthalmol*. May 2005;139(5):795–801.

20. Polito A, Del Borrello M, Polini G, Furlan F, Isola M, Bandello F. Diurnal variation in clinically significant diabetic macular edema measured by the Stratus OCT. *Retina*. January 2006;26(1):14–20.

21. Kang SW, Sa HS, Cho HY, Kim JI. Macular grid photocoagulation after intravitreal triamcinolone acetonide for diffuse diabetic macular edema. *Arch Ophthalmol*. May 2006;124(5):653–658.

22. Chan A, Duker JS. A standardized method for reporting changes in macular thickening using optical coherence tomography. *Arch Ophthalmol*. July 2005;123(7):939–943.

23. Goebel W, Franke R. Retinal thickness in diabetic retinopathy: comparison of optical coherence tomography, the retinal thickness analyzer, and fundus photography. *Retina*. January 2006;26(1):49–57.

24. Giovannini A, Amato G, Mariotti C, Scassellati-Sforzolini B. Optical coherence tomography findings in diabetic macular edema before and after vitrectomy. *Ophthalmic Surg Lasers*. May–June 2000;31(3):187–191.

25. Schaudig UH, Glaefke C, Scholz F, Richard G. Optical coherence tomography for retinal thickness measurement in diabetic patients without clinically significant macular edema. *Ophthalmic Surg Lasers*. May–June 2000;31(3):182–186.

26. Rivellese M, George A, Sulkes D, Reichel E, Puliafito C. Optical coherence tomography after laser photocoagulation for clinically significant macular edema. *Ophthalmic Surg Lasers*. May–June 2000;31(3):192–197.

27. Panozzo G, Parolini B, Gusson E, et al. Diabetic macular edema: an OCT-based classification. *Semin Ophthalmol*. March–June 2004;19(1–2):13–20.

28. Panozzo G, Gusson E, Parolini B, Mercanti A. Role of OCT in the diagnosis and follow up of diabetic macular edema. *Semin Ophthalmol*. June 2003;18(2):74–81.

29. Massin P, Duguid G, Erginay A, Haouchine B, Gaudric A. Optical coherence tomography for evaluating diabetic macular edema before and after vitrectomy. *Am J Ophthalmol.* February 2003;135(2):169–177.
30. Ciardella AP, Klancnik J, Schiff W, Barile G, Langton K, Chang S. Intravitreal triamcinolone for the management of refractory diabetic macular oedema with hard exudates: an optical coherence tomography study. *Br J Ophthalmol.* September 2004;88(9):1131–1136.
31. Shimura M, Yasuda K, Nakazawa T, Kano T, Ohta S, Tamai M. Quantifying alterations of macular thickness before and after panretinal photocoagulation in patients with severe diabetic retinopathy and good vision. *Ophthalmology.* December 2003;110(12):2386–2394.
32. Chan A, Duker JS, Ko TH, Fujimoto JG, Schuman JS. Normal macular thickness measurements in healthy eyes using Stratus optical coherence tomography. *Arch Ophthalmol.* February 2006;124(2):193–198.
33. Optical coherence tomography of ocular disease, 2nd Ed., Schuman JS, Puliafito CA, Fujimoto JG (Eds.), Thorofare, NJ: Slack Incorporated; 2004.
34. Brancato R, Lumbroso B. Guide to coherence tomography interpretation. Innovative-News-Corporation, Rome, Italy, 2004, 54–61.
35. Villegas VC, Flynn Jr. HW. Diabetic retinopathy. In: Schuman JS, Puliafito CA, Fujimoto JG, eds., *Optical Coherence Tomography of Ocular Disease*, 2nd ed. Thorofare, NJ: Slack Incorporated; 2004:158–214.
36. Moshfeghi AA, Mavrofrides EC, Puliafito CA. Optical coherence tomography and retinal thickness assessment for diagnosis and management. In: Ryan SJ, ed., *Retina*, 4th ed., Vol. 2. Schachat A (Ed.), Philadelphia, PA: Elsevier Mosby; 2006:1533–1556.
37. Budenz DL, Chang RT, Huang X, Knighton RW, Tielsch JM. Reproducibility of retinal nerve fiber thickness measurements using the stratus OCT in normal and glaucomatous eyes. *Invest Ophthalmol Vis Sci.* July 2005;46(7):2440–2443.
38. Budenz DL, Michael A, Chang RT, McSoley J, Katz J. Sensitivity and specificity of the Stratus OCT for perimetric glaucoma. *Ophthalmology.* January 2005;112(1):3–9.
39. Brown JC, Solomon SD, Bressler SB, Schachat AP, DiBernardo C, Bressler NM. Detection of diabetic foveal edema: contact lens biomicroscopy compared with optical coherence tomography. *Arch Ophthalmol.* March 2004;122(3):330–335.
40. Strom C, Sander B, Larsen N, Larsen M, Lund-Andersen H. Diabetic macular edema assessed with optical coherence tomography and stereo fundus photography. *Invest Ophthalmol Vis Sci.* January 2002;43(1):241–245.
41. Browning DJ, McOwen MD, Bowen RM Jr, O'Marah TL. Comparison of the clinical diagnosis of diabetic macular edema with diagnosis by optical coherence tomography. *Ophthalmology.* April 2004;111(4):712–715.
42. Browning DJ. Interobserver variability in optical coherence tomography for macular edema. *Am J Ophthalmol.* June 2004;137(6):1116–1117.
43. Browning DJ, Fraser CM. Intraobserver variability in optical coherence tomography. *Am J Ophthalmol.* September 2004;138(3):477–479.
44. Massin P, Vicaut E, Haouchine B, Erginay A, Paques M, Gaudric A. Reproducibility of retinal mapping using optical coherence tomography. *Arch Ophthalmol.* August 2001;119(8):1135–1142.
45. Larsen M, Wang M, Sander B. Overnight thickness variation in diabetic macular edema. *Invest Ophthalmol Vis Sci.* July 2005;46(7):2313–2316.
46. Frank RN, Schulz L, Abe K, Iezzi R. Temporal variation in diabetic macular edema measured by optical coherence tomography. *Ophthalmology.* February 2004;111(2):211–217.

47. Browning DJ, Altaweel MM, Bressler NM, et al. Diabetic macular edema: what is focal and what is diffuse? *Am J Ophthalmolol.* Nov 2008;146(5):649–655,655. e1–6.
48. Diabetic Retinopathy Clinical Research Network. Relationship between optical coherence tomography-measured central retinal thickness and visual acuity in diabetic macular edema. *Ophthalmology.* 2007;114:525–536.
49. Bressler NM, Edwards AR, Antosyzk AN, et al. Retinal thickness on Stratus optical coherence tomography in people with diabetes and minimal or no diabetic retinopathy. *Am J Ophthalmolol.* 2008;145:894–901.
50. Forooghian F, Cukras C, Meyerle CB, Chew EY, Wong WT. Evaluation of time domain and spectral domain optical coherence tomography in the measurement of diabetic macular edema. *Invest Ophthalmol Vis Sci.* October 2008;49(10):4290–4296.
51. Davis MD, Bressler SB, Aiello LP, et al. Comparison of time-domain OCT and fundus photographic assesments of retinal thickening in eyes with diabetic macular edema. *Invest Ophthalmol Vis Sci.* 2008;49:1745–1752.
52. Diabetic Retinopathy Clinical Research Network. Reproducibility of macular thickness and volume using Zeiss optical coherence tomography in patients with diabetic macular edema. *Ophthalmology.* 2007;114:1520–1525.
53. Martidis A, Duker JS, Greenberg PB, et al. Intravitreal triamcinolone for refractory diabetic macular edema. *Ophthalmology.* May 2002;109(5):920–927.
54. Browning DJ, Fraser CM. Regional patterns of sight-threatening diabetic macular edema. *Am J Ophthalmol.* July 2005;140(1):117–124.
55. Larsson J, Zhu M, Sutter F, Gillies MC. Relation between reduction of foveal thickness and visual acuity in diabetic macular edema treated with intravitreal triamcinolone. *Am J Ophthalmol.* May 2005;139(5):802–806.
56. Lewis H, Abrams GW, Blumenkranz MS, Campo RV. Vitrectomy for diabetic macular traction and edema associated with posterior hyaloidal traction. *Ophthalmology.* 1992;99:753–759.
57. Kaiser PK, Riemann CD, Sears JE, Lewis H. Macular traction detachment and diabetic macular edema associated with posterior hyaloidal traction. *Am J Ophthalmol.* January 2001;131(1):44–49.
58. Gaucher D, Tadayoni R, Erginay A, Haouchine B, Gaudric A, Massin P. Optical coherence tomography assessment of the vitreoretinal relationship in diabetic macular edema. *Am J Ophthalmol.* May 2005;139(5):807–813.
59. Karatas M, Ramirez JA, Ophir A. Diabetic vitreopapillary traction and macular oedema. *Eye.* June 2005;19(6):676–682.
60. Kay CN, Mohamed GG, Lujan B, Punjabi OS, Gregori G, Flynn HW Jr. Composite spectral domain optical coherence tomography images of diabetic tractional retinal detachment. *Ophthalmic Surg Lasers Imaging.* July–August 2008;39(4 Suppl):S99–S103.
61. Browning DJ, Glassman AR, Aiello LP, et al. Optical coherence tomography measurements and analysis methods in optical coherence tomography studies of diabetic macular edema. *Ophthalmology.* 2008;115:1366–1371.
62. Diabetic Retinopathy Clinical Research Network. A randomized trial comparing intravitreal triamcinolone acetonide and focal/grid laser photocoagulation for diabetic macular edema. *Ophthalmology.* 2008;115:1447–1459.

9

Clinical Studies on Treatment for Diabetic Retinopathy

FREDERICK L. FERRIS III, MD,
MATTHEW D. DAVIS, MD,
LLOYD M. AIELLO, MD,
AND EMILY Y. CHEW, MD

CORE MESSAGES

- Clinical trials provide evidence regarding the safety and efficacy of various management options for treatment of diabetic retinopathy.
- In patients with proliferative diabetic retinopathy (PDR) or severe nonproliferative diabetic retinopathy (NPDR), scatter laser photocoagulation reduces the rate of severe visual loss by 50%.
- In patients with clinically significant macular edema, focal/grid laser photocoagulation reduces the rate of moderate visual acuity loss by 50%.
- Clinical trial data have documented the value of vitrectomy in eyes with very severe PDR or severe vitreous hemorrhage.
- Improved glycemic control has been demonstrated to be associated with reduced incidence and progression of diabetic retinopathy.

Diabetic retinopathy has been, and probably remains, one of the four major causes of blindness in the United States [1,2]. Without treatment, eyes that develop proliferative diabetic retinopathy (PDR) have at least a 50% chance of becoming blind within 5 years [3–5]. Appropriate application of treatments that have been developed in the last three decades can reduce this risk of blindness to less than 5% [6]. Medical treatments designed to maximize blood glucose control and reduce the development and progression of retinopathy can further reduce the risk of blindness [7]. This chapter discusses the treatments available, the evidence that the treatments are effective and whether the treatments are widely used.

PHOTOCOAGULATION

Blindness from PDR was recognized as a growing public health problem in the 1960s. Although a number of possible treatments were tried, there was general uncertainty as to the best approach for treating diabetic retinopathy [8]. Introduced by Meyer-Schwickerath, photocoagulation was initially used to coagulate patches of new vessels on the surface of the retina [9]. During the 1960s, it became apparent that extensive retinal photocoagulation seemed to have a beneficial, but unexplained, indirect effect on both neovascularization and macular edema [10]. By the early 1970s, a few small clinical trials had indicated that photocoagulation might be an effective treatment [11].

Diabetic Retinopathy Study, 1971–1978. Because of the public health importance of the disease and the collective doubt as to its treatment, the Diabetic Retinopathy Study (DRS) was organized in 1971 to test the effect of photocoagulation on diabetic retinopathy (Table 9.1). This was the first randomized, multicenter, collaborative clinical trial sponsored by the newly formed National Eye Institute of the National Institutes of Health. The DRS enrolled 1742 patients with PDR or severe nonproliferative diabetic retinopathy (SNPDR) and visual acuity of 20/100 or better in each eye [12]. The age distribution of the population was bimodal, with 23% in the 20 to 29 years age group and 27% in the 50 to 59 group. The majority of DRS patients were male (56%) and white (94%).

One eye of each patient was randomly assigned to receive photocoagulation, and the fellow eye was observed without treatment. One of two photocoagulation techniques, using either the xenon arc or the newly developed argon laser, was randomly selected. All treated eyes received both direct and scatter (panretinal) photocoagulation and the treatment techniques, using either photocoagulation modality, were similar.

Table 9.1. Diabetic Retinopathy Study

Study Question
Is photocoagulation (argon or xenon) effective for treating diabetic retinopathy?
Eligibility
Proliferative diabetic retinopathy or bilateral severe nonproliferative diabetic retinopathy, with visual acuity 20/100 or better in each eye
Randomization
1742 participants, one eye randomly assigned to photocoagulation (argon or xenon), and one eye assigned to no photocoagulation
Outcome Variable
Visual acuity less than 5/200 for at least 4 months
Result
Photocoagulation (argon or xenon) reduces risk of severe visual loss compared with no treatment

Direct treatment involved the placement of photocoagulation burns over abnormal new vessels. All neovascularization elsewhere (NVE) was treated directly with either modality, but neovascularization of the disc (NVD) was treated directly only with the argon laser. Direct treatment was also applied to microaneurysms or other lesions thought to be causing macular edema. Scatter photocoagulation consisted of photocoagulation burns that avoided the macula and optic nerve, with each burn separated from its neighbors by one-half burn width. This resulted in a polka-dot pattern of burns in the retina that extended from the temporal vascular arcades to beyond the equator. In general, the argon laser burns were smaller and less intense than the xenon arc burns.

Analysis of follow-up data from that study demonstrated a 50% reduction in severe visual loss in eyes that had received photocoagulation (Fig. 9.1) [13]. Severe visual loss was defined as visual acuity <5/200 at two or more consecutively completed follow-up visits, which were scheduled at 4-month intervals. In addition to demonstrating that photocoagulation was effective, the DRS identified retinopathy features associated with a particularly high risk of severe visual loss [14–17]. Treatment was recommended for eyes with these high-risk characteristics, which can be summarized as either neovascularization accompanied by vitreous hemorrhage or obvious neovascularization on or near the optic disc (Fig. 9.2), even in the absence of vitreous hemorrhage.

After 24 months of follow-up in the DRS, the rates of severe visual loss for eyes with high-risk characteristics in the control group and treated groups were 26% and 11%, respectively. Eyes with PDR but without high-risk characteristics had a much lower risk of developing severe visual loss by 2 years in both the control group and the treated group (7% and 3%, respectively); these rates were even lower for the eyes with nonproliferative diabetic retinopathy (NDPR).

Harmful effects of treatment were greater in the xenon group, as shown in Table 9.2. Of the xenon-treated eyes, 25% suffered a modest loss of visual field, and an additional 25% suffered a more severe loss. Loss of visual field was much less in the argon-treated group, with only 5% of eyes suffering a modest or severe loss as measured using the largest test object (Goldmann IVe4). About 19% of

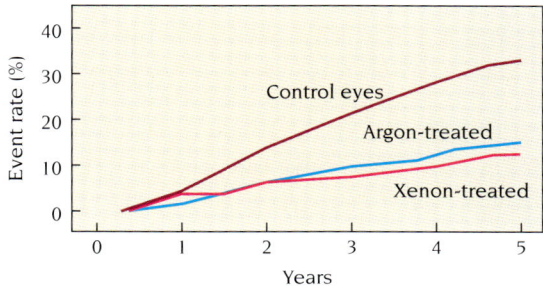

Figure 9.1. Diabetic Retinopathy Study results: Cumulative incidence of severe visual loss (visual acuity worse than 5/200 at two consecutive 4-month follow-up visits) for untreated eyes ($N = 1681$), argon-treated eyes ($N = 835$), and xenon-treated eyes ($N = 847$); $P < 0.001$ for both treated groups versus control group.

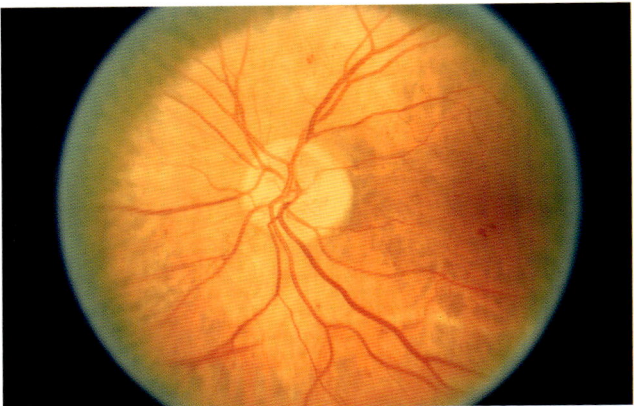

Figure 9.2. Diabetic Retinopathy Study standard photograph 10A demonstrating definite disc neovascularization. (Source: Published with permission form Diabetic Retinopathy Study Research Group: Photocoagulation treatment of proliferative diabetic retinopathy: the second report of Diabetic Retinopathy Study findings. *Ophthalmology.* 1978;85:82–106.)

Table 9.2. Estimated Percentages of Eyes with Harmful Effects Attributable to Treatment in Diabetic Retinopathy Study

Constriction of Visual Field (Goldman IVe4) to the average of	Argon	Xenon
# 45° but > 30° per meridian	5%	25%
# 30° per meridian	0%	25%
Decrease in Visual Acuity	**Argon**	**Xenon**
1 line	11%	19%
≥2 lines	3%	11%

xenon-treated eyes had a persistent visual acuity decrease of one line, which was possibly due to treatment, and an additional 11% had a persistent decrease or two or more lines. Comparable estimates for the argon-treated group were 11% and 3%, respectively. Subjectively, many patients noticed difficulties with dark adaptation and driving at night after either argon or xenon scatter photocoagulation.

Based on DRS results and clinical experience, mild to moderate intensity argon laser is recommended, rather than more intense lesions created by the xenon arc, because of similar benefits but fewer side effects. Direct treatment of neovascularization, although part of the original DRS protocol, has generally been discontinued based on the comparison of xenon and argon treatment in eyes with NVD. In the DRS, the argon treatment included direct photocoagulation of NVD, whereas this was not possible with xenon. There was no increase in regression of NVD in the argon group, but there was an increased risk of hemorrhage at the time of direct treatment.

Early Treatment Diabetic Retinopathy Study, 1980–1989. Although scatter photo-coagulation was shown by the DRS to be beneficial for patients with high-risk retinopathy, the question remained as to whether treatment at an earlier stage (non-high-risk PDR or severe NPDR) would be more helpful. The Early Treatment Diabetic Retinopathy Study (ETDRS) was designed to address this question, as well as questions related to the treatment of diabetic macular edema and the use of aspirin (Table 9.3) [18,19]. The 3711 ETDRS patients had mild-to-severe NDPR or early PDR, with or without diabetic macular edema. Compared with patients in the DRS, patients in the ETDRS were somewhat older (70% classified as type 2 and 52% over age 50), were less predominantly white (76%), and were equally likely to be male (56%).

All ETDRS patients were randomly assigned to 650 mg aspirin per day or placebo in order to assess whether the antiplatelet effects of aspirin would affect the microcirculation of the retina and slow the development of PDR [20–24]. One eye of each patient was randomly assigned to immediate photocoagulation, while the fellow eye was assigned to deferral of photocoagulation, that is, careful follow-up and prompt scatter photocoagulation if high-risk retinopathy developed. Eyes assigned to immediate photocoagulation received different treatments depending on the severity of the retinopathy: (1) eyes without DME were randomly assigned to full or mild scatter; (2) eyes with DME and severe NPDR or early PDR were randomly assigned to full or mild scatter and focal/grid treatment; (3) eyes with mild to moderate NPDR (for which it was thought that scatter could be deferred safely) were randomly assigned to either immediate focal/grid treatment (with deferred

Table 9.3. Early Treatment Diabetic Retinopathy Study

Study Questions

1. Is photocoagulation effective for treating diabetic macular edema?
2. Is early photocoagulation effective for treating diabetic retinopathy?
3. Is aspirin effective for preventing progression of diabetic retinopathy?

Eligibility

Mild nonproliferative diabetic retinopathy through early proliferataive diabetic retinopathy, with visual acuity 20/200 or better in each eye.

Randomization

3711 participants: one eye randomly assigned to photocoagulation (scatter and/or focal), and one eye assigned to no photocoagulation; patients randomly assigned to 650 mg/d aspirin or placebo.

Outcome Variables

Visual acuity less than 5/200 for at least 4 months; visual acuity worsening by doubling of initial visual angle (for example, 20/40 to 20/80); retinopathy progression.

Results

1. Macular edema: Table 9.4
2. Early photocoagulation: Table 9.5
3. Aspirin: Table 9.6

scatter—mild or full) or immediate scatter—mild or full (with deferred focal/grid treatment).

Aspirin use did not affect the progression of retinopathy (Table 9.4 and Fig. 9.3), nor did it affect the risk of visual loss. Perhaps surprisingly, aspirin use did not increase the risk of vitreous hemorrhage in patients with PDR [25]. In addition, aspirin use was associated with a 17% reduction in morbidity and mortality from cardiovascular disease [26]. Therefore, aspirin use should be considered for persons with diabetes, not because of any effect on their diabetic retinopathy, but because of their increased risk of cardiovascular disease. The presence of PDR should not be considered a contraindication to aspirin use.

The ETDRS utilized a factorial study design of aspirin (persons randomized) and photocoagulation (eyes randomized). Because aspirin use had little if any effect on any of the ETDRS ocular outcome variables and aspirin use was not associated with any statistically significant interactions with photocoagulation treatment, all randomized comparisons of photocoagulation treatment versus control combined the aspirin and placebo groups.

The comparison of early photocoagulation versus deferral in the ETDRS revealed a small reduction in the incidence of severe visual loss in the early-treated eyes (Table 9.5 and Fig. 9.4), but 5-year rates were low in both the early-treatment group and the deferral group (2.6% and 3.7%), respectively [27]. For eyes with only mild-to-moderate NPDR, rates of progression to severe vision loss were even

Table 9.4. Early Treatment Diabetic Retinopathy Study: Aspirin Use Results

1. Aspirin use did not alter progression of diabetic retinopathy
2. Aspirin use did not increase risk of vitreous hemorrhage
3. Aspirin use did not affect visual acuity
4. Aspirin use reduced risk of cardiovascular morbidity and mortality
5. Aspirin use did not increase rates of vitrectomy

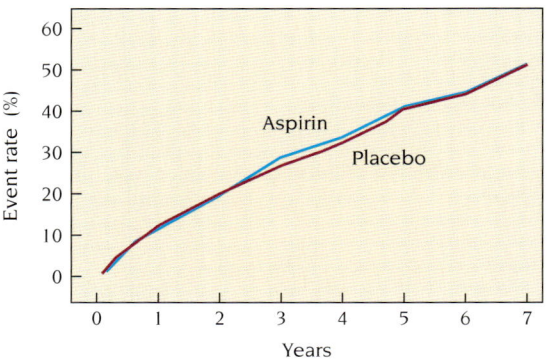

Figure 9.3. Early Treatment Diabetic Retinopathy Study results: Cumulative incidence of development of high-risk proliferative diabetic retinopathy for eyes assigned to deferral of photocoagulation in patients given placebo ($N = 1855$) and in aspirin-treated patients ($N = 1856$); $P = 0.58$.

lower; early photocoagulation benefits were not sufficient to compensate for the unwanted side effects. However, with very severe nonproliferative (Fig. 9.5) or early proliferative stages, the risk–benefit ratio was more favorable and consideration of initiating scatter photocoagulation before the development of high-risk PDR is suggested.

Recent analyses of ETDRS data suggest that early scatter treatment for eyes with severe NPDR or early PDR is especially effective in reducing severe visual loss in patients with type 2 diabetes (Fig. 9.6) [28]. These data provide an additional reason to recommend early scatter photocoagulation in older patients with very severe NPDR or early PDR.

The ETDRS results also provide clinically important information to guide the treatment of diabetic macular edema [29–32]. In the ETDRS, eyes that were assigned to immediate focal/grid photocoagulation, compared with those assigned to no focal laser treatment even if the macular edema progressed or vision was lost, had a reduced risk of moderate visual acuity loss of about 50% (Table 9.6 and Fig. 9.7). Moderate visual acuity loss was defined as a doubling of the visual angle from baseline to follow-up (e.g., 20/20 to 20/40 or 20/50 to 20/100). This benefit was greatest for eyes in which the center of the macula was already involved with edema, but eyes with edema that either involves or threatens the center of the macula also benefited. Side effects of treatment include scotomas related to

Table 9.5. Early Treatment Diabetic Retinopathy Study: Early Scatter Photocoagulation Results

1. Early scatter photocoagulation resulted in small reduction in risk of severe visual loss (<5/200 for at least 4 months)
2. Early scatter photocoagulation is not indicated for eyes with mild-to-moderate diabetic retinopathy
3. Early scatter photocoagulation may be most effective in patients with type 2 diabetes

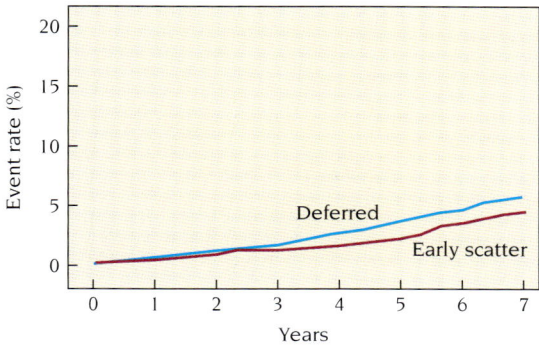

Figure 9.4. Early Treatment Diabetic Retinopathy Study results: Cumulative incidence of severe visual loss (<5/200 for at least 4 months) for eyes assigned to early scatter photocoagulation ($N = 3711$) and eyes assigned to deferral of treatment ($N = 3711$); $P < 0.01$.

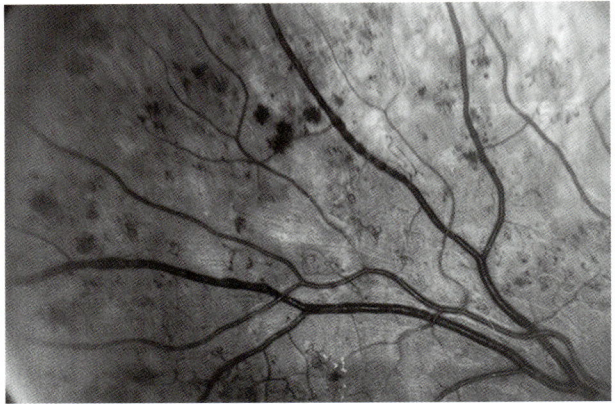

Figure 9.5. Red-free photograph of eye with severe nonproliferative diabetic retinopathy.

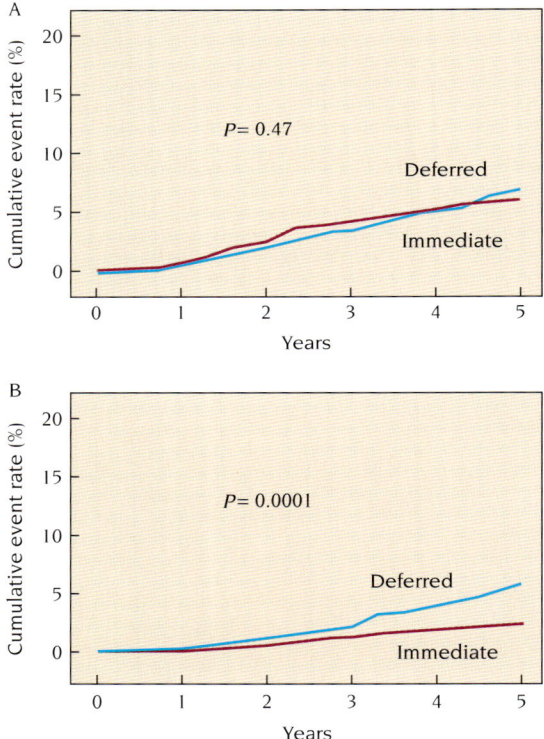

Figure 9.6. Early Treatment Diabetic Retinopathy Study results: Cumulative incidence of severe visual loss (<5/200 for at least 4 months) for eyes with severe nonproliferative diabetic retinopathy or early proliferative diabetic retinopathy in patients with (A) type 1 or (B) type 2 diabetes assigned to early scatter photocoagulation or deferral of photocoagulation (N in each group > 500); P< 0.01 for interaction of diabetes type and treatment effect.

Table 9.6. Early Treatment Diabetic Retinopathy Study: Macular Edema Results

1. Focal photocoagulation for diabetic macular edema decreased risk of moderate visual loss (doubling of initial visual angle)
2. Focal photocoagulation for diabetic macular edema increased chance of moderate visual gain (halving of initial visual angle)
3. Focal photocoagulation for diabetic macular edema reduced retinal thickening

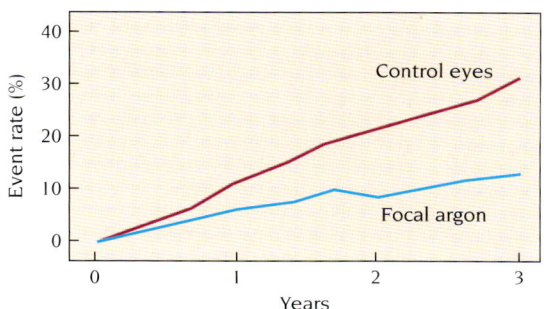

Figure 9.7. Early Treatment Diabetic Retinopathy Study results: Proportion of eyes with mild-to-moderate nonproliferative diabetic retinopathy and macular edema involving center of macula that has loss of three lines of visual acuity from baseline (doubling of initial visual angle, for example, 20/20 to 20/40) for eyes assigned to no treatment ($N = 607$) or to immediate focal treatment for macular edema ($N = 292$); $P < 0.01$ for each visit after 4 months.

the focal laser burns, although there was limited documentation of this using the visual fields as measured during the ETDRS. However, longer follow-up has demonstrated that photocoagulation scars enlarge over time and may eventually cause a decrease in visual acuity. For eyes in which involvement of the center of the macula was equivocal and there was little or no decrease in visual acuity, the ETDRS did not compare immediate photocoagulation versus careful follow-up, withholding photocoagulation until central involvement was definite and/or visual acuity has started to decrease. This would seem to be an appealing strategy to reduce the risk of visual loss while limiting the number of patients exposed to the risks of treatment.

VITRECTOMY

While photocoagulation treatment was being developed, another major advance was added to the practice of ophthalmology. New instrumentation and techniques made it possible to remove the vitreous gel and operate in the posterior aspect of the eye. This vitreous surgery offered hope of dramatic visual improvement in patients with severe vitreous hemorrhage [33–35].

Diabetic Retinopathy Vitrectomy Study, 1976–1983. The Diabetic Retinopathy Vitrectomy Study (DRVS) provides randomized clinical trial data demonstrating the benefits and risks of vitrectomy in eyes with severe vitreous hemorrhage or very severe neovascularization even in the absence of severe hemorrhage (Table 9.7) [36–40]. Results from the DRVS showed that conventional management at that time (deferring vitrectomy for 1 year in patients with severe vitreous hemorrhage or until tractional retinal detachment involved the macula) reduced the chance of obtaining good vision compared with doing early (<6 months) vitrectomy [37,40]. After 2 years of follow-up, 25% of the early-vitrectomy group had visual acuity of 20/40 or better, compared with 15% in the deferral group ($P = 0.01$). For patients with type 1 diabetes, who were on the average younger and had more severe PDR, this difference at 2 years was even greater (35% versus 12%, $P = 0.001$).

Early vitrectomy was also effective in saving good visual acuity in patients without severe vitreous hemorrhage, but with severe or very severe PDR [38,39]. The early-treated group had a higher percentage of eyes with 20/40 or better visual acuity at each of the 6-month visits during the 4 years of follow-up. About one third of treated eyes with more severe retinopathy had good vision at these 6-month visits, compared to less than 20% of the deferral eyes ($P < 0.05$ at every visit except the 6- and 24-month visits).

In both trials, the proportion of eyes with no light perception vision reached about 20% to 25% at 4 years in both the treated and the control groups, but there were more patients with no light perception in the treated group during the first several years of follow-up, especially in those eyes with the least severe retinopathy. Complications during follow-up included phthisis, endophthalmitis or uveitis, and corneal epithelial problems or neovascular glaucoma. Up to one third of treated eyes had at least one of these complications [37–40].

Table 9.7. Diabetic Retinopathy Vitrectomy Study

Study Questions

Is early vitrectomy preferable to deferral of vitrectomy in eyes with:

1. Severe vitreous hemorrhage from proliferative diabetic retinopathy?
2. Very severe proliferative diabetic retinopathy?

Eligibility

Recent severe vitreous hemorrhage from proliferative diabetic retinopathy (616 eyes); advanced, active, severe proliferative diabetic retinopathy (370 eyes, 240 with prior scatter photocoagulation)

Randomization

Early vitrectomy versus conventional management

Outcome Variable

Visual acuity 20/40 or better

Results

Visual acuity 20/40 or better was more frequent in early-vitrectomy groups (1–6 months from baseline); benefit of early vitrectomy was seen only in eyes with most severe proliferative diabetic retinopathy

Vitrectomy techniques have progressed considerably since this clinical trial. Instrumentation is markedly improved and photocoagulation can be done at the time of vitrectomy. Side effects have been reduced [41–44]. These clinical trial data, supported by additional case series, document the value of vitrectomy in eyes with very severe PDR or severe vitreous hemorrhage.

MEDICAL APPROACHES

Although photocoagulation, in combination with vitrectomy when necessary, is markedly effective in reducing the risk of blindness in persons with diabetic retinopathy, prevention of the development of retinopathy would be even more effective in preserving vision.

Blood Glucose Control. For years, there was debate as to whether improved control of blood glucose would reduce the chronic complications of diabetes, including diabetic retinopathy. Definitive studies have confirmed the benefit of blood glucose control.

Diabetes Control and Complications Trial, 1983–1989, Epidemiology of Diabetes Interventions and Complications. The Diabetes Control and Complications Trial (DCCT) was initiated to address this important clinical and scientific question [45]. The DCCT enrolled 1441 patients with type 1 diabetes (726 with no retinopathy and 715 with mild-to-moderate NPDR at baseline). These patients were randomly assigned to either intensive or conventional insulin therapy. Not only was there a remarkable reduction in the rate of development or progression of retinopathy in those patients assigned to intensive treatment (Table 9.8 and Fig. 9.8), there was also a reduction in the progression of diabetic nephropathy and neuropathy [46–48].

At the completion of the DCCT, 95% of the study patients were enrolled in the follow-up study called the Epidemiology of Diabetes Interventions and Complications (EDIC) study [49]. All patients were instructed in intensive insulin treatment and were all encouraged to achieve optimal control of blood sugar. By 5 years after entry, the 2% point difference in hemoglobin A_1C levels between the former intensive treatment group and the conventional treatment group had narrowed to virtually no difference between the two groups (persons in the intensive group could not maintain their former level of good blood glucose control and persons in the conventional treatment group improved their average hemoglobin A_1C). Despite the similar blood glucoses over the four years after the end of the clinical trial, further progression of diabetic retinopathy continued to be 66% to 77% less in the former intensive treatment group than in the former conventional treatment group. The benefit derived from the years of difference in diabetes control during the DCCT persists even at 7 years after the randomly assigned groups reverted to "standard care." It appears to take time for improvements in control to negate the long-lasting effects of prior prolonged hyperglycemia, and once the biological effects of prolonged improved control

Table 9.8. Diabetes Control and Complications Trial

Study Questions

1. Primary prevention study: Will intensive control of blood glucose slow development and subsequent progression of diabetic retinopathy?
2. Secondary prevention study: Will intensive control of blood glucose slow progression of diabetic retinopathy?

Eligibility

1. 726 patients with insulin-dependent diabetes mellitus (1–5 years' duration) and no diabetic retinopathy
2. 715 patients with insulin-dependent diabetes mellitus (1–15 years' duration) and mild-to-moderate diabetic retinopathy

Randomization

Intensive control of blood glucose (multiple daily insulin injections or insulin pump) versus conventional management

Outcome Variables

Development of diabetic retinopathy or progression of retinopathy by three steps using modified Airlie House classification scale; neuropathy, nephropathy, and cardiovascular outcomes were also assessed

Results

Intensive control reduced risk of developing retinopathy by 76% and slowed progression of retinopathy by 54%; intensive control also reduced risk of clinical neuropathy by 60% and albuminuria by 54%

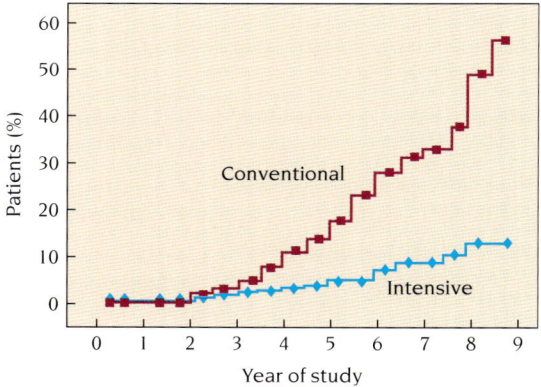

Figure 9.8. Diabetic Control and Complications Trial results: Cumulative incidence of sustained worsening of retinopathy (three steps on modified Airlie House scale for at least 6 months) in patients with type 1 diabetes and no diabetic retinopathy at baseline receiving intensive ($N = 342$) or conventional ($N = 375$) insulin therapy. $P < 0.001$. (Source: Redrawn with permission form Diabetes Control and Complications Trial Research Group: The effect of intensive treatment of diabetes on the development and progression of long-term complications in insulin-dependent diabetes mellitus. *N Engl J Med.* 1993;329:977–986. Copyright 10993 Massachusetts Medical Society. All rights reserved.)

are manifest, the benefits are long lasting. Furthermore, the total glycemic exposure of the patient (i.e., degree and duration) determines the degree of retinopathy observed at any one time.

A smaller randomized clinical trial of 102 patients with type 1 diabetes, observed for more than 7 years, also found that intensified insulin treatment reduced all three of the major microvascular complications of diabetes [50]. These consistent clinical trial results, combined with the strong observational study results [51], directly implicate elevated blood glucose in the development of the chronic microvascular complications of diabetes.

Evidence is accumulating to confirm the impression that microvascular complications are the result of chronic elevations of blood glucose levels. These complications take years to develop and are directly associated with long-term elevations of glycosylated hemoglobin. It also appears that it may take several years to realize the benefits of effective interventions to lower blood glucose.

Early studies of the effect of intensified glucose control on retinopathy actually demonstrated an unanticipated and paradoxical worsening of retinopathy in patients whose blood glucose control was rapidly markedly improved [46,52–58]. However, in patients with mild-to-moderate NPDR, this early worsening is not usually associated with visual loss, and the long-term benefits of intensive insulin treatment greatly outweighed this risk in the DCCT [59]. When intensive insulin treatment is to be instituted in patients who have PDR or severe NPDR, ophthalmologic consultation is desirable because photocoagulation may be desirable prior to initiating intensive insulin treatment.

The effect of glycemic control on the incidence and progression of diabetic microvascular complications, as assessed in observational studies, is similar in both type 1 and type 2 patients [60]. Randomized studies of the effect of intensive glucose control on type 2 patients in Japan and the United Kingdom have demonstrated benefits from reduced blood glucose similar to those found for type 1 patients by the DCCT [61–63].

The clinical implications of the DCCT results have been extensively discussed and the evidence is compelling that better blood glucose control lowers the risk of the chronic complications of diabetes. Data exist to suggest that avoiding prolonged blood glucose elevations may be useful for most patients with diabetes. Unfortunately, although the risk is significantly reduced with intensive effort, it is not yet eliminated for many patients. The search for additional methods of preventing and treating the chronic complications of diabetes, including retinopathy, therefore continues.

Serum Lipid Lowering. Some currently available treatments may be effective in slowing the progression of diabetic retinopathy or reducing its complications. Higher serum lipids are associated with a greater risk of developing high-risk PDR, as well as with a greater risk of developing vision loss from diabetic macular edema and associated retinal hard exudates. Therefore, in addition to reducing the risk of cardiovascular disease, lowering elevated serum lipids may also reduce the risk of vision loss from diabetic retinopathy [64].

Blood Pressure Lowering. A randomized clinical trial of lisinopril, an inhibitor of angiotensin-converting enzyme (ACE) suggested that ACE inhibitor or blood pressure lowering, even in normotensive persons, may slow the progression of diabetic retinopathy [65].

United Kingdom Prospective Diabetes Study 1981–1998. Date from another randomized clinical trial, the United Kingdom Prospective Diabetes Study (UKPDS), suggest that it may be the blood pressure lowering that is responsible for slowing the progression of retinopathy and not a specific retina-vascular response to ACE inhibitor [66,67]. The UKPDS showed that both captopril, an ACE inhibitor, and atenolol, a beta blocker, were effective in slowing the progression of retinopathy compared with the control group and that there was no statistically significant difference between the two treatment groups.

Patients allocated to tight BP control showed benefit in many different aspects of diabetic retinopathy. They were less likely to undergo photocoagulation (RR, 0.65; $P = .03$) and less likely to have their retinopathy progress. Macular edema was less likely in the tight BP group and these patients were less likely to need photocoagulation for macular edema (RR, 0.58; $P = .02$). Blindness (defined as 20/200 or worse) was also reduced by tight blood pressure when compared with the conventional blood pressure control ($P = .046$; RR, 0.76; 99% confidence interval, 0.29–1.99) [68].

ACCORD Study. An NIH sponsored trial will evaluate these three important medical factors. The Action to Control Cardiovascular Risk in Diabetes (ACCORD) is a randomized clinical trial with three components, determining the cardiovascular disease (CVD) effects of blood glucose lowering, blood pressure lowering, and lowering of serum triglycerides plus raising serum high density lipoprotein cholesterol levels in patients with type 2 diabetes. 10,251 participants were randomly assigned in equal numbers to two glycemic management treatment arms, while 4733 of the 10,251 were also randomly assigned to the blood pressure management trial and the remainder, 5518, were randomly assigned to strategies of treatment dyslipidemia. Follow-up of at least 5 years is expected to be completed by May of 2009. An ACCORD Eye Substudy [69] was conducted on 3537 participants who had comprehensive eye exams with stereoscopic fundus photography of seven standard fields at baseline and at the 4 year follow-up visit. Study results will be available in fall of 2009 (http://www.accordtrial.org).

Aldose-Reductase Inhibitor. A medical approach for preventing the development of retinopathy that has been hypothesized for decades involves blocking the effects of aldose reductase [70]. This enzyme facilitates the conversion of glucose to sorbitol, which accumulates in cells during hyperglycemia and may result in cell death [71,72]. Animal experiments suggest that an aldose-reductase inhibitor could slow the development of diabetic retinopathy [73,74]. Clinical trials in patients with diabetes have not yet demonstrated any slowing of the progression of retinopathy.

Sorbinil Retinopathy Trial, 1983–1985. The Sorbinil Retinopathy Trial (SRT) enrolled 497 patients with type 1 diabetes and little or no retinopathy. After 3 to 4 years of follow-up, administration of the drug sorbinil showed no apparent effect on progression of diabetic retinopathy or neuropathy (Table 9.9 and Fig. 9.9) [75,76]. However, interest continues in developing more potent inhibitors, which may slow the progression of diabetic retinopathy or neuropathy.

Other Medical Investigations. Other medical approaches to reduce the secondary complications of diabetes are currently under evaluation. Drugs with antiangiogenic activity, such as inhibitors of vascular endothelial growth factor (VEGF), protein kinase C inhibitors, and growth hormone antagonists are in early clinical trials, as are inhibitors of advanced glycosylated end products [77–80]. Prevention will inevitably be more effective than treatment, and methods to prevent the development of diabetes and improved techniques for blood glucose control are also being tested.

Table 9.9. Sorbinil Retinopathy Study

Study Question

Does aldose-reductase inhibitor sorbinil reduce rate of progression of diabetic retinopathy?

Eligibility

Type 1 diabetes of 1–15 years' duration and no more than 5 microaneurysms in either eye

Randomization

497 patients randomly assigned to sorbinil (250 mg/d) or placebo

Outcomes Variable

Progression of retinopathy

Result

No significant reduction in progression of retinopathy in treated eyes compared with placebo

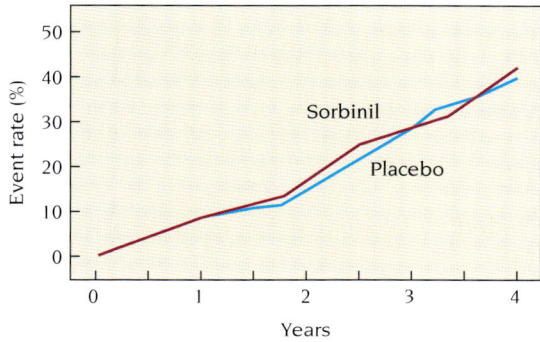

Figure 9.9. Sorbinil Retinopathy Trial results: Cumulative incidence of sustained worsening of retinopathy (two steps on modified Airlie House scale for at least 6 months) in patients with type 1 diabetes with mild or no retinopathy at baseline receiving placebo or 250 mg/d sorbinil.

The DRCR Network was established in 2003 for the purpose of conducting multicenter clinical research of diabetic retinopathy and associated disorders. The DRCR Network involves community-based practices as well as academic medical centers. This National Eye Institute sponsored cooperative agreement has conducted multiple studies (see Appendix) including laser photocoagulation, pharmacotherapy, and vitrectomy. The DRCR Network has industry collaboration as well as foundation support from the Juvenile Diabetes Research Foundation and the International Diabetes Foundation. DRCR Network clinical studies incorporate optical coherence tomography as well as both monotherapies and combined therapies for both diabetic macular edema and proliferative diabetic retinopathy.

CONCLUSION

The history of treatments for diabetic retinopathy is one of the best examples of the use of evidence-based patient care. From developing methods of preventing retinopathy to treatment with photocoagulation or vitrectomy, there are clinical trial results that reveal which treatments are more effective, who is most at risk, and who will benefit most from intervention.

Diabetic retinopathy is probably still the leading cause of visual loss in the United States among working-age Americans. This is surprising because, when retinopathy is properly treated, the 5-year risk of blindness for patients with PDR is reduced by 90% and the risk of visual loss from macular edema is reduced by 50%. Unfortunately, only 50% of patients with diabetes receive regular dilated eye examinations and many patients go blind without treatment [81–83], despite the fact that the value of screening eye examinations has been well documented [84].

Many professional groups, including the American Diabetes Association, the American College of Physicians, the American Academy of Ophthalmology, and the American Optometric Association, have provided guidelines for their members as to when eye examinations should be performed (Table 9.10). Emphasis on identifying patients at risk and new screening methods will, hopefully, reduce the number of patients who do not have regular eye examinations, appropriate medical care and careful follow-up.

Table 9.10. Recommended Eye Examination Schedule

Time of Onset of Diabetes	Recommended Time for First Examination	Routine Minimum Follow-up
<30 years of age	5 years after onset or at puberty	Yearly
≥ 30 years of age	At time of diagnosis	Yearly
Prior to Pregnancy	Just prior to, or soon after, conception	Every 3 months or at discretion of ophthalmologist

Improved patient education programs, such as the National Eye Health Education Program, can motivate patients to take better care of themselves [85–87]. Access to the educational materials and facilities that will enable patients to improve the control of their diabetes will lead to fewer secondary complications.

Prevention is cost effective [88–91]. The record of carefully developing new treatments for diabetic retinopathy is a good one. With continued careful research, the risk of blindness from diabetic retinopathy can be further reduced and the life-long preservation of vision a reality.

REFERENCES

1. Kahn HA, Hiller R. Blindness caused by diabetic retinopathy. *Am J Ophthalmol.* 1974;78:58–67.
2. Kahn HA. Bradley RF. Prevalence of diabetic retinopathy: age, sex, and duration of diabetes. *Br J Ophthalmol.* 1975;59:345–349.
3. Beetham WP. Visual prognosis of proliferating diabetic retinopathy. *Br J Ophthalmol.* 1963;47:611–619.
4. Caird FI. Burditt AF, Draper GJ. Diabetic retinopathy: a further study of prognosis for vision. *Diabetes.* 1968;17:121–123.
5. Deckert T, Simonsen SE, Poulson JE. Prognosis of proliferative retinopathy in juvenile diabeties. *Diabetes.* 1967;16:728–733.
6. Ferris FL III. How effective are treatments for diabetic retinopathy? *J Am Med Assoc.* 1993;269:1290–1291.
7. Diabetes Control and Complications Trial Research Group. The effect of intensive treatment of diabetes on the development and progression of long-term complications in insulin-dependent diabetes mellitus. *N Engl J Med.* 1993;329:977–986.
8. Goldberg MF, Fine SL (eds). *Symposium on the Treatment of Diabetic Retinopathy* (Airlie House, 1968) Public Health Service Publ. No. 1890. Washington, DC: US Govt Printing Office; 1969.
9. Meyer-Schwickerath G. *Light Coagulation.* Translated by Drance SM. St. Louis: CV Mosby Co; 1960.
10. Beetham WP, Aiello LM, Balodimos MC, Koncz L. Ruby-laser photocoagulation of early diabetic neovascular retinopathy: preliminary report of a long-term controlled study. *Trans Am Ophthalmol Soc.* 1969;67:39–67.
11. Ederer F, Hiller R. Clinical trials, diabetic retinopathy and photocoagulation: a reanalysis of five studies. *Surv Ophthalmol.* 1975;19:267–286.
12. Diabetic Retinopathy Study Research Group: Design, methods, and baseline results. DRS Report Number 6. *Invest Ophthalmol.* 1981;21:149–209.
13. Diabetic Retinopathy Study Research Group. Preliminary report on effects of photocoagulation therapy. *Am J Ophthalmol.* 1976;81:383–396.
14. Diabetic Retinopathy Study Research Group. Photocoagulation treatment of proliferative diabetic retinopathy: clinical application of diabetic retinopathy study (DRS) findings. DRS Report Number 8. *Ophthalmology.* 1981;88:583–600.
15. Diabetic Retinopathy Study Research Group: Photocoagulation treatment of proliferative diabetic retinopathy: the second report of Diabetic Retinopathy Study findings. *Ophthalmology.* 1978;85:82–106.
16. Diabetic Retinopathy Study Research Group. Four risk factors for severe visual loss in diabetic retinopathy: the third report from the Diabetic Retinopathy Study. *Arch Ophthalmol.* 1979;97:654–655.

17. Diabetic Retinopathy Study Research Group. Photocoagulation treatment of prolif- erative diabetic retinopathy: relationship of adverse treatment effects to retinopathy severity. DRS Report Number 5. *Dev Ophthalmol*. 1981;248–261.

18. Early Treatment Diabetic Retinopathy Study Research Group: Early Treatment Diabetic Retinopathy Study design and baseline patient characteristics. ETDRS Report Number 7. *Ophthalmology*. 1991;98(suppl):741–756.

19. Early Treatment Diabetic Retinopathy Study Research Group: Effects of aspi- rin treatment on diabetic retinopathy. ETDRS Report Number 8. *Ophthalmology*. 1991;98(suppl):757–765.

20. Sagel J, Colwell JA, Crook L, Laimins M. Increased platelet aggregation in early dia- betes mellitus. *Ann Intern Med*. 1975;82:733–738.

21. Dobbie JG, Kwaan HC, Colwell JA, Suwanwela N. The role of platelets in path- ogenesis of diabetic retinopathy. *Trans Am Acad Ophthalmol Otolaryngol*. 1973;77:OP43–OP47.

22. Regnault F. The role of platelets in the pathogenesis of diabetic retinopathy. *Sem Hop (Paris)*. 1972;48:893–902.

23. Powell ED, Field RA. Diabetic retinopathy and rheumatoid arthritis. *Lancet*. 1964;42:17–18.

24. Carroll WW, Geeraets WJ. Diabetic retinopathy and salicylates. *Ann Ophthalmol*. 1972;4:1019–1045.

25. Chew EY, Klein ML. Murphy RP, et al. Effects of aspirin on vitreous/preretinal hemorrhage in patients with diabetes mellitus. ETDRS Report Number 20. *Arch Ophthalmol*. 1995;113:52–55.

26. Early Treatment Diabetic Retinopathy Study Research Group. Aspirin effects on mor- tality and morbidity in patients with diabetes mellitus. ETDRS Report Number 14. *J Am Med Assoc*. 1992;268:1292–1300.

27. Early Treatment Diabetic Retinopathy Study Research Group. Early photocoagulation for diabetic retinopathy ETDRS Report Number 9. *Ophthalmology*. 1991;98(suppl): 766–785.

28. Ferris F. Early photocoagulation in patients with either type I or type II diabetes. *Trans Am Ophthalmol Soc*. 1996;94:505–537.

29. Early Treatment Diabetic Retinopathy Study Research Group. Photocoagulation for diabetic macular edema. ETDRS Report Number 1. *Arch Ophthalmol*. 1985;103: 1796–1806.

30. Early Treatment Diabetic Retinopathy Study Research Group. Treatment techniques and clinical guidelines for photocoagulation of diabetic macular edema. ETDRS Report Number 2. *Ophthalmology*. 1987;94:761–774.

31. Early Treatment Diabetic Retinopathy Study Research Group. Techniques for scatter and local photocoagulation treatment of diabetic retinopathy. ETDRS Report Number 3. *Int Ophthalmol Clin*. 1987;27:254–264.

32. Early Treatment Diabetic Retinopathy Study Research Group. Photocoagulation for diabetic macular edema. ETDRS Report Number 4. *Int Ophthalmol Clin*. 1987;27: 265–272.

33. Machemer R, Parel JM, Buettner H. A new concept for vitreous surgery, I: instrumen- tation. *Am J Ophthalmol*. 1972;73:1–7.

34. Machemer R. A new concept for vitreous surgery, 2: surgical technique and complica- tions. *Am J Ophthalmol*. 1972;74:1022–1033.

35. Machemer R, Norton EW. A new concept for vitreous surgery, 3: indications and results. *Am J Ophthalmol*. 1972;74:1034–1056.

36. Diabetic Retinopathy Vitrectomy Study Research Group. Two-year course of visual acuity in severe proliferative diabetic retinopathy with conventional management. DRVS Report Number 1. *Ophthalmology.* 1985;92:492–502.

37. Diabetic Retinopathy Vitrectomy Study Research Group. Early vitrectomy for severe vitreous hemorrhage in diabetic retinopathy: two year results of a randomized trial. DRVS Report Number 2. *Arch Ophthalmol.* 1985;103:1644–1652.

38. Diabetic Retinopathy Vitrectomy Study Research Group. Early vitrectomy for severe proliferative diabetic retinopathy in eyes with useful vision: results of a randomized trial. DRVS Report Number 3. *Ophthalmology.* 1988;95:1307–1320.

39. Diabetic Retinopathy Vitrectomy Study Research Group. Early vitrectomy for severe proliferative diabetic retinopathy in eyes with useful vision: clinical application of results of a randomized trial. DRVS Report Number 4. *Ophthalmology.* 1988;95:1321–1334.

40. Diabetic Retinopathy Vitrectomy Study Research Group. Early vitrectomy for severe vitreous hemorrhage in diabetic retinopathy: four-year results of a randomized trial. DRVS Report Number 5. *Arch Ophthalmol.* 1990;108:958–964.

41. Smiddy WE, Feuer W, Irvine WD, et al. Vitrectomy for complications of proliferative diabetic retinopathy: functional outcomes. *Ophthalmology.* 1995;102:1688–1695.

42. Smiddy W. Vitrectomy for complications of diabetic retinopathy. *Int Ophthalmol Clin.* 1998;38:155–167.

43. Early Treatment Diabetic Retinopathy Study Research Group. Pars Plana vitrectomy in the Early Treatment Diabetic Retinopathy Study. ETDRS Report Number 17. *Ophthalmology.* 1992;99:1351–1357.

44. Smiddy WE, Flynn HW Jr. Vitrectomy in the management of diabetic retinopathy. *Surv Ophthalmol.* 1999;43:491–507.

45. Diabetes Control and Complications Trial Research Group. The Diabetes Control and Complications Trial (DCCT): design and methodologic considerations for the feasibility phase. *Diabetes.* 1986;35:530–545.

46. Diabetes Control and Complications Trial Research Group. The effect of intensive treatment of diabetes on the development and progression of long-term complications in insulin-dependent diabetes mellitus. *N Engl J Med.* 1993;329:977–986.

47. Diabetes Control and Complications Trial Research Group. Effect of intensive therapy on the development and progression of diabetic nephropathy in the Diabetes Control and Complications Trial. *Kidney Int.* 1995;47:1703–1720.

48. Diabetes Control and Complications Trial Research Group. Effect of intensive diabetes treatment on nerve conduction in the Diabetes Control and Complications Trial. *Ann Neurol.* 1995;38:869–880.

49. The Diabetes Control and Complications Trial/Epidemiology of Diabetes Interventions and Complications Research Group. Effect of intensive therapy on the microvascular complications of type 1 diabetes mellitus. *JAMA.* 2002;287:2563–2569.

50. Reichart P, Nilsson BY, Rosenqvist U. The effect of long-term intensified insulin treatment on the development of microvascular complications of diabetes mellitus. *N Engl J Med.* 1993;329:304–309.

51. Klein R, Klein BE, Moss SE, et al. Glycosylated hemoglobin predicts the incidence and progression of diabetic retinopathy. *J Am Med Assoc.* 1988;260:2864–2871.

52. Dahl-Jorgensen K, Brinchmann-Hansen O, Hanssen KF, et al. Rapid tightening of blood glucose control leads to transient deterioration of retinopathy in insulin dependent diabetes mellitus: the Oslo Study. *Br Med J.* 1985;290:811–815.

53. Daneman D, Drash A, Lobes LA, et al. Progressive retinopathy with improved control in diabetic dwarfism (Mauriac's syndrome). *Diabetes Care.* 1981;4:360–365.

54. Puklin JE, Tamborlane WV, Felig P, et al. Influence of long-term insulin infusion pump treatment of type 1 diabetes on diabetic retinopathy. *Ophthalmology.* 1982;89:735–747.

55. Lauritzen T, Frost_Larson K, Larsen HW, Deckert T. Effect of 1 year of near-normal blood glucose levels on retinopathy. *Lancet.* 1983;1:200–204.

56. Lauritzen T, Frost-Larsen K, Larsen HW, Deckert T. Two-year experience with continuous subcutaneous insulin infusion in relation to retinopathy and neuropathy. *Diabetes.* 1985;34(suppl):74–79.

57. Kroc Collaborative Study Group. Blood glucose control and the evolution of diabetic retinopathy and albuminuria: a multicenter trial. *N Engl J Med.* 1984;311:365–372.

58. Kroc Collaborative Study Group. Diabetes retinopathy after two years of intensified insulin treatment: follow-up of the Kroc Collaborative Study. *JAMA.* 1988;260:37–41.

59. Diabetes Control and Complications Trial Research Group. Early worsening of diabetic retinopathy in the Diabetes Control and Complications Trial. *Arch Ophthalmol.* 1998;116:874–886.

60. Klein R, Klein BE, Moss SE. Relation of glycemic control to diabetic microvascular complications in diabetes mellitus. *Ann Intern Med.* 1996;124:90–96.

61. Ohkubo Y, Kishikawa H, Araki E, et al. Intensive insulin therapy prevents the progression of diabetic microvascular complications in Japanese patients with non-insulin-dependent diabetes mellitus: a randomized prospective 6-year study. *Diabetes Res Clin Pract.* 1995;28:103–117.

62. United Kingdom Prospective Diabetes Study Group. Intensive blood-glucose control with sulphonylureas of insulin compared with conventional treatment and risk of complications in patients with type 2 diabetes. UKPDS 33. *Lancet.* 1998;352:837–853.

63. United Kingdom Prospective Diabetes Study Group. Effect of intensive blood-glucose control with metformin on complications in overweight patients with type 2 diabetes. UKPDS 34. *Lancet.* 1998;352:854–865.

64. Chew EY, Klein ML, Ferris FL III, et al. Association of elevated serum lipid levels with retinal hard exudates in diabetic retinopathy. ETDRS Report Number 22. *Arch Ophthalmol.* 1996;114:1079–1084.

65. Chaturvedi N, Sjolie AK, Stephenson JM, et al. Effect of lisinopril on progression of retinopathy in normotensive people with type 1 diabetes. EUCLID Study Group. EURODIAB Controlled Trial of Lisinopril in Insulin-Dependent Diabetes Mellitus. *Lancet.* 1998;351:28–31.

66. United Kingdom Prospective Diabetes Study Group. Tight blood pressure control and risk of macrovascular and microvascular complications in type 2 diabetes. UKPDS 38. *Br Med J.* 1998;317:703–713.

67. United Kingdom Prospective Diabetes Study Group. Efficacy of atenolol and captopril in reducing risk of macrovascular and microvascular complications in type 2 diabetes. UKPDS 39. *Br Med J.* 1998;317:713–720.

68. Risks of progression of retinopathy and vision loss related to tight blood pressure control in type 2 diabetes mellitus: UKPDS 69. *Arch Ophthalmol.* 2004;122(11):1631–1640.

69. Chew EY, Ambrosius WT, Howard LT, et al. Rationale, design, and methods of the Action to Control Cardiovascular Risk in Diabetes Eye Study (ACCORD-EYE). *Am J Cardiol.* 2007;99(12A):103i–111i.

70. Frank RN. The aldose reductase controversy. *Diabetes.* 1994;43:169–172.

71. Kinoshita JH. Mechanisms initiating cataract formation. [Proctor Lecture]. *Invest Ophthalmol.* 1974;13:713–724.

72. Gabbay KH. Hyperglycemia, polyol metabolism, and complications of diabetes mellitus. *Ann Rev Med*. 1975;26:521–536.
73. Kador PF, Akagi Y, Takahashi Y, et al. Prevention of retinal vessel changes associated with diabetic retinopathy in galactose-fed dogs by aldose reductase inhibitors. *Arch Ophthalmol*. 1990;108:1301–1309.
74. Robinson WG Jr, Laver NM, Jacot JL, et al. Diabetic-like retinopathy ameliorated with the aldose reductase inhibitor WAY-121, 509. *Invest Ophthalmol Vis Sci*. 1996;37:1149–1156.
75. Sorbinil Retinopathy Trial Research Group. A randomized trial of sorbinil, an aldose reductase inhibitor, in diabetic retinopathy. *Arch Ophthalmol*. 1990;108:1234–1244.
76. Sorbinil Retinopathy Trial Research Group. The sorbinil retinopathy trial: neuropathy results. *Neurology*. 1993;43:1141–1149.
77. Aiello KP, Pierce EA, Foley ED, et al. Suppression of retinal neovascularization in vivo by inhibition of vascular endothelial growth factor (VEGF) using soluble VEGF-receptor chimeric proteins. *Proc Natl Acad Sci USA*. 1995;92:10457–10461.
78. Smith LE, Kopchick JJ, Chen W, et al. Essential role of growth hormone in ischemia-induced retinal neovascularization. *Science*. 1997;276:1706–1709.
79. Brownlee M, Cerami A, Vlassara H. Advanced glucosylation end products in tissue and the biochemical basis of diabetic complications. *N Engl J Med*. 1988;318:1315–1321.
80. Brownlee M, Vlassara H, Kooney A, et al. Aminoguanidine prevents diabetes-induced arterial wall protein cross-linking. *Science*. 1986;232:1629–1632.
81. Moss SE, Klein R, Klein BE. Factors associated with having eye examinations in persons with diabetes. *Arch Fam Med*. 1995;4:529–534.
82. Sprafka JM, Fritsche TL, Baker R, et al. Prevalence of undiagnosed eye disease in high-risk diabetic individuals. *Arch Intern Med*. 1990;150:857–861.
83. Will JC, German RR, Schuman E, et al. Patient adherence to guidelines for diabetes eye care: results from the diabetic eye disease follow-up study. *Am J Public Health*. 1994;84:1669–1671.
84. Javitt JC, Canner JK, Sommer A. Cost effectiveness of current approaches to the control of retinopathy in type 1 diabetes. *Ophthalmology*. 1989;96:255–264.
85. Kupfer C. The challenge of transferring research results into patient care. *Ophthalmology*. 1989;96:737–738.
86. Klein R. Eye-care delivery for people with diabetes: an unmet need. *Diabetes Care*. 1994;17:614–615.
87. Klein R. Barriers to prevention of vision loss caused by diabetic retinopathy. *Arch Ophthalmol*. 1997;115:1073–1075.
88. Diabetes Control and Complications Trial Research Group. Lifetime benefits and costs of intensive therapy as practiced in the Diabetes Control and Complications Trial. *J Am Med Assoc*. 1996;276:1409–1415.
89. Ackerman SJ. Benefits of preventive programs in eye care are visible on the bottom line: a new nationwide effort to improve eye care for people with diabetes gets backing from a study on the cost-effectiveness of screening for retinopathy. *Diabetes Care*. 1992;15:580–581.
90. Javitt JC, Aiello LP, Chiang Y, et al. Preventive eye care in people with diabetes is cost-saving to the federal government: implications for health-care reform. *Diabetes Care*. 1994;17:909–917.
91. Javitt JC, Aiello LP. Cost-effectiveness of detecting and treating diabetic retinopathy. *Ann Intern Med*. 1996;124:164–169.

10

Photocoagulation for Diabetic Macular Edema and Diabetic Retinopathy

MITCHELL J. GOFF, MD,
H. RICHARD McDONALD, MD,
AND EVERETT AI, MD

CORE MESSAGES

- The indications and techniques, as well as the safety and efficacy, of laser photocoagulation for diabetic retinopathy and diabetic macular edema are well established by the Diabetic Retinopathy Study (DRS) and the Early Treatment Diabetic Retinopathy Study (ETDRS).
- Focal laser photocoagulation should be considered for *all* eyes with clinically significant macular edema (CSME).
- Laser re-treatment sessions may be necessary for macular edema.
- Scatter (panretinal) photocoagulation treatment is performed promptly for proliferative diabetic retinopathy (PDR) with high-risk characteristics and may be considered for severe nonproliferative retinopathy.
- Laser photocoagulation has potential complications, including foveal burn, choroidal detachment, and secondary glaucoma.

Advances in the understanding of the natural history of diabetic retinopathy and simultaneous advances in laser technology have enabled the development and refinement of safe and effective laser photocoagulation treatments. Large, prospective, randomized clinical trials such as the Diabetic Retinopathy Study (DRS) in 1976, which reported that severe visual loss could be reduced by as much as 60% with timely laser treatment, and the Early Treatment Diabetic Retinopathy Study (ETDRS) in 1985, which showed that laser treatment of clinically significant macular edema (CSME) reduced the risk of moderate visual loss, have made laser photocoagulation the standard of care for various manifestations of diabetic retinopathy [1–8].

LASER PHOTOCOAGULATION FOR DIABETIC MACULAR EDEMA

Macular edema is a major cause of vision loss in patients with diabetes, occurring in approximately 10% of all diabetics [9]. The development of macular edema is related to both the duration of diabetes (as many as 29% of patients with diabetes for more than 20 years having macular edema), and to the severity of diabetic retinopathy (as many as 74% of patients with proliferative diabetic retinopathy (PDR) having macular edema). The development of macular edema is also related to elevated glycosolated hemoglobin levels and proteinuria [9,10]. Diabetic macular edema may be categorized as localized or diffuse. Localized macular edema is characterized by discrete areas of retinal thickening associated with specific points of leakage on fluorescein angiography, usually microaneurysms (Fig. 10.1). Diffuse macular edema represents a generalized breakdown of the inner blood–retinal

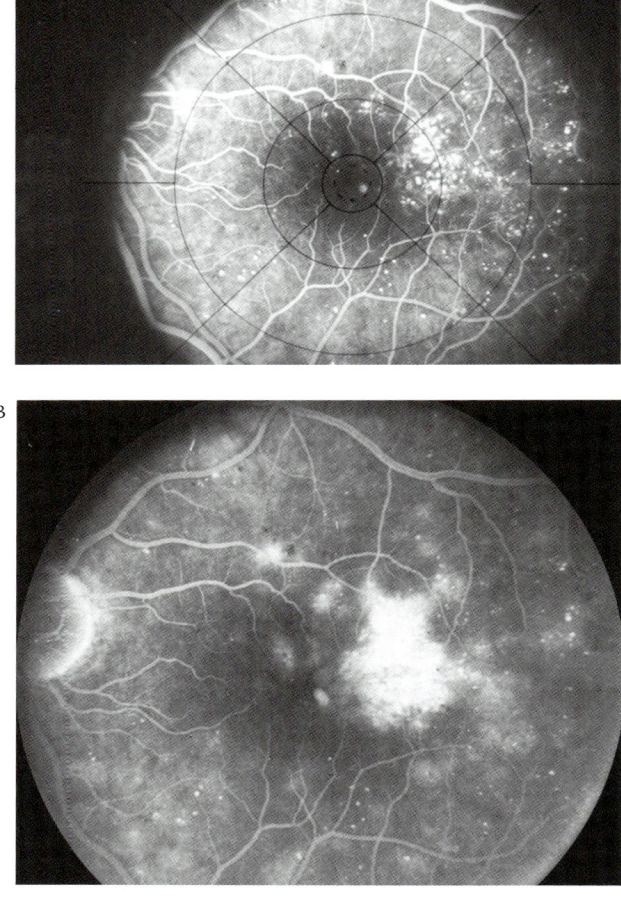

Figure 10.1. (A) Early phase fluorescein angiogram demonstrating a cluster of microaneurysms. Note the standardized grid, which can be used for measurements. (B) Later phase of angiogram demonstrating leakage from microaneurysms.

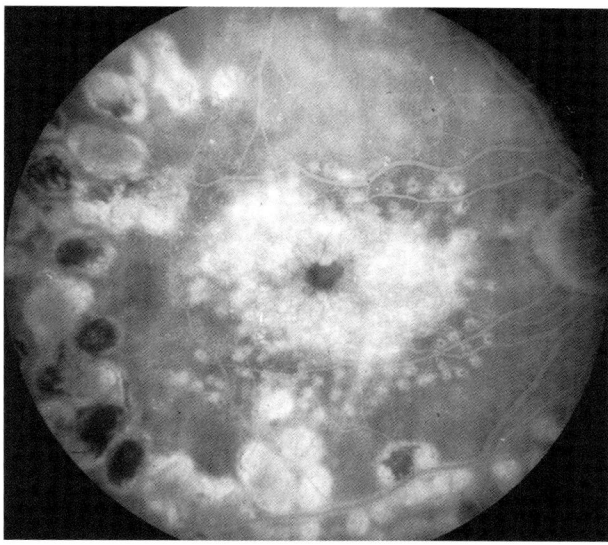

Figure 10.2. Fluorescein angiogram demonstrating a grid pattern of prior laser therapy applied to an area of diffuse macular edema.

barrier and is defined as two or more disc areas of retinal thickening involving the foveal avascular zone [11] (Fig. 10.2). The treatment approach for diabetic macular edema may be altered, depending on whether there is localized or diffuse edema. Focal laser photocoagulation for diabetic macular edema, as described by the ETDRS, includes focal (direct) photocoagulation, directed at specific areas of focal leakage, and grid photocoagulation, in which a grid pattern of burns is applied to areas of diffuse macular edema or nonperfusion (Table 10.1).

Although recovery of reduced vision is relatively unlikely after treatment, the goal of focal laser photocoagulation is to achieve modest improvement or stabilization of vision. Accordingly, even patients with macular edema and excellent visual function should be considered for treatment before visual acuity is affected [4,12,13].

Management recommendations, as prescribed by the American Academy of Ophthalmology, Preferred Practice Patterns, for patients with diabetes, including those with diabetic macular edema, are summarized in Table 10.2 and are more fully described in the following sections.

Indications for Treatment. The ETDRS demonstrated a 50% reduction in moderate visual loss (a loss of 15 or more letters, or a doubling of the visual angle) in eyes with CSME. CSME was defined by any one of the following: (1) Retinal thickening within 500 microns of the center of the macula (Fig. 10.3), (2) hard exudates within 500 microns of the center of the macula with associated thickening (Fig. 10.4), or (3) zone or zones of thickening larger than one disc area in size, any part of which is within one disc diameter of the center of the macula (Fig. 10.5). The three-year risk of moderate visual loss was 24% in untreated eyes compared with 12% in photocoagulation-treated eyes ($p = 0.01$) [4,14]. Adverse effects on

Table 10.1. Modified ETDRS and MMG Laser Photocoagulation Techniques

Burn Characteristic	Modified ETDRS Technique (Direct/ Grid Photocoagualtion)	MMG Photocoagulation Technique
Direct treatment	Directly treat all leaking microaneurysms in areas of retinal thickening 500–3000 microns from the center of the macula (but not within 500 microns of the disc).	NA
Change in MA color with direct treatment	Not required, but at least a mild gray-white burn should be evident beneath all microaneurysms.	NA
Burn size for direct treatment, microns	50	NA
Burn duration for direct treatment, s	0.05–0.10	NA
Grid treatment	Applied to all areas with diffuse leakage or nonperfusion within area considered for grid treatment.	Applied to entire area considered for grid treatment (including unthickened retina).
Area considered for grid treatment	500–3000 microns superiorly, nasally, and inferiorly from center of macula	500–3000 microns superiorly, nasally, and inferiorly from center of macula
	500–3500 microns temporally from macular center	500–3500 microns temporally from macular center
	No burns are placed within 500 microns of the disc	No burns are placed within 500 microns of the disc
Burn size for grid treatment, microns	50	50
Burn duration for grid treatment, s	0.05–0.10	0.05–0.10
Burn intensity for grid treatment	Barely visible (light gray)	Barely visible (light gray)
Burn separation for grid treatment	2 visible burn widths apart	200–300 total burns evenly distributed over the area considered for grid treatment, approximately 2–3 burns widths apart
Wavelength (grid and focal treatment)	Green to yellow	Green to yellow

Source: Comparison of modified-ETDRS and mild macular grid laser photocoagulation strategies for diabetic macular edema. Arch Ophthalmol 2007; 125: 469–480.
Note: This study showed that the modified ETDRS technique was preferable to the mild macular grid technique.
Abbreviations: ETDRS, Early Treatment Diabetic Retinopathy Study; MA, microaneurysm; MMG, mild macular grid; NA, Not applicable.

central vision or color vision were not found compared to eyes assigned to deferral of focal laser [2]. In the ETDRS, eyes without CSME at baseline had low rates of visual loss, and the differences between the treatment and the deferral groups were not statistically significant. Visual acuity and fluorescein angiographic characteristics were not included in the ETDRS definitional criteria for CSME. In fact, the

Table 10.2. Management Recommendations for Patients with Diabetes

Severity of Retinopathy	Presence of CSME*	Follow-up (Months)	Scatter (Panretinal) photocoagulation	Fluorescein Angiography	Focal laser
Normal or minimal NPDR	No	12	No	No	No
Mild to moderate NPDR	No	6–12	No	No	No
	Yes	2–4	No	Usually	Usually[a,b]
Severe or very severe NPDR	No	2–4	Sometimes[c]	Rarely	No
	Yes	2–4	Sometimes[c]	Usually	Usually[d]
Non–high-risk PDR	No	2–4	Sometimes[c]	Rarely	No
	Yes	2–4	Sometimes[c]	Usually	Usually[‡]
High-risk PDR	No	3–4	Usually	Rarely	No
	Yes	3–4	Usually	Usually	Usually[d]
High-risk PDR not amenable to photocoagulation (e.g., media opacities)	—	1–6	Not possible[e]	Occasionally	Not Possible[e]

Source: From: American Academy of Ophthalmology, Preferred Practice Patterns, 2008.

[a]Exceptions include: hypertension or fluid retention associated with heart failure, renal failure, pregnancy, or any other causes that may aggravate macular edema. Deferral of photocoagulation for a brief period of medical treatment may be considered in these cases. Also, deferral of CSME treatment is an option when the center of the macula is not involved, visual acuity is excellent, close follow-up is possible, and the patient understands the risks.

Focal photocoagulation refers to focal laser to leaking microaneurysms or grid photocoagulation to areas of diffuse leakage or nonperfusion seen on fluorescein angiography.

[b]Deferring focal photocoagulation for CSME is an option when the center of the macula is not involved, visual acuity is excellent, close follow-up is possible, and the patient understands the risks. However, initiation of treatment with focal photocoagulation should also be considered because although treatment with focal photocoagulation is less likely to improve the vision, it is more likely to stabilize the current visual acuity.

[c]Scatter (panretinal) photocoagulation surgery may be considered as patients approach high-risk PDR. The benefit of early scatter photocoagulation at the severe nonproliferative or worse stage of retinopathy is greater in patients with type 2 diabetes than in those with type 1. Treatment should be considered for patients with severe NPDR and type 2 diabetes. Other factors, such as poor compliance with follow-up, impending cataract extraction or pregnancy, and status of the fellow eye will help in determining the timing of the scatter photocoagulation.

[d]Some experts feel that it is preferable to perform focal photocoagulation first, prior to scatter photocoagulation, to minimize scatter laser-induced exacerbation of the macular edema.

[e]Vitrectomy is indicated in selected cases.

Note: The Diabetic Retinopathy Clinical Research Network study (*Arch Ophthalmol* 2009; 127:132–140) showed that outcomes were similar following application of PRP in one sitting compared with four sittings in eyes with no or mild center involved macular edema.

low rates of visual improvement in the ETDRS may be due to the fact that a large number of treated patients had 20/20 vision or better at the time of treatment [4]. Based on the reduced rates of moderate visual loss by 50%, and the low complication rate with laser treatment, the ETDRS recommended that focal laser photocoagulation be considered for all eyes with CSME [14].

It is important to note that retinal thickening is an ophthalmoscopic, not an angiographic finding (Fig. 10.6). In addition, hard exudates may be found without associated retinal thickening and are not necessarily indicative of CSME, as defined by the ETDRS.

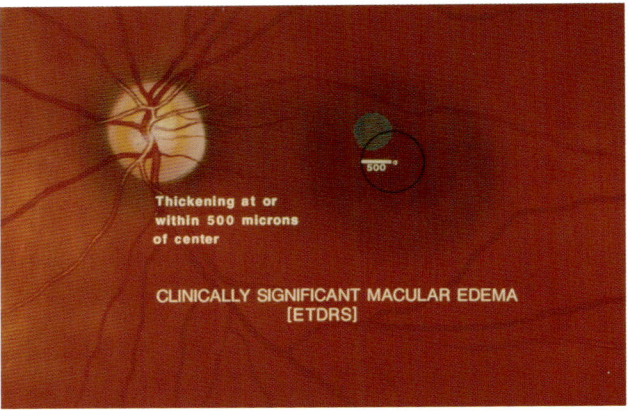

Figure 10.3. Clinically significant macular edema defined as retinal thickening within 500 microns of the center of the macula. ETDRS, Early Treatment Diabetic Retinopathy Study.

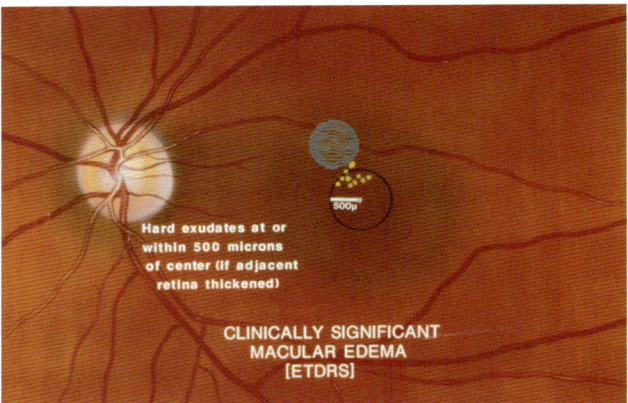

Figure 10.4. Clinically significant macular edema defined as hard exudates at or within 500 microns of the center of the macula if there is adjacent retinal thickening. ETDRS, Early Treatment Diabetic Retinopathy Study.

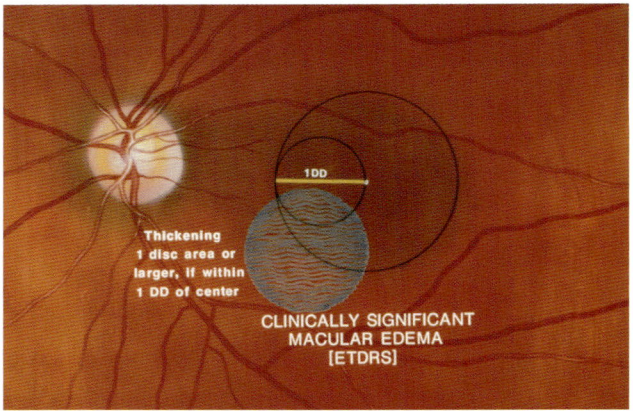

Figure 10.5. Clinically significant macular edema defined as retinal thickening one disc area or larger in size if within one disc diameter of the center of the macula. ETDRS, Early Treatment Diabetic Retinopathy Study.

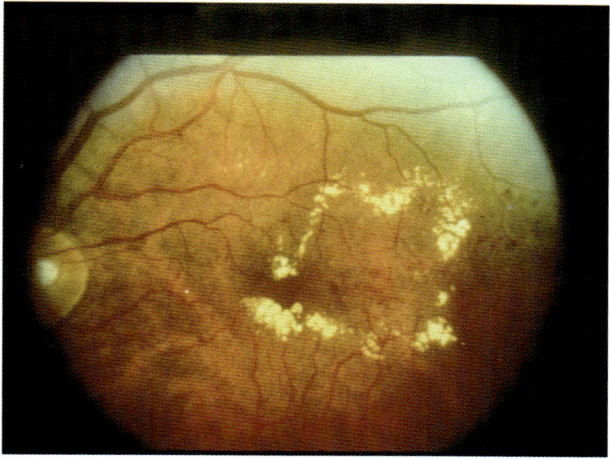

Figure 10.6. Clinically significant macular edema with a circinate ring of hard exudate formation.

Many clinicians choose to follow patients with 20/20 vision, unless the center of the macula is threatened or involved. An additional analysis of ETDRS data considering only eyes with macular edema and 20/20 or better vision, demonstrated that photocoagulation reduced the occurrence of moderate visual loss from 23% to 11% at 3 years among eyes in which the edema involved the center of the macula. If the edema did not involve the center of the macula, rates of moderate visual loss were low in both the treated and the untreated groups (2.5% and 7%, respectively) [13]. While not statistically significant, this data suggests that involvement of the central macula favors treatment. When treatment is deferred for such patients, close follow-up (every 3–4 months) is warranted to monitor for disease progression [15]. Although the ETDRS only included eyes with vision of 20/200 or better, eyes with lower levels of visual acuity may be considered for treatment because resolution of macular edema may stabilize or improve whatever visual function remains.

Treatment. Mechanism of Action. There are several postulated mechanisms by which laser photocoagulation decreases macular edema. The precise mechanism is unknown and may be a combination of the following: (1) direct closure of retinal vascular anomalies, (2) photocoagulation debridement of dysfunctional (or replacement with newly proliferated) pigment epithelium resulting in an enhanced outer blood–retinal barrier, (3) destruction of photoreceptors leading to improved inner retinal oxygenation and compensatory vasoconstriction with decreased blood flow and decreased vascular leakage, (4) stimulation of vascular endothelial proliferation resulting in restoration of the inner blood–retinal barrier, and (5) reduction of the total surface area of leaking retinal vessels (by their destruction) [16–19].

Wavelength Considerations. Yellow and blue wavelengths have several theoretical advantages including high absorption by hemoglobin that may make them useful for closing microaneurysms in the treatment of diabetic macular edema. Blue light, in addition to being absorbed well by hemoglobin, is also absorbed well by macular xanthophyll and may cause neurosensory retinal damage not only to the patient, but also to the treating physician [20,21]. Both argon green and argon blue-green wavelengths were used in the ETDRS trials. While there was no direct evidence that one was preferable to the other, many investigators switched to argon green, particularly when treating near the fovea, to avoid excess uptake of the blue wavelengths by macular xanthophylls in the inner retina. Krypton red was not used because it makes direct photocoagulation of microaneurysms difficult [4]. With these considerations, argon green is the wavelength of choice in most cases of diabetic macular edema.

Focal (Direct) Photocoagulation. Focal (direct) photocoagulation involves application of laser spots to all leaking microaneurysms between 500 and 3000 microns (two disc diameters) from the center of the macula (Table 10.3). Although the ETDRS did not require fluorescein angiographic confirmation of CSME, treating physicians used a baseline angiogram at the time of treatment to facilitate identification of focal points of leakage, usually microaneurysms, and to identify perifoveal capillary dropout with enlarged foveal avascular zones. Treatment of focal points of leakage in the retina farther than two disc diameters from the center of the macula is optional, but it was recommended if they leak prominently and were associated with retinal thickening or hard exudates rings that extended into the area of the retina within two disc diameters of the center of the macula [2].

Individual microaneurysms are treated with a spot size of 50 to 100 microns, and an exposure time of 0.1 s or less. Power is set low and titrated upward until a therapeutic effect is obtained. The ETDRS recommended increasing power until a whitening of the microaneurysm was observed. However, this often required energy sufficient to cause rupture of Bruch's membrane. Whitening the microaneurysm is not necessary to achieve the goal of leakage cessation. In general, a very low intensity burn is required to affect microaneurysm closure (Fig. 10.7).

Treatment of focal leaks between 300 and 500 microns from the center of the macula can be performed if (1) previous treatment has been applied and CSME persists, (2) vision is less than 20/40, and (3) treatment is not likely to destroy the remaining perifoveal capillary network. For these lesions closer to the center of the macula, a smaller spot size of 50 microns and a shorter exposure time of 0.05 s were

Table 10.3. Parameters for Focal (Direct) Photocoagulation

Spot size	50–100 microns
Duration	0.1 s or less
Endpoint	Barely visible color change
Extent	All leaking microaneurysms between 500 and 3000 microns from the center of the macula
Wavelength	Argon-green

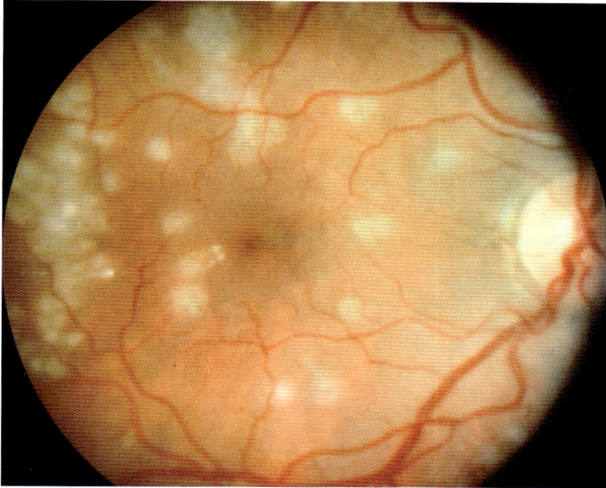

Figure 10.7. Immediate posttreatment photograph of focal (direct) photocoagulation to leaking microaneurysms.

recommended by the ETDRS [2]. Effective laser intensity (i.e., uptake) is increased by decreasing spot size and exposure time without decreasing power, so great care must be taken not to rupture Bruch's membrane by decreasing the power to the lowest level required to observe mild retinal whitening.

Grid Photocoagulation. Grid photocoagulation is used for diffuse macular edema and involves the application of uniformly spaced laser burns to areas of diffuse leakage and occasionally to areas of capillary nonperfusion associated with areas of leakage (Table 10.4). Angiographic leakage does not always correspond to ophthalmoscopically evident retinal thickening. To avoid over treatment, only clinically observable thickening should be treated. ETDRS guidelines for grid photocoagulation consist of placing light burns, 50 to 200 microns in size, at the level of the retinal pigment epithelium in areas of diffuse leakage that are more than 500 microns from the center of the macula and more than 500 microns from the temporal edge of the optic nerve. The spacing of the spots is dependent on the amount of leakage and should be one burn width apart for areas of intense leakage and slightly farther for areas of less intense leakage. Exposure time should be 0.1 s or less. Power should be started low and titrated upward until a barely visible light gray outer retinal lesion is visualized (Fig. 10.8). This helps to avoid over treatment and "spread" of laser burns over time, which can lead to coalescence of the laser scars in the macula (retinal pigment epithelial creep) with resultant paracentral scotomas.

Other Treatment Strategies. The ETDRS technique of meticulous focal (direct) photocoagulation of individual microaneurysms combined with grid photocoagulation to areas of diffuse leakage has been proven beneficial. Other techniques may also be beneficial, but have not been proven in large clinical trials. One technique

Table 10.4. Parameters for Grid Photocoagulation

Spot size	50–200 microns
Duration	0.1 s or less
Endpoint	Barely-visible light gray outer retinal lesion
Spacing	One burn width apart or more
Extent	All areas of diffuse thickening 500 microns from the center of macula and more than 500 microns from the temporal edge of the optic nerve, extending in all directions up to 3000 microns from the center of the macula
Wavelength	Argon-green

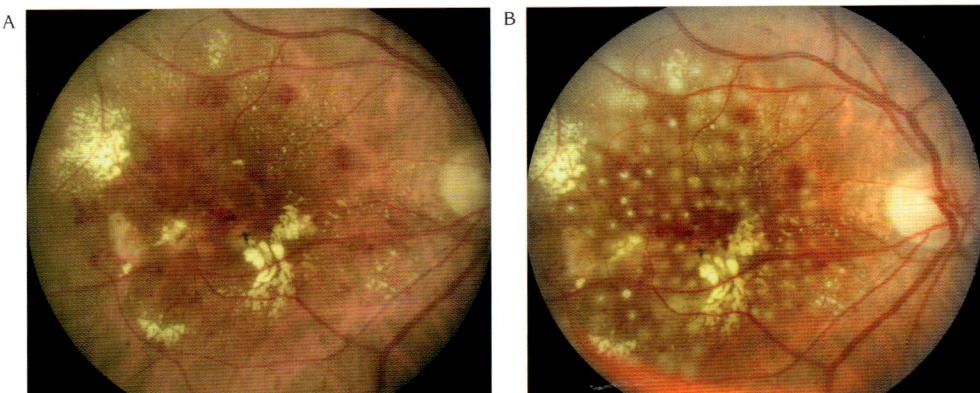

Figure 10.8. Example of diffuse macular edema prior to treatment (A), and 4 days after grid laser photocoagulation (B).

involves the application of two to three rows of grid laser around the fovea, as well as grid laser to all areas of thickened retina, followed by confluent laser to all areas of focal leakage [11]. This technique, termed modified grid photocoagulation, has not been shown to be favorable to ETDRS guidelines and may lead to over treatment.

The Diabetic Retinopathy Clinical Research Network, funded by the National Eye Institute, conducted a randomized controlled clinical trial to compare two laser photocoagulation techniques for treatment of diabetic macular edema: the modified ETDRS direct/grid photocoagulation technique and a potentially milder (but potentially more extensive) mild macular grid (MMG) laser technique in which microaneurysms were not treated directly and small mild burns were placed throughout the macula, whether or not edema was present [22]. At 12 months after treatment, the MMG technique was reported to be less effective at reducing optical coherence tomography-measured retinal thickening than the more extensively evaluated current modified ETDRS laser photocoagulation approach. However, the visual acuity outcome with both approaches was not substantially different.

Many pharmacologic treatments for diabetic macular edema have been proposed in recent years. The pathogenesis of diabetic macular edema has been attributed in part to inflammation, making corticosteroids a potential therapeutic option. The Diabetic Retinopathy Clinical Research Network conducted a randomized, prospective clinical trial to compare the efficacy of intravitreal triamcinolone to focal/grid laser photocoagulation for diabetic macular edema [23]. At 4 months, mean visual acuity was better in the intravitreal triamcinolone treated eyes. This was not sustained however, and at 1 year, there was no difference between treatment groups. At the end of the 2-year follow-up period, the focal/grid laser photocoagulation treatment group had better visual acuity outcomes. In addition, complications including cataract formation and glaucoma, were less frequent in the laser-treated group. The investigators concluded that focal/grid laser photocoagulation for diabetic macular edema remains the benchmark against which other treatments should be compared.

Follow-up and Re-treatment. It may take 3 to 4 months for the maximum effect of edema resorption to occur after a session of focal (direct) or grid photocoagulation. Therefore, follow-up intervals of 2 to 4 months are recommended for most patients. If there is persistent CSME present at 4 months, angiography should be repeated and additional treatment offered for selected areas of new or persistent leakage. These consist of leaking microaneurysms 500 to 3000 microns from the center of the macula, leaking microaneurysms 300 to 500 microns from the center of the macula if vision is less than 20/40 and there is no perifoveal capillary dropout. Grid treatment can be administered to areas of diffuse leakage 500 microns from the center of the macula if not treated previously. Treatment over areas of prior laser photocoagulation is not recommended as excessive spread and coalescence of laser scars can ensue.

Multiple laser sessions over many months are often necessary to accomplish the goals of treatment. In fact, most patients require three to four sessions 2 to 4 months apart for macular edema to resolve [12]. While ophthalmoscopically evident thickening was the treatment criterion subjected to the definitive clinical trial, optical coherence tomography may be a useful adjunct to monitor resolution of macular edema or to identify vitreomacular traction in patients with macular edema caused by a taut posterior hyaloid who are unresponsive to laser treatment [24–26].

Prognosis. The goal of laser photocoagulation treatment for diabetic macular edema is modest improvement or stabilization of vision. Patients should be counseled to avoid unrealistic expectations of visual improvement. Visual prognosis or response to treatment is related to several factors. Young age and diet-controlled diabetes mellitus have been associated with a more favorable prognosis [27]. Eyes that exhibit diffuse leakage appear to have a worse prognosis [4,28–32]. Additional factors associated with a worse prognosis include ischemic maculopathy, extensive perifoveal capillary nonperfusion, cystoid changes, hard exudates in the fovea, older age of the patient, and systemic treatment for hypertension [27,28].

LASER PHOTOCOAGULATION FOR PROLIFERATIVE
DIABETIC RETINOPATHY

PDR is characterized by extraretinal fibrovascular proliferation in response to chronic, widespread retinal ischemia. This fibrovascular tissue has the propensity to differentiate into fibroblasts and form firm adhesions at the interface of the retina and vitreous. Consequently, vitreous contraction may lead to vitreous hemorrhage or tractional retinal detachment, resulting in marked visual loss. Anteriorly, neovascular tissue arising from the iris can obstruct the trabecular meshwork causing neovascular glaucoma. The development of PDR is related to the duration of diabetes. Among type 1 diabetics, 50% develop PDR after 20 years. Among type 2 diabetics, 10% develop PDR after 20 years [33].

Scatter (panretinal) photocoagulation is a type of laser surgery for PDR, in which laser is delivered in a scatter pattern throughout the peripheral fundus and is intended to lead to regression of neovascularization [34]. The primary goal of laser photocoagulation for PDR is to prevent vision loss from tractional retinal detachment, vitreous hemorrhage and neovascular glaucoma.

Management considerations, as prescribed by the American Academy of Ophthalmology, Preferred Practice Patterns, for patients with diabetic retinopathy are summarized in Table 10.2 and described more fully in the following sections.

Indications for Treatment. The DRS clearly demonstrated that timely scatter photocoagulation to eyes with high-risk proliferative changes reduces the incidence of severe visual loss (defined as visual acuity of 5/200 or less on two consecutive exams, four months apart) and inhibits the progression of retinopathy. The rate of severe vision loss after 2 years was 15.9% among untreated eyes compared to 6.4% in treated eyes, a reduction of 60% [8]. Further analysis identified specific proliferative features, known as high-risk characteristics, which were present among those who benefited most from laser photocoagulation. These include: (1) any neovascularization located on or within one disc diameter of the disc (NVD) associated with preretinal or vitreous hemorrhage, (2) moderate to severe degree of NVD (greater than or equal to one-fourth to one-third disc diameter, without associated preretinal or vitreous hemorrhage, or (3) neovascularization elsewhere (NVE), greater than or equal to one-half disc area, associated with preretinal or vitreous hemorrhage [5,6,35] (Fig. 10.9). The DRS demonstrated that the risk of severe vision loss was related to the degree of retinopathy and that treatment was beneficial in all groups, but to a lesser extent in eyes without high-risk characteristics. In fact, after 24 months of follow-up, the rate of severe vision loss for control eyes with high-risk characteristics was 26% and was reduced to 11% in treated eyes. In eyes without high-risk characteristics, a similar treatment effect was seen, but both control and treatment group rates of severe vision loss were low, 7% and 3% respectively [5]. The DRS investigators concluded that laser photocoagulation should be performed promptly for eyes with high-risk characteristics, because the benefits appear to outweigh the risks in this subgroup of patients [3]. The DRS findings did not provide a clear choice between prompt photocoagulation and deferral for eyes without high-risk characteristics.

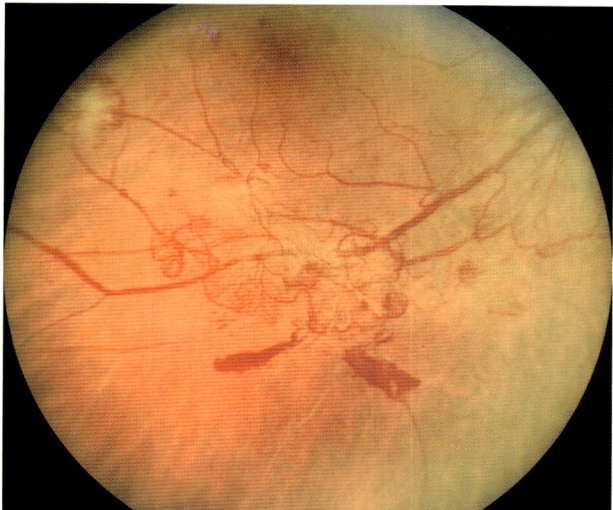

Figure 10.9. Fundus photograph demonstrating neovascularization elsewhere with preretinal hemorrhage.

The ETDRS Research Group attempted to determine the benefit of laser photocoagulation prior to the development of high-risk characteristics. They found that the rates of severe vision loss were low among all groups, whether assigned to treatment or deferral, 2.6% and 3.7% respectively. In addition, the severity of retinopathy and the presence of macular edema were found to be associated with the development of severe vision loss. In fact, the 5-year rate of severe vision loss in eyes with macular edema and "more severe retinopathy," defined as severe nonproliferative or proliferative without high-risk characteristics, was 6.5%. This risk was reduced with early photocoagulation treatment to between 3.8% and 4.7%. While no statistically significant differences were found between any of the treatment or deferral groups, or between any of the treatment strategies employed, the most effective strategy was immediate scatter photocoagulation combined with immediate focal laser photocoagulation for eyes with macular edema and more severe retinopathy. Conversely, deferral of photocoagulation for this group of eyes was the least effective strategy, associated with the highest rates of severe vision loss [36]. With these considerations, the ETDRS recommended that, provided careful follow-up can be maintained, scatter photocoagulation is not recommended for eyes with mild or moderate nonproliferative diabetic retinopathy (NPDR). When retinopathy is more severe, scatter photocoagulation should be considered and usually should not be delayed if the eye has reached the high-risk proliferative stage [4,36]. The benefit of early scatter photocoagulation appears to be greater in patients with type 2 diabetes and may be considered in these patients with severe nonproliferative or worse retinopathy [34,37]. Additional factors that may favor early treatment include medical conditions that increase the risk of retinopathy progression such as impending or recent cataract surgery or pregnancy, the status of the fellow eye, and poor compliance [34].

Neovascularization elsewhere (NVE) and neovascularization of the iris (NVI) were not found to be high-risk characteristics by the DRS Group. However, in clinical practice, scatter photocoagulation is generally administered once any neovascularization occurs rather than waiting for disease progression. In such patients, ocular changes may occur while waiting for high-risk characteristics to develop that could compromise future therapy and lead to vision loss. NVI can lead to rapid synechial closure of the anterior chamber angle with subsequent neovascular glaucoma. Laser photocoagulation of these eyes can result in regression of angle neovascularization, particularly if neovascular glaucoma has not occurred, and may improve the success of filtering surgeries [38,39].

Treatment

Mechanism of Action. The mechanism of action for scatter photocoagulation for the treatment of PDR is incompletely understood. Possible theories include: (1) ablation of ischemic retina leading to decreased production of vasoproliferative factors such as vascular endothelial growth factor (VEGF), (2) ablation of oxygen-consuming photoreceptors and pigment epithelium may lead to improved inner retinal oxygenation and a decreased stimulus for vasoproliferative factors, and (3) stimulation of release of neovascular inhibitors normally found in the retinal pigment epithelium [40–43].

Wavelength Considerations. A wide variety of wavelengths are available for scatter photocoagulation; when tested, several seem to have similar efficacy [44,45]. The DRS used argon-blue laser and xenon arc light. Blue light from the blue-green laser is absorbed by macular xanthophyll and may potentially damage the retina of the patient and the administering surgeon. For these reasons, green-only laser is preferred in clinical practice for macular treatments. Patients treated with xenon experienced higher rates of central and peripheral visual loss compared to patients treated with argon [3]. For this reason, as well as logistical constraints, xenon is no longer used. Yellow wavelengths are presumed to be of equal efficacy and may have theoretical advantages as discussed previously. Red wavelengths have the advantage of penetrating media opacities such as mild to moderate vitreous hemorrhage and cataract. Red wavelengths are absorbed by the choroid more deeply, causing more pain and potentially increasing the risk of choroidal hemorrhage [46]. Experience with diode laser is limited, but it presumably has properties similar to krypton red with respect to its interaction with the retina, media opacities, and retinal pigment epithelium. Similarly, it may produce a deeper, more painful burn [47,48].

Scatter (Panretinal) Photocoagulation. Full scatter photocoagulation, according to DRS and ETDRS protocol, consists of the application of 1200 to 1600 moderate intensity burns, 500 microns in size, spaced one-half burn width apart, using an exposure time of 0.1 s (Table 10.5) [2,5,49]. Care must be taken to adjust the spot size setting for the contact lens being used. For example, if using the Rodenstock lens, the spot size setting is reduced to approximately 250 to 300 microns to obtain a 500-micron burn. The burns appear to enlarge slightly within several minutes after application and allowance is made for this by slightly widening the spacing as they are applied, up to one burn width apart. The power setting should be titrated upward until a moderately intense gray-white burn is seen. If media opacity or a lightly pigmented fundus prevents this with powers up to one watt, smaller spot size and longer exposure times may be used. The posterior border of initial scatter photocoagulation treatment should be two disc diameters temporal, superior and inferior to the center of the macula and 500 microns from the nasal edge of the disc. From this border, burns extend peripherally to or beyond the equator avoiding direct treatment of major vessels (Fig. 10.10).

Treatment was applied in two or more sessions in the DRS and ETDRS protocols, with no more than 900 burns applied in a single episode. If two treatment sessions were used, they were separated by at least two weeks. If three or more sessions were required, they were at least 4 days apart. The order in which specific parts of the fundus are treated was optional. The technique of avoiding the posterior pole by treating the midperiphery to anterior to the equator in an effort to decrease the incidence of posttreatment macular edema may leave significant areas of nonperfusion untreated posteriorly. Accordingly, DRS and ETDRS guidelines should be followed in most cases.

Local Photocoagulation of Neovascularization. Both the DRS and the ETDRS included local photocoagulation treatment of neovascular foci less than two disc areas in size. Local treatment of NVD and elevated NVE did not prove to be beneficial, demonstrated increased rates of hemorrhage and was ultimately abandoned. Today, local photocoagulation has little role in current practice and is usually used primarily in combination with full scatter photocoagulation [5,50].

Local photocoagulation of small, flat NVE is considered when judged likely to be effective and free of complications (i.e., when new vessel patches are flat, less than two disc areas in size, and their direct treatment is uncomplicated by proximity to the macula, large retinal vessels, chorioretinal scars, or preretinal hemorrhage). Under less favorable circumstances, local treatment is optional and full scatter treatment alone may be used [49]. Treatment consists of 200 to 1000 micron confluent burns over the NVE and extending 500 microns beyond its borders. Exposure times are 0.1 to 0.5 s. Power is titrated to achieve moderately intense whitening of retina (Table 10.6).

Table 10.5. Parameters for Scatter (Panretinal) Photocoagulation

Spot size	500 microns
Duration	0.1–0.5 s
Endpoint	Moderately intense gray-white burn
Spacing	One burn width apart
Extent	Two disc diameters superiorly, inferiorly, and temporally from the center of the macula and 500 microns from the edge of the disc, extending to the equator or beyond
Wavelength	Argon-green, tunable dye yellow or red, krypton red, diode

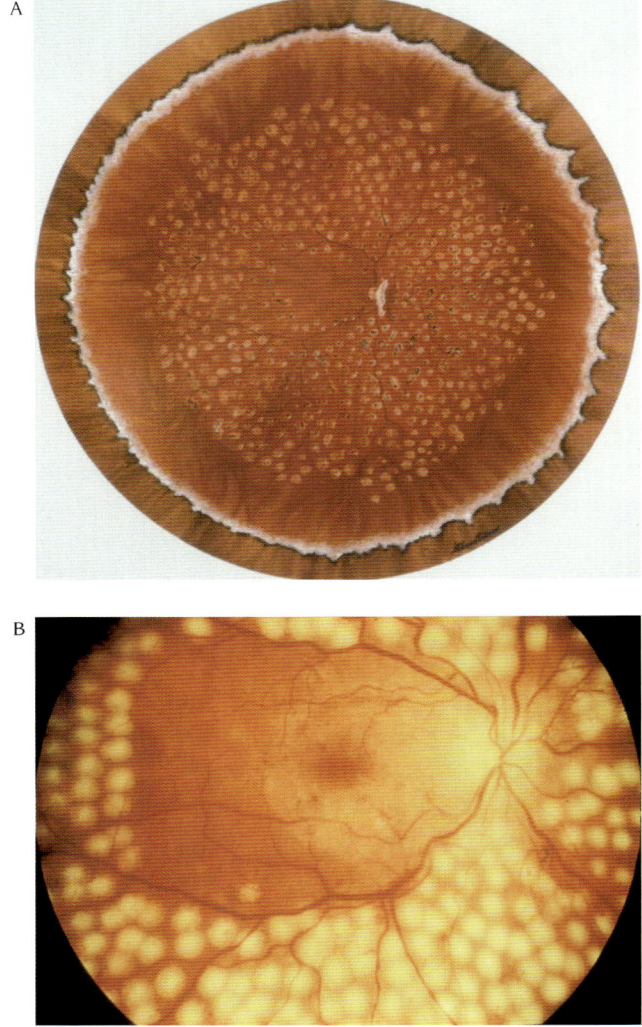

Figure 10.10. (A) Illustration demonstrating full panretinal photocoagulation extending from the vascular arcades to the equator. (B) Clinical photograph demonstrating full panretinal photocoagulation with the temporal margin approximately three disc diameters temporal to the fovea.

Special Considerations. Special considerations with scatter photocoagulation include the number of treatment sessions and the timing of treatment in the presence of macular edema. In the ETDRS, initial scatter photocoagulation was separated into two or more sessions (Fig. 10.11). Multiple sessions may decrease the risk of macular edema development or exacerbation, exudative retinal detachment, choroidal detachment, and angle closure glaucoma [49,51–53]. However, these complications are usually transient and resolve spontaneously. Furthermore, there has been no conclusive evidence that single-session treatment results in a greater rate of permanent vision loss than multiple-session treatment. Therefore, while multiple sessions may have advantages including decreased complications, decreased pain, and less need for retrobulbar anesthesia, single-session scatter photocoagulation should not be avoided if follow-up is not ensured. In the DRCR network, the results of single session versus divided four sessions treatments with PRP showed no significant difference in eyes with no or mild diabetic macular edema.

In eyes with CSME and high-risk PDR, scatter photocoagulation may exacerbate macular edema. For this reason, focal laser photocoagulation of CSME can be considered at the same time or prior to initiating scatter photocoagulation [28,49,52]. Delaying scatter photocoagulation for several weeks in patients without high-risk characteristics is unlikely to increase the risk of severe vision loss from PDR. However, if the retinopathy demonstrates high-risk characteristics, delaying scatter photocoagulation treatment is undesirable. In the ETDRS, patients with both CSME and high-risk PDR received combined focal photocoagulation and scatter photocoagulation to the nasal quadrants; scatter photocoagulation to the remaining temporal quadrants was applied approximately 2 weeks later [49]. The simultaneous application of focal photocoagulation and scatter photocoagulation did not appear to have a detrimental effect on visual acuity outcomes in the ETDRS or in other studies, and may be the best sequence for CSME in the presence of high-risk characteristics [27].

Table 10.6. Parameters for Local Treatment of Neovascularization

Spot size	200–1000 microns
Duration	0.1–0.5 s
Endpoint	Moderately intense gray-white burn
Spacing	Confluent
Extent	Cover NVE and 500 microns beyond its border
Wavelength	Argon-green, tunable dye yellow or red, krypton red, diode

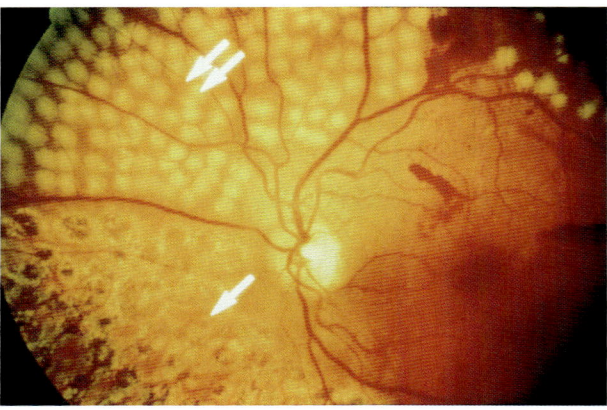

Figure 10.11. Full panretinal photocoagulation therapy in a patient with high-risk characteristics. Note prior laser scars from earlier treatment session (single arrow), and fresh laser scars from recent treatment session (double arrows).

Follow-up and Re-treatment. Follow-up examinations at 2 to 4 month intervals are recommended following complete scatter photocoagulation therapy. The decision to apply more treatment is multifactoral and must be individualized. Factors favoring additional treatment include enlarging neovascularization, increasing activity of neovascularization, (e.g., the formation of tight vascular networks with a paucity of associated fibrous tissue), or an increase in the frequency or extent of vitreous hemorrhage if active neovascularization is present. In many cases, recurrence of mild vitreous hemorrhages (i.e., following posterior vitreous detachment) after adequate scatter photocoagulation and regression of neovascularization, is not a definitive indication for additional treatment. Because the presence of a posterior vitreous detachment decreases the visual complications of vitreoretinal traction, it is also a consideration. If repeated vitreous hemorrhages or tractional macular detachment occurs despite full scatter photocoagulation, surgical intervention should be considered. Finally, the extent and completeness of prior laser treatment should be considered. All of these considerations must be weighed against the risk of producing confluent scars with resulting peripheral visual field loss, and the possibility of retinal-choroidal anastamoses [3,54].

Strategies for applying additional scatter photocoagulation include (1) photocoagulation anterior to, or between prior laser scars, (2) local photocoagulation of areas of small, flat NVE, or (3) photocoagulation in the posterior pole to within 500 microns of the center of the macula. Between 1500 and 500 microns from the center of the macula, burns no larger than 200 microns in size should be used [49]. It was the clinical impression of some ETDRS investigators that the area temporal to the center of the macula, where extensive capillary loss is common and the posterior extent of treatment is often farther than the prescribed two disc diameters from the center of the macula, should be given priority [49].

Prognosis. The DRS identified four risk factors for severe vision loss. These included (1) presence of vitreous or preretinal hemorrhage, (2) presence of new vessels, (3) location of new vessels on or near the optic disc, and (4) moderate or severe extent of new vessels [6]. Scatter photocoagulation provides a 50% reduction in the presence of these retinopathy risk factors over 6 months. Furthermore, only 32% of patients exhibit no change or an increase in the number of retinopathy risk factors over six months of follow-up [53].

COMPLICATIONS OF LASER PHOTOCOAGULATION

As with any procedure, laser photocoagulation may result in side effects and complications. Minor anterior segment complications that may occur with either focal or scatter photocoagulation include corneal abrasions or burns, lenticular burns, iris burns or iritis. These complications are avoided by proper placement and minimal manipulation of contact lenses, and by careful focusing of the aiming beam through a well-dilated pupil.

Some pain, reported to occur in the majority of patients undergoing scatter photocoagulation and 27% of patients undergoing focal photocoagulation, despite topical anesthesia, may be a factor during or after photocoagulation [55]. More pain may occur in the location of the ciliary nerves running in the suprachoroidal space along the horizontal meridian. Strategies to help minimize pain include using low intensity burns and short exposure times. Retrobulbar, subconjunctival, or subtenons administration of local anesthesia is occasionally required and effectively reduce pain [56]. Topical nonsteroidals have also been reported to reduce pain [55].

Complications Related to Focal Laser Photocoagulation. It is important to recognize that a transient increase in macular edema is often observed after focal laser photocoagulation and this should not be considered an indication for re-treatment [11]. Patients often experience a transient corresponding decrease in vision during the first several weeks following treatment, and should, therefore, be made aware of this possibility in advance. In patients with extensive subretinal hard exudates in the macula and elevated serum lipid levels, there is a small risk of subretinal fibrosis and permanent visual loss. Subretinal fibrosis may occur with or without focal laser photocoagulation and is attributed to treatment in only 8% of cases [57–59].

Enlargement of photocoagulation scars over time can lead to confluence of laser scars and may cause paracentral scotoma or central visual loss [60] (Fig. 10.12). The extent of "spread" over the long term is unpredictable. Immediately following a laser application, thermal conduction may contribute to enlargement of the spot beyond the spot size setting, especially with longer duration burns (greater than 0.1 s) [61,62]. Therefore, adequately spacing burns and minimizing exposure times may be important to prevent "spread" and confluence of laser scars.

Accidental foveal burns can occur with dramatic effect on vision. Foveal photocoagulation can be avoided by accurately and repeatedly identifying the fovea during treatment.

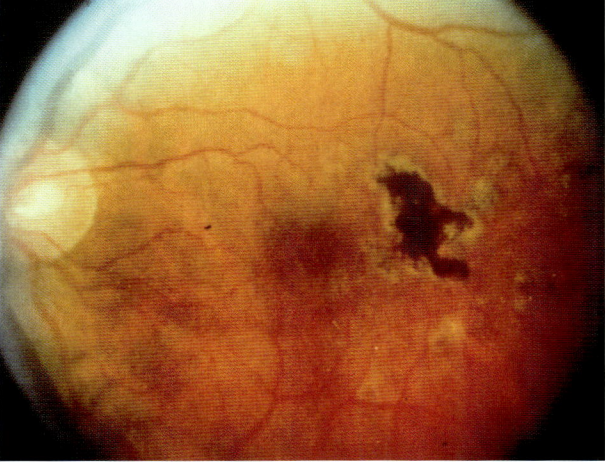

Figure 10.12. Focal photocoagulation treatment with high intensity burns may result in future coalescence of laser scars and paracentral scotomas.

Complications Related to Scatter Photocoagulation. Elevated intraocular pressure may result because of choroidal effusions with anterior displacement of the lens-iris diaphragm or to a transient decrease in facility of outflow after treatment. Generally, the peak intraocular pressure is seen 1 day after treatment and returns to normal within 1 week. Though rarely necessary, topical medications are usually sufficient for treatment [63–65].

Internal ophthalmoplegia with pupillary abnormalities resulting from damage to parasympathetic nerves in the suprachoroidal space has also been reported [66]. This generally resolves spontaneously without sequela.

High intensity burns can cause choroidal, subretinal, or vitreous hemorrhage by rupturing Bruch's membrane. If bleeding occurs, choroidal blood flow should be slowed by applying pressure on the globe with the contact lens. Vitreochoroidal neovascularization may occur later as a result of breaks in Bruch's membrane.

Decreased visual acuity, constricted visual fields, decreased color vision, and decreased dark adaptation were observed by the DRS and the ETDRS groups following scatter photocoagulation. With at least two years of follow-up in the DRS, permanent losses of two or more lines of vision were attributed to scatter photocoagulation in 3% of the argon-treated group and 11% in the xenon-treated group [3]. In most cases, decreased visual acuity is related to a transient increase in macular edema following scatter photocoagulation [67]. A retrospective study reviewed 175 eyes treated with scatter photocoagulation for PDR with high-risk characteristics and found that 43% showed an increase in macular edema at 6 to 10 weeks following treatment. Macular edema persisted in 27%, and had an associated two line decrease in visual acuity in 8% of patients [68].

CONCLUSION

Over the last century, laser photocoagulation has become an integral part of the treatment for many ocular diseases, especially diabetic eye disease. Innovations in laser technology have allowed for more selective and reproducible delivery to specific ocular tissues, and safer and more controlled delivery systems. Landmark studies such as the DRS and the ETDRS have solidified the purpose and place of laser therapeutics in diabetic eye disease. Further technological innovations and public health measures are necessary to make this safe, effective treatment widely available to those who need it.

SUMMARY FOR CLINICIANS

- All eyes with CSME, even those with 20/20 vision, may be considered for focal laser photocoagulation.
- Close follow-up is necessary as several treatment sessions are often required for resolution of diabetic macular edema.
- PDR with high-risk characteristics is an indication for scatter photocoagulation.

- For patients with CSME and PDR with high-risk characteristics, focal laser photocoagulation and scatter photocoagulation may be administered at the same treatment session.
- Scatter photocoagulation may be considered in patients with severe NPDR, particularly in patients with type 2 diabetes.
- Vision loss is possible with laser photocoagulation for diabetic retinopathy. It is usually transient and related to an exacerbation of macular edema following scatter photocoagulation treatment.

REFERENCES

1. Early Treatment Diabetic Retinopathy Study (Research) Group. Photocoagulation for diabetic macular edema: Early Treatment diabetic Retinopathy Study report no. 4. *Int Ophthalmol Clin*. 1987;27:265–272.
2. Early Treatment Diabetic Retinopathy Study (Research) Group. Treatment techniques and clinical guidelines for photocoagulation of diabetic macular edema: Early Treatment Diabetic Retinopathy Study report number 2. *Ophthalmology*. 1987;94:761–774.
3. Diabetic Retinopathy Study Group. Indications for photocoagulation treatment of diabetic retinopathy: Diabetic Retinopathy Study report no. 14. *Int Ophthalmol Clin*. 1987;27:239–253.
4. Early Treatment Diabetic Retinopathy Study (Research) Group. Photocoagulation for diabetic macular edema: Early Treatment Diabetic Retinopathy Study report number 1. *Arch Ophthalmol*. 1985;103:1796–1806.
5. Diabetic Retinopathy Study Group. Photocoagulation treatment of proliferative diabetic retinopathy: Clinical applications of Diabetic Retinopathy Study (DRS) findings, DRS report number 8. *Ophthalmology*. 1981;88:583–600.
6. Diabetic Retinopathy Study Group. Four risk factors for severe visual loss in diabetic retinopathy: the third report from the Diabetic Retinopathy Study. *Arch Ophthalmol*. 1979;97:654–655.
7. Diabetic Retinopathy Study Group. Photocoagulation treatment of proliferative diabetic retinopathy: the second report of Diabetic Retinopathy Study findings. *Ophthalmology*. 1978;85:82–106.
8. Diabetic Retinopathy Study Group. Preliminary report on the effects of photocoagulation therapy. *Am J Ophthalmol*. 1976;81:383–396.
9. Klein R, Klein BEK, Moss SE, Davis MD, DeMets DL. The Wisconsin Epidemiologic Study of Diabetic Retinopathy: IV. Diabetic macular edema. *Ophthalmology*. 1984; 91:1464–1474.
10. Klein R, Moss SE, Klein BEK, Davis MD, DeMets DL. The Wisconsin Epidemiologic Study of Diabetic Retinopathy: the incidence of macular edema. *Ophthalmology*. 1989;96:1501–1510.
11. Olk R. Modified grid argon (blue-green) laser photocoagulation for diffuse diabetic macular edema. *Ophthalmology*. 1986;93:938–950.
12. Early Treatment Diabetic Retinopathy Study (Research) Group. Focal photocoagulation treatment of diabetic macular edema. Relationship of treatment effect to fluorescein angiographic and other retinal characteristics at baseline: ETDRS report no. 19. *Arch Ophthalmol*. 1985;113:1144–1155.
13. Ferris F III, Davis MD. Treating 20/20 eyes with diabetic macular edema. *Arch Ophthalmol*. 1999;117:675–676.
14. Early Treatment Diabetic Retinopathy Study (Research) Group. Results from the Early Treatment diabetic Retinopathy Study. *Ophthalmology*. 1991;98:739–840.

15. American Academy of Ophthalmology Retina Panel. Preferred Practice Pattern Guidelines. Diabetic Retinopathy. San Francisco, CA: American Academy of Ophthalmology;2008. Available at http//www.aao.org/ppp.

16. Wilson DJ, Finkelstein D, Quigley HA, Green WR. Macular grid photocoagulation: an experimental study of the primate retina. *Arch Ophthalmol.* 1988;106:100–105.

17. Marshall J, Clover G, Rothery S. Some new findings on retinal irradiation by krypton and argon lasers. *Doc Ophthalmol Proc Ser.* 1984;36:21–37.

18. Weiter J, Zuckerman R. The influence of the photoreceptor-RPE complex on the inner retina: an explanation for the beneficial effects of photocoagulation. *Ophthalmology.* 1980;87:1133–1139.

19. Bresnick G. Diabetic maculopathy: a critical review highlighting diffuse macular edema. *Ophthalmology.* 1983;90:1301–1317.

20. Marshall J, Hamilton AM, Bird AC. Intra-retinal absorption of argon laser irradiation in human and monkey retinae. *Experientia.* 1974;30:1355–1357.

21. Arden G, Berninger T, Hogg CR, Perry S. A survey of color discrimination in German ophthalmologists. *Ophthalmology.* 1991;98:567–575.

22. Diabetic Retinopathy Clinical Research Network. Comparison of the modified Early Treatment Diabetic Retinopathy Study and mild macular grid laser photocoagulation strategies for diabetic macular edema. *Arch Ophthalmol.* 2007;125:469–480.

23. Diabetic Retinopathy Clinical Research Network. A randomized trial comparing intravitreal triamcinolone acetonide and focal/grid photocoagulation for diabetic macular edema. *Ophthalmology.* 2008;115:1447–1459.

24. Kaiser P, Riemann CD, Sears JE, Lewis H. Macular traction detachment and diabetic macular edema associated with posterior hyaloidal traction. *Am J Ophthalmol.* 2001;131:44–49.

25. Martidis A, Duker JS, Greenberg PG, et al. Intravitreal triamcinolone for refractory diabetic macular edema. *Ophthalmology.* 2002;109:920–927.

26. Strom C, Sander B, Larsen N, et al. Diabetic macular edema assessed with optical coherence tomography and stereo fundus photography. *Invest Ophthalmol Vis Sci.* 2002;43:241–245.

27. Browning DJ, Zhang Z, Benfield JM, Scott AQ. The effect of patient characteristics on response to focal laser treatment for diabetic macular edema. *Ophthalmology.* 1997;104:446–472.

28. McDonald HR, Schatz H. Grid photocoagulation for diffuse macular edema. *Retina.* 1985;5:65–72.

29. Blankenship G. Diabetic macular edema and laser photocoagulation. *Ophthalmology.* 1979;86:69–75.

30. British MSG. Photocoagulation for diabetic maculopathy: a randomized controlled clinical trial using xenon arc. *Diabetes.* 1983;32:1010–1016.

31. Patz A, Schatz H, Berkow JW, et al. Macular edema: an overlooked complication of diabetic retinopathy. *Ophthalmology.* 1979;77:34–42.

32. Whitelocke R, Kearns M, Black RK, et al. The diabetic maculopathies. *Trans Ophthalmol Soc UK.* 1979;99:314–320.

33. Klein R, Klein BEK, Moss SE, Davis MD, DeMets DL. The Wisconsin Epidemiological Study of Diabetic Retinopathy. III. Prevalence and risk of diabetic retinopathy when age at diagnosis is 30 or more years. *Arch Ophthalmol.* 1984;102:527–532.

34. American Academy of Ophthalmology Retina Panel. Preferred Practice Pattern Guidelines. Diabetic Retinopathy. San Francisco, CA: American Academy of Ophthalmology;2008. Available at http//www.aao.org/ppp.

35. Diabetic Retinopathy Study Group. Clinical application of Diabetic Retinopathy Study (DRS) findings: DRS report number 8. *Ophthalmology.* 1981;88:583–600.
36. Early Treatment Diabetic Retinopathy Study (Research) Group. Early photocoagulation for diabetic retinopathy: ETDRS report number 9. *Ophthalmology.* 1991;98: 766–785.
37. Ferris F. Early photocoagulation in patients with either type I or type II diabetes. *Trans Am Ophthalmol Soc.* 1996;94:505–537.
38. Pavan PR, Folk JC, Weingeist TA, et al. Diabetic rubeosis and panretinal photocoagulation: a prospective, controlled, masked trial using fluorescein angiography. *Arch Ophthalmol.* 1983;101:882–884.
39. Jacobson D, Murphy RP, Rosenthal AR. The treatment of angle neovascularization with panretinal photocoagulation. *Ophthalmology.* 1979;86:1270–1275.
40. Glaser B. Extracellular modulatory factors and the control of intraocular neovascularization: an overview. *Ophthalmology.* 1988;106:603–607.
41. Glaser B. Retinal pigment epithelial cells release an inhibitor of neovascularization. *Arch Ophthalmol.* 1985;103:1870–1875.
42. Patz A. Retinal neovascularization: early contributions of Professor Michaelson and recent observations. *Br J Ophthalmol.* 1984;68:42–46.
43. Landers M, Stefanson E, Wolbarsht ML. Panretinal photocoagulation and retinal oxygenation. *Retina.* 1982;2:167–175.
44. Singerman LJ, Ferris FL III, Mowery RP, et al. Krypton laser for proliferative diabetic retinopathy: the Krypton Argon Regression of Neovascularization Study. *J Diabet Complications.* 1988;2:189–196.
45. The Krypton Argon Regression Neovascularization Study Research Group. Randomized comparison of krypton versus argon scatter photocoagulation for diabetic disc neovascularization. The Krypton Argon Regression Neovascularization Study Report Number 1. *Ophthalmology.* 1993;100:1655–1664.
46. Khairallah M, Chachia N. Post laser choroidal hematoma in a diabetic treated with an oral anticoagulant. *J Fr Ophthalmol.* 1994;17:138–140.
47. Ulbig M, Hamilton AM. Comparative use of diode and argon laser for panretinal photocoagulation in diabetic retinopathy. *Ophthalmologe.* 1993;90:457–462.
48. Bandello F, Brancato R, Trabucchi G, Lattazio R, Malegori A. Diode versus argon-green laser panretinal photocoagulation in proliferative diabetic retinopathy: a randomized study in 44 eyes with a long follow-up time. *Graefes Arch Clin Exp Ophthalmol.* 1993;231:491–494.
49. Early Treatment Diabetic Retinopathy Study (Research) Group. Techniques for scatter and local photocoagulation: Early Treatment Diabetic Retinopathy Study report no. 3. *Int Ophthalmol Clin.* 1987;27:254–264.
50. Ferris F III, Davis MD, Aiello LM. Treatment of diabetic retinopathy. *NEJM.* 1999;341:667–678.
51. Blankenship G. A clinical comparison of central and peripheral argon laser panretinal photocoagulation for proliferative diabetic retinopathy. *Ophthalmology.* 1988;95:170–177.
52. Ferris F III, Podgor MJ, Davis MD, The Diabetic Retinopathy Study Research Group. Macular edema in Diabetic Retinopathy Study patients: diabetic Retinopathy Study report number 12. *Ophthalmology.* 1987;95:754–760.
53. Doft B, Blankenship GW. Single versus multiple treatment sessions of argon laser panretinal photocoagulation for proliferative diabetic retinopathy. *Ophthalmology.* 1982;89:772–779.

54. Aylward GW, Pearson RV, Jagger JD, Hamilton AM. Extensive argon laser photocoagulation in the treatment of proliferative diabetic retinopathy. *Br J Ophthalmol.* 1989;73:197–201.

55. Weinberger D, Ron Y, Lichter H, Rosenblat I, Axer-Siegel R, Yassur Y. Analgesic effect of topical sodium diclofenac 0.1% drops during retinal laser photocoagulation. *Br J Ophthalmol.* 2000;84:135–137.

56. Stevens JD, Foss AJ, Hamilton AM. No-needle one-quadrant sub-tenon anaesthesia for panretinal photocoagulation. *Eye.* 1993;7:768–771.

57. Han D, Mieler WF, Burton TC. Subretinal fibrosis after laser photocoagulation for diabetic macular edema. *Am J Ophthalmol.* 1992;113:513–521.

58. Guyer D, D'Amico DJ, Smith CW. Subretinal fibrosis after laser photocoagulation for diabetic macular edema. *Am J Ophthalmol.* 1992;113:652–656.

59. Lewis H, Schachat AP, Haimann, MH, et al. Choroidal neovascularization after laser photocoagulation for diabetic macular edema. *Ophthalmology.* 1990;97:503–510.

60. Schatz H, Madeira D, McDonald HR, Johnson RN. Progressive enlargement of laser scars following grid laser photocoagulation for diffuse diabetic macular edema. *Arch Ophthalmol.* 1991;109:1549–1551.

61. Mainster M, White TJ, Tips JH, Wilson PW. Retinal temperature increases produced by intense light sources. *J Opt Soc Am.* 1970;60:264–270.

62. Mainster M. Wavelength selection in macular photocoagulation: tissue optics, thermal effects and laser systems. *Ophthalmology.* 1986;93:952–958.

63. Blondeau P, Pavan PR, Phelps CD. Acute pressure elevation following panretinal photocoagulation. *Arch Ophthalmol.* 1981;99:1239–1241.

64. Mensher J. Anterior chamber depth alteration after retinal photocoagulation. *Arch Ophthalmol.* 1977;95:113–116.

65. Huamonte FU, Peyman GA, Goldberg MF, Locretz A. Immediate fundus complications after retinal scatter photocoagulation. 1. Clinical picture and pathogenesis. *Ophthalmic Surg.* 1976;7:88–89.

66. Lobed L, Bourgon P. Pupillary abnormalities induced by argon laser photocoagulation. *Ophthalmology.* 1985;92:234–236.

67. McDonald HR, Schatz H. Visual loss following panretinal photocoagulation for proliferative diabetic retinopathy. *Ophthalmology.* 1985;92:388–393.

68. McDonald HR, Schatz H. Macular edema following panretinal photocoagulation. *Retina.* 1985;5:5–10.

11

Vitrectomy for Diabetic Retinopathy

WILLIAM E. SMIDDY, MD,
AND HARRY W. FLYNN, JR., MD

CORE MESSAGES

- Indications for pars plana vitrectomy in the management of complications from diabetic retinopathy have changed substantially since the inception of vitrectomy.
- Generally, vitrectomy is recommended early in the disease process, especially for type 1 diabetic patients, before irreversible changes occur.
- Panretinal laser photocoagulation (PRP) is recommended before vitrectomy whenever the clinical presentation and course allow it.
- New instrumentation and techniques, including high-speed vitrectomy instruments, wide-field viewing systems, and transconjunctival systems, have facilitated the objectives of diabetic vitrectomy.
- There are many different surgical approaches, but all allow for acceptably good results.
- Visual acuity outcomes of diabetic vitrectomy are best for clearance of media opacities and diminish as increasing traction causes retinal detachment.

The hallmark of proliferative diabetic retinopathy is ischemia-driven retinal vascular changes including neovascularization (NV). The most efficient strategies to preserve vision in diabetic patients are to prevent or mitigate complications through population screening and early detection, and timely and appropriate treatment of complications [1–3]. Prevention of retinopathy or reduction in rates of retinopathy progression via optimal glucose control [4,5] and laser treatment at earlier stages have been advocated and implemented [3]. Prospective clinical trial results have largely defined the management of complications of diabetic retinopathy. Timely application (and reapplication as needed) of panretinal laser photocoagulation (PRP) is the mainstay of treatment to reduce visual loss and to avoid the need for vitrectomy in patients with more advanced diabetic retinopathy complications [6–14]. Javitt has shown the cost-effectiveness of implementation of guidelines obtained from the results of collaborative, National Eye Institute sponsored laser studies to the diabetic population at risk [15].

However, despite timely treatment and preventative regimens, substantial numbers of eyes will develop complications of progressive retinopathy and may become candidates for vitrectomy [16]. Clinical trials together with case series form the foundation for defining treatment by vitrectomy [17,18].

SURGICAL INDICATIONS

The initial indications and surgical rationale for pars plana vitrectomy in diabetic patients were largely established by the mid-1980s [17–29]. As instrumentation and surgical techniques evolved, these indications have been refined. General categories of surgically approachable complications from diabetic retinopathy include eyes with media opacities and vitreoretinal traction (Table 11.1). The timing for vitrectomy has been generally accelerated as improvements in surgical instrumentation have resulted in better visual acuity outcomes. An addition to surgical indications is certain subsets of eyes with macular edema [29,30]. Optimal application for this indication is still undergoing definition and evaluation, but seems to be most effective if vitreomacular traction is present [31]. The DRCR network has recently reported that pars plana vitrectomy for eyes with vitreomacular traction and clinically significant macular edema was associated with significant improvement in

Table 11.1. Indications for Vitrectomy due to Complications of Severe
Diabetic Retinopathy

A. Media Opacities:
  1) Nonclearing hemorrhage
    a) Vitreous hemorrhage
    b) Subhyaloid, premacular hemorrhage
    c) Anterior segment neovascularization with posterior segment opacity
  2) Cataract preventing treatment of severe proliferative diabetic retinopathy
B. Tractional Defects:
  1) Progressive fibrovascular proliferation
  2) Traction retinal detachment involving the macula
  3) Combined tractional and rhegmatogenous retinal detachment
  4) Macular edema associated with taut, persistently attached posterior hyaloid
C. Other Miscellaneous Indications (often following previous vitrectomy):
  1) Vitreous hemorrhage/ghost cell glaucoma
  2) Anterior hyaloidal fibrovascular proliferation
  3) Fibrinoid syndrome
  4) Epiretinal membrane (nonvascularized)
  5) Macular heterotopia
  6) Macular hole
  7) Macular edema without traction

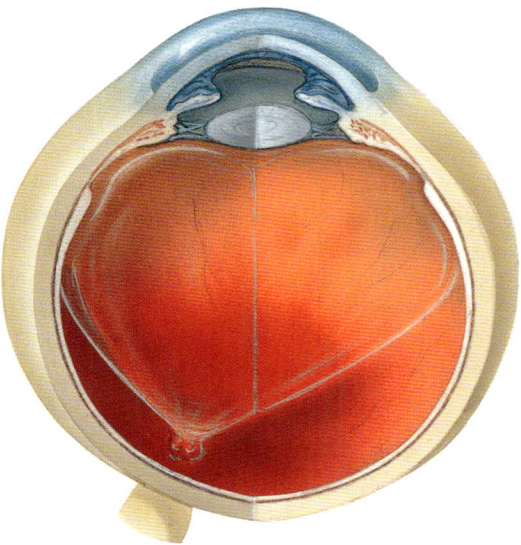

Figure 11.1. Diabetic vitreous hemorrhage most commonly presents as a fairly sudden decrease in vision. Depending upon the degree of hemorrhage, the posterior pole may not be visible. The hemorrhage is usually due to vitreous traction on elevated neovascularization. The neovascularization can be isolated or more broadly distributed. This schematic illustrates the subhyaloid hemorrhage in all areas except at the optic nerve head where a stump of neovascularization is present. (Source: Redrawn with permission of Johns Hopkins University from Michels RG: Proliferative diabetic retinopathy: pathophysiology of extraretinal complications and principles of vitreous surgery. *Retina* 1981;1:1–17.)

optical coherence tomography (OCT) outcomes but visual acuity outcomes were relatively unchanged at six months follow-up.

Media Opacities. Severe nonclearing diabetic vitreous hemorrhage was the first indication for diabetic vitrectomy [32,33] (Fig. 11.1). Vitreous hemorrhage probably results from vitreous traction on the vascular stalk of fibrovascular complexes [34–36]. Timely application of PRP has decreased the incidence of dense vitreous hemorrhage by truncating the extent of retinal NV. Newer vitrectomy techniques and instrumentation now allow successful surgery on more complex cases, expanding the indications for diabetic vitrectomy.

Probably the greatest change in clinical practice during the last decade is the timing for vitrectomy, which has generally come to be undertaken after a shorter waiting period. Several clinical features may influence the decision on timing of vitrectomy for diabetic vitreous hemorrhage. Surgical intervention is usually considered within several weeks to a few months after onset of symptoms. However, a substantial proportion of such cases will have spontaneous clearing, and careful clinical assessment is necessary during the initial observation period. Earlier surgical intervention is generally recommended for type 1 diabetic patients, especially when no previous PRP has been performed, when the proliferative complexes are more extensive, and when the retinopathy in the fellow eye has been more aggressive. Conversely, surgical intervention may be more appropriately deferred, at least temporarily, when there is a posterior vitreous detachment (PVD), when extensive prior PRP has been delivered, and when other labile medical conditions coexist. Patients with sustained hypertension or elevated levels of glycosylated hemoglobin should have prompt and appropriate treatment for these systemic conditions. Echographic monitoring for retinal detachment is important when media opacities prohibit visualization of the fundus.

Other coexisting clinical features define subsets of vitrectomy indications for vitreous hemorrhage. Rubeosis iridis in an eye with a recent vitreous hemorrhage, especially when no PRP has been applied, constitutes an urgent indication for intervention (Fig. 11.2). An extensive subhyaloid macular hemorrhage (SHMH) constitutes another surgical indication (Fig. 11.3). The confinement of blood in the subhyaloid space indicates that the posterior hyaloid has not fully separated and remains as a scaffold for progressive fibrovascular proliferation (FVP) [35–37]. Although the hemorrhage may clear over several months, this SHMH is often associated with broad-based areas of vitreoretinal adhesions. Because of the relatively poor visual prognosis in eyes with substantial SHMH even with spontaneous clearing, surgical intervention should be considered relatively early in the course (probably within 2 months of onset). As with the conventional form of

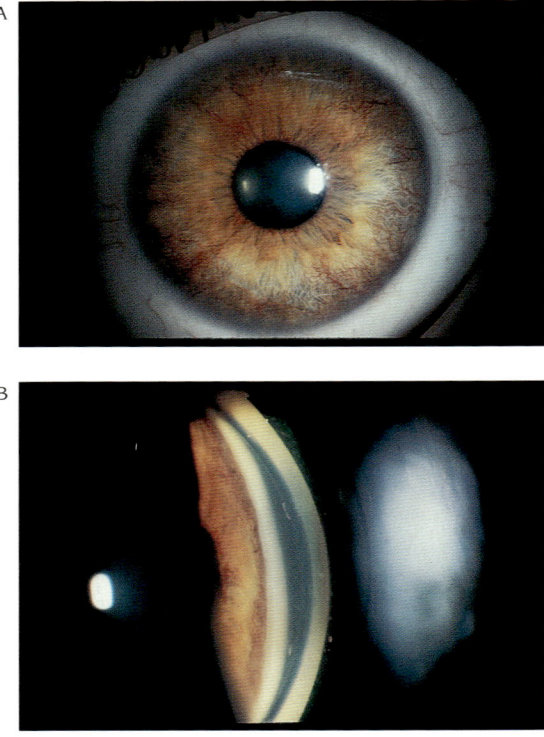

Figure 11.2. Rubeosis iridis characteristically appears first at the pupillary border and then extends onto the iris surface, but in progressive cases, may be visible in the anterior chamber angle. Subsequent neovascular glaucoma and precipitous loss of vision may result, especially without prompt and extensive panretinal photocoagulation treatment.

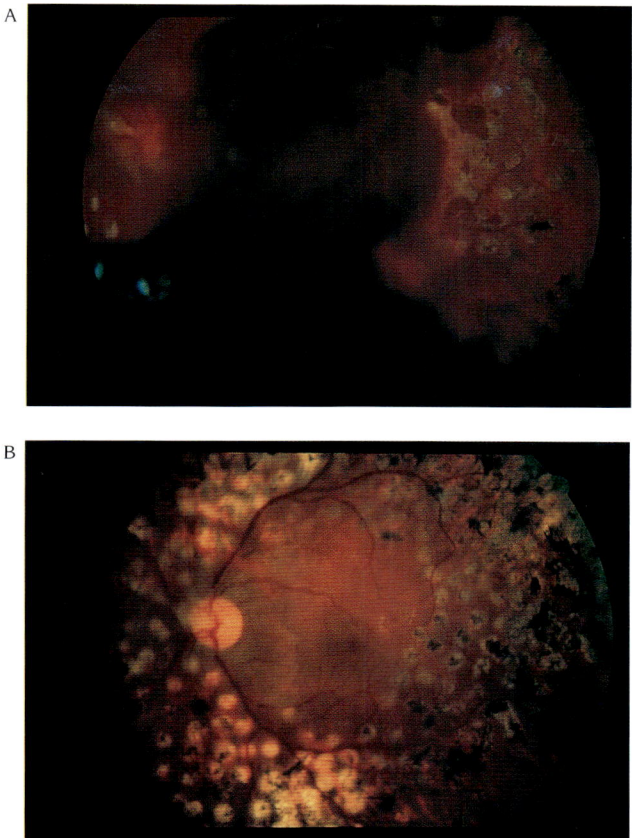

Figure 11.3. (A) This patient presented with extensive subhyaloid hemorrhage and vision of 2/200. (B) Postoperative appearance following vitrectomy with supplementation of panretinal photocoagulation. Vision is 20/40.

vitreous hemorrhage, intervention is generally recommended earlier for type 1 diabetic patients compared to type 2 diabetic patients. While waiting for clearing of SHMH, however, PRP should be applied in more peripheral areas, as breakthrough bleeding into the central vitreous may later prevent this.

Lens opacities may be sufficient to impair not only the patient's vision but also the physician's ability to diagnose, monitor, and apply laser treatment to the retina. In such cases, cataract removal may be considered either as a separate procedure or in combination with vitrectomy. In eyes with vitreous hemorrhage, the accurate assessment of the degree of cataract may be difficult. Reports before the availability of endolaser photocoagulation documented a substantial rate of rubeosis iridis and poor visual prognosis in aphakic eyes, or in those eyes undergoing lensectomy at the time of vitrectomy [38–41]. However, more recent experience with better techniques for lens removal and the ability to deliver intraoperative photocoagulation have improved outcomes with combined lens removal and intraocular lens (IOL) implantation during vitrectomy in selected cases [42–44].

Two general approaches for combined vitrectomy and cataract surgery have been reported. In the first approach, pars plana lensectomy is combined with vitrectomy maneuvers, and the anterior capsule (with central capsulotomy) is preserved for posterior chamber (PC) IOL support. Using this approach, the visual acuity has been reported to improve in over 75% of eyes, including about 25% with ≥20/40 vision [42,43]. In the second approach, a standard clear corneal phacoemulsification is performed, with IOL insertion into the capsular bag, followed by the vitrectomy. Using that approach, visualization was reported to be excellent, but visual acuity outcomes were not as good in one study [44]; the discrepancy in visual results between the two approaches is most probably accounted for by case selection. Modern techniques for cataract surgery allow successful outcomes even in the presence of rubeosis iridis [45].

Vitreoretinal Traction. Vitreoretinal traction constitutes the second general indication category for diabetic vitrectomy. The spectrum of tractional involvement includes macular heterotopia [46], progressive FVP without retinal detachment, tractional retinal detachment, and rhegmatogenous retinal detachment where the retinal break formed because of progressive traction. Frequently, tractional elements and media opacities coexist, and a dual set of indications for vitrectomy must be assessed (Fig. 11.4).

Progressive FVP may occur despite appropriate PRP and may be especially aggressive in type 1 diabetics (Fig. 11.5). Although FVP may be very extensive in some cases, visual loss may only be slight in its early- to mid-stages. Ultimately, FVP usually progresses and induces marked visual loss, and a more guarded prognosis for vitrectomy. The lack of a complete PVD is commonly the determining factor influencing anatomic extent and visual prognosis. Broad-based posterior hyaloid attachment usually allows the FVP to be more extensive, requiring more prolonged scissors dissection. In general, the more chronic the FVP, the more adherent its retinal attachment. On the other hand, more acute onset is frequently associated with a more active vascular component that allows more complete removal, but leads to more intraoperative and postoperative vitreous hemorrhage. Incomplete removal may form a nidus for reproliferation. Surgical relief of traction is accomplished with fewer complications when the zone of vitreoretinal attachment is less extensive, extends less anteriorly, and is of recent onset.

The pathogenesis of retinal detachment involves progressive vitreoretinal traction (Fig. 11.6). Since peripheral or mid-peripheral tractional retinal detachments progress to involve the macula in only about 15% of cases per year [47], caution is advised in recommending vitrectomy for localized, non–macular-involving detachments; they may never lead to visual loss, whereas surgical removal might accelerate visual loss. Vitrectomy is generally reserved for cases in which the macula is involved or clearly threatened by progressive tractional retinal detachment. Currently, tractional retinal detachment is probably the most common specific indication for vitrectomy in patients with progressive FVP.

As with cases of nonclearing diabetic vitreous hemorrhage, additional factors may influence the timing of surgical intervention. Patients with type 1 diabetes, coexisting media opacities (which may have prevented delivery of adequate PRP),

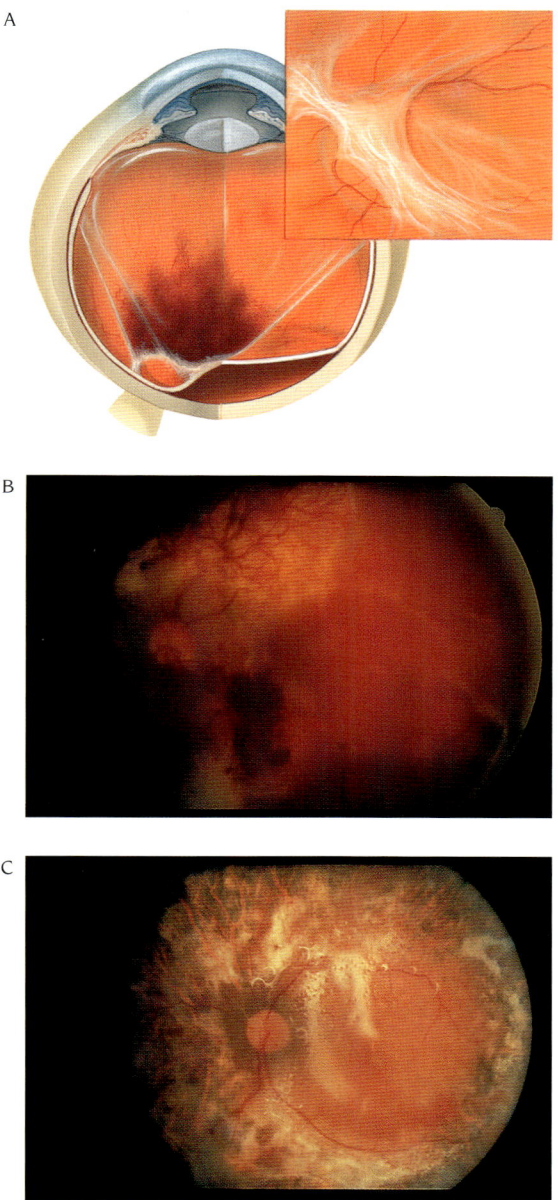

Figure 11.4. (A) Frequently, media opacities and tractional components coexist. In this schematic representation, there is vitreous hemorrhage admixed with fibrovascular proliferation, which is causing a tractional retinal detachment. However, this may not be clinically evident due to the obscuration of the posterior pole by the media opacities. (B) This patient presented with vision of hand motions. Clearly, there is vitreous hemorrhage, but the view is clear enough to depict fibrovascular proliferation along the superotemporal arcade. (C) Appearance postoperatively following vitrectomy with extensive membrane peeling and silicone oil infusion. Vision is 20/400. (Source: Part A redrawn with permission of Johns Hopkins University from Michels RG: Proliferative diabetic retinopathy: pathophysiology of extraretinal complications and principles of vitreous surgery. *Retina* 1981;1:1–17.)

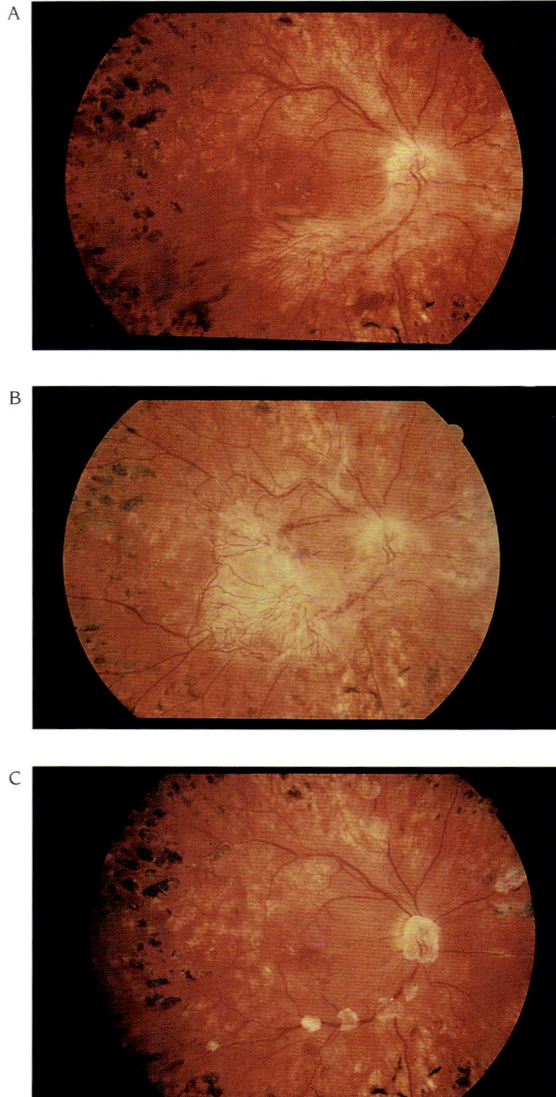

Figure 11.5. (A) Fibrovascular proliferation typically progresses from neovascularization of the nerve head and along the arcade with, initially, relatively good visual acuity. This 29-year-old woman presented with vision of 20/30. (B) With further progression over the ensuing three months, the visual acuity dropped to 20/200 as the fibrovascular proliferation enveloped the posterior pole. (C) After vitrectomy, the vision returned to 20/30.

and patients with severe retinopathy in the fellow eye should be considered for earlier vitrectomy. Chronic macular detachment leads to thinner, more atrophic retina, with more extensive and more tightly adherent fibrovascular membranes. Consequently, the anatomic and visual prognoses are poorer in such patients; macular detachment for 6 months or more has a poor visual prognosis and may not be recommended for surgery [19,25].

A third traction-related indication for diabetic vitrectomy is combined tractional and rhegmatogenous retinal detachment (Fig. 11.7). The rhegmatogenous component results from progressive contraction of FVP. Pathognomonic of a rhegmatogenous etiology is the appearance of hydration lines, and usually the retina is more mobile and elevated. Compared to tractional retinal detachment, more sudden and

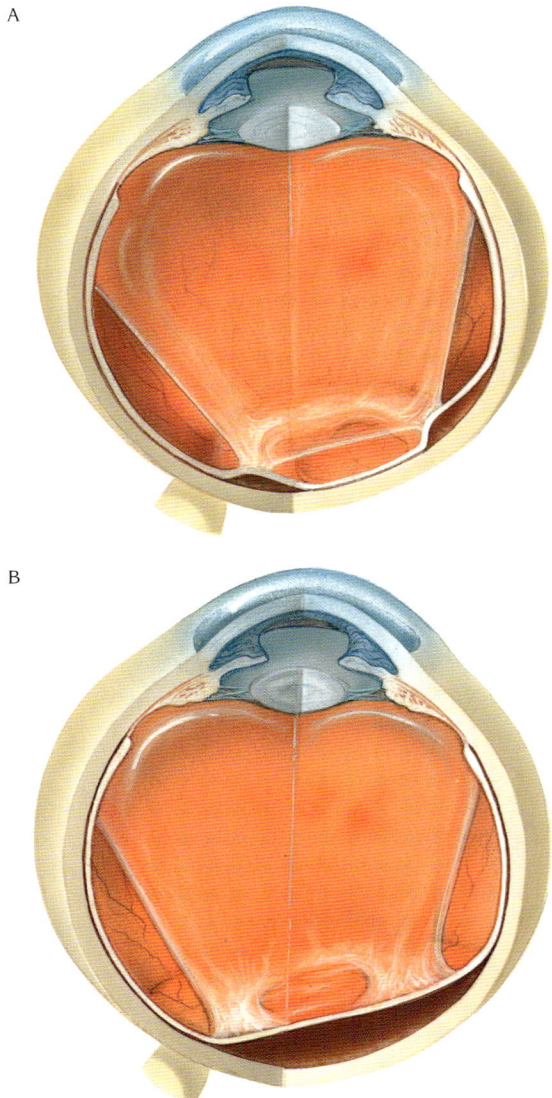

Figure 11.6. (A) This schematic representation demonstrates tractional retinal detachment beginning outside of the fovea due to traction from fibrovascular proliferation along the arcades and disc. (B) With further progression, a "table-top" configuration ensues in which the macula is additionally affected. (C) This is illustrated by this 39-year-old man who presented with 2/200 vision. (D) Postoperatively, the vision improved to 20/60. (Source: Part A and B redrawn with permission of Johns Hopkins University from Michels RG: Proliferative diabetic retinopathy: pathophysiology of extraretinal complications and principles of vitreous surgery. *Retina* 1981;1:1–17.)

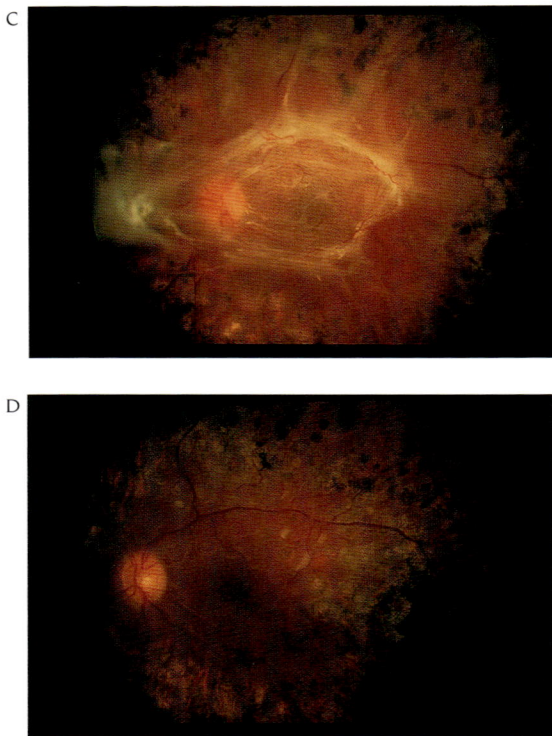

Figure 11.6. (Continued)

profound visual loss usually occurs soon after the rhegmatogenous component occurs. While some cases with a rhegmatogenous component may be only slowly progressive and could be monitored closely without surgery, more commonly, prompt surgery is indicated. The pathogenic retinal break typically occurs posterior to the equator, but may be obscured by FVP and not be appreciable during the preoperative examination. Common sites for retinal breaks include areas adjacent to previous chorioretinal scars or at the base of vitreoretinal adhesions.

A more subtle traction-induced complication is macular edema induced by the traction of a taut, persistently attached posterior hyaloid. While this is uncommon, it is demonstrated readily on OCT. This subtype of diabetic macular edema characteristically does not respond to focal laser photocoagulation or intravitreal corticosteroids. The vast majority of diabetic macular edema cases are not induced by traction and should be considered for photocoagulation in accordance with the results of the Early Treatment Diabetic Retinopathy Study [48] or, in selected cases, for intravitreal corticosteroids. Selected cases with this configuration respond to surgical release of the traction [24,29]. A subsequent study corroborated those results but also emphasized both the rarity of the condition and the difficulty in accurately assessing such cases during the preoperative examination [30]. Other techniques that involve internal limiting membrane removal in cases with even less apparent traction are still being evaluated.

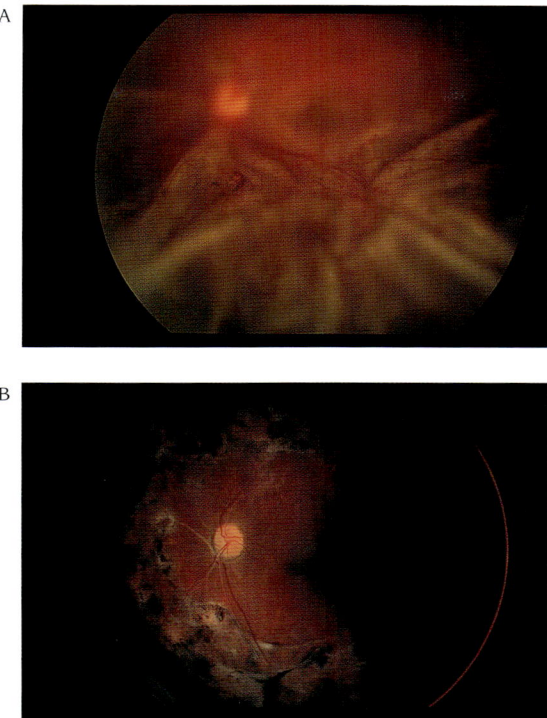

Figure 11.7. (A) With continued traction, especially with more broad-based fibrovascular enti-ties, a rhegmatogenous component may develop in the retina. This leads to a more generalized retinal detachment, which may be apparent as rapid onset of decreased vision, extensive retinal detachment, and hydration lines. (B) Postoperative appearance of this patient. Visual acuity remained 20/400.

Complications of Previous Vitrectomy. A third, miscellaneous category of vitrectomy indications includes complications from a previous vitrectomy. As in primary cases, there are two broad subcategories: media opacities and traction. Severe recurrent vitreous hemorrhage not only constitutes a media opacity but may also induce a secondary glaucoma through a ghost cell mechanism [49–52]. Most such cases are self-limited (spontaneous clearing of hemorrhage) or respond to medi-cal therapy (glaucoma), but selected cases will respond to vitrectomy by debulk-ing the substrate for outflow blockage [53]. In some cases, office-based fluid–gas exchange may provide sufficient elimination of blood, avoiding repeat vitrectomy in the operating room [54,55]. In most cases, however, recurrent severe vitreous hemorrhage after vitrectomy is a manifestation of reproliferation, retinal break formation, or other more severe complications that require operative repair.

Retinal detachment—either tractional or rhegmatogenous—after previous vit-rectomy may constitute an indication for repeat vitrectomy. Such cases usually have a guarded visual prognosis because of coexisting proliferative vitreoretinopa-thy (PVR). Silicone oil may be considered for retinal tamponade.

An especially difficult condition to control is progressive anterior hyaloid FVP that typically occurs several weeks following vitrectomy. These cases are usually managed by lensectomy and extensive anterior vitreous dissection similar to techniques used for PVR [56].

Intravitreal injection of bevacizumab may be useful preoperatively in eyes with extensive FVP in order to reduce intraoperative bleeding [57,58]. Although no randomized prospective study has been conducted, the use of preoperative bevacizumab has gained considerable popularity. However, progressive traction retinal detachment following intravitreal bevacizumab has being described in patients with severe proliferative diabetic retinopathy and these cases may have very poor visual outcomes [59].

A rare entity after vitrectomy is the fibrinoid syndrome, which involves extensive fibrinous membrane cross-linking of the vitreous [60]. The fibrinoid syndrome may reflect ischemia and increased vascular permeability. Minor degrees of postoperative fibrin formation usually resolve spontaneously, but when severe degrees of fibrin occur, as is characteristic of fibrinoid syndrome cases, tissue plasminogen activator [61] or streptokinase [62] may be useful. The visual prognosis is guarded, but pretreatment with intravitreal triamcinolone acetonide has been suggested to attempt to reduce the severity of this complication. Similarly, intraoperative use of intravitreal triamcinolone may reduce this complication.

SURGICAL OBJECTIVES AND TECHNIQUES

The surgical objectives of vitrectomy for complications of diabetic retinopathy are to neutralize and, when possible, to eliminate the components that have led to the visual loss (Table 11.2). These objectives are usually interrelated and involve removal of axial media opacities, relief of preretinal traction, and delivery of appropriate laser treatment. New instruments and techniques have emerged in response to the need to achieve these objectives more safely and reproducibly.

Media Opacities. Endoillumination, an operating microscope, and an optical viewing system provide standard visualization of the vitreous strands and surfaces.

Removal of axial opacities involves the vitreous cutter, the extrusion needle, and lensectomy instruments. Newer instruments now offer better control of cutting rates, suction pressure, and fragmentation power and mode. Removal of vitreous

Table 11.2. Objectives of Vitrectomy for Severe Diabetic Retinopathy

1. Remove axial opacities
2. Relieve anteroposterior traction
3. Relieve tangential traction
4. Segment or peel epiretinal membranes
5. Effect hemostasis
6. Treat all retinal breaks
7. Deliver laser treatment
   a. Limited or full panretinal photocoagulation
   b. Local treatment of flat neovascularization elsewhere
8. Use retinal tamponade if necessary
   a. Air or gas
   b. Silicone oil

and FVP is facilitated with more complete posterior vitreous separation. In eyes not requiring extensive membrane dissection, 23- or 25-gauge transconjunctival vitrectomy is a useful option for clearing media opacities and applying endolaser PRP. Improving ancillary instrumentation has allowed the application of 23- or 25-gauge surgery to increasingly complex vitreoretinal traction in diabetic retinopathy.

Vitreoretinal Traction. Elimination of traction involves removal of anteroposterior and tangential vitreoretinal traction, as well as removal of membrane-induced surface traction. At least three conceptually different surgical techniques have been developed to achieve these goals [63–71]. While each technique seems to represent a different approach, all achieve the same objectives albeit in a different sequence:

1. Segmentation: the traction is sequentially dissected by removing anterior to posterior traction (Fig. 11.8A), scissors dissection of bridging epiretinal traction (Fig. 11.8B) and, finally, removal of residual islands of surface traction including epiretinal membranes [63,64] (Fig. 11.8C).
2. Delamination: the anteroposterior traction is commonly removed first. Preretinal tissue is removed using horizontal scissors and multifunction instruments (such as lighted picks or lighted forceps) at the retinal plane as one or more large pieces [65,66] (Fig. 11.9). In this regard, it is similar to the "en bloc" technique except that the anterior to posterior traction of the vitreous has been removed previously. Delamination techniques are reported to induce less intraoperative bleeding than segmentation techniques.
3. "En bloc": the surface traction is removed with scissors as a large, confluent piece using the anteroposterior traction for countertraction before relief of anteroposterior traction [68–72] (Fig. 11.10). The theoretical advantage of this technique is that the anteroposterior traction serves as a "third hand" function by retracting tissue from the retinal surface so that subsequent surface dissection is facilitated. The anteroposterior traction and the bulk of the vitreous are removed as the last step. Initial reports suggested that this technique was associated with more intraoperative retinal breaks (35% in an early report) [70], but further experience yields a rate equivalent to other techniques (20%) [71]. The consequences of an iatrogenic retinal break (as long as it is appropriately treated) when the traction has been relieved more fully are minimal compared to leaving traction unrelieved. In many cases, the selected surgical technique is a hybrid of all three techniques. Use of high-speed vitrectomy probes (e.g., 2500 cuts per minute) and 23- or 25-gauge surgery may reduce the need for scissors or other ancillary instrumentation [72,73].

Scleral buckling may be necessary to neutralize peripheral retinal traction from unreachable or undissectable membranes [74], especially in cases with combined tractional and rhegmatogenous retinal detachment.

Control of Hemorrhage and Reproliferation. Intraoperative hemostasis facilitates completion of the other surgical objectives and optimizes the chance for surgical success by reducing postoperative fibrin and blood. While the latter are most apparent as media opacities, a potentially more deleterious factor is that they may contain promoters of cellular proliferation or serve as a template for reproliferation.

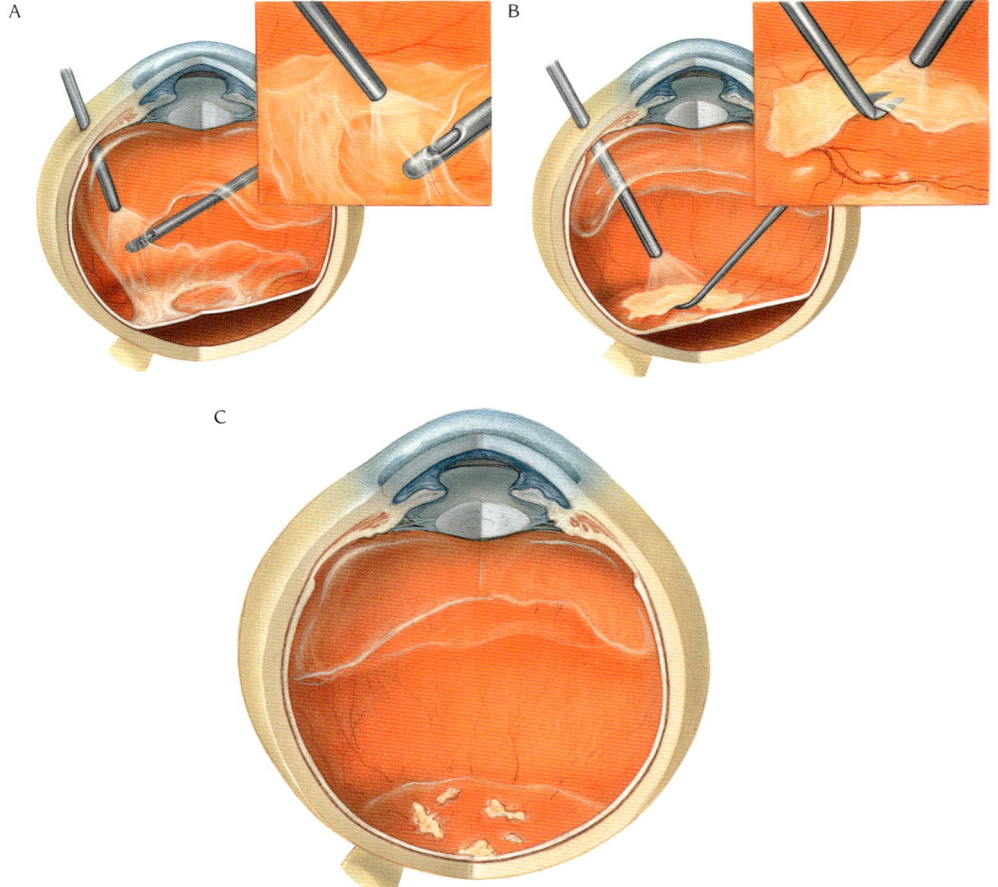

Figure 11.8. This series of illustrations demonstrates the technique of vitreoretinal surgery in which first media opacities and anterior to posterior traction is relieved (A), followed by relief of bridging traction (B), typically with the vitreous cutter (C). Vitreoretinal picks and scissors are used to segment preretinal membrane components. The final result is one of removal of all posterior segment traction with remnant stumps of fibrovascular proliferation. Sometimes, the fibrovascular proliferation is extensive and the posterior hyaloid is well defined. In such cases, the hyaloid may be peeled up in a relatively confluent fashion and fewer fibrovascular stumps ensue. This is more similar to the delamination technique. (Source: Redrawn with permission of Johns Hopkins University from Michels RG: Proliferative diabetic retinopathy: pathophysiology of extraretinal complications and principles of vitreous surgery. *Retina* 1981;1:1–17.)

Strategies to control bleeding include using intravitreal diathermy, increasing the infusion pressure, or using intraocular thrombin [75,76]. Optimal intraoperative control of systemic blood pressure lessens intraoperative and postoperative bleeding. Preoperative treatment with an anti-VEGF agent such as bevacizumab has been reported to reduce intraoperative bleeding [77–79]; the scope of its recommended use is being widely investigated.

An important surgical objective is control of reproliferation. With the advent of improved endolaser [80–84] and indirect laser ophthalmoscopic delivery systems

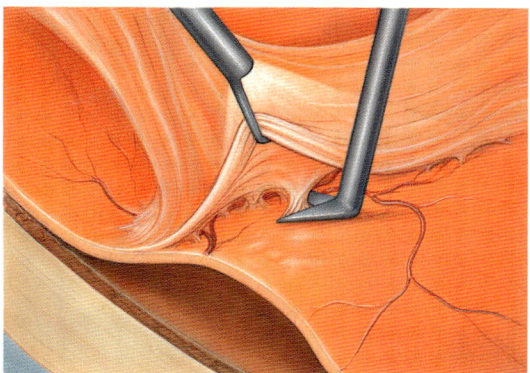

Figure 11.9. This schematic illustrates the delamination technique. Although similar to the en bloc technique, the horizontal scissors are more commonly supplemented by the use of lighted instruments such as lighted picks and lighted forceps to shave the fibrovascular proliferation from its retinal attachments. The end result characteristically shows fewer fibrovascular stumps.

[85,86], this objective can now be achieved reproducibly. Endolaser, even if PRP treatment has been applied, is usually delivered intraoperatively as it has been reported to reduce rates of postoperative vitreous hemorrhage [80]. Preoperative anterior segment NV often regresses after infusing silicone oil, possibly via blocking diffusion of a vasoproliferative substance, and may constitute an indication for the use of silicone oil in selected cases [87]. Lensectomy may lead to an increased risk of postoperative rubeosis, but this rate is reduced after application

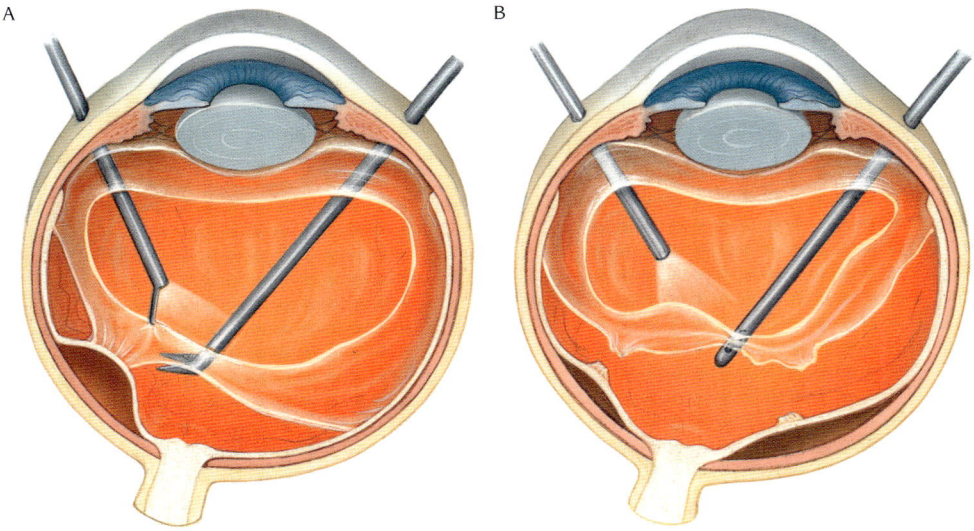

Figure 11.10. (A) These two illustrations depict the "en bloc" technique. Initially, a small core vitrectomy is performed. The posterior hyaloid space is entered and, typically, horizontal scissors are used to dissect the vitreous from the fibrovascular attachment. (B) Once this has been accomplished, the vitreous cutter is used to remove the remaining vitreous and fibrovascular proliferations in one "en bloc" fashion.

of intraoperative PRP. The illuminated laser probes allow endophotocoagulation with certain logistical conveniences [88,89]. Elevated pressure may persist despite regression of rubeosis iridis, and combined vitrectomy and glaucoma seton surgery may stabilize more advanced cases [90–92].

Management of Severe Conditions. A necessary surgical objective is treatment of pre-existing or iatrogenic retinal breaks. Intraoperative retinal breaks may occur during up to 20% of diabetic vitrectomy cases and may lead to retinal detachment if untreated [93]. Most intraoperative breaks can be managed successfully by performing fluid–gas exchange and applying endolaser photocoagulation. Silicone oil may play a role in effecting long-term internal tamponade, especially when there are multiple retinal breaks, as may be encountered in the setting of a reoperation for recurrent retinal detachment due to reproliferation of fibrovascular tissues causing PVR [94–97]. With anterior hyaloidal FVP, removal of the lens may allow more complete peripheral membrane dissection; lens removal is usually reserved for reoperations, and silicone oil is commonly utilized [98].

A final, but concurrent surgical objective is to treat and avoid future complications. Endolaser PRP, even if previous treatment has been applied, is usually delivered intraoperatively to reduce the likelihood of anterior segment NV, to treat retinal breaks, and to maintain retinal reattachment. Intraoperative PRP has also been reported to reduce rates of postoperative vitreous hemorrhage. Preoperative anterior segment NV often regresses in eyes with silicone oil, possibly by blocking diffusion of a vasoproliferative substance, and may constitute an indication for the use of silicone oil in selected cases [98]. Lensectomy may lead to an increased risk of postoperative rubeosis, but this rate is reduced after application of intraoperative PRP in more recent reports.

Instrumentation. A host of multifunction intraocular instruments has been developed to facilitate achieving the surgical objectives. The earliest vitreous cutter

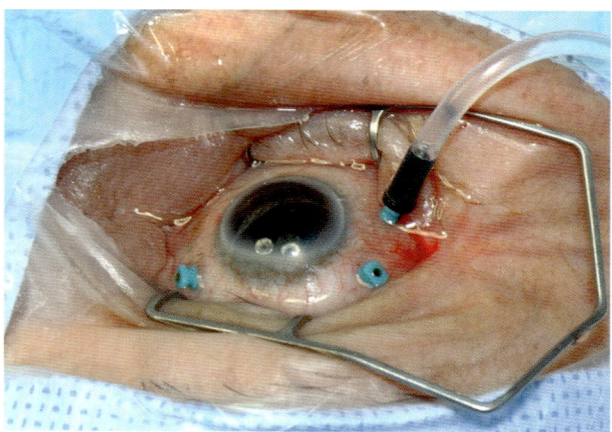

Figure 11.11. Transconjunctival 25-gauge ports for sutureless pars plana vitrectomy.

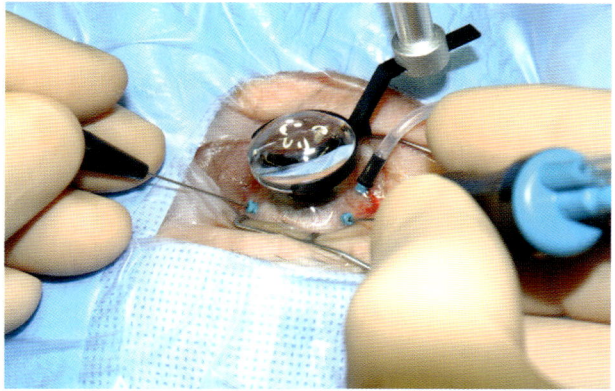

Figure 11.12. Noncontact wide-field viewing system for pars plana vitrectomy using 25-gauge instruments.

probes combined the functions of infusion, suction, and cutting. Later generations of instruments separated these three essential tasks and allowed smaller sclerotomies, which may have lowered the risk of iatrogenic retinal dialysis. The light probe has been modified to allow additional functions, including the illuminated pick or forceps or illuminated endolaser probe, while preserving a normal-sized sclerotomy. A multiport illumination system freeing up the second hand to use a pick or forceps has also been developed. The transconjunctival 23- or 25-gauge instrumentation system (Fig. 11.11) can achieve the surgical objectives and the small incisions may decrease morbidity and speed up postoperative recovery [72,73].

Wide-field viewing systems (Fig. 11.12) have been developed and are now commonly used to facilitate the global view of the posterior segment, thereby lessening the risk of inducing unintended traction and retinal breaks in distant areas [99,100]. Another useful innovation has been iris retractors [100–102]. Usually reserved for pseudophakic or aphakic patients, iris retractors facilitate achieving surgical objectives by allowing a maximum view of the posterior segment in patients with fixed, small pupils.

OUTCOMES OF VITRECTOMY

Concomitant traction, capillary nonperfusion, retinal detachment and macular edema influence visual acuity outcomes in patients with diabetic retinopathy. Thus, very few cases present with vitreous hemorrhage as the sole cause of visual loss because concurrent diabetic maculopathy and extensive capillary nonperfusion frequently coexist. With improvements in instrumentation, the complications of vitrectomy have decreased, allowing surgical intervention in patients with better preoperative visual acuity.

Media Opacities. The results of vitrectomy for nonclearing diabetic hemorrhage have been reviewed extensively [19,20,32–34,37,103,104]. The vision improves in

59% to 83% with a final visual acuity of ≥20/200 in 40% to 62%. The Diabetic Retinopathy Vitrectomy Study (DRVS) demonstrated that early vitrectomy (1–6 months after the onset of severe vitreous hemorrhage) for type 1 diabetics yields final visual acuity ≥20/40 at two years in 36% of this subgroup compared to only 12% with conventional management defined by the DRVS as deferral of vitrectomy until 12 months of hemorrhage ($p = 0.001$) [37]. The larger treatment differential is postulated to be due to the tendency for type 1 diabetic patients to have more extensive and aggressive NV at an earlier stage. However, the rate of no light perception, ≥5/200, and ≥20/200 were similar for both groups. Eyes with especially dense vitreous hemorrhage, particularly without previous PRP, are usually operated after a shorter waiting period [13].

Excellent surgical results have been reported for subhyaloid hemorrhage removal [105,106]. All patients with preoperative visual acuity ≥20/100 achieved a visual acuity of ≥20/40 after vitrectomy.

Combined cataract removal, vitrectomy, and endolaser has been studied in relatively small series with the finding that removal of the cataract does not increase the risk of rubeosis iridis or compromise the anatomic objectives [40–42].

Vitreoretinal Traction. The first report of the DRVS showed that observation over a year for patients with progressive FVP involved a nearly 50% rate of severe visual loss [107]. Those results justified a prospective study of 370 patients with severe NV randomized to early (within a few weeks) vitrectomy or conventional management (deferral of vitrectomy to 1 year unless tractional detachment involved the macula). The rate of final vision ≥20/40 was 44% for the early vitrectomy group compared to 28% in the conventional group with 4 years of follow-up ($p = <0.05$) [18]. Other investigators have found that preoperative factors indicating a more favorable postoperative result include age less than 40 years, preoperative vision ≥5/200, absence of iris NV, and application of preoperative photocoagulation [24]. One study involving a series of 50 eyes, many with relatively good visual acuity, reported that 72% had improvement and only 10% lost vision after vitrectomy [108]. Thus, vitrectomy can be considered even with only moderate visual loss (20/40–20/80 range) caused by progressive FVP [105,109].

The outcomes of vitrectomy for macula-involving tractional retinal detachment are, as expected, worse than those for vitreous hemorrhage. Visual improvement of greater than or equal to two lines or more has been reported in 59% to 80% of cases, but postoperative visual acuity of ≥20/200 results in only 21% to 58% [19,25,65,110–116].

The outcomes of vitrectomy for combined tractional and rhegmatogenous retinal detachment are generally worse. Visual improvement is reported in 32% to 53% and ≥20/200 final vision in 25% to 36% [22,115,116,117,118].

All too often, final visual acuity is limited despite successful achievement of the surgical and anatomic objectives. This outcome is usually attributable to generalized retinal ischemia, which may be evident as attenuated arterioles, capillary nonperfusion, and retinal thinning (featureless) (Fig. 11.13).

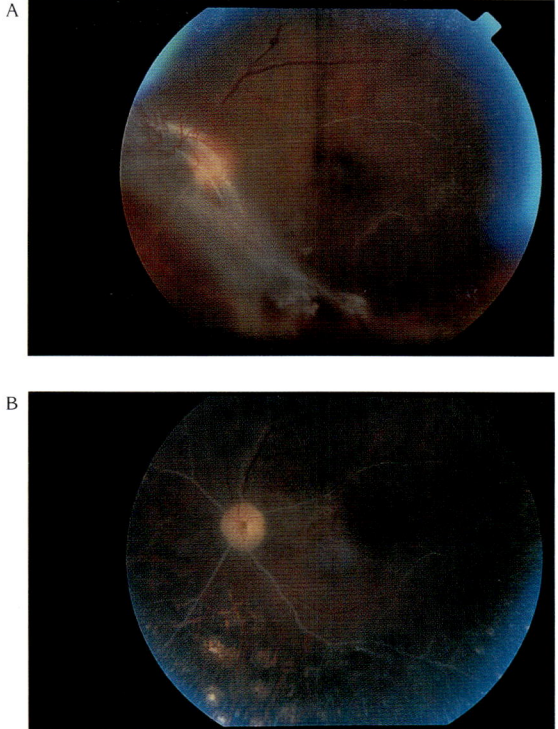

Figure 11.13. (A) This patient presented with vision of 20/400 and tractional elevation extending from the disc and inferotemporal arcade into the macula. Even preoperatively, marked vascular sclerosis extending into the macula is evident. (B) Postoperative appearance demonstrates a total removal of preretinal components and supplementary panretinal photocoagulation. However, the vascular sclerosis is now more evident and is the probable cause of the limited vision (postoperative vision was 20/200).

Complications of Previous Vitrectomy. The outcomes of repeat vitrectomy for complications after initial vitrectomy are often poor but visual acuity can be maintained or improved in many patients. A report of 41 reoperated eyes found that the reason for reoperation determined the visual prognosis, with rhegmatogenous retinal detachment carrying the worst prognosis [119]. Overall, 56% had a final visual acuity of light perception or no light perception, including 32% with phthisis and 94% with rubeosis iridis. It is this group that most frequently requires silicone oil to achieve even modest degrees of success [94–98].

COMPLICATIONS

The principal complications of vitrectomy in diabetic patients include recurrent vitreous hemorrhage, retinal detachment, and rubeosis irides [120–123]. Postoperative vitreous hemorrhage occurs to some degree in virtually all cases, but is severe in up to 30% of cases [121]. Management options include office-based fluid–gas exchange [54,124] or vitreous lavage. Before reoperation, a waiting period ranging from weeks to months is generally recommended to allow spontaneous clearing. The rates of postoperative retinal detachment and neovascular glaucoma vary with the preoperative diagnoses, and occur in up to 20% of cases. In severe cases with uncontrollable glaucoma, combined procedures such as pars plana vitrectomy, endolaser PRP, and Baerveldt glaucoma implants may be considered, since standard glaucoma filtering surgery is usually unsuccessful in such cases [123,124]. The risk of endophthalmitis after vitrectomy is higher in diabetic compared to nondiabetic patients [123,124], but is still very low. Other potential vitrectomy complications such as lens touch, peripheral retinal breaks or detachment, and choroidal hemorrhage are not unique to diabetic cases.

Public Health Considerations. As the technical upper limits in treating certain conditions are asymptotically approached, much attention has been directed toward optimal application of preventive therapies [2,3,125]. Javitt and associates have shown the cost-effectiveness of proper application of subsequent collaborative laser studies sponsored by the National Eye Institute to the diabetic population at risk [126]. With appropriate and timely laser photocoagulation, disability and associated expenses can be minimized.

Currently, medical care expenditures are being increasingly examined. The high costs for complex surgical cases, such as pars plana vitrectomy, have come under particular scrutiny and, indeed, have been a target of significant reimbursement reductions. The field of evidence-based medicine has emerged to evaluate the effectiveness of various treatment resources. These studies have been mostly focused on the functional outcomes of patients undergoing cataract surgery [127]. Outcomes research relies heavily on "patient satisfaction" and patients' perceptions of their functional status, which are difficult to quantify because of their subjective nature.

Objective measures of functional status were developed and studied in a series of 213 diabetic patients who underwent vitrectomy for complications of proliferative diabetic retinopathy [128]. In this series, the operated eye became the better-seeing eye in 32% of patients and equal to the fellow eye in 16%. These patients had an average of 61% disability of the visual system preoperatively (as determined by guidelines of the American Medical Association) because of the high frequency of disease in the fellow eye, but improved postoperatively to 50% disability. Improvements were greater in eyes without preoperative retinal detachment. Similar outcomes were found in analyses of nondiabetic vitreoretinal procedures [129] and in the same study, cohort outcomes were found to be worthwhile as measured by patient satisfaction surveys [130–132].

CONCLUSION

The indications and timing of pars plana vitrectomy for diabetic retinopathy continue to evolve but have not changed conceptually. The thresholds for doing surgery for established indications have generally been lowered and a few additional indications have been established. The lowered threshold is attributable to improvements in both instrumentation and surgical techniques. Accordingly, more difficult cases are now being considered and postoperative recovery of vision is more consistent.

Although the postoperative visual prognosis is favorable compared to the natural history, it is still poor compared to the potential efficacy of preventative measures, such as tight control of blood glucose, and timely application of laser treatment. Despite optimal medical and ophthalmological management, substantial numbers of eyes will have progressive retinopathy leading to the need for laser treatment and pars plana vitrectomy [16]. Since the long-term stability of initially successful treatment is good [133], and the life expectancy following diabetic vitrectomy is relatively favorable [134], pars plana vitrectomy remains an essential tool in the management of complications from diabetic retinopathy. Most recently, the increased understanding of the biochemical mediators of NV have led to preliminary reports of success with adjunctive pharmacotherapy for eyes undergoing vitrectomy, an area that is likely to be further developed in future years [77–79].

REFERENCES

1. Aiello LP, Gardner TW, King GL, et al. Diabetic retinopathy. *Diabetes Care.* 1998;21:143–156.
2. American Diabetes Association (Position Statement) Diabetic retinopathy. *Diabetes Care.* 2004;27(suppl.):84–87.
3. Patz A, Smith RE. The ETDRS and Diabetes 2000. *Ophthalmology.* 1991;98: 739–740.
4. The Diabetes Control and Complications Trial Research Group. The effect of intensive treatment of diabetes on the development and progression of long-term complications in insulin-dependent diabetes mellitus. *N Engl J Med.* 1993;329:977–986.
5. The Diabetes Control and Complications Trial Research Group. The effect of intensive diabetes treatment on the progression of diabetic retinopathy in insulin-dependent diabetes mellitus. *Arch Ophthalmol.* 1995;113:36–51.
6. Aiello LM, Beetham WP, Balodimos MC, et al. Ruby laser photocoagulation in treatment of diabetic proliferating retinopathy: preliminary report. In: Goldberg MI, Fine SL, eds. *Symposium on the Treatment of Diabetic Retinopathy.* US Public Health Service publication No. 1890. Washington DC: US Government Printing Office; 1968.
7. The Diabetic Retinopathy Study Research Group. Preliminary report on effects of photocoagulation therapy. *Am J Ophthalmol.* 1976;81:383–396.
8. The Diabetic Retinopathy Study Research Group. Photocoagulation treatment of proliferative diabetic retinopathy: the second report of the Diabetic Retinopathy Study findings. *Ophthalmology.* 1978;85:82–106.
9. The Diabetic Retinopathy Study Research Group. Four risk factors for severe visual loss in diabetic retinopathy. *Arch Ophthalmol.* 1979;97:654–655.
10. The Diabetic Retinopathy Study Research Group. Photocoagulation treatment of proliferative diabetic retinopathy: Relationship of adverse treatment effects to retinopathy severity. The Diabetic Retinopathy Study report No. 5. *Dev Ophthalmol.* 1981;2:248–261.

11. L'Esperance FA. The treatment of ophthalmic vascular disease by argon laser photocoagulation. *Ophthalmology.* 1968;72:1077–1096.

12. Doft BH, Metz DJ, Kelsey SF. Augmentation laser for proliferative diabetic retinopathy that fails to respond to initial panretinal photocoagulation. *Ophthalmology.* 1992;99:1728–1735.

13. Chew EY, Chair, Macula Society and Retina Society Representative, Benson WE, MD, Blodi BA. *Diabetic retinopathy. Preferred Practice Pattern.* San Francisco American Academy of Ophthalmology; 2008.

14. Vine AK. The efficacy of additional argon laser photocoagulation for persistent, severe proliferative diabetic retinopathy. *Ophthalmology.* 1985;92:1532–1537.

15. Javitt JC, Aiello LP, Bassi LJ, et al. Detecting and treating retinopathy in patients with Type 1 diabetes mellitus: savings associated with improved implementation of current guidelines. *Ophthalmology.* 1991;98:1565–1574.

16. Flynn HW Jr, Chew EY, Simons BD, et al. Pars plana vitrectomy in the Early Treatment Diabetic Retinopathy Study. *Ophthalmology.* 1992;99:1351–1357.

17. The Diabetic Retinopathy Study Research Group. Early vitrectomy for severe vitreous hemorrhage in diabetic retinopathy: two-year results of randomized trial. DRVS report No. 2. *Arch Ophthalmol.* 1985;03:1644–1652.

18. The Diabetic Retinopathy Study Research Group. Early vitrectomy for severe proliferative diabetic retinopathy in eyes with useful vision: results of a randomized trial. DRVS report No. 3. *Ophthalmology.* 1988;95:1307–1320.

19. Aaberg TM. Pars plana vitrectomy for diabetic traction retinal detachment. *Ophthalmology.* 1981;88:639–642.

20. Michels RG, Rice TA, Rice EF. Vitrectomy for diabetic vitreous hemorrhage. *Am J Ophthalmol.* 1983;95:12–21.

21. Blankenship GW. Preoperative prognostic factors in diabetic pars plana vitrectomy. *Ophthalmology.* 1982;89:1246–1249.

22. Sigurdsson H, Baines PS, Roxburgh STD. Vitrectomy for diabetic eye disease. *Eye.* 1988;2:418–423.

23. Rice TA, Michels RG, Rice EF. Vitrectomy for diabetic rhegmatogenous retinal detachment. *Am J Ophthalmol.* 1983;95:34–44.

24. de Bustros S, Thompson JT, Michels RG, Rice TA. Vitrectomy for progressive proliferative diabetic retinopathy. *Arch Ophthalmol.* 1987;105:196–199.

25. Hutton WL, Bernstein I, Fuller DG. Diabetic traction retinal detachment. *Ophthalmology.* 1980;87:1071–1077.

26. Machemer R, Norton EWD. A new concept for vitreous surgery, 3. Indications and results. *Am J Ophthalmol.* 1972;74:1034–1055.

27. Michels RG. Vitrectomy for complications of diabetic retinopathy. *Arch Ophthalmol.* 1978;96:237–246.

28. Ho T, Smiddy WE, Flynn HW Jr. Vitrectomy in the management of diabetic eye disease. *Surv Ophthalmol.* 1992;37:190–202.

29. Lewis H, Abrams GW, Blumenkranz MS, Campo RV. Resolution of diabetic macular edema associated with a thickened and taut premacular posterior hyaloid after vitrectomy. *Ophthalmology.* 1991;98(S):146.

30. Harbour W, Smiddy WE, Flynn HW Jr, Rubsamen PE. Vitrectomy for diabetic macular edema associated with posterior hyaloid thickening and contraction. *Am J Ophthalmol.* 1996;121:405–413.

31. Hartley KL, Smiddy WE, Flynn HW Jr, Murray TG. Pars plana vitrectomy with internal limiting membrane peeling for diabetic macular edema. *Retina.* 2008;28:410–419.

32. Machemer R, Blankenship G. Vitrectomy for proliferative diabetic retinopathy associated with vitreous hemorrhage. *Ophthalmology.* 1981;88:643–646.
33. Aaberg TM, Abrams GW. Changing indications and techniques for vitrectomy in management of complications of diabetic retinopathy. *Ophthalmology.* 1987;94:775–779.
34. Machemer R. Pathogenesis of proliferative neovascular retinopathies and the role of vitrectomies: a hypothesis. *Int Ophthalmol.* 1978;1:1–3.
35. Davis MD. Vitreous contraction in proliferative diabetic retinopathy. *Arch Ophthalmol.* 1965;74:741.
36. Fallborn J, Bowald S. Micro-proliferations in proliferative diabetic retinopathy and their relationship to the vitreous: corresponding light and electron microscopic studies. *Graefe's Arch Clin Exp Ophthalmol.* 1985;223:130–136.
37. The Diabetic Retinopathy Study Research Group. Early vitrectomy for severe vitreous hemorrhage in diabetic retinopathy. Four-year results of a randomized trial: the Diabetic Retinopathy Study Report No. 5. *Arch Ophthalmol.* 1990;108:958–964.
38. Blankenship GW. The lens influence on diabetic vitrectomy results. Report of a prospective randomized study. *Arch Ophthalmol.* 1980;98:2196–2198.
39. Aiello RC, Wand M, Liang G. Neovascular glaucoma and vitreous hemorrhage following cataract surgery in patients with diabetes mellitus. *Ophthalmology.* 1983;90:814–820.
40. Blankenship GW, Cortez R, Machemer R. The lens and pars plana vitrectomy for diabetic retinopathy complications. *Arch Ophthalmol.* 1979;97:1263–1267.
41. Rice TA, Michels RG, Maguire MG, Rice EF. The effect of lensectomy on the incidence of iris neovascularization and neovascular glaucoma after vitrectomy for diabetic retinopathy. *Am J Ophthalmol.* 1983;95:1–11.
42. Blankenship GW, Flynn HW Jr, Kokame G. Posterior chamber intraocular lens insertion during pars plana lensectomy and vitrectomy for complications of proliferative diabetic retinopathy. *Am J Ophthalmol.* 1989;108:1–5.
43. Kokame GT, Flynn HW Jr, Blankenship GW. Posterior chamber intraocular lens implantation during diabetic pars plana vitrectomy. *Ophthalmology.* 1989;96:603–610.
44. Benson WE, Brown GC, Tasman W, McNamara JA. Extracapsular cataract extraction, posterior chamber lens insertion, and pars plana vitrectomy in one operation. *Ophthalmology.* 1990;97:918–921.
45. Küchle M, Händel A, Naumann GOH. Cataract extraction in eyes with diabetic iris neovascularization. *Ophthalmic Surg Lasers.* 1998;29(1):28–32.
46. Sato Y, Hiroyuki S, Shinichi A, Matsui M. Vitrectomy for diabetic macular heterotopia. *Ophthalmology.* 1994;101(1):63–67.
47. Charles S, Flinn CE. The natural history of diabetic extramacular traction retinal detachment. *Arch Ophthalmol.* 1981;99:66–68.
48. Early Treatment Diabetic Retinopathy Study Research Group. Photocoagulation for diabetic macular edema. ETDRS report No. 1. *Arch Ophthalmol.* 1985;103:1796–1806.
49. Campbell DG, Simmons RJ, Tolentino FI, McMeel JW. Glaucoma occurring after closed vitrectomy. *Am J Ophthalmol.* 1977;83:63–69.
50. Campbell DG, Simmons RJ, Grant WM. Ghost cells as a cause of glaucoma. *Am J Ophthalmol.* 1976;81:441–450.
51. Han DP, Lewis H, Lambrou FH Jr, et al. Mechanisms of intraocular pressure elevation after pars plana vitrectomy. *Ophthalmology.* 1989;96:1357–1362.
52. Weinberg RS, Peyman GA, Huamonte FJ. Elevation of intraocular pressure after pars plana vitrectomy. *Albrecht von Graefes Arch Klin Exp Ophthalmol.* 1976;200:157–161.

53. Singh H, Grand MG. Treatment of blood-induced glaucoma by trans plana vitrectomy. *Retina*. 1981;1:255.
54. Miller JA, Chandra SR, Stevens TS. A modified technique for performing outpatient fluid-air exchange following vitrectomy surgery. *Am J Ophthalmol*. 1986;101: 116–117.
55. Blankenship GW. Management of vitreous cavity hemorrhage following pars plana vitrectomy for diabetic retinopathy. *Ophthalmology*. 1986;93:39–44.
56. Lewis H, Abrams GW, Williams GA. Anterior hyaloidal fibrovascular proliferation after diabetic vitrectomy. *Am J Ophthalmol*. 1987;104:607–613.
57. Chen E, Park CH. Use of intravitreal bevacizumab as a preoperative adjunct for tractional retinal detachment repair in severe proliferative diabetic retinopathy. *Retina*. 2006;26:699–700.
58. Avery RL, Pearlman J, Pieramici DJ, et al. Intravitreal bevacizumab (Avastin) in the treatment of proliferative diabetic retinopathy. *Ophthalmology*. 2006;113:1695, e1–e15.
59. Arevalo, JF, Maia, M, Flynn HW Jr, et al. Traction retinal detachment following intravitreal bevacizumab (Avastin) in patients with severe proliferative diabetic retinopathy. *Br J Ophthalmol*. 2008;92:213–216.
60. Sebestyen JG. Fibrinoid syndrome: a severe complication of vitrectomy in diabetics. *Ann Ophthalmol*. 1982;14:853–856.
61. Williams GA, Lambrou FH, Jaffe GA, et al. Treatment of post-vitrectomy fibrin formation with intraocular tissue plasminogen activator. *Arch Ophthalmol*. 1988;106:1055–1058.
62. Cherfan GM, Maghraby AE, Tabbara KF, et al. Dissolution of intraocular fibrinous exudate by streptokinase. *Ophthalmology*. 1991;98:870–874.
63. Michels RG. Proliferative diabetic retinopathy: pathophysiology of extraretinal complications and principles of vitreous surgery. *Retina*. 1981;1:1–17.
64. Meredith TA, Kaplan HJ, Aaberg TM. Pars plana vitrectomy techniques for relief of epiretinal traction by membrane segmentation. *Am J Ophthalmol*. 1980;89: 408–413.
65. Charles S. *Vitreous Microsurgery*. Baltimore: Williams & Wilkins; 1981:107–120.
66. Meredith TA. Epiretinal membrane delamination with a diamond knife. *Arch Ophthalmol*. 1997;115:1598–1599.
67. Abrams GW, Williams GA: "En bloc" excision of diabetic membranes. *Am J Ophthalmol*. 1987;103:302–308.
68. McCuen BW II, Hickingbotham D. Fiberoptic diathermy tissue manipulator for use in vitreous surgery. *Am J Ophthalmol*. 1984;98:803–804.
69. Abrams GW. Dissection methods in vitrectomy for diabetic retinopathy. In: Franklin RM, editor. *Retina and Vitreous*. Amsterdam/New York: Kugler Publication; 1993:101–113.
70. Williams DF, Williams GA, Hartz A, et al. Results of vitrectomy for diabetic traction retinal detachments using the en bloc excision technique. *Ophthalmology*. 1989;96:752–758.
71. Han DP, Murphy ML, Mieler WF. A modified en bloc excision technique during vitrectomy for diabetic traction retinal detachment. *Ophthalmology*. 1994;101: 803–808.
72. Fujii GY, de Juan E Jr, Humayun MS, et al. Initial experience using the transconjunctival sutureless vitrectomy system for vitreoretinal surgery. *Ophthalmology*. 2002;109:1814–1820.

73. Ibarra MS, Hermel M, Prenner JL, Hassan TS. Longer-term outcomes of transconjunctival sutureless 25-gauge vitrectomy. *Am J Ophthalmol*. 2005;139:831–836.
74. Han DP, Pulido JS, Mieler WF, Johnson MW. Vitrectomy for proliferative diabetic retinopathy with severe equatorial fibrovascular proliferation. *Am J Ophthalmol*. 1995;119:563–570.
75. de Bustros S, Glaser BM, Johnson MA. Thrombin infusion for the control of intraocular bleeding during vitreous surgery. *Arch Ophthalmol*. 1985;103:837–839.
76. Thompson JT, Glaser BM, Michels RG, de Bustros S. The use of intravitreal thrombin to control hemorrhage during vitrectomy. *Ophthalmology*. 1986;93:279–282.
77. Spaide RF, Fisher YL. Intravitreal bevacizumab (Avastin) treatment of proliferative diabetic retinopathy complicated by vitreous hemorrhage. *Retina*. March 2006;26(3):275–278.
78. Avery RL. Regression of retinal and iris neovascularization after intravitreal bevacizumab (Avastin) treatment. *Retina*. March 2006;26(3):352–354.
79. Bakri SJ, Donaldson MJ, Link TP. Rapid regression of disc neovascularization in a patient with proliferative diabetic retinopathy following adjunctive intravitreal bevacizumab. *Eye*. December 2006;20(12):1474–1475.
80. Charles S. Endophotocoagulation. *Retina*. 1981;1:117–120.
81. Fleischman JA, Swartz M, Dixon JA. Argon laser endophotocoagulation, an intraoperative trans-pars plana technique. *Arch Ophthalmol*. 1981;99:1610–1612.
82. Liggett PE, Lean JS, Barlow WE, Ryan SJ. Intraoperative argon endophotocoagulation for recurrent vitreous hemorrhage after vitrectomy for diabetic retinopathy. *Am J Ophthalmol*. 1987;103:146–149.
83. Landers MB III, Trese MT, Stefansson E, Bessler M. Argon laser intraocular photocoagulation. *Ophthalmology*. 1982;89:785–788.
84. Parke DW III, Aaberg TM. Intraocular argon laser photocoagulation in the management of severe proliferative vitreoretinopathy. *Am J Ophthalmol*. 1984;97:434–443.
85. Friberg TR. Clinical experience with a binocular indirect ophthalmoscope laser delivery system. *Retina*. 1987;7:28–31.
86. Whitacre MM, Manoukian N, Mainster MA. Argon indirect ophthalmoscopic photocoagulation: reduced potential phototoxicity with a fixed safety filter. *Br J Ophthalmol*. 1990;74:233–234.
87. McCuen BW II, Rinkoff JS Silicone oil for progressive anterior ocular neovascularization after failed diabetic vitrectomy. *Arch Ophthalmol*. 1989;107:677–682.
88. Smiddy WE. Diode endolaser photocoagulation. *Arch Ophthalmol*. 1992;110:1172–1176.
89. Sasoh M, Smiddy WE. Diode endolaser photocoagulation. *Retina*. 1995;15:388–393.
90. Smiddy WE, Rubsamen PE, Grajewski A. Vitrectomy for pars plana placement of Molteno implant tube. *Ophthalmic Surg*. 1994;25:532–535.
91. Lloyd MA, Heuer DK, Baerveldt G, et al. Combined Molteno implantation and pars plana vitrectomy for neovascular glaucomas. *Ophthalmology*. 1991;98:1401–1405.
92. Varma R, Heuer DK, Lundy DC, et al. Pars plana Baerveldt tube insertion with vitrectomy in glaucomas associated with pseudophakia and aphakia. *Am J Ophthalmol*. 1995;119:401–407.
93. Oyakawa RT, Schachat AP, Michels RG, Rice TA. Complications of vitreous surgery for diabetic retinopathy. *Ophthalmology*. 1983;90:517–521.

94. Rinkoff JS, de Juan E Jr, McCuen BW. Silicone oil for retinal detachment with advanced proliferative vitreoretinopathy following failed vitrectomy for proliferative diabetic retinopathy. *Am J Ophthalmol.* 1986;101:181–186.

95. Yeo JH, Glaser BM, Michels RG. Silicone oil in the treatment of complicated retinal detachments. *Ophthalmology.* 1987;94:1109–1113.

96. Heimann K, Dahl B, Dimopoulos S, Lemmen KD. Pars plana vitrectomy and silicone oil injection in proliferative diabetic retinopathy. *Graefe's Arch Clin Exp Ophthalmol.* 1989;227:152–156.

97. Brourman ND, Blumenkranz MS, Cox MS, Trese MT. Silicone oil for the treatment of severe proliferative diabetic retinopathy. *Ophthalmology.* 1989;96:759–764.

98. Douglas MJ, Scott IU, Flynn HW Jr. Pars plana lensectomy, pars plana vitrectomy, and silicone oil tamponade as initial management of cataract and combined traction/rhegmatogenous retinal detachment involving the macula associated with severe proliferative diabetic retinopathy. *Ophthalmic Surg.* 2003;34:270–278.

99. Spitznas M. A binocular indirect ophthalmomicroscope (BIOM) for non-contact wide-angle vitreous surgery. *Graefe's Arch Clin Exp Ophthalmol.* 1987;225:13–15.

100. Spitznas M, Reiner J. A stereoscopic diagonal inverter (SDI) for wide-angle vitreous surgery. *Graefe's Arch Clin Exp Ophthalmol.* 1987;225:9–12.

101. DeJuan E Jr, Hickingbotham D. Flexible iris retractor. *Am J Ophthalmol.* 1991; 111(6):776–777.

102. Arpa P. A new device for pupillary dilatation in vitreous surgery. *Retina.* 1992;12: S87–S89.

103. Blankenship GW. Proliferative diabetic retinopathy: Principles and techniques of surgical treatment. In: Ryan SJ, ed. *Retina.* St. Louis: CV Mosby Co.; 1989:51–539.

104. Peyman GA, Raichand M, Huamonte F, et al. Vitrectomy in 125 eyes with diabetic vitreous haemorrhage. *Br J Ophthalmol.* 1976;60:752–755.

105. The Diabetic Retinopathy Study Research Group. Early vitrectomy for severe proliferative diabetic retinopathy in eyes with useful vision. Clinical application of results of a randomized trial. DRVS report No. 4. *Ophthalmology.* 1988;95:1321–1334.

106. Packer AJ. Vitrectomy for progressive macular traction associated with proliferative diabetic retinopathy. *Arch Ophthalmol.* 1987;105:1679–1683.

107. The Diabetic Retinopathy Vitrectomy Study Research Group. Two-year course of visual acuity in severe proliferative diabetic retinopathy with conventional management. DRVS Report No. 1. *Ophthalmology.* 1985;92:492–502.

108. Rice TA, Michels RG. Long-term anatomic and functional results of vitrectomy for diabetic retinopathy. *Am J Ophthalmol.* 1980;90:297–303.

109. Grewing R, Mester U. Early vitrectomy for progressive diabetic proliferations covering the macula. *Br J Ophthalmol.* 1994;78:433–436.

110. Thompson JT, de Bustros S, Michels RG, Rice TA, Glaser BM. Results of vitrectomy for proliferative diabetic retinopathy. *Ophthalmology.* 1986;93:1571–1574.

111. Miller SA, Butler JB, Myers FL, Bresnick GH. Pars plana vitrectomy. Treatment for tractional macular detachment secondary to proliferative diabetic retinopathy. *Arch Ophthalmol.* 1980;98:659–664.

112. Rice TA, Michels RG, Rice EF. Vitrectomy for diabetic traction retinal detachment involving the macula. *Am J Ophthalmol.* 1983;95:22–33.

113. Thompson JT, de Bustros S, Michels RG, Rice TA. Results and prognostic factors in vitrectomy for diabetic traction retinal detachment of the macula. *Arch Ophthalmol.* 1987;105:497–502.

114. Tolentino FI, Freeman HM, Tolentino FL. Closed vitrectomy in the management of diabetic traction retinal detachment. *Ophthalmology*. 1980;87:1078–1089.
115. Nakae R, Saito Y, Nishikawa N, Ikeda T, Tano Y. Results of vitrectomy for diabetic traction retinal detachment involving the macula: A comparison of six-month and three-year postoperative findings. *Nippon Ganka Gakkai Zasshi-Acta Societatis Ophthalmologicae Japonica*. 1989;93:271–275.
116. Meier P, Weidemann P. Vitrectomy for traction macular detachment in diabetic retinopathy. *Graefe's Arch Clin Exp Ophthalmol*. 1997;235:569–574.
117. Rice TA, Michels RG, Rice EF. Vitrectomy for diabetic rhegmatogenous retinal detachment. *Am J Ophthalmol*. 1983;95:34–44.
118. Thompson JT, de Bustros S, Michels RG, Rice TA. Results and prognostic factors in vitrectomy for diabetic traction rhegmatogenous retinal detachment. *Arch Ophthalmol*. 1987;105:503–507.
119. Brown GC, Tasman WS, Benson WE, et al. Reoperation following diabetic vitrectomy. *Arch Ophthalmol*. 1992;110:506–510.
120. Aaberg TM, Van Horn DL. Late complications of pars plana vitreous surgery. *Ophthalmology*. 1978;85:126–140.
121. Schachat AP, Oyakawa RT, Michels RG, Rice TA. Complications of vitreous surgery for diabetic retinopathy. II. Postoperative complications. *Ophthalmology*. 1983;90:522–530.
122. Novak MA, Rice TA, Michels RG, Auer C. Vitreous hemorrhage after vitrectomy for diabetic retinopathy. *Ophthalmology*. 1984;91:1485–1489.
123. Wand M, Madigan JC, Gaudio AR, Sorokanich S. Neovascular glaucoma following pars plana vitrectomy for complications of diabetic retinopathy. *Ophthalmic Surg*. 1990;21:113–117.
124. Martin DF, McCuen BW II. Efficacy of fluid-air exchange for postvitrectomy diabetic vitreous hemorrhage. *Am J Ophthalmol*. 1992;114:457–463.
125. Cohen SM, Flynn HW Jr, Murray TG, Smiddy WE. Endophthalmitis after pars plana vitrectomy. *Ophthalmology*. 1995;102:705–712.
126. Eifrig CWM, Scott IU, Flynn HW Jr., Smiddy WE, Newton J. Endophthalmitis after pars plana vitrectomy: incidence, causative organisms, and visual acuity outcomes. *Am J Ophthalmol*. 2005;138:183–184.
127. Chew EY, Chair, Macula Society and Retina Society Representative, Benson WE, MD, Blodi BA. *Diabetic Retinopathy. Preferred Practice Pattern*. San Francisco. American Academy of Ophthalmology; 2008.
128. Javitt JC, Aiello LP, Bassi LJ, et al. Detecting and treating retinopathy in patients with type 1 diabetes mellitus; savings associated with improved implementation of current guidelines. *Ophthalmology*. 1991;98:1565–1574.
129. Steinberg EP, Tielsch JM, Schein OD, et al. National study of cataract surgery outcomes: variation in 4-month postoperative outcomes as reflected in multiple outcome measures. *Ophthalmology*. 1994;101:1131–1141.
130. Smiddy WE, Feuer W, Irvine WD, et al. Vitrectomy for complications of proliferative diabetic retinopathy: functional outcomes. *Ophthalmology*. 1995;102:1688–1695.
131. Scott IU, Smiddy WE, Merikansky A, Feuer W. Vitreoretinal surgery outcomes: impact on bilateral visual function. *Ophthalmology*. 1997;104:1041–1048.
132. Scott IU, Smiddy WE, Feuer W, Merikansky A. Vitreoretinal surgery outcomes results of a patient satisfaction/functional status survey. *Ophthalmology*. 1998;105:795–803.

133. Blankenship GW, Machemer R. Long-term diabetic vitrectomy results: report of a 10-year follow-up. *Ophthalmology.* 1985;92:503–506.
134. Gollamudi SR, Smiddy WE, Schachat AP, et al. Long-term survival rate after vitreous surgery for complications of diabetic retinopathy. *Ophthalmology.* 1991;98:18–22.

12

Intravitreal Pharmacotherapies for Diabetic Retinopathy

SOPHIE J. BAKRI, MD,
AND PETER K. KAISER, MD

CORE MESSAGES

- Intravitreal pharmacotherapies are now being used as an adjunct to traditional laser treatments in diabetic retinopathy.
- The most common complication of intravitreal triamcinolone is an intraocular pressure elevation.
- Other complications of intravitreal triamcinolone include infectious and non-infectious endophthalmitis, cataract, and retinal detachment.
- Trials of sustained-release steroid implants in diabetic macular edema are under way.
- Intravitreal anti-vascular endothelial growth factor (anti-VEGF) agents are also under clinical testing for diabetic macular edema, and have shown early promise.

*I*n the past few years, delivering medication to the eye via the intravitreal route has become increasingly utilized. Intravitreal corticosteroids have played an increasing role in the treatment of macular edema owing to a variety of causes, and intravitreal anti-VEGF agents are currently in clinical trials.

INTRAVITREAL CORTICOSTEROIDS

History of Intravitreal Corticosteroids in Retinal Disease. The use of intravitreal corticosteroids was first reported by Machemer in 1979 [1] in an effort to halt cellular proliferation after retinal detachment surgery. Graham [2], McCuen [3], Tano [4], and others have studied its use in both animal and human models.

Several corticosteroids have been evaluated; however, triamcinolone acetonide was chosen because of its long half-life of 18.6 days in the nonvitrectomized eye [5], lack of toxicity, and the fact that it was generally well tolerated [3,6]. In addition, there is a considerable body of literature describing the efficacy of triamcinolone administration in various ocular diseases including uveitis [7,8], macular edema secondary to ocular trauma or retinal vascular disease [9], proliferative diabetic retinopathy (PDR) [10], intraocular proliferation such as proliferative vitreoretinopathy [11], and choroidal neovascularization from age-related macular degeneration [12,13].

The Rationale for Using Intravitreal Triamcinolone Acetonide in Diabetic Retinopathy. Aiello et al. [14] reported increased levels of VEGF in eyes with PDR, and Funatsu et al. [15] have reported increased levels of VEGF in eyes with diabetic macular edema (DME). The cause of DME is believed to be multifactorial, because of breakdown of the blood–retinal barrier secondary to alterations of various antipermeability factors, such as interleukin-6 and VEGF.

Corticosteroids have antiangiogenic, antifibrotic, and antipermeability properties. The principal effects of corticosteroids are stabilization of the blood–retinal barrier, resorption of exudation, and down-regulation of inflammatory stimuli [16–20].

Experimentally, corticosteroids have been shown to reduce inflammatory mediators including interleukin-5, interleukin-6, interleukin-8, prostaglandins, interferon-gamma, and tumor necrosis factor [16–18]; decrease levels of VEGF, a potent permeability factor [19,20]; and improve blood–retinal barrier function [21]. Several known mechanisms of action of corticosteroids could explain the stabilization of the blood–retinal barrier including stabilization of cell and lysosomal membranes [22], reduction of the release [22] or synthesis [23] of prostaglandins, inhibition of cellular proliferation [24], blockage of macrophage recruitment in response to macrophage inhibitory factor, inhibition of phagocytosis by mature macrophages, and decreased polymorphonuclear infiltration into injured tissues [25]. Triamcinolone acetonide in particular has been shown to have an antiangiogenic effect. It has been shown to inhibit basic fibroblast growth factor–induced migration and tube formation in choroidal microvascular endothelial cells and down-regulate metalloproteinase-2 (MMP-2) [26], decrease permeability and down-regulate intercellular adhesion molecule-1 (ICAM-1) expression in vitro [27], and decrease major histocompatibility complex-II (MHC-II) antigen expression [28].

Penfold and associates found that triamcinolone acetonide significantly decreased MHC-II expression consistent with immunocytochemical observations, which revealed condensed microglial morphology [28]. The modulation of subretinal edema and microglial morphology correlated with in vitro observations suggesting that down-regulation of inflammatory markers and endothelial cell permeability are significant features of the mode of action of triamcinolone acetonide. In another study, Penfold et al. investigated the capacity of triamcinolone to modulate the expression of adhesion molecules and permeability using a human epithelial cell line (ECV304) as a model of the outer blood–retinal barrier [27]. They found that triamcinolone modulated transepithelial resistance of TER and ICAM-1 expression in vitro, suggesting that reestablishment of the blood–retinal barrier and down-regulation of inflammatory markers are the principal effects of intravitreal triamcinolone in vivo. These studies indicate that triamcinolone has the potential to influence cellular permeability, including the barrier function of the retinal pigment epithelium.

Why Deliver Triamcinolone by Intravitreal Injection? Topical corticosteroids have been shown to penetrate the anterior segment [29], but not the posterior segment. Topical corticosteroids sometimes reduce cystoid macular edema occurring after cataract extraction, by reducing the anterior segment inflammation causing the cystoid macular edema. Posterior subtenon corticosteroids may be useful in the treatment of DME [30], but they take longer to diffuse into the posterior segment, and placement over the macula may be variable. In addition, there is considerable systemic absorption with a subtenon injection, which may adversely influence blood sugar levels in diabetic patients. The best way to circumvent the blood–ocular barrier is by direct intravitreal injection. Intravitreal triamcinolone has been shown to deliver high initial concentrations to the target tissue and provide effective levels for at least 3 months [5].

Preclinical Evaluation of the Safety of Intravitreal Triamcinolone. A single, pure, intravitreal triamcinolone acetonide injection has been shown to be well tolerated in rabbit eyes [3]. Electroretinographic data showed no significant differences between treated and control eyes and both light and electron microscopy were normal in both groups. Hida and associates [6] investigated the vehicles of six commercially available depot corticosteroids in rabbit eyes and found no toxic effect on the retina and lens with the vehicle in Kenalog (commercially available triamcinolone acetonide) at levels two times higher than in the marketed drug. However, preservatives present in the vehicle for Kenalog including benzyl alcohol were shown in the same report to have toxic effects on the retina in other steroid preparations. Triescence (Alcon, Fort Worth, TX) is a preservative-free preparation of triamcinolone acetonide that is approved by the Food and Drug Administration (FDA) for intraocular use. It comes as a 1-mL vial containing a suspension of triamcinolone acetonide with concentration of 40 mg/mL. Recommended dosing is 1 to 4 mg (25–100 mL) administered intravitreally. Trivaris (Allergan, Irvine, CA) was also recently approved as a preservative-free gel for intravitreal injection. It was used in the National Eye Institute-sponsored clinical trials evaluating intraocular corticosteroids for macular edema (e.g., SCORE, DRCR.net trials). It comes in a blister pack as a 0.1-mL vial with 8 mg of triamcinolone acetonide; therefore, the concentration is 8 mg/0.1 mL. As an off-label use, Kenalog (Bristol-Myers Squibb, Peapack, NJ) can be administered for the same indication. Kenalog contains benzyl alcohol as a preservative; many retinal surgeons prefer to use nonpreserved Kenalog, after a compounding pharmacy removes the preservative [31]. The standard concentration of this preparation is 40 mg/mL.

Efficacy of Intravitreal Triamcinolone for Diabetic Macular Edema. In the first report of intravitreal corticosteroids for DME, Martidis and colleagues [32] injected 4 mg of intravitreal triamcinolone into 16 eyes with clinically significant macular edema (CSME) that failed to respond to at least two previous sessions of laser photocoagulation. With all patients in this retrospective study completing 1- and 3-month follow-up, and 50% completing 6 or more months, the mean improvement in visual acuity was 2.4, 2.4, and 1.3 Snellen lines at the 1-, 3-, and 6-month follow-up intervals, respectively. The central macular thickness measured by optical coherence tomography (OCT) decreased by 55%, 57.5%, and 38%, respectively, from a baseline mean thickness of 540 microns. Reinjection was performed in three of eight eyes after 6 months because of recurrence of macular edema.

Another interventional case series included 26 eyes of 20 patients who received 25 mg of intravitreal triamcinolone acetonide by repeatedly filtering and concentrating the standard triacminolone acetonide preparation, for treatment of diffuse DME [33]. Visual acuity improved from 20/166 at baseline to 20/105 over a mean of 6.64 months follow-up ($P < 0.001$), compared with a control group of 16 patients who underwent macular grid laser photocoagulation. Seventeen (81%) of 21 injected eyes with a follow-up period of more than 1 month had improved visual acuity; in contrast, the visual acuity of the control group did not change significantly.

In the Intravitreal Steroid Injection Study (ISIS) [34], a prospective, pilot study, 30 eyes of 30 patients were randomized to receive either 2 or 4 mg intravitreal triamcinolone for CSME present at least 3 months and refractory to focal laser treatment. Mean change in visual acuity at 3 months compared to baseline was 7.1 letters ($P = 0.01$) in the 2-mg group and 12.5 letters in the 4-mg group ($P < 0.0001$). There was no significant difference in visual gain between the 2- and 4-mg dose groups ($P = 0.11$). Vision improved >15 letters at 3 months in 23% (3/13) of the 2-mg group and in 33% (5/15) of the 4-mg group ($P = 0.69$), and 0% (0/11) and 21% (3/14) at 6 months, respectively ($P = 0.23$). Visual improvement was more likely in cystoid-type DME than diffuse DME.

In a small, randomized study, Massin and associates [35] evaluated 12 patients with bilateral DME unresponsive to laser photocoagulation. One eye was randomized to receive 4 mg intravitreal triamcinolone, and the other eye was observed. All patients were followed for at least 3 months; seven had a follow-up of 6 months. The baseline central macular thickness measured by OCT was 510 microns in injected eyes and 474 microns in control eyes. Retinal thickness improved to 207 microns ($P < 0.001$) in injected eyes and was not improved in control eyes (506 microns) at 4 weeks after injection. Retinal thickness remained improved in the injected eyes after 12 weeks (207 microns) and was significantly ($P = 0.005$) different from the control eyes (469 microns). The difference between the central macular thickness of injected and control eyes was no longer significant at 24 weeks because of the recurrence of macular edema in 5 of 12 (42%) injected eyes. Despite the improved anatomic results demonstrated by OCT, at no time was the difference between the visual acuity scores measured on the Early Treatment Diabetic Retinopathy Study (ETDRS) chart for injected and control eyes significant.

The Diabetic Retinopathy Clinical Research network (DRCR.net) conducted a prospective randomized trial comparing laser treatment with intravitreal injection of either 1- or 4-mg doses of Trivaris (Allergan, Irvine, CA), a new formulation of preservative-free triamcinolone acetonide for DME. Eight hundred forty study eyes of 693 subjects with DME involving the fovea and with visual acuity of 20/40 to 20/320 were randomized to focal/grid photocoagulation ($n = 330$), 1 mg intravitreal triamcinolone ($n = 256$), or 4 mg intravitreal triamcinolone ($n = 254$). Retreatment was given for persistent or new edema at 4-month intervals. At 4 months, mean visual acuity was better in the 4-mg triamcinolone group than in either the laser group ($P < 0.001$) or the 1-mg triamcinolone group ($P = 0.001$). However, by 1 year, there were no significant differences among groups in mean visual acuity. At the 16-month visit and extending through the primary outcome at 2 years, the mean change in visual acuity was better in the laser group than in the other two groups (at 2 years, $P = 0.02$ comparing the laser and 1-mg groups, $P = 0.002$ comparing the laser and 4-mg groups, and $P = 0.49$ comparing the 1- and 4-mg groups). Treatment group differences in the visual acuity outcome could not be attributed solely to cataract formation. Optical coherence tomography results generally paralleled the visual acuity results.

The DRCR.net study concluded that over a 2-year period, focal/grid photocoagulation is more effective and has fewer side effects than 1- or 4-mg doses of preservative-free intravitreal triamcinolone for most patients with DME who have characteristics similar to the cohort in this clinical trial. However, 40% of eyes in the study had received no previous focal laser treatment and 79% of eyes were phakic. In addition, the preparation of triamcinolone used was a gel and may have different diffusion characteristics compared to the triamcinolone suspensions used in the other studies. In the ISIS study, patients with a cystoid component of macular edema did better with triamcinolone than eyes with diffuse DME. This finding was not replicated in the DRCR.net. We also do not know what the visual results of the DRCR.net would be if those phakic eyes had cataract extraction—in the study, cataract grading was subjective, and cataract may have accounted for more of the vision loss than was believed to be the case. In addition, the treatments were given every 4 months, and perhaps visual results would have been better had they been given at 3-month intervals or even more frequently. Nevertheless, the DRCR.net study does suggest that focal laser is the first line treatment for DME, with consideration of the addition of triamcinolone if a large cystoid component is present, or if two or three focal laser sessions fail to produce the desired visual or OCT outcome.

Dosage of Intravitreal Triamcinolone. Reported doses of triamcinolone used for the treatment of macular edema include 2, 4, and 20 to 25 mg. The optimal dose of intravitreal triamcinolone is not known. In the United States, 4 mg (in 0.1 cc) is the most commonly used dosage. In Germany, the literature reports using 20 to 25 mg, which is prepared by repeatedly filtering and concentrating the triamcinolone preparation. Studies comparing the efficacy, complications, and duration of different doses of triamcinolone in different diseases are necessary to determine the optimum dose. In the ISIS trial, the 4-mg dose was found to be more effective than the 2-mg dose.

Safety of Intravitreal Triamcinolone. Potential complications of intravitreal steroid injections include endophthalmitis, retinal detachment, retinal tears, vitreous hemorrhage, increased intraocular pressure, and cataract formation [36].

Intraocular Pressure (IOP) Rise. The most common adverse effect of intravitreal triamcinolone is increased IOP [37–39]. Bakri et al. reported a pressure rise of 5 mmHg or greater in 49% of 43 eyes, and a pressure rise of 10 mmHg or greater in 28%, within 12 weeks after a 4-mg intravitreal triamcinolone injection (Table 12.1) [38]. The mean time for an IOP rise of 5 mmHg or greater to occur was 4.1 weeks, and the mean time to reach maximum IOP was 6.6 weeks, although the follow-up interval was variable. The difference between the mean preinjection IOP (15.12 mmHg, $n = 43$) and the maximum postinjection IOP (20.74 mmHg, $n = 43$) was statistically significant ($P < 0.0001$). All eyes in this study responded adequately tc topical ocular hypotensive medications within 6 months [38]. Jonas [37] reported that after intravitreal injection of a higher dose of 25 mg of triamcinolone acetonide, an IOP elevation developed in about 50% of eyes, starting 1 to 2 months after the injection. In the vast majority, IOP was normalized by topical medications, and returned to normal values without further medication about 6 months after the injection. Wingate [36] reviewed 113 patients at a single time point (3 months) after a 4-mg intravitreal triamcinolone injection and found that 32% had a rise of 5 mmHg or greater, and 11% had a pressure rise of 10 mmHg or greater. In most of these series, IOP was controlled with topical medications; however, there have been reports [40] of eyes with uncontrolled IOP elevations undergoing trabeculectomy, or even vitrectomy to remove the triamcinolone. In the DRCR.net study, IOP increased from baseline by 10 mmHg or more at any visit in 4% in the focal laser group, 16% in the 1-mg triamcinolone group, and 33% of eyes in the 4-mg triamcinolone group.

Infectious Endophthalmitis. Acute-onset bacterial endophthalmitis was reported in 0.87% of 922 intravitreal triamcinolone acetonide injections (95% confidence interval of 0.38–1.70%) in a retrospective, multicenter review [41]. Potential predisposing risk factors in these eight patients included non-insulin dependent diabetes mellitus ($n = 5$), injection from a multi-use Kenalog bottle ($n = 2$), filtering blebs ($n = 1$), and blepharitis ($n = 1$). The median time to presentation was 7.5 days (range, 1–15 days). *Mycobacterium chelonae* endophthalmitis has also been reported

Table 12.1. Intraocular pressure elevation after 4 mg intravitreal triamcinolone

Reference	Number of eyes	IOP rise ≥ 5	IOP rise ≥ 10	Comment
Bakri et al.	43	49%	28%	At any time within 3 months
Wingate et al.	113	32%	11%	At the 3 month time-point
DRCR.net	254	NA	33%	Any study visit

after intravitreal steroid injections [42]; the eye eventually underwent enucleation. In the DRCR.net study, there were no cases of endophthalmitis or inflammatory pseudoendophthalmitis after 1649 intravitreal injections performed in the trial.

Noninfectious Endophthalmitis with Pseudohypopyon. Acute, noninfectious endophthalmitis has been reported following intravitreal triamcinolone injection in 0.87% to 5% of cases [43–46]. Features differentiating inflammatory vitritis from true endophthalmitis include earlier onset, better visual acuity at presentation, lack of growth on culture or organisms on gram stain, and better final visual acuity, all associated with inflammatory vitritis. Median time to presentation in noninfectious endophthalmitis was 1.5 days [44] versus 7.5 days in infectious endophthalmitis [40]. A pseudohypopyon consisting of triamcinolone acetonide particles may occur after intravitreal injection [47]. One technique to help differentiate a pseudohypopyon from true endophthalmitis is to place the patient on their side. If the hypopyon settles in the dependent region, then it is more likely pseudo and not real.

Other Complications. Intravitreal triamcinolone accelerates cataractogenesis and intravitreal injection may cause retinal detachment and vitreous hemorrhage. The sudden onset of cataract after needle entry into the lens is uncommon but it did occur in reported series [48]. Retinal detachment can occur if the needle penetrates through the retina and causes a retinal break, or if an induced posterior vitreous detachment precipitates a retinal tear. Injecting the triamcinolone acetonide slowly may decrease this risk.

SUSTAINED-RELEASE INTRAVITREAL CORTICOSTEROIDS

Several extended-release steroid preparations are currently undergoing clinical trials. The Retisert implant (developed by Bausch and Lomb and Control Delivery Systems), which is implanted surgically in a similar fashion to the ganciclovir sustained-release implant, releases fluocinolone acetonide in a linear release pharmacokinetics over 3 years. In the phase 3 trial for DME, 80 patients were randomized to receive standard of care (macular grid laser or observation) ($n = 28$) or either a 0.5-mg ($n = 11$) or a 2-mg ($n = 41$) Retisert implant. Enrollment for the 2-mg dose was discontinued early because of an increased incidence of steroid related complications (e.g., IOP, cataract). The 12-month results (Pearson et al. Association for Research and Vision in Ophthalmology, Fort Lauderdale, FL, 2004) reported that more patients randomized to the 0.5-mg group than the standard of care group had resolution of central macular edema (48.8% vs. 25.0%; $P = 0.047$) and improvement in central retinal thickness ($P = 0.003$). More patients treated with 0.5 mg Retisert than standard of care gained 15 letters from baseline (19.5% vs. 7.1%; not statistically significant). More patients receiving standard of care lost 15 letters from baseline (14.3% vs. 4.7%). Overall, 70% of patients in the Retisert group, compared with 50% in the standard of care group, had stable visual acuity ($P = 0.08$).

The overall incidence of serious ocular adverse events (e.g., increased IOP, cataracts, retinal detachment, vitreous hemorrhage) in the study eye over 12 months was 58.5% in patients receiving the 0.5 mg implant and 10.7% in the standard of care group. The proportion of patients with an increase in IOP ≥30 mmHg in the study eye was higher in the 0.5 mg-group (19.5%) than in the standard of care group (0.0%) with three of eight patients in the 0.5-mg group undergoing a trabeculectomy. In addition, cataract progression at 12 months was 0.0% in the standard of care group versus 54.8% of the 31 patients in the 0.5-mg implant group who had not undergone cataract surgery prior to enrollment in the study. No patients required implant removal or withdrew from the study due to an adverse event.

The Posurdex implant (Allergan, Irvine, CA) is a biodegradable copolymer consisting of 70% dexamethasone (350 or 700 µg) and 30% polylactic–glycolic acid. The copolymer hydrolyzes to lactic and glycolic acids. Lactic acid is metabolized to H_2O and CO_2; glycolic acid is either excreted or enzymatically converted to other metabolized species. The implant is delivered via an applicator as an in-office procedure. A phase 2 trial randomized patients with macular edema due to a variety of causes to receiving placebo, or the 350- or 700-µg Posurdex implant. Three-month results in the subgroup of patients with DME ($n = 172$) showed a two or more line visual improvement in 34% of eyes receiving the 700 µg implant, compared with 24.5% receiving the 350 µg implant and 12.7% undergoing observation (Haller JA, American Academy of Ophthalmology, New Orleans, LA, October 2004). The retinal thickness was comparable in all three groups at baseline. At day 90, the observation group had an average increase in thickness of 0.31 microns, while the 350-µg group had an average decrease in thickness of 72 microns and thickness in the 700-µg group decreased on average 157 microns.

ANTIANGIOGENIC AGENTS

The antiangiogenic and antipermeability properties of anti-VEGF agents could potentially be useful in the treatment of diabetic retinopathy. Since DME is a VEGF-mediated disease, intravitreal anti-VEGF may be useful in the treatment of DME. The advantage of intravitreal anti-VEGF agents over intravitreal triamcinolone is that they do not cause cataract or glaucoma, whereas triamcinolone does. However, the half-life of anti-VEGF agents is considerably less than that of triamcinolone; thus patients may need more frequent injections. Ranibizumab (Lucentis, Genentech, San Francisco, CA) is currently in phase 3 clinical testing for DME. Another anti-VEGF agent, Macugen (pegaptanib sodium, formerly NX1838; Eyetech Pharmaceuticals), has completed phase 2 testing for diabetic macular edema.

Ranibizumab is a humanized, antigen-binding fragment (Fab) of a second-generation, recombinant mouse monoclonal antibody directed toward VEGF. It consists of two parts: a nonbinding human sequence (humanized), making it less antigenic in humans, and a high-affinity binding epitope (Fab fragment) derived from the mouse, which serves to bind the antigen [49]. It is produced via a plasmid, containing the appropriate gene sequence, inserted into an *Escherichia coli* expression vector that undergoes large-scale fermentation. This is drained, and the supernatant collected and purified to produce the active drug. Ranibizumab is FDA approved for choroidal neovascularization due to age-related macular degeneration and there are ongoing clinical trials using Ranibizumab for diabetic macular edema.

In a pilot study [50], 10 eyes of 10 patients with DME involving the center of the macula and best-corrected visual acuity (BCVA) in the study eye between 20/63 and 20/400 were treated with ranibizumab. Three intravitreal injections of ranibizumab (0.3 or 0.5 mg each injection) were administered on day 0, month 1, and month 2, and observation until month 24. Of the 10 patients enrolled, 5 received 0.3 mg and 5 received 0.5 mg ranibizumab. At month 3, 4 of 10 patients gained 15 letters or more, 5 of 10 gained 10 letters or more, and 8 of 10 gained 1 or more letters. At month 3, the mean decrease in retinal thickness of the center point of the central subfield was 45.3 ± 196.3 microns for the 0.3-mg group and 197.8 ± 85.9 microns for the 0.5-mg group.

The anti-VEGF pegylated aptamer Macugen is a polyethylene-glycol (PEG) conjugated oligonucleotide with high specificity and affinity for the major soluble human VEGF isoform, VEGF165. Pegylation decreases the clearance of the drug from the vitreous following intravitreal injection. Aptamers are chemically synthesized short strands of RNA or DNA (oligonucleotides) designed to bind to specific molecular targets based on their three-dimensional structure, and are made using SELEX technology (Systematic Evolution of Ligands by EXponential enrichment). Macugen is an aptamer composed of 28 nucleotide bases that avidly binds and inactivates VEGF165 [51]. Macugen is FDA approved for treatment of choroidal neovascularization in age-related macular degeneration and has completed phase 2 testing for diabetic macular edema [52].

In the Macugen for diabetic macular edema phase 2 trial, 172 patients were randomized to receive intravitreal pegaptanib (0.3, 1, and 3 mg) or sham injections at study entry, week 6, and week 12. Additional injections and/or focal photocoagulation were performed as needed for another 18 weeks. Median visual acuity was better at week 36 with 0.3 mg pegaptanib (20/50), as compared with sham (20/63) ($P = 0.04$). More patients receiving 0.3 mg pegaptanib gained 10 or more letters of vision (34% vs. 10%, $P = 0.003$) and 15 or more letters (18% vs. 7%, $P = 0.12$). Mean central retinal thickness decreased by 68 microns with 0.3 mg pegaptanib, versus an increase of 4 microns with sham ($P = 0.02$). Focal laser treatment was necessary in fewer subjects in each pegaptanib arm (0.3 mg vs. sham, 25% vs. 48%; $P = 0.04$).

A retrospective analysis of this trial identified patients with retinal neovascularization [53]. Changes in retinal neovascularization were assessed on fundus photographs and fluorescein angiograms graded at a reading center. Scatter panretinal photocoagulation (PRP) before study enrollment was permitted, but not within 6 months of randomization and study entry. Of the 172 participants, 19 had retinal neovascularization in the study eye at baseline. Excluding 1 who had PRP 13 days before randomization and 2 with no follow-up photographs, 1 of the remaining 16 subjects had PRP during study follow-up. Of these 16 subjects, 8 of 13 (62%) in a pegaptanib treatment group (including the one who received PRP), 0 of 3 in the sham group, and 0 of 4 fellow eyes showed either regression of neovascularization on fundus photographs or regression or absence of fluorescein leakage from neovascularization (or both) at 36 weeks. In 3 of 8 with regression, neovascularization progressed at week 52 after cessation of pegaptanib at week 30. Although a retrospective analysis, these findings implied an effect of pegaptanib upon retinal neovascularization in patients with diabetic retinopathy.

Bevacizumab (Avastin, Genentech, San Francisco, CA) is a full-length monoclonal antibody against VEGF. It is FDA approved for intravenous administration with intravenous 5-fluorouracil (5-FU)-based chemotherapy for the treatment of metastatic colorectal cancer. It has been shown to be nontoxic to the retina, retinal pigment epithelium, and optic nerve when injected intravitreally [54,55], and has been shown to penetrate the retina [56]. After the first report of the off-label use of intravitreal bevacizumab in treating choroidal neovascularization [57], its use has rapidly gained popularity among ophthalmologists and is now widespread.

It is used off-label, intravitreally, for the treatment of VEGF-mediated ocular diseases, such as choroidal neovascularization [55,58], central retinal vein occlusion [59,60], and PDR [61–63]. It has been shown to reduce leakage and cause regression of retinal and iris neovascularization in eyes with PDR [60,61]. Intravitreal bevacizumab is useful in eyes that have vitreous hemorrhage with actively bleeding neovascularization, where the view is inadequate to perform PRP. Injection of bevacizumab may promote faster reabsorption of the vitreous hemorrhage, by stopping active leakage, and may allow the view to clear enough for PRP to be performed. It is also useful to inject in eyes with PDR that have active neovascularization and require vitrectomy, as it makes for much less bleeding during delamination of fibrovascular tissue. Intravitreal bevacizumab is also beneficial in the treatment of neovascular glaucoma, by reducing iris neovascularization [64]. However, the half-life of intravitreal avastin in the vitreous is short: approximately 4.3 days in a rabbit model [65], and 5.6 days in a monkey model. It is therefore a temporary treatment for PDR, and must be followed up by proven long-term therapy such as PRP or pars plana vitrectomy.

In one prospective study, 28 eyes of 14 patients with bilateral DME participated. In each patient, one eye received an intravitreal injection of 4 mg triamcinolone acetonide and the other eye received 1.25 mg bevacizumab. The triamcinolone-injected eye showed significantly better improvement in central retinal thickness than the bevacizumab-injected eye, and the improvement lasted longer than the bevacizumab-injected eye. Triamcinolone (410.4 ± 82.4 microns and 0.47 ± 0.25 microns) kept better results than bevacizumab (501.6 ± 92.5 microns and 0.61 ± 0.17 microns). This suggests that DME benefits not only from VEGF-suppression but also from other mechanisms of action of corticosteroids.

In another study [66], 126 patients with chronic diffuse diabetic macular edema were treated with repeated intravitreal injections of bevacizumab (1.25 mg). Patients were observed in intervals of 4 to 12 weeks for a period of up to 6 to 12 months. Within this period, 48% received at least three intravitreal injections of bevacizumab. Visual acuity changes were significant with ± 5.1 ETDRS letters improvement from baseline after 12 months. Moreover, the mean central retinal thickness on OCT decreased to 374 microns after 6 months ($P < 0.001$) and to 357 microns after 12 months ($P < 0.001$).

The most commonly used dose for intravitreal bevacizumab injection is currently 1.25 mg (0.05 cc) in the USA, although up to 2.50 mg (0.1 cc) may be used. Since such a small amount of drug from a large vial is required to treat ocular disease, ophthalmologists have been obtaining the drug from compounding pharmacies that fractionate the vial into smaller amounts, at a lower cost. The anti-VEGF activity has been shown to degrade minimally over 6 months when bevacizumab is withdrawn into a syringe and refrigerated or frozen [67]. Current reports of the use of intravitreal bevacizumab are limited to small series and anecdotal reports, and the optimum dose for each disease has not been established.

SUMMARY

Data concerning the effectiveness of intravitreal triamcinolone acetonide in macular edema for retinal diseases has come from small, interventional case series and the recent DRCR.net trial. Certainly, a dramatic response on OCT has been noted with cases demonstrating resolution of macular edema with large cystoid spaces and return of normal retinal contours after intravitreal triamcinolone injections. However, the visual results are commonly less impressive. Whether this is due to permanent photoreceptor damage by the time of injection in these refractory cases or a lack of efficacy still needs to be determined. In patients with long-standing macular edema unresponsive to conventional treatments such as focal or grid laser, or posterior subtenon triamcinolone, intravitreal triamcinolone acetonide injection can be considered. We also await the results of the ongoing trials of ranibizumab for diabetic macular edema.

REFERENCES
1. Machemer R, Sugita G, Tano Y. Treatment of intraocular proliferations with intravitreal corticosteroids. *Trans Am Ophthalmol Soc.* 1979;77:171–180.
2. Graham RO, Peyman GA. Intravitreal injection of dexamethasone. Treatment of experimentally induced endophthalmitis. *Arch Ophthalmol.* August 1974;92(2):149–154.
3. McCuen BW 2nd, Bessler M, Tano Y, Chandler D, Machemer R. The lack of toxicity of intravitreally administered triamcinolone acetonide. *Am J Ophthalmol.* June 1981;91(6):785–788.
4. Tano Y, Chandler D, Machemer R. Treatment of intraocular proliferation with intravitreal injection of triamcinolone acetonide. *Am J Ophthalmol.* December 1980;90(6): 810–816.
5. Beer PM, Bakri SJ, Singh RJ, Liu W, Peters GB 3rd, Miller M. Intraocular concentration and pharmacokinetics of triamcinolone acetonide after a single intravitreal injection. *Ophthalmology.* April 2003;110(4):681–686.
6. Hida T, Chandler D, Arena JE, Machemer R. Experimental and clinical observations of the intraocular toxicity of commercial corticosteroid preparations. *Am J Ophthalmol.* February 15, 1986;101(2):190–195.

7. Antcliff RJ, Spalton DJ, Stanford MR, Graham EM, ffytche TJ, Marshall J. Intravitreal triamcinolone for uveitic cystoid macular edema: an optical coherence tomography study. *Ophthalmology*. April 2001;108(4):765–772.

8. Young S, Larkin G, Branley M, Lightman S. Safety and efficacy of intravitreal triamcinolone for cystoid macular oedema in uveitis. *Clin Experiment Ophthalmol*. February 2001;29(1):2–6.

9. Martidis A, Duker JS, Greenberg PB, et al. Intravitreal triamcinolone for refractory diabetic macular edema. *Ophthalmology*. 2002;109:920–927.

10. Jonas JB, Hayler JK, Sofker A, Panda-Jonas S. Intravitreal injection of crystalline cortisone as adjunctive treatment of proliferative diabetic retinopathy. *Am J Ophthalmol*. April 2001;131(4):468–471.

11. Jonas JB, Hayler JK, Panda-Jonas S. Intravitreal injection of crystalline cortisone as adjunctive treatment of proliferative vitreoretinopathy. *Br J Ophthalmol*. September 2000;84(9):1064–1067.

12. Danis RP, Ciulla TA, Pratt LM, Anliker W. Intravitreal triamcinolone acetonide in exudative age-related macular degeneration. *Retina*. 2000;20(3):244–250.

13. Challa JK, Gillies MC, Penfold PL, Gyory JF, Hunyor AB, Billson FA. Exudative macular degeneration and intravitreal triamcinolone: 18 month follow up. *Aust N Z J Ophthalmol*. 1998;26(4):277–281.

14. Aiello LP, Avery RL, Arrigg PG, et al. Vascular endothelial growth factor in ocular fluid of patients with diabetic retinopathy and other retinal disorders. *N Engl J Med*. December 1, 1994;331(22):1480–1487.

15. Funatsu H, Yamashita H, Ikeda T, Mimura T, Eguchi S, Hori S. Vitreous levels of interleukin-6 and vascular endothelial growth factor are related to diabetic macular edema. *Ophthalmology*. 2003;110(9):1690–1696.

16. Kang BS, Chung EY, Yun YP, et al. Inhibitory effects of anti-inflammatory drugs on interleukin-6 bioactivity. *Biol Pharm Bull*. 2001;24(6):701–703.

17. Umland SP, Nahrebne DK, Razac S, et al. The inhibitory effects of topically active glucocorticoids on IL-4, IL-5, and interferon-gamma production by cultured primary CD4± T cells. *J Allergy Clin Immunol*. 1997;100:511–519.

18. Floman N, Zor U. Mechanism of steroid action in ocular inflammation: inhibition of prostaglandin production. *Invest Ophthalmol*. 1977;16:69–73.

19. Bandi N, Kompella UB. Budesonide reduces vascular endothelial growth factor secretion and expression in airway (Calu-1) and alveolar (A549) epithelial cells. *Eur J Pharmacol*. 2001;425:109–116.

20. Fischer S, Renz D, Schaper W, Karliczek GF. In vitro effects of dexamethasone on hypoxia-induced hyperpermeability and expression of vascular endothelial growth factor. *Eur J Pharmacol*. January 12, 2001;411(3):231–243.

21. Wilson CA, Berkowitz BA, Sato Y, et al. Treatment with intravitreal steroid reduces blood-retinal barrier breakdown due to retinal photocoagulation. *Arch Ophthalmol*. 1992;110:1155–1159.

22. Naveh N, Weissman C. Prolonged corticosteroid treatment exerts transient inhibitory effect on prostaglandin E2 release from rabbits' eyes. *Prostaglandins Leukot Essent Fatty Acids*. February 1991;42(2):101–105.

23. Lewis GD, Campbell WB, Johnson AR. Inhibition of prostaglandin synthesis by glucocorticoids in human endothelial cells. *Endocrinology*. July 1986;119(1):62–69.

24. Heffernan JT, Futterman S, Kalina RE. Dexamethasone inhibition of experimental endothelial cell proliferation in retinal venules. *Invest Ophthalmol Vis Sci*. June 1978;17(6):565–568.

25. Bhattacherjee P, Williams RN, Eakins KE. A comparison of the ocular anti-inflammatory activity of steroidal and nonsteroidal compounds in the rat. *Invest Ophthalmol Vis Sci.* August 1983;24(8):1143–1146.

26. Wang YS, Friedrichs U, Eichler W, Hoffmann S, Wiedemann P. Inhibitory effects of triamcinolone acetonide on bFGF-induced migration and tube formation in choroidal microvascular endothelial cells. *Graefes Arch Clin Exp Ophthalmol.* 2002; 240(1): 42–48.

27. Penfold PL, Wen L, Madigan MC, Gillies MC, King NJ, Provis JM. Triamcinolone acetonide modulates permeability and intercellular adhesion molecule-1 (ICAM-1) expression of the ECV304 cell line: implications for macular degeneration. *Clin Exp Immunol.* September 2000;121(3):458–465.

28. Penfold PL, Wong JG, Gyory J, Billson FA. Effects of triamcinolone acetonide on microglial morphology and quantitative expression of MHC-II in exudative age-related macular degeneration. *Clin Experiment Ophthalmol.* June 2001;29(3):188–192.

29. Leibowitz HM, Berrospi AR, Kupferman A, Restropo GV, Galvis V, Alvarez JA. Penetration of topically administered prednisolone acetate into the human aqueous humor. *Am J Ophthalmol.* March 1977;83(3):402–406.

30. Bakri SJ, Kaiser PK. Posterior subtenon triamcinolone acetonide for refractory diabetic macular edema. *Am J Ophthalmol.* February 2005;139(2):290–294.

31. Bakri SJ, Shah A, Falk NS, Beer PM. Intravitreal preservative-free triamcinolone acetonide for the treatment of macular oedema. *Eye.* June 2005;19(6):686–688.

32. Martidis A, Duker JS, Greenberg PB, et al. Intravitreal triamcinolone for refractory diabetic macular edema. *Ophthalmology.* May 2002;109(5):920–927.

33. Jonas JB, Kreissig I, Sofker A, Degenring RF. Intravitreal injection of triamcinolone for diffuse diabetic macular edema. *Arch Ophthalmol.* January 2003;121(1):57–61.

34. Kim JE, Pollack JS, Miller DG, Mittra RA, Spaide RF, Isis Study Group. ISIS-DME: a prospective, randomized, dose-escalation intravitreal steroid injection study for refractory diabetic macular edema. *Retina.* May 2008;28(5):735–740.

35. Massin P, Audren F, Haouchine B, et al. Intravitreal triamcinolone acetonide for diabetic diffuse macular edema: preliminary results of a prospective controlled trial. *Ophthalmology.* February 2004;111(2):218–224; discussion 224–225.

36. Aiello LP, Brucker AJ, Chang S, et al. Evolving guidelines for intravitreous injections. *Retina.* 2004;24:S3–S19.

37. Wingate RJ, Beaumont PE. Intravitreal triamcinolone and elevated intraocular pressure. *Aust N Z J Ophthalmol.* 1999;27:431–432.

38. Jonas JB, Kreissig I, Degenring R. Intraocular pressure after intravitreal injection of triamcinolone acetonide. *Br J Ophthalmol.* January 2003;87(1):24–27.

39. Bakri SJ, Beer PM. The effect of intravitreal triamcinolone acetonide on intraocular pressure. *Ophthalmic Surg Lasers Imaging.* September–October 2003;34(5):386–390.

40. Kaushik S, Gupta V, Gupta A, Dogra MR, Singh R. Intractable glaucoma following intravitreal triamcinolone in central retinal vein occlusion. *Am J Ophthalmol.* April 2004;137(4):758–760.

41. Moshfeghi DM, Kaiser PK, Scott IU, et al. Acute endophthalmitis following intravitreal triamcinolone acetonide injection. *Am J Ophthalmol.* November 2003;136(5):791–796.

42. Benz MS, Murray TG, Dubovy SR, Katz RS, Eifrig CW. Endophthalmitis caused by Mycobacterium chelonae abscessus after intravitreal injection of triamcinolone. *Arch Ophthalmol.* February 2003;121(2):271–273.

43. Roth DB, Chieh J, Spirn MJ, Green SN, Yarian DL, Chaudhry NA. Noninfectious endophthalmitis associated with intravitreal triamcinolone injection. *Arch Ophthalmol.* September 2003;121(9):1279–1282.

44. Nelson ML, Tennant MT, Sivalingam A, Regillo CD, Belmont JB, Martidis A. Infectious and presumed noninfectious endophthalmitis after intravitreal triamcinolone acetonide injection. *Retina*. October 2003;23(5):686–691.

45. Moshfeghi DM, Kaiser PK, Bakri SJ, et al. Presumed sterile endophthalmitis following intravitreal triamcinolone acetonide injection. *Ophthalmic Surg Lasers Imaging*. January–February 2005;36(1):24–29.

46. Moshfeghi AA, Scott IU, Flynn HW Jr, Puliafito CA. Pseudohypopyon after intravitreal triamcinolone acetonide injection for cystoid macular edema. *Am J Ophthalmol*. September 2004;138(3):489–492.

47. Sharma MC, Lai WW, Shapiro MJ. Pseudohypopyon following intravitreal triamcinolone acetonide injection. *Cornea*. May 2004;23(4):398–399.

48. Jager RD, Aiello LP, Patel SC, Cunningham ET Jr. Risks of intravitreous injection: a comprehensive review. *Retina*. October 2004;24(5):676–698.

49. Mordenti J, Cuthbertson RA, Ferrara N, et al. Comparisons of the intraocular tissue distribution, pharmacokinetics, and safety of 125I-labeled full-length and Fab antibodies in rhesus monkeys following intravitreal administration. *Toxicol Pathol*. September–October 1999;27(5):536–544.

50. Chun DW, Heier JS, Topping TM, Duker JS, Bankert JM. A pilot study of multiple intravitreal injections of ranibizumab in patients with center-involving clinically significant diabetic macular edema. *Ophthalmology*. October 2006;113(10):1706–1712.

51. Eyetech Study Group. Preclinical and phase 1A clinical evaluation of an anti-VEGF pegylated aptamer (EYE001) for the treatment of exudative age-related macular degeneration. *Retina*. April 2002;22(2):143–152.

52. Cunningham ET Jr, Adamis AP, Altaweel M, et al. A phase II randomized double-masked trial of pegaptanib, an anti-vascular endothelial growth factor aptamer, for diabetic macular edema. *Ophthalmology*. October 2005;112(10):1747–1757.

53. Adamis AP, Altaweel M, Bressler NM, et al. Changes in retinal neovascularization after pegaptanib (Macugen) therapy in diabetic individuals. *Ophthalmology*. January 2006;113(1):23–28.

54. Bakri SJ, Cameron J D, McCannel CA, Pulido JS, Marler RJ. Absence of histologic retinal toxicity of intravitreal bevacizumab in a rabbit model. *Am J Ophthalmol*. July 2006;142(1):162–164.

55. Manzano RP, Peyman GA, Khan P, Kivilcim M. Testing intravitreal toxicity of bevacizumab (Avastin). *Retina*. March 2006;26(3):257–261.

56. Shahar J, Avery RL, Heilweil G, et al. Electrophysiologic and retinal penetration studies following intravitreal injection of bevacizumab (Avastin). *Retina*. March 2006;26(3):262–269.

57. Rosenfeld PJ, Moshfeghi AA, Puliafito CA. Optical coherence tomography findings after an intravitreal injection of bevacizumab (avastin) for neovascular age-related macular degeneration. *Ophthalmic Surg Lasers Imaging*. 2005;36:331–335.

58. Spaide RF, Laud K, Fine HF, et al. Intravitreal bevacizumab treatment of choroidal neovascularization secondary to age-related macular degeneration. *Retina*. April 2006;26(4):383–390.

59. Rosenfeld PJ, Fung AE, Puliafito CA. Optical coherence tomography findings after an intravitreal injection of bevacizumab (avastin) for macular edema from central retinal vein occlusion. *Ophthalmic Surg Lasers Imaging*. July–August 2005;36(4):336–339.

60. Iturralde D, Spaide RF, Meyerle CB, et al. Intravitreal bevacizumab (Avastin) treatment of macular edema in central retinal vein occlusion: a short-term study. *Retina*. March 2006;26(3):279–284.

61. Spaide RF, Fisher YL. Intravitreal bevacizumab (Avastin) treatment of proliferative diabetic retinopathy complicated by vitreous hemorrhage. *Retina*. March 2006;26(3):275–278.

62. Avery RL. Regression of retinal and iris neovascularization after intravitreal bevacizumab (Avastin) treatment. *Retina*. March 2006;26(3):352–354.

63. Bakri SJ, Donaldson MJ, Link TP. Rapid regression of disc neovascularization in a patient with proliferative diabetic retinopathy following adjunctive intravitreal bevacizumab. *Eye*. December 2006;20(12):1474–1475.

64. Kahook MY, Schuman JS, Noecker RJ. Intravitreal bevacizumab in a patient with neovascular glaucoma. *Ophthalmic Surg Lasers Imaging*. March–April 2006;37(2):144–146.

65. Bakri SJ, Snyder MR, Reid JM, Pulido JS, Singh RJ. Pharmacokinetics of intravitreal bevacizumab (Avastin). *Ophthalmology*. May 2007;114(5):855–859.

66. Kook D, Wolf A, Kreutzer T, et al. Long-term effect of intravitreal bevacizumab (avastin) in patients with chronic diffuse diabetic macular edema. *Retina*. October 2008;28(8):1053–1060.

67. Bakri SJ, Snyder M, Pulido JS, McCannel CA, Weiss WT, Singh RJ. Six-month stability of bevacizumab (avastin) after withdrawal into a syringe and refrigeration or freezing. *Retina*. May–June 2006;26(5):519–522.

Evolving Algorithms for Managing Diabetic Macular Edema

DIANA V. DO, MD,

AND JULIA A. HALLER, MD

CORE MESSAGES

- Optimal treatment of diabetic macular edema requires attention to both systemic and ocular factors.
- Typically, Early Treatment Diabetic Retinopathy Study (ETDRS)-type laser is first-line therapy, with options for further treatment including additional laser photocoagulation, adjuvant pharmacological therapy, combined photocoagulation and pharmacological intervention, vitrectomy, or referral of the patient to a clinical trial.

The optimal management of diabetic macular edema (DME), the most common cause of moderate vision loss in individuals with diabetes mellitus, is complicated by the many systemic and ocular issues that impact on its therapy, the variable responses of individual eyes to treatment, and the increasing number of therapeutic approaches available to the clinician [1]. Because of this complex web of multifactorial and interrelated considerations, the disease is resistant to simple algorithmic formulations for its management. With that caveat, it is nevertheless possible to devise a systematic, practical, step-by-step approach to evaluating and treating a patient with DME, which may provide an organizational management framework for the busy clinician. The six steps in this management framework are as follows:

1. Complete ocular evaluation
2. Optimization of metabolic control

Note: The authors have no proprietary interests in any aspect of this report.

3. Exclusion of other treatable causes of macular edema
4. Early Treatment Diabetic Retinopathy Study (ETDRS) laser photocoagulation
5. Careful follow-up and reassessment
6. Further treatment if indicated: either additional laser photocoagulation, use of adjuvant pharmacological therapy, combined photocoagulation and pharmacological intervention, vitrectomy, or referral of the patient to a clinical trial.

STEP 1: COMPLETE OCULAR EVALUATION

Emphasis on a complete and careful ocular evaluation is important because many factors other than the presence of thickening in the macula alone impact on the clinician's decision-making when treating DME. To pick just a few examples, the patient's visual acuity affects numerous decisions including the recommendation for treatment and discussion of the relative risks, side effects, and benefits of various management strategies. A small, mobile anterior chamber intraocular lens could be responsible for iris irritation and inflammation, which, in turn, may exacerbate edema. Iris neovascularization, if present, signals the presence of more emergent issues than edema alone. The lens examination impacts on the consideration of corticosteroid therapies or vitrectomy surgery, both of which cause cataract progression. Evaluation of intraocular pressure (IOP) and optic nerve cupping also factors into consideration of corticosteroid use with its attendant glaucoma risk. And retinal examination is important not only from the standpoint of assessing presence or absence of macular edema but also in terms of grading the level of retinopathy. Patients with more severe levels of retinopathy have a less favorable response to laser therapy and worse visual prognosis than those with milder levels. The patient deserves a complete overview of his or her ocular condition at the time of initial evaluation.

STEP 2: OPTIMIZE METABOLIC CONTROL

As important as the ocular evaluation in the ophthalmologist's care of the diabetic patient, is the discussion about metabolic control and its impact on the eye. The ophthalmologist has a crucial role here as a communicator with the patient and also with the patient's medical care team, including endocrinologist, primary care physician, internist and/or other personnel. The ophthalmologist needs to make it clear that optimization of metabolic control will impact significantly on the patient's DME. This "tuning up" is the first important step in the management of DME, and has occasionally been sufficient to result in edema resolution (Fig. 13.1A and B) [2]. Although these cases are the exception, certainly levels of glycemia, hypertension, and blood lipid abnormalities are crucial to assess and at least begin to control before committing patients to invasive treatment regimens.

Glycemia. The first step to reduce the progression of diabetic retinopathy is glycemic control. The Diabetes Control and Complications Trial (DCCT) [3] provided

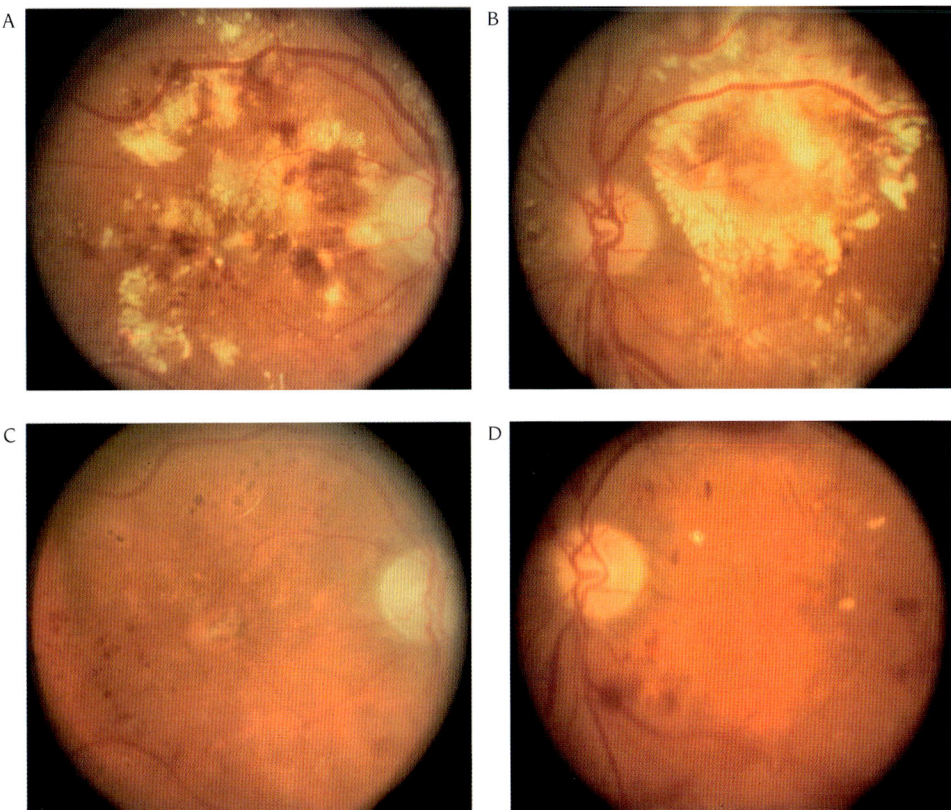

Figure 13.1. (A and B) Fundus photograph from a patient with type 2 diabetes and bilateral diabetic macular edema with severe hard exudates. Initial laboratory examination revealed a total cholesterol of 421 mg/dL and triglyceride of 1272 mg/dL. One session of focal laser photocoagulation was performed in each eye and medical treatment for his elevated serum lipids was initiated. (Source: Reprinted from *Ophthalmology*, Cusick M, Chew EY, Chan CC, et al. Histopathology and regression of retinal hard exudates in diabetic retinopathy after reduction of elevated serum lipid levels, 110:2126–2133 © 2003 with permission from the American Academy of Ophthalmology.) (C and D) Twelve months after presentation, serum lipids normalized and fundus examination revealed regression of hard exudates and resolving diabetic macular edema. (Source: Reprinted from *Ophthalmology*, Cusick M, Chew EY, Chan CC, et al. Histopathology and regression of retinal hard exudates in diabetic retinopathy after reduction of elevated serum lipid levels, 110:2126–2133 © 2003 with permission from the American Academy of Ophthalmology.)

incontrovertible evidence that intensive management of hyperglycemia, as demonstrated by a reduction in the HbA1c to 7.0%, is associated with decreased rates of development and progression of retinopathy in type 1 diabetic persons. In addition, the United Kingdom Prospective Diabetes Study (UKPDS) [4] showed that intensive control of blood glucose (reducing the HbA1C to 7.0%) in type 2 diabetics resulted in a 25% risk reduction in microvascular endpoints, such as the need for retinal laser photocoagulation. Data from these landmark studies have resulted in the recommendation for achieving intense glycemic control with HbA1C level below 7% in order to reduce the risk and progression of retinopathy, which may translate to preservation of vision among individuals with diabetes.

Hypertension and Serum Lipids. In addition to glycemic control, blood pressure control also plays an important role in diabetic retinopathy. The UKPDS demonstrated that intensive blood pressure control was associated with a decreased risk of retinopathy progression and resulted in a 37% reduction in microvascular diseases [5]. Control of hypertension is essential in the management of diabetic retinopathy and collaboration with an internist is recommended.

Observational studies have also shown that elevated levels of serum lipids are associated with increased severity of hard exudates and decreased visual acuity. Among the participants in the DCCT, triglyceride levels were associated with severity of retinopathy while high-density lipoprotein cholesterol levels were inversely associated [6,7]. Data from the DCCT also revealed that, in models controlling for randomized treatment assignment, HbA1c levels and other factors (both total-to-high density lipoprotein (HDL) cholesterol ratio and low density lipoprotein (LDL) predicted the development of clinically significant macular edema (CSME) [8]. Lowering of lipid levels, recommended to prevent cardiovascular disease, may also reduce the risk of CSME, which is an important cause of vision loss.

Pregnancy. Several studies have demonstrated that diabetic retinopathy may be accelerated during pregnancy [9,10]. This increase in retinopathy severity may be due to changes in metabolic control during pregnancy or to the pregnancy itself. In addition to optimizing metabolic control, women with diabetes who are planning a pregnancy should have a baseline ophthalmic examination before attempting to conceive, and have a follow-up examination during the first trimester. Depending on the level of diabetic retinopathy, additional examinations throughout the pregnancy are recommended.

Other less common systemic entities such as sleep apnea, which may impact on the diabetic patient's ocular status, should also be evaluated and treated as necessary [11].

STEP 3: EXCLUDE OTHER TREATABLE CAUSES OF MACULAR EDEMA

Although most cases of macular edema among diabetic individuals are due to the effect of their systemic disease, a thorough ophthalmic examination may reveal other treatable causes of central retinal thickening. There may be coexisting ocular disorders that are the primary, or a contributing secondary, cause of decreased visual acuity. Vitreomacular interface abnormalities such as an epiretinal membrane (ERM) or vitreomacular traction (VMT) may cause retinal edema and distorted vision (Figs. 13.1C and D and 13.2A). These conditions can be diagnosed with careful biomicroscopic fundus examination, but additional imaging modalities are helpful. Optical coherence tomography (OCT) imaging in particular is valuable in identifying DME due to traction from an ERM or from a partially detached posterior hyaloid, both conditions that may benefit from surgical intervention (Fig. 13.2B) [12]. OCT is also more accurate than clinical examination in grading macular edema, and can detect the thickening earlier [13]. Particularly in situations where the degree of edema and visual loss seem out of proportion to the amount of leakage seen on fluorescein angiography, vitreomacular interface abnormalities should be suspected. Patients with suspected vitreomacular interface abnormalities may benefit from OCT imaging to evaluate the macula. If ERM or VMT is at least in part responsible for the macular edema and decreased vision, pars plana vitrectomy may be an initial therapy to be considered.

Another possible cause of vision loss among individuals with diabetes is postsurgical cystoid macular edema (CME). Postsurgical CME has a characteristic petalloid pattern of leakage on fluorescein angiography and is accompanied by optic disc staining. Although diffuse DME may also present in a cystoid pattern on angiography, postsurgical CME should be suspected in diabetic patients who have undergone recent ocular surgery. Treatment with topical nonsteroidal and/or steroidal anti-inflammatory eye drops may help resolve all or some component of the CME without

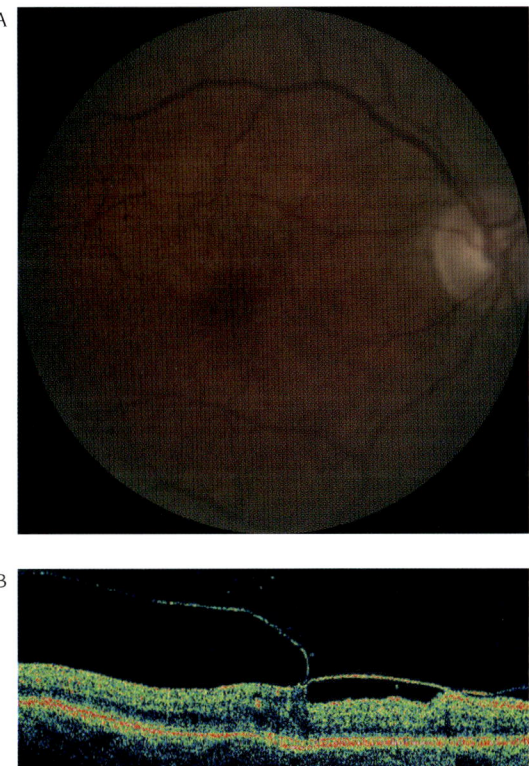

Figure 13.2. (A) Fundus photograph of an eye with mild nonproliferative diabetic retinopathy and suspected diabetic macular edema. (B) Corresponding optical coherence tomography (OCT) image demonstrated vitreomacular traction as the cause of the macular edema.

the need for more invasive therapy. Similarly, eyes with vitreous incarcerated in a cataract surgical incision, patients with mobile anterior chamber intraocular lenses, or patients with retained posteriorly dislocated lens fragments potentially responsible for low-grade inflammation and macular edema may benefit from correction of these anatomic problems as a first step before other therapies are instituted.

STEP 4: LASER PHOTOCOAGULATION

Laser photocoagulation has been the gold standard for treatment of DME since the ETDRS [14]. This type of photocoagulation has been adjusted in clinical practice over the years since the trial results were initially published, so that the type of treatment commonly applied employs lighter burns. This "modified ETDRS" laser photocoagulation is the type used in the Diabetic Retinopathy Clinical Research (DRCR) Network protocols (Table 13.1) [15].

Two strategies for laser treatment are used in this type of therapy. Focal laser involves direct treatment of individual microaneurysms in the areas of retinal edema. A spot size of 50 to 100 microns is typically used with an exposure time of 0.05 to 0.1 s. The power is set low and increased to obtain a mild whitening or darkening of the microaneurysm, or subjacent retinal pigment epithelium (RPE) effect. Grid laser is commonly used in areas of retinal thickening, particularly if the fluorescein angiogram demonstrates a diffuse leakage pattern and few microaneurysms. The laser burns, usually 50 to 100 microns in size, are equally spaced and placed more than one burn-width apart to produce light intensity laser marks in edematous retina.

STEP 5: CAREFUL FOLLOW-UP AND REASSESSMENT

Following focal laser therapy, patients are, in general, followed at approximately 3-month intervals to assess their response to therapy. Tools used to evaluate this response include clinical examination with biomicroscopy, OCT imaging, and fluorescein angiography, although all of these are not always necessary. At the time of evaluation, the level of retinopathy is also carefully assessed for progression, and the overall state of the eye and the patient's metabolic control reviewed.

STEP 6: FURTHER TREATMENT IF INDICATED

Re-treatment with Laser. Eyes with diminishing edema may continue to be followed even if they still have some degree of persistent thickening, or re-treatment may be considered. Eyes with no response to laser photocoagulation are, in general, re-treated with further laser photocoagulation. Eyes unresponsive to laser photocoagulation, or eyes in which further laser photocoagulation is considered relatively contraindicated (such as eyes with leaking microaneuryms very close to the foveal center or eyes with extensive fibrotic or pigmentary reaction to previous laser) may be considered for other types of therapy.

Table 13.1. Laser Treatment Techniques for Diabetic Macular Edema

Burn Characteristic	Focal/Grid Photocoagulation (modified ETDRS technique)	Mild Macular Grid Photocoagulation Technique
Focal Treatment	Focally treat all leaking MAs in areas of retinal thickening between 500 and 3000 microns from center of macula (but not within 500 microns of disk)	Not applicable
Change in MA Color with Focal Treatment	Not required, but at least a mild gray-white burn should be evident beneath all MAs	Not applicable
Burn Size for Focal Treatment	50 microns	Not applicable
Burn Duration for Focal Treatment	0.05 to 0.10 s	Not applicable
Grid Treatment	Applied to all areas with diffuse leakage or nonperfusion within area described below for treatment	Applied to entire area described below for treatment (including unthickened retina)
Area Considered for Grid Treatment	500 to 3000 microns from center of macula (no burns placed within 500 microns of disk)	500 to 3000 microns superiorly, nasally, and inferiorly from center of macula (no burns placed within 500 microns of disk)
Burn Size for Grid Treatment	50 microns	50 microns
Burn Duration for Grid Treatment	0.05 to 0.10 s	0.05 to 0.10 s
Burn Intensity for Grid Treatment	Barely visible (light gray)	Barely visible (light gray)
Burn Separation for Grid Treatment	2 visible burn widths apart	200–300 total burns evenly distributed over the treatment area outlined above (approximately 2–3 burn widths apart)
Wavelength (Grid and Focal Treatment)	Green to yellow wavelengths	Green to yellow wavelengths

Adapted from the Diabetic Retinopathy Clinical Research Network Protocol #1A: A Pilot Study of Laser Photocoagulation for Diabetic Macular Edema.

MA = microaneurysm

Other Options: Pharmacological Agents, Combination Therapy, Referral to Prospective Clinical Trials. Options for eyes unresponsive to laser photocoagulation continue to expand, and any list is bound to become out of date rapidly. At this writing, all drugs are used off-label for DME, and include the anti-vascular endothelial growth factor (VEGF) agents pegaptanib, ranibizumab, and bevacizumab, and steroids that can be introduced in and around the eye, specifically triamcinolone acetonide (Kenalog) and the fluocinolone implant Retisert. Finally, numerous new drugs in the investigational pipeline offer promise for DME treatment in the future.

Trials of these drugs as monotherapy or in combination with other pharmacological agents and/or laser photocoagulation and/or surgery are frontiers that remain to be fully and carefully explored. Referral of the appropriately informed, eligible, motivated diabetic patient to a prospective study is an important and beneficial option for the management of DME.

Anti-VEGF Agents. Several studies have shown that VEGF plays an important role in vascular permeability and contributes to diabetic retinopathy and DME [16,17]. Pegaptanib (Macugen, Eyetech Pharmaceuticals Inc.), an aptamer that blocks the effects of the 165 isomer of VEGF and has already been approved for use in neovascular age-related macular degeneration (AMD), is being evaluated for the treatment of DME. A phase 2 study has shown that subjects assigned to intravitreal injections of pegaptanib had better visual acuity outcomes, were more likely to show reduction in central retinal thickness, and were deemed less likely to need additional therapy with photocoagulation compared to subjects assigned to sham injections at 36 weeks of follow-up [18].

In addition to pegaptanib, several studies are underway to investigate other anti-VEGF agents for the treatment of DME. Ranibizumab (Lucentis, Genentech Inc.), a humanized monoclonal antibody to VEGF which has been approved for the treatment of neovascular AMD, has also shown promise for the treatment of DME in a small single center study [19]. Bevacizumab (Avastin, Genentech, Inc.), a full-length monoclonal antibody to VEGF, which is Food and Drug Administration (FDA) approved as an intravenous therapy for patients with metastatic colorectal cancer, has been reported to effect resolution of DME in some eyes when injected intravitreally [20]. VEGF-Trap (Regeneron, Inc.), a humanized protein against the VEGF molecule, and other novel agents are also being tested in phase 1 clinical trials for efficacy and safety in DME [21]. Results from these and other randomized clinical trials will help determine the safety and efficacy of anti-VEGF agents and other novel therapies in the treatment of DME.

Steroids and Other Pharmacologic Agents. Several studies have also investigated the role of intraocular steroids for DME. Steroids have a host of effects on processes that result in leakage from retinal blood vessels, notably stabilizing tight junctions between vascular endothelial cells. Intravitreal and posterior sub-Tenon's injection of steroids, principally the commercially available formulation of triamcinolone acetonide, Kenalog, have been widely used to treat DME that has not responded to laser therapy [20,22]. Although results from these case series have shown a beneficial effect of intraocular steroids in the treatment of DME, steroids are also known to have significant side effects, including cataract progression and an increase in IOP with development of glaucoma (Fig. 13.3). In addition, the beneficial effects of intraocular steroids when given as an intravitreal or sub-Tenon's injection often wane several months after the injection.

The DRCR Network has investigated the role of a new ocular-specific formulation of triamcinolone administered in the sub-Tenon's space in a pilot study as well as that of the drug injected intravitreally in a larger randomized study to help elucidate the role of these drugs in treating DME [15]. In a phase 2 study of

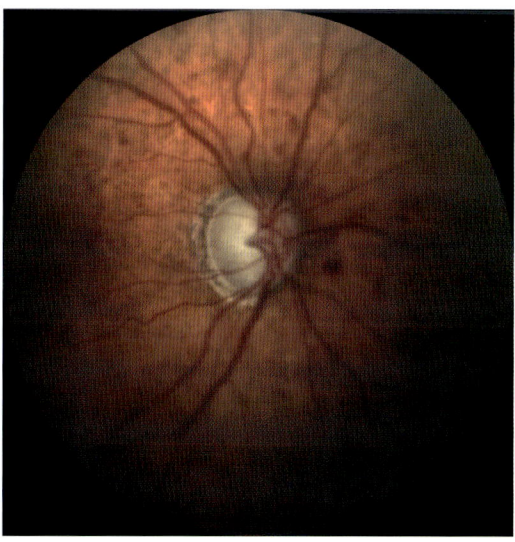

Figure 13.3. Fundus photograph of an optic disc with significant glaucomatous cupping due to increased intraocular pressure after intravitreal injection of triamcinolone acetonide.

sub-Tenon's injections of triamcinolone either alone or in combination with focal photocoagulation in the treatment of mild DME [23], 129 eyes with mild DME and a visual acuity of 20/40 or better were randomized to receive either focal photocoagulation, a 20-mg anterior sub-Tenon's injection of triamcinolone, a 20-mg anterior sub-Tenon's injection followed by focal photocoagulation after 4 weeks, a 40-mg posterior sub-Tenon's injection of triamcinolone, or a 40-mg posterior sub-Tenon's injection followed by focal photocoagulation after 4 weeks. Changes in visual acuity and OCT retinal thickness were not significantly different among the five treatment groups at 34 weeks ($P = 0.94$ and $P = 0.46$, respectively). Elevated IOP and ptosis were adverse effects related to the injections. On the basis of these results, the DRCR investigators concluded that peribulbar triamcinolone, with or without focal photocoagulation, is unlikely to be of substantial benefit in eyes with DME and good visual acuity comparable to those studied.

The DRCR also conducted a phase 3 clinical trial evaluating the efficacy and safety of 1- and 4-mg doses of preservative-free intravitreal triamcinolone in comparison with focal/grid photocoagulation for the treatment of DME [24]. The primary outcome of this study was ETDRS visual acuity at 2 years. Eight hundred forty study eyes of 693 subjects with DME with visual acuity of 20/40 to 20/320 were randomized to focal/grid photocoagulation, 1 mg intravitreal triamcinolone, or 4 mg intravitreal triamcinolone. Re-treatment was given for persistent or new edema at 4-month intervals. Although at 4 months, the mean visual acuity was better in the 4-mg triamcinolone group than in either the laser group ($P < 0.001$) or the 1-mg triamcinolone group ($P = 0.001$), this benefit was not sustained, and at 1 year, there were no significant differences among the three treatment groups in mean visual acuity. At the primary outcome visit at 2 years, mean visual acuity was better in the laser group than in the other two groups ($P = 0.02$ comparing the laser and 1-mg groups, $P = 0.002$ comparing the laser and 4-mg groups, and $P = 0.49$ comparing the 1- and 4-mg groups). The mean change $\pm$ standard deviation in visual acuity letter score from baseline was $+1 \pm 17$ in the laser group, -2 ± 18 in the 1-mg triamcinolone group, and -3 ± 22 in the 4-mg triamcinolone group. Although cataract progression was more common in eyes randomized to triamcinolone injection, the differences in the 2-year visual acuity outcome could not be attributed solely to cataract formation. Cataract surgery was performed in 13%, 23%, and 51% of eyes in the three treatment groups. In addition, IOP increased from baseline by 10 mmHg or more at any visit in 4%, 16%, and 33% of eyes in the three treatment groups, respectively. This phase 3 randomized clinical trial has shown that focal/grid photocoagulation is more effective and has fewer side effects than 1- or 4-mg doses of preservative-free intravitreal triamcinolone for eyes with DME through 2 years of follow-up for eyes similar to those included in this study.

In order to increase the duration of steroid effects, scientists have developed sustained delivery devices that release steroids into the eye at a constant rate over months to years. A fluocinolone acetonide sustained delivery device sutured intravitreally to the sclera at the pars plana has been shown to decrease macular edema and improve visual acuity in patients with diabetic retinopathy, although its use was associated with significant risks of cataract and glaucoma [25]. In a randomized controlled trial, 97 patients were assigned to receive either a fluocinolone implant or standard care (defined as laser treatment or observation). At 3 years, 58% of implanted eyes had no evidence of edema compared to 30% of standard-of-care eyes ($p < 0.001$) and 45% of implanted eyes had 2 steps of retinal thickness improvement relative to 24% of standard-of-care eyes. In addition, 28% of implanted eyes experienced visual acuity improvements of 3 or more lines compared to 15% of standard of care eyes ($P < 0.05$). Of interest was the finding that steroid implant-treated eyes had a reduced rate of retinopathy progression compared with the standard-of-care-group. However, the intravitreal fluocinolone acetonide-implanted eyes were at higher risk of developing serious adverse events than non-implanted eyes; 95% of phakic implanted eyes underwent cataract surgery over the three year study period. In addition 35% of implanted eyes developed intraocular pressure elevation, among whom 28% required a filtering procedure and 5% required removal of the implant to manage the increased intraocular pressure.

A dexamethasone sustained-release biodegradable implant currently being evaluated in a phase 3 trial for DME was shown in a phase 2 study to significantly improve visual acuity, fluorescein angiographic leakage, and OCT-measured macular thickness when compared to placebo. In a 6-month, phase 2 randomized controlled trial, 315 patients with persistent macular edema (55% of whom had macular edema secondary to diabetic retinopathy, 45% had macular edema secondary to retinal vein occlusion, Irvine-Gass syndrome, or uveitis) were randomized to treatment with 350 µg or 700 µg dexamethasone implant or observation [26]. At 3 months (primary end point of the study), an improvement of 10 letters or more was achieved by a greater proportion of patients treated with the dexamethasone implant, 700 µg (35%) or 350 µg (24%), than observed patients (13%; $P < .001$ vs 700 µg group; $P = .04$ vs 350 µg group). In addition, an improvement of 15 letters or more was achieved in 18% of patients treated with dexamethasone implant, 700 µg versus 6% of observed patients ($P = .006$). Of note, 33% of implanted patients within the diabetic retinopathy subgroup had at least a 10-letter improvement compared to 12% in the observation group. The improvements from dexamethasone treatment relative to observation were also significant on the physiologic and anatomic levels. Twenty percent, and 34% of the 350 and 700 µg dexamethasone groups, respectively, had reductions of 2 or more levels of improvement on fluorescein leakage (an indication of vascular permeability) compared to 5% from the observation group. In addition, OCT-analyses revealed a mean reduction of −53.19 and −106.57 microns respectively in the 350 and 700 µg dexamethasone groups, respectively, compared to a mean increase in thickness of +20.67 microns in the observation group. At 6 months, 12% and 17% of the 350 and 700 µg dexamethasone groups developed an increase in intraocular pressure of 10 mmHg or more from baseline, relative to 3% in the observation arm. All subjects with intraocular pressure increases were managed with observation or topical IOP-lowering medications, and no significant increase in cataract formation was observed in the treatment group versus, the control at 6 months.

In addition to the fluocinolone and dexamethasone implants mentioned here, other sustained delivery steroid devices are in development. Results from randomized clinical trials with long-term follow-up are needed to better evaluate the potential role and safety of steroids in macular edema.

Vitrectomy surgery is an option for the treatment of DME not uncommonly proposed in situations where the edema is resistant to other therapies. Maneuvers including peeling of epiretinal membranes, peeling of internal limiting membrane, concomitant injection of pharmacological agents, and supplementary endolaser have all been advocated, although none proven to be valuable. In cases where clearcut traction on the macula is observed, whether from epiretinal membrane contracture or vitreomacular traction, the rationale for this approach is much more straightforward than in cases where no such traction is documented. Although numerous papers, many in the preOCT era and most retrospective, have been published on this topic [27–29], the reported results are variable and in many cases contradictory, and this treatment modality remains at this point one of last resort, with incompletely understood indications, benefits and longterm risks.

Because of the changing landscape in the DME therapy field, new options and new data are emerging continually. The most accurate statement seems to be that our approach to this disease requires continual reevaluation. Although pharmacologic therapy appears promising, laser photocoagulation remains the standard treatment for DME and our armamentarium will still require close collaboration with our medical colleagues.

SUMMARY

Optimal treatment of DME requires a multipronged battle plan with both systemic and ocular fronts (Table 13.2). An algorithm for approaching these patients includes a complete ocular evaluation, maximization of metabolic control, and

Table 13.2. Algorithm for Managing Diabetic Macular Edema

1. Complete Ocular Evaluation
2. Metabolic Control
3. Exclude Other Treatable Causes of Edema
4. Start with ETDRS Laser Photocoagulation
5. Follow the patient carefully
6. Re-treat with laser or consider other options: New drugs, combination of drugs and laser photocoagulation, referral to clinical trial

identification and correction of other treatable causes of macular edema. This is typically followed by ETDRS-type laser photocoagulation with subsequent careful follow-up and reassessment. Options for further treatment, if indicated, include additional laser photocoagulation, use of adjuvant pharmacological therapy, combined photocoagulation and pharmacological intervention, vitrectomy, or referral of appropriate patients to clinical trials.

REFERENCES

1. Kahn HA, Hiller R. Blindness caused by diabetic retinopathy. *Am J Ophthalmol.* 1974;78:58–67.
2. Cusick M, Chew EY, Chan CC, Kruth HS, Murphy RP, Ferris FL 3rd. Histopathology and regression of retinal hard exudates in diabetic retinopathy after reduction of elevated serum lipid levels. *Ophthalmology.* 2003;110(11):2126–2133.
3. The Diabetes Control and Complications Trial Research Group. The effect of intensive treatment of diabetes on the development and progression of long-term complications in insulin-dependent diabetes mellitus. *N Engl J Med.* 1993;329:977–986.
4. The United Kingdom Prospective Diabetes Study Group. Intensive blood-glucose control with sulphonylureas or insulin compared with conventional treatment and risk of complications in patients with type 2 diabetes (UKPDS 33). *Lancet.* 1998;352: 837–853.
5. The United Kingdom Prospective Diabetes Study Group. Tight blood pressure control and risk of macrovascular and microvascular complications in type 2 diabetes (UKPDS 38). *Br Med J.* 1998;317:703–713.
6. Chew EY, Klein ML, Ferris FL III, et al. Association of elevated serum lipid levels with retinal hard exudates in diabetic retinopathy. *Arch Ophthalmol.* 1996;114: 1079–1084.
7. Lyons TJ, Jenkins AJ, Zhen D, et al. Diabetic retinopathy and serum lipoprotein subclasses in the DCCT/EDIC cohort. *Invest Ophthalm Vis Sci.* 2004;45:910–918.
8. Miljanovic B, Glynn RJ, Nathan DM, Manson JE, Schaumberg DA. A prospective study of serum lipids and risk of diabetic macular edema in type 1 diabetes. *Diabetes.* 2004;53:2883–2892.
9. Chew EY, Mills JL, Metzger BE, et al. Metabolic control and progression of retinopathy. The Diabetes in Early Pregnancy Study. National Institute of Child Health and Human Development Diabetes in Early Pregnancy Study. *Diabetes Care.* 1995;18: 631–637.

10. Klein BEK, Moss SE, Klein R. Effect of pregnancy on progression of diabetic retinopathy. *Diabetes Care*. 1990;13:34–40.

11. Duh EJ, Finkelstein D, Schneider T, Malouf A, Kaplan G. Bilateral iris neovascularization as the initial sign of obesity-hypoventilation (pickwickian) syndrome: hypoxia/hypercapnea as a stimulus for angiogenesis. *Arch Ophthalmol*. 2000;118:1297–1298.

12. Kaiser PK, Rieman CD, Sears JE, et al. Macular traction detachment and diabetic macular edema associated with posterior hyaloidal traction. *Am J Ophthalmol*. 2001;131: 44–49.

13. Brown JC, Solomon SD, Bressler SB, et al. Detection of diabetic foveal edema: contact lens biomicroscopy compared with optical coherence tomography. *Arch Ophthalmol*. 2004;122:330–335.

14. Early Treatment Diabetic Retinopathy Study Research Group. Photocoagulation for diabetic macular edema. ETDRS Report Number 1. *Arch Ophthalmol*. 1985;103: 1796–1806.

15. Diabetic Retinopathy Clinical Research Network: www.drcr.net

16. Ozaki H, Hayashi H, Vinores SA, et al. Intravitreal sustained release of VEGF causes retinal neovascularization in rabbits and breakdown of the blood-retinal barrier in rabbits and primates. *Exp Eye Res*. 1997;64:505–517.

17. Derevjanik NL, Vinores SA, Xiao W-H, et al. Quantitative assessment of the integrity of the blood-retinal barrier in mice. *Invest Ophthalmol Vis Sci*. 2002;43:2462–2467.

18. Cunningham ET Jr, Adamis AP, Altaweel M, et al. A phase II randomized double-masked trial of pegaptanib, an anti-vascular endothelial growth factor aptamer, for diabetic macular edema. *Ophthalmology*. 2005;112(10):1747–1757.

19. Nguyen QD, Tatlipinar S, Shah SM, et al. Vascular endothelial growth factor is a critical stimulus for diabetic macular edema. *Am J Ophthalmol*. 2006;142(6):961–969.

20. Diabetic Retinopathy Clinical Research Network. A phase II randomized clinical trial of intravitreal bevacizumab for diabetic macular edema. *Ophthalmology*. 2007;114: 1860–1867.

21. Do DV, Nguyen QD, Shah SM, et al. An exploratory study of the safety, tolerability and bioactivity of a single intravitreal injection of vascular endothelial growth factor Trap-Eye in patients with diabetic macular oedema. *Br J Ophthalmol*. February 2009;93(2):144–149.

22. Chieh JJ, Roth DB, Liu M, et al. Intravitreal triamcinolone acetonide for diabetic macular edema. *Retina*. 2005;25(7):828–834.

23. Diabetic Retinopathy Clinical Research Network, Chew E, Strauber S, et al. Randomized trial of peribulbar triamcinolone acetonide with and without focal photocoagulation for mild diabetic macular edema: a pilot study. *Ophthalmology*. June 2007;114(6):1190–1196.

24. Diabetic Retinopathy Clinical Research Network. A randomized trial comparing intravitreal triamcinolone acetonide and focal/grid photocoagulation for diabetic macular edema. *Ophthalmology*. September 2008;115(9):1447–1449, 1449. e1–1449.10. July 26, 2008. www.aaojournal.org

25. Pearson P, Levy B, Comstock T. Fluocinolone acetonide intravitreal implant to treat diabetic macular edema: 3-year results of a multi-center clinical trial. Poster presented at the Association for Research in Vision and Ophthalmology, April 30–May 4, 2006, Fort Lauderdale, FL. Abstract 5442.

26. Kuppermann B, Blumenkranz M, Haller J, et al. Randomized controlled study of an intravitreous dexamethasone drug delivery system in patients with persistent macular edema. *Arch Ophthalmol*. 2007;125:309–317.

27. Harbour JW, Smiddy WE, Flynn HW Jr, Rubsamen PE. Vitrectomy for diabetic macular edema associated with a thickened and taut posterior hyaloid membrane. *Am J Ophthalmol*. April 1996;121(4):405–413.
28. Kaiser PK, Riemann CD, Sears JE, Lewis H. Macular traction detachment and diabetic macular edema associated with posterior hyaloidal traction. *Am J Ophthalmol*. January 2001;131(1):44–49.
29. Hartley KL, Smiddy WE, Flynn HW Jr, Murray TG. Pars plana vitrectomy with internal limiting membrane peeling for diabetic macular edema. *Retina*. March 2008;28(3):410–419.

14

Management of Diabetic Retinopathy: Evidence-based Systematic Review

QURESH MOHAMED, MD,
AND TIEN Y. WONG, MD, PhD

CORE MESSAGES

- Diabetic retinopathy is the leading cause of blindness in the working-age population in the United States.
- Intensive glycemic and blood pressure controls in patients with type 1 and 2 diabetes remain the cornerstone for prevention of diabetic retinopathy and its progression.
- Laser photocoagulation reduces severe visual loss in people with proliferative diabetic retinopathy or clinically significant macular edema by at least 50%.
- Early surgical vitrectomy increases the chance of restoring or maintaining good vision in eyes known or suspected to have very severe proliferative diabetic retinopathy (with fibrovascular proliferation or nonclearing vitreous hemorrhage).
- Aspirin does not reduce the risk of developing diabetic retinopathy, and it does not increase the incidence of retinal or vitreous hemorrhage.
- More data are needed on intravitreal or retinal implants and intravitreal anti-angiogenic agents before general clinical application.

There are 200 million persons with diabetes mellitus worldwide [1], with 20 million in the United States alone [2]. The most specific microvascular complication of diabetes is diabetic retinopathy, the leading cause of visual impairment in working-age persons. The prevalence of diabetic retinopathy increases with disease duration [3], so that after 20 years, nearly all persons with type 1 diabetes and 60% of those with type 2 have some retinopathy. The major risk factors for diabetic retinopathy include hyperglycemia, hypertension, and hyperlipidemia [3,4], and have been summarized in Chapter 5.

Control for these risk factors can reduce the incidence of diabetic retinopathy (primary prevention), while laser photocoagulation may prevent further progression of diabetic retinopathy and vision loss (secondary interventions). While there are many new interventions, the evidence to support their use is uncertain. This chapter provides a systematic review of the literature to determine the best evidence for primary and secondary interventions for diabetic retinopathy.

METHODOLOGY AND DATA SOURCES

A systematic literature search to identify English-language randomized controlled trials or meta-analyses evaluating interventions for diabetic retinopathy was conducted. Articles were retrieved using MEDLINE (1966 through August 2007), EMBASE, Cochrane Collaboration and NIH Clinical Trials Database through August 2007. Search terms included variations of keywords for retinopathy, diabetes, diabetic retinopathy, diabetic macular edema, retinal neovascularization, controlled clinical trial, and randomized clinical trial. This was supplemented by hand searching the reference lists of major review articles. Because the primary interest was in longer-term outcomes, studies with less than 12 months of follow-up and studies failing to separate data of different retinal conditions (e.g., macular edema from diabetes vs. retinal vein occlusion) were excluded. Where duplicate results were published, the most recent or complete source was used. Secondary complications of proliferative diabetic retinopathy such as neovascular glaucoma and tractional detachments were excluded as they were beyond the scope of this review. A total of 831 citations were accessed, of which 45 studies (including three meta-analyses) on interventions for diabetic retinopathy met our inclusion criteria. Additional references up to 31st December 2008 were included in the current review.

The quality of studies was assessed via the Delphi consensus criteria list [5]. Studies were evaluated on a standardized data extraction form for (1) valid method of randomization, (2) concealed allocation of treatment, (3) similarity of groups at baseline regarding the most important prognostic indicators, (4) clearly specified eligibility criteria, (5) blinding of the outcome assessor, (6) care provider, (7) patient, (8) reporting of point estimates and measures of variability for outcomes, (9) intention-to-treat analysis, and (10) acceptable loss to follow-up rate unlikely to cause bias. Studies were scored out of a maximum of 10, and studies with a score >5 were considered as higher quality studies. The overall strength of evidence (levels I, II, and III) and ratings for clinical recommendations (levels A, B, and C) were based on previously reported criteria [6].

For primary interventions, measures included incidence of diabetic retinopathy in patients with diabetes with no retinopathy at baseline, and rate of adverse effects of intervention. For secondary interventions, outcome measures included progression of diabetic retinopathy, changes in visual acuity and macular thickness, and rates of legal blindness and adverse effects. Emphasis was given to studies where best-corrected visual acuity was measured in a masked fashion using Early Treatment Diabetic Retinopathy Study (ETDRS) protocol. For some randomized controlled trials (RCTs), both primary (incidence of diabetic retinopathy) and secondary (progression of diabetic retinopathy) interventions were evaluated.

There were significant variations between studies. For example, studies used different methods to ascertain retinopathy, including clinical ophthalmoscopy, retinal photography, and/or fluorescein angiography [7]. Studies also classified diabetic retinopathy differently, with most using the Airlie House classification with some modifications [8,9]; diabetic macular edema was usually classified as absent or present. Definitions for progression of diabetic retinopathy also varied. The Diabetes Control and Complications Trial (DCCT) [10,11] defined progression as at least three steps worsening from baseline, while the United Kingdom Prospective Diabetes Study (UKPDS) [12] defined progression as a two-step change from baseline. Other studies used increases in number of microaneurysms or the need for laser photocoagulation as indicators of progression.

Primary Interventions

Glycemic Control. A consistent relationship between glycated hemoglobin (HbA1c) levels and the incidence of diabetic retinopathy has been demonstrated in epidemiological studies [13,14]. This key observation has been confirmed in large randomized clinical trials demonstrating that tight glycemic control reduces both the incidence and progression of diabetic retinopathy (Table 14.1). For type 1 diabetes, the DCCT [10,11,15,16] conducted between 1983 and 1993, randomized 1441 patients with type 1 diabetes to receive intensive glycemic or conventional therapy. Over 6 years of follow-up, intensive treatment (median HbA1c, of 7.2%) reduced the incidence of diabetic retinopathy by 76% (95% confidence interval [CI], 62–85%) and progression of diabetic retinopathy by 54% (95% CI, 39–66%), as compared with conventional treatment (median HbA1c, of 9.1%) [10,11,15,16].

For type 2 diabetes, similar findings were reported in the UKPDS [18]. The UKPDS randomized 3867 newly diagnosed persons with type 2 diabetes to intensive or conventional therapy. Intensive therapy reduced microvascular endpoints by 25% (95% CI, 7–40%) and the need for laser photocoagulation by 29%. Data from a subgroup of participants' retinal photographic grading showed a similar association [32]. These findings have been replicated in other studies [20,33], including a meta-analysis prior to the DCCT [21] (Table 14.1).

Long-term observational data from the DCCT, with participants followed up in the Epidemiology of Diabetes Intervention and Complications study (EDIC), showed that despite gradual equalization of HbA1c values after study termination, the rate of diabetic retinopathy progression in the former intensively treated group in DCCT remained significantly lower than the former conventional group [11,17], emphasizing the importance of instituting tight glycemic control early in the course of diabetes. This concept is supported in another randomized clinical trial [34] in which participants initially assigned to intensive glucose control had lower 10-year incidence of severe retinopathy as compared to conventional treatment [35].

While the benefits of tight glycemic control are apparent, this intervention has two clinically important adverse effects. First, there is risk of early worsening of diabetic retinopathy. In the DCCT, this occurred in 13.1% of the intensive as compared to 7.6% of the conventional treatment group [36]. However, this effect was

Table 14.1. Randomized Controlled Controlled Trials Evaluating Role of Glycemic Control in Diabetic Retinopathy

Study	N	Diabetes Type	Intervention	Outcome	Comments	Follow up
Diabetes Control and Complications Trial (DCCT) [10,11,16,17]	1441	Type 1 DM (726 No DR and 715 Mild-mod NPDR)	Intensive vs conventional treatment	Median HbA1c 7.2% IT vs 9.1% CT (P < 0.001) IT ↓ risk of developing DR by 76%. IT ↓ risk of progression DR by 54% IT ↓ risk of maculopathy by 23%* IT ↓ risk of severe NPDR/PDR by 47% IT ↓ risk of laser photocoagulation for macular edema or PDR by 51%	43 extra episodes of hypoglycemia requiring assistance per 100 patient yrs with IT 3.4 extra cases of being "overweight" per 100 patient yrs with IT	6.5 yrs
United Kingdom Prospective Diabetes Study (UKPDS) [18,19]	3867	Newly diagnosed type 2 DM	Intensive (sulphonylurea or insulin, aiming for fasting plasma glucose <6 mmol/L) vs conventional (fasting plasma glucose <15 mmol/L) treatment	Mean HbA1c 7% IT vs 7.9% CT. IT ↓ risk in microvascular endpoints by 25% IT ↓ risk retinal photocoagulation by 29% IT ↓ risk progression DR by 17% IT ↓ risk VH by 23%* IT ↓ risk legal blindness by 16%*		10 yrs
Kumamoto Study [20] (Japan)	110	Japanese patients with type 2 DM (55 No DR, 55 with NPDR)	Intensive vs conventional treatment	Mean HbA1c 7.2% IT vs 9.4% CT. IT ↓ risk of developing DR by 32% IT ↓ risk of progression DR by 32% IT ↓ progression to pre-proliferative and PDR compared to CT (1.5 vs 3.0 events/100 patient-yrs)	No patient in the primary cohort developed pre-proliferative or PDR	8 yrs
Wang et al. [21,22] Meta analysis	529	Type 1 DM	Intensive vs conventional treatment	Mean HbA1c for IT groups 7% to 10.5% across included RCTs IT ↓ risk of progression DR by 51% IT ↓ risk of progression to PDR or changes requiring laser reduced by 56% Trend towards progression of DR after	Hypoglycemia episodes requiring assistance 9.1 extra cases per 100 patient years with IT.	2 to 5 yrs

Study	N	Population	Intervention	Results	Comments	Duration
Lauritzen T, et al. [23]§	30	Type 1 DM with advanced NPDR	CSII vs conventional treatment	PDR developed in 4 patients in the CSII group vs 5 in the CT group* Trend towards more frequent improvement of retinal morphology in the CSII group (47%) than in the CT group (13%)*	Small numbers, study underpowered for any firm conclusion.	2 yrs
Kroc collaborative study group [24,25]§	70	Type 1 DM with low C-peptide level with NPDR	CSII vs conventional injection treatment	Mean HbA1c 8.1% CSII vs 10.0% CT. Retinopathy ↑ in both groups. Trend towards progression DR with CSII (↑ soft exudates and IRMA) in first 8 months,* which was reversed by 2 yrs	The study continued after the initial 8 months with 23/34 CSII group and 24/34 CT group followed for a further 16 months.	8 months to 2 yrs
Beck-Nielsen H, et al. [26] Olsen T, et al. [27] (1987 3 year results)§	24	Type 1 DM without proteinuria with minimal/No DR	CSSI with a portable pump vs conventional insulin treatment	Mean HbA1c 7.4% CSII vs 8.6% CT (P <0.01). Trend for progression of DR in CIT patients than in CSII (P > 0.1)*	Small sample. 1 loss to follow-up in CSII group	5 yrs
The Stockholm Diabetes Intervention Study [28]	96	Type 1 DM with NPDR	Intensive vs conventional treatment	Median HbA1c 7.2% IT vs 8.7% CT Retinopathy ↑ in both groups (P < 0.001) OR for serious retinopathy was 0.4 in the IT group as compared with CT (P = 0.04)	242 vs 98 episodes hypoglycemia in IT and CT groups (P < 0.05) IT ↑ BMI by 5.8%	5 yrs
Oslo Study [29–31]	45	Type 1 DM	CSII vs multiple insulin injections (5–6/day) vs conventional treatment (twice daily injections)	A transient ↑ in MA and hemorrhage in CSII and multiple insulin group compared with CT (P < 0.01)	A transient ↑ in MA and hemorrhages was seen at 3 months in CSII group	2 yrs

* Effect was not statistically significant, § included in Meta-analysis by Wang et al. [21].

DM = diabetes mellitus; NPDR = nonproliferative diabetic retinopathy; vs = versus, HbA1c = glycosylated hemoglobin; IT = intensive treatment; CT = conventional treatment, DR = diabetic retinopathy; PDR = proliferative diabetic retinopathy;NPDR = nonproliferative diabetic retinopathy; RCTs = randomized clinical trials; CSII = continuous subcutaneous insulin infusion, IRMA = intraretinal microvascular abnormalities; MA = microaneurysms; HEx = hard exudates; OR = odds ratio.

reversed by 18 months and no case of early worsening resulted in serious visual loss. Similar adverse event rates were reported in a meta-analysis [22]. Participants at risk of this early worsening had higher HbA1c levels at baseline and a more rapid reduction of HbA1c levels in the first 6 months, suggesting that physicians should avoid rapid reductions of HbA1c levels where possible. Second, tight glycemic control is a known risk factor for hypoglycemic episodes and diabetic ketoacidosis [21]. A meta-analysis of 14 randomized clinical trials, including the DCCT [37], indicated that intensive treatment is associated with a three-fold increased risk of hypoglycemia and 70% higher risk of ketoacidosis as compared with conventional treatment. The risk of ketoacidosis was seven-fold higher among patients exclusively using insulin pumps [37], suggesting that multiple daily insulin injections might be a safer strategy.

Blood Pressure Control. Blood pressure has not been shown to be a consistent risk factor for diabetic retinopathy incidence and progression in epidemiological studies [38–41]. However, evidence from randomized clinical trials indicates that tight blood pressure control is a major modifiable factor for the incidence and progression of diabetic retinopathy (Table 14.2). The UKPDS [12] randomized 1048 patients with hypertension to tight control (target blood pressure <150/<85 mmHg) or conventional control (target blood pressure <180/<105 mmHg). After 9 years of follow-up, patients having tight control had a 34% reduction (99% CI, 11–50%) in diabetic retinopathy progression, 47% reduction (99% CI, 7–70%) in visual acuity deterioration, and 35% reduction in laser photocoagulation therapies (primarily due to a reduction in the incidence of diabetic macular edema) compared with those having conventional control. In fact, the magnitude of benefit with tighter blood pressure control outweighed the magnitude of the benefits seen with tight glucose control in the UKPDS.

The Appropriate Blood Pressure Control in Diabetes (ABCD) trial [43,47], which randomized 470 people with type 2 diabetes and hypertension to receive intensive control (target diastolic blood pressure of 75 mmHg) or moderate blood pressure control (target diastolic blood pressure of 80–89 mmHg), found somewhat different findings as compared to the UKPDS. In the ABCD, over 5 years, there was no difference in diabetic retinopathy progression between the groups. The lack of efficacy in this study may be related to poorer glycemic control, shorter follow-up and lower blood pressure levels at baseline as compared to the UKPDS. It is unclear if there is a threshold effect beyond which further blood pressure lowering no longer influences diabetic retinopathy progression.

The effects of therapy with antihypertensive agents are also apparent among people with diabetes who are normotensive. In another arm of the ABCD trial [47], among 480 patients with type 2 diabetes without hypertension, intensive blood pressure control (10 mmHg below the baseline diastolic) significantly reduced diabetic retinopathy progression over 5 years as compared to moderate blood pressure control. The EURODIAB Controlled Trial of Lisinopril in Insulin-Dependent Diabetes Mellitus (EUCLID) [45] evaluated the effects of the angiotensin-converting enzyme (ACE) inhibitor lisinopril on diabetic retinopathy progression in normotensive, normoalbuminuric patients with type 1 diabetes. Lisinopril reduced the

Table 14.2. Randomized Controlled Trials Evaluating Role of Blood Pressure Control in Diabetic Retinopathy

Study	N	Diabetes Type	Intervention	Outcome	Comments	Follow up
United Kingdom Prospective Diabetes Study (UKPDS) [42]	1148	Type 2 DM with hypertension (mean BP of 160/94 mmHg)	Tight BP control (<150/85 mmHg) vs. less tight BP control (<180/105 mm Hg (Randomized to beta-blocker or angiotensin-converting enzyme (ACE) inhibitor)	IT ↓ risk of progression DR (≥2 ETDRS steps) by 34% (99% CI; 11–50% P = 0.004) IT ↓ risk VA loss 3 ETDRS lines by 47% (7–70%, P = 0.004) IT ↓ risk of laser photocoagulation by 35%. (P = 0.02) IT ↓ risk of >5 MA (RR, 0.66; P < .001), Hex (RR, 0.53; P < .001), and CWS (RR, 0.53; P < .001) at 7.5 yrs.	Observational data suggest 13% ↓ in microvascular complications for each 10 mmHg ↓ in mean systolic BP. No difference in outcome between ACE inhibitor and beta-blockade	8.4 yrs
Appropriate Blood Pressure Control in Diabetes trial (ABCD) [43]	470	Hypertensive type 2 DM (mean baseline diastolic BP >90 mmHg)	Intensive BP control (aiming for a DBP of 75 mmHg) vs. moderate control (DBP 80–89 mmHg)	No difference in progression of DR between IT (mean BP 132/78 mmHg) and CT (mean BP 138/86 mmHg).	No difference in progression of DR with nisoldipine vs enalapril.	5.3 yrs
Appropriate Blood Pressure Control in Diabetes trial (ABCD) [44]	480	Normotensive type 2 DM (BP <140/90 mm Hg)	Intensive (10 mm Hg below the baseline DBP) vs. moderate (80–89 mm Hg) DBP control	IT (mean BP 128/75mm Hg) ↓ progression of DR compared to CT (mean BP 137/81mm Hg) (P = 0.019).	Results were the same regardless of the initial antihypertensive agent used	5.3 yrs

(*Continued*)

Table 14.2. (Continued)

Study	N	Diabetes Type	Intervention	Outcome	Comments	Follow up
The EURODIAB Controlled Trial of Lisinopril in Insulin-Dependent Diabetes Mellitus (EUCLID) [45]		Normotensive and normoalbuminuric Type 1 DM	Lisinopril treatment	Lisinopril ↓ progression DR (2 ETDRS steps) by 50% and ↓ progression to PDR by 80%.	Concern about possibility of inadequate randomization (Lisinopril group had lower HbA1c levels)	2 yrs
Action in Diabetes and Vascular disease study (ADVANCE) [46]	11140	Normotensive and Hypertensive type 2 DM	Additional treatment with fixed perindopril/ indapamide combination vs placebo	No difference in eye events between additional treatment (mean BP 140.3/77 mm Hg) and CT (mean BP 134.7/74.8 mm Hg) Visual deterioration in 2446/5569 treated vs 2524/5571 placebo RR 5% (95% CI; -1–10%) New/worsening eye disease in 289 treated vs 286 placebo RR -1% (95%CI; -18–15%)	Treatment reduced macrovascular events, but no effect on vision loss or eye disease. Participants had excellent glycemic control and were allowed additional anti-HT agents.	4.3 yrs

DM = diabetes mellitus, BP = blood pressure, DM = diabetes mellitus, NPDR = nonproliferative diabetic retinopathy, vs.= versus, HbA1c = glycosylated hemoglobin A levels, IT = intensive treatment, CT = conventional treatment, DR = diabetic retinopathy, PDR = proliferative diabetic retinopathy, NPDR = nonproliferative diabetic retinopathy, RR = relative risk, MA = microaneurysms; Hex = hard exudates; BP = Blood pressure; HbA1c = glycosylated hemoglobin.

progression of diabetic retinopathy by 50% (95% CI, 0.28–0.89) and progression to proliferative diabetic retinopathy by 80% over 2 years [45]. EUCLID was limited by differences in baseline glycemic levels between groups (treatment group had lower HbA1c) and a short follow-up of 2 years. This study, along with another smaller randomized clinical trial [48] suggested that ACE inhibitors may have an additional benefit on diabetic retinopathy progression independent of blood pressure lowering. However, data from the UKPDS [42] and the ABCD study [43,47] did not find ACE inhibitors to be superior to other blood pressure medications.

The Action in Diabetes and Vascular Disease (ADVANCE) [49] study evaluated a low dose perindopril-indapamide combination in 11,140 hypertensive and normotensive persons with type 2 diabetes. Although additional treatment with perindopril-indapamide reduced mean blood pressure (140.3/77 mmHg compared to 134.7/74.8 mmHg with placebo) and macrovascular events, there was no significant reduction in eye events or visual deterioration with treatment [46]. Whether newer blood pressure medications have additional beneficial effects is unclear. A recent small randomized clinical trial ($n = 24$) with short follow-up (4 months) reported a worsening of diabetic macular edema among patients treated with angiotensin-II receptor blocker losartan compared with controls [50].

The Diabetic Retinopathy Candesartan Trial (DIRECT) randomized 5231 normotensive or mildly hypertensive patients with type 1 or type 2 diabetes to daily placebo or 32 mg candesartan, an angiotensin II receptor blocker [51,52] After 6 years' follow-up, use of candesartan in patients with type 1 diabetes modestly reduced the incidence of retinopathy by 18% but had no effect on the progression of existing retinopathy. In patients with type 2 diabetes, candesartan significantly increased the regression of existing retinopathy by 34% and reduced its progression by 13%, although the latter finding was not statistically significant. In both DIRECT studies, these modest effects were achieved in participants with early retinopathy only and could be related to the blood pressure lowering effects of candesartan. Thus, although DIRECT indicates that candesartan reduces retinopathy in both type 1 and 2 diabetes, whether this effect is independent of tight blood pressure control and whether it translates into significant prevention of vision loss is still unclear.

Finally, the Action to Control Cardiovascular Risk in Diabetes Eye Study (ACCORD-EYE), which is evaluating development and progression of diabetic retinopathy with target systolic blood pressure of <120 and <140 mmHg, respectively, will be reporting results in 2010 [53].

Lipid-Lowering Therapy. There are several epidemiological studies suggesting that dyslipidemia increases the risk of diabetic retinopathy, particularly diabetic macular edema [38,54]. Observational data from the DCCT and ETDRS both linked higher LDL cholesterol levels with increased risk of hard exudates [55]. A small randomized clinical trial in 50 patients with diabetic retinopathy and short follow up found a nonsignificant trend in visual acuity improvement in patients on simvastatin treatment [56], while another study reported a reduction in hard exudates but no improvement in visual acuity in clinically significant diabetic macular edema treated with clobifrate [57].

In the Fenofibrate Intervention and Event Lowering in Diabetes (FIELD) study (Table 14.3) [58], among 9795 participants with type 2 diabetes, those treated with fenofibrate were less likely than controls to need laser treatment (5.2% vs. 3.6%, $P < 0.001$). However, the severity of diabetic retinopathy, indications for laser treatment, and type of laser treatment (focal or pan-retinal) were not reported.

The Collaborative Atorvastatin Diabetes Study (CARDS), a randomized clinical trial of 2830 patients with type 2 diabetes, did not find atorvastatin to be effective in reducing diabetic retinopathy progression [68,69]. The study was limited by substantial missing data (only 65% had retinopathy status at baseline) and lack of photographic grading for diabetic retinopathy. There are several ongoing RCTs that may clarify the role of lipid reduction in diabetic retinopathy. The Atorvastatin Study for Prevention of Coronary Endpoints in NIDDM (ASPEN) [70] will evaluate the effects of atorvastatin in diabetic retinopathy and the ACCORD-EYE study [53] will compare treatment to increase high density lipoprotein (HDL) and reduce low density lipoprotein (LDL) (fibrate + statin) with LDL reduction only (statin and placebo) on diabetic retinopathy.

SECONDARY INTERVENTION

Medical Interventions. Various other medical interventions for diabetic retinopathy are described in Table 14.3 and summarized below.

Antiplatelet Agents. With regards to the efficacy and safety of aspirin, the ETDRS showed that aspirin (650 mg/day) had no beneficial effect on diabetic retinopathy progression or loss of visual acuity in patients with diabetic macular edema or severe nonproliferative diabetic retinopathy during 9-years of follow-up [59,60]. Aspirin treatment was not associated with an increased rate of vitrectomy [59,60]. A smaller randomized clinical trial evaluating aspirin alone and in combination with dipyridamole reported a reduction in microaneurysms on fluorescein angiograms in both groups as compared to placebo [61]. A similar trend was seen in a small randomized clinical trial [62] evaluating ticlodipine although results were not statistically significant.

Protein Kinase C Inhibitors. In recent years, there has been significant interest in the use of protein kinase C (PKC) inhibitors for treatment of diabetic retinoipathy. Hyperglycemia induces synthesis of diacylglycerol in vascular cells, leading to activation of PKC isozymes, particularly PKC-ß. Excessive PKC activation is thought to be a key pathophysiological mechanism of diabetic retinopathy. The PKC-Diabetic Retinopathy Study evaluated the effects of ruboxistaurin, an orally active, selective PKC-ß inhibitor [63]. The study randomized 252 patients with moderate to severe nonproliferative diabetic retinopathy to receive ruboxistaurin (8, 16, or 32 mg) or placebo. No significant difference in diabetic retinopathy progression was seen after 36 months of follow-up, although patients treated with 32 mg of ruboxistaurin had a significant reduction in the risk of moderate visual loss. Treatment was well tolerated with few adverse events, largely mild gastrointestinal symptoms. A larger study, which randomized 685 patients, showed similar results [71].

Table 14.3. Randomized Controlled Trials of Medical Interventions in Diabetic Retinopathy

Author	Diagnosis	Intervention	N	Outcome	Comment	Follow up
Fenofibrate Intervention and Event Lowering in Diabetes (FIELD study) [58]	Type 2 DM Total cholesterol 3 to 6.5 mmol/L and no lipid-lowering Rx at baseline	Fenofibrate vs placebo	9795	Treatment ↓ reported need for retinal laser photocoagulation (5.2%vs 3.6%, P = 0.0003).	Not main endpoint. Large loss of data. Severity of DR, indication for laser and the type of laser (focal or panretinal) not reported.	5 yrs
ETDRS [59] Chew E, et al. [60]	Mild-to-severe NPDR or early PDR	Aspirin 650 md/day vs placebo	3711	VH in 32% aspirin vs. 30% placebo, P = 0.48)*. No difference in the severity of vitreous/ preretinal hemorrhages (P = 0.11)* or rate of resolution (P = 0.86)	Aspirin had no effect on DR incidence/progression, VH, or need for vitrectomy.	3 yrs
The DAMAD Study Group [61]	Early diabetic retinopathy (type 1 and type 2 DM)	Aspirin (330 mg tds) alone vs Aspirin + dipyridamole (75 mg tds) vs placebo	475	Aspirin alone and aspirin + dipyridamole ↓ mean yearly increases in MA on FFA (Aspirin-alone group (0.69 ± 5.1); aspirin + dipyridamole (0.34 ± 3.0), placebo (1.44 ± 4.5) (P = 0.02)	Loss to follow-up of 10% patients.	3 yrs
The Ticlopidine Microangiopathy of Diabetes study (TIMAD) [62]	NPDR	Ticlopidine hydrochloride (antiplatelet agent) vs. placebo	435	Treatment ↓ yearly MA progression on FFA (0.23 ± 6.66 vs 1.57 ± 5.29; P = 0.03). Treatment ↓ progression to PDR (P = 0.056)*	Adverse reactions included neutropenia (severe in one case), diarrhea, and rash.	3 yrs

(Continued)

Table 14.3. (Continued)

Author	Diagnosis	Intervention	N	Outcome	Comment	Follow up
Cullen JF, et al. [57]	Exudative diabetic maculopathy	Atromid-S (clofibrate)		↓ hard exudates but no statistical improvement in VA	Lacked power.	1 yr
The PKC-DRS Study Group [63]	Moderately severe to very severe NPDR (ETDRS severity level between 47B - 53E), VA ≥20/125 and no previous scatter photocoagulation	Ruboxistaurin RBX (8, 16, or 32 mg/day) vs placebo	252	No significant effect on progression DR. 32 mg RBX delayed occurrence of MVL (P = 0.038) and SMVL (P = 0.226).* In multivariable Cox proportional hazard analysis, RBX 32 mg ↓ risk of MVL vs. placebo (hazard ratio 0.37 [95% CI 0.17–0.80], P = 0.012).	RBX ↓ of SMVL was only seen in eyes with definite DME at baseline (10% RBX vs. 25% placebo, P = 0.017).	36 to 46 months
PKC-DRS2 Study Group	Moderately severe to very severe NPDR (ETDRS severity level between 47B - 53E), VA ≥20/125 and no previous scatter photocoagulation)	Ruboxistaurin 32 mg/day vs placebo	685	No significant effect on progression DR. Treatment ↓ risk of sustained MVL (5.5% treated vs 9.1% placebo, P = 0.034)		3 yrs
PKC-DME Study [64]	DME > 300 microns from center. (ETDRS severity level 20–47A, VA ≥75 ETDRS letters and no previous laser)	Ruboxistaurin 32 md/day	686	No significant effect on progression to sight threatening DME or need for focal laser.	Variation in application focal laser between centers. 32 mg RBX reduced progression of DME vs placebo in secondary analysis (P = 0.054 unadjusted)	3 yrs

Study	Population	Treatment	N	Results	Comments	Follow-up
The Sorbinol Retinopathy Trial [65]	Type I diabetics	oral sorbinil 250 mg vs placebo	497	No significant effect on progression DR (28% sorbinil vs. 32% placebo; P = 0.344)*.	Hypersensitivity reaction in 7% sorbinil treated group.	41 months
Gardner TW, et al. [66]	DME (no previous macular photocoagulation)	astemizole, an antihistamine, versus placebo	63	No effect on retinal thickening or HEx (photographs graded by modified ETDRS protocol)	54/63 patients (86%) completed 1 year of follow up	1-yr
Grant MB, et al. [67]	Severe NPDR or early non-high-risk PDR	Max tolerated doses octreotide (200–5,000 µg/day subcutaneously vs conventional treatment	23	Treatment ↓ progression to high risk PDR needing PRP (1/22 eyes treated vs 9/24 controls, P<0.006) Octreotide ↓ progression DR (27% vs 42% controls; P = 0.0605)*.	Thyroxine replacement therapy needed in all treated patients	15 months

VH = vitreous hemorrhage; NPDR = nonproliferative diabetic retinopathy; NV = neovascularization; NVD = neovascularization of the disk; PDR = proliferative diabetic retinopathy; DME = diabetic macular edema, PRP = panretinal photocoagulation; RR = risk reduction; MVL = moderate visual loss, SVL = severe visual loss; Hex = hard exudates, vs. = versus; BP = blood pressure.

The PKC-Diabetic Macular Edema Study reported no significant reduction in progression of diabetic retinopathy or incidence of diabetic macular edema in 686 patients with mild to moderate nonproliferative diabetic retinopathy with no prior laser therapy [64,72]. However, there was a trend for a reduction in clinically significant diabetic macular edema among patients treated with 32 mg ruboxistaurin ($P = 0.041$), with a larger effect when patients with HbA1c levels of 10% or greater were excluded ($P = 0.019$).

Aldose Reductase Inhibitors. The rate controlling enzyme in the polyol pathway of glucose metabolism is aldose reductase. Excess glucose is converted into fructose and sorbitol in the retina and may play a key role in the pathogenesis of diabetic retinopathy. Two aldose reductase inhibitors, sorbinil (Pfizer, New York, NY) and tolrestat (Wyeth-Ayerst, St. Davids, PA) showed no statistically significant effect in reducing diabetic retinopathy incidence or progression in RCTs of 3 to 5 years duration [65]. About 7% of the patients assigned to sorbinil in one randomized clinical trial developed a hypersensitivity reaction in the first 3 months [65].

Growth Hormone/Insulin-like Growth Factor Inhibitors. Studies showing improvements in diabetic retinopathy following surgical hypophysectomy [73,74], and of elevated serum and ocular levels of insulin-like growth factor in patients with severe diabetic retinopathy led to researchers investigating the use of agents inhibiting the growth hormone–insulin-like growth factor pathway for prevention of diabetic retinopathy [75]. A small randomized clinical trial over 15 months among 23 patients reported reduction in retinopathy severity with octreotide, a synthetic analogue of somatostatin that blocks growth hormone [67], but another trial conducted over 1 year among 20 patients [76] evaluating continuous subcutaneous infusion of octreotide found no significant benefits. Two larger trials currently evaluating extended release octreotide injection [77,78] have reported inconclusive preliminary results [79], with significant adverse effects (e.g., diarrhoea, cholelithiasis, hypoglycemic episodes).

Laser and Surgical Interventions for Severe Nonproliferative Diabetic Retinopathy and Proliferative Diabetic Retinopathy

Panretinal Laser Photocoagulation. There is strong evidence that panretinal laser photocoagulation (PRP) is useful for treating severe nonproliferative diabetic retinopathy and proliferative diabetic retinopathy [80] (Table 14.4). Two landmark clinical trials, the Diabetic Retinopathy Study (DRS) [80,81] and the ETDRS [82], provide high-quality data on the effectiveness and safety of PRP on clinically relevant outcomes.

The DRS randomized 1758 patients with proliferative diabetic retinopathy in at least one eye or bilateral severe nonproliferative diabetic retinopathy to PRP or no treatment. At 2 years, severe visual loss (visual acuity <5/200 on two successive visits) was seen in 6.4% of treated versus 15.9% of untreated eyes, with the greatest benefit in eyes with high-risk characteristics (new vessels at the optic disc or vitreous hemorrhage with new vessels elsewhere), in which the risk of severe visual

Table 14.4. Randomized Controlled Trials of Laser Treatment in Nonproliferative and Proliferative Diabetic Retinopathy and Diabetic Macular Edema

Study	N	Retinopathy severity	Intervention	Outcome	Comments	Follow up
NonProliferative and Proliferative Diabetic Retinopathy						
Rohan et al. Review/Meta-analysis of 5 trials [83]	2243	NPDR/PDR (± DME)	Peripheral PRP ± focal laser vs observation	PRP ↓ risk of blindness in eyes with PDR by 61% (combined "best estimate" based on 5 RCTs including Diabetic Retinopathy Study and British Multicenter Study)	Criteria for study inclusion, quality assessment, baseline comparability and adverse effects of included studies not described	1 to 5 yrs
Diabetic Retinopathy Study (DRS) [81]	1742	Severe NPDR (bilateral) or PDR (± DME	Peripheral PRP ± focal laser vs observation	PRP ↓ risk of SVL by 52% at 2 yrs 90/650 (14%) treated vs 171/519 (33%) deferred treatment RR 0.42 (0.34 to 0.53) Eyes with "high risk" features had most benefit (57% ↓ risk SVL)	Decreased VA and constriction of peripheral visual field in some eyes	5 yrs
Early Treatment Diabetic Retinopathy Study (ETDRS) [84,85]	3711	mild-to-severe NPDR or early PDR (± DME in both eyes)	One eye of each patient assigned to early PRP ± focal vs deferral of treatment	SVL in 2.6% treated vs 3.7% deferred treatment PRP ↓ risk vitrectomy (2.3% treated vs 4% deferred) ↓ risk of SVL or vitrectomy 4% with early photocoagulation vs 6% in deferred group	Eyes assigned to deferral of PRP did not receive any focal laser for any coexsistant DME, until the positive results of macular treatment were released	5 yrs
British Multicenter study [86]	107	PDR (bilateral symmetrical)	Xenon-arc laser photocoagulation vs observation	PRP ↓ risk of blindness 5% vs 17% observed RR 0.29 (0.11 to 0.77)	Large loss to FU (28%) Only 77 completed the 5 yr follow-up. No intention to treat analysis	5 to 7 yrs

(Continued)

Table 14.4. (Continued)

Study	N	Retinopathy severity	Intervention	Outcome	Comments	Follow up
				Patients with NVD at entry had greatest difference. Treated eyes that became blind had less treatment than those that retained vision.		
British Multicenter Study [87]	99	NPDR	Peripheral xenon arc laser vs observation	PRP ↓ visual deterioration 32% treated vs 55% controls RR 0.49 (0.32 to 0.74)	Large loss to FU No intention to treat analysis	5 yrs
Hercules BL, et al. [88]	94	Symmetrical PDR involving optic disc	PRP vs observation	PRP ↓ risk of blindness 7%(7/94) compared to 38% (36/94) RR 0.19 (0.09 to 0.41)	Incomplete masking No ITA	3 yrs
Patz A, et al. [89]	66	NPDR (+ DME)	PRP vs observation	Treatment ↓ visual deterioration (6% treated vs 63% controls) RR 0.10 (0.04 to 0.26)	Poorly specified criteria Loss not specified	26 months
Lövestam-Adrian, M [90] (2003)	81	Severe NPDR and PDR in type 1 diabetes patients	All participants treated with PRP. (one randomly selected eye per patient entered into study)	35% (14/40) eyes treated for severe NPDR developed NV. VH less frequent in treated eyes with severe NPDR vs PDR (2/40 vs 12/41; P = 0.007). ↓ vitrectomy for VH in eyes treated for severe NPDR (1/40 versus 6/41; P = 0.052). ↓ visual impairment in eyes treated for severe NPDR compared to PDR (4/40 vs 10/40; P = 0.056).	Time-point for PRP not randomly assigned. Adverse outcomes not assessed. Inclusion/exclusion criteria, blinding, intention to treat analysis not specified. Coexistent CSME was treated with macular laser	2.9 ± 1.5 yrs

Diabetic Macular Edema

Study	No.	Condition	Intervention	Results	Comments	Duration
ETDRS [91]	2244	Bilateral DME (mild-to-moderate NPDR)	Focal argon laser (754 eyes) vs observation (1490 eyes).	Treatment ↓ moderate visual loss (RR 0.50 (0.47 to 0.53). Benefits most marked in eyes with CSME, particularly if the center of the macula was involved or imminently threatened (subgroup analysis)		3 yrs
Blankenship GW, et al. [93]	39	Bilateral symmetrical DME (mod-severe NPDR)	Grid argon laser vs observation	Visual deterioration in 7/30 (23%) eyes with laser vs 13/30 (43%) eyes with no treatment; RR 0.54, (CI 0.25 to 1.16)*		2 yrs
Olk RJ, et al. [94]	92	Diffuse DME ± CSME	Modified grid argon laser vs observation	Treatment ↓ risk of moderate visual loss by 50% to 70%. Loss of VA reduced compared with no treatment at 1 yr (RR 0.84) and at 2 yrs (RR 0.78, CI 0.60 to 0.96)		2 yrs
Interim report of a multicenter controlled study [95]	76	Bilateral symmetrical DME	Xenon-arc laser vs observation	8 treated vs 18 control eyes blind. Prognosis was best in those with initial VA ≥ 6/24	Only 44 patients at 2 yrs, and 25 after 3yrs	3 yrs
Ladas ID, et al. [96]	42	Diffuse DME (NPDR)	Modified grid argon laser vs observation	Trend for improved VA with treatment at 1 and 2yrs. No difference in VA at 3 years. *	No masking. Poor characterization of groups.	3 yrs

DME = diabetic macular edema; CSME = clinically significant macular edema; PRP = panretinal laser photocoagulation; VA = visual acuity; VF = visual fields; MVL = moderate visual loss, SVL = severe visual loss; VH = vitreous hemorrhage; NPDR = nonproliferative diabetic retinopathy, NV = neovascularization; NVD = neovascularization of the disk, PDR = proliferative diabetic retinopathy, RR = risk reduction; CI = confidence intervals (95%); vs. = versus; BP = blood pressure.

loss was reduced by 50% [80]. The ETDRS [82] randomized 3711 patients with less severe diabetic retinopathy and visual acuity >20/100 to early PRP or deferral (4-monthly observation, and treatment if high-risk proliferative diabetic retinopathy developed). Early PRP treatment decreased the risk of high-risk proliferative diabetic retinopathy by 50% as compared to deferral, although the incidence of severe visual loss was low in both early and deferral groups (2.6% vs. 3.7%).

The effectiveness of PRP has been confirmed by other RCTs [86–88] and a meta-analysis with a combined data of 2243 patients [83].

There are well-known adverse effects of PRP. These include visual field constriction (important for driving [97,98]), reduced night vision, color vision changes, reduced contrast sensitivity, inadvertent laser burn, macular edema exacerbation, acute glaucoma, and traction retinal detachment [99]. The possibility of visual loss immediately following PRP is also well recognized. The DRS reported vision loss of 2 to 4 lines within 6 weeks of PRP in 10% to 23% of patients versus 6% for controls [100].

Surgical Vitrectomy for Proliferative Diabetic Retinopathy. Vitrectomy is used for treatment of eyes with advanced diabetic retinopathy, including proliferative diabetic retinopathy with nonclearing vitreous hemorrhage or fibrosis, areas of traction involving or threatening the macula, and more recently, persistent diabetic macular edema with vitreous traction (Table 14.5) [101]. The Diabetic Retinopathy Vitrectomy Study (DRVS) randomized 616 eyes with recent vitreous hemorrhage and visual acuity ≤5/200 for at least 1 month to early vitrectomy within 6 months or observation [102–105]. After 2 years follow-up, 25% of the early vitrectomy group versus 15% of the observation group had ≥20/40 vision, with the benefits maintained at 4 years and longer in type 1 diabetes. The DRVS also randomized 381 eyes with severe proliferative diabetic retinopathy and visual acuity >10/200 to early vitrectomy or conventional management. Treatment increased the probability of visual acuity ≥20/40.

The indications of vitrectomy have expanded in the last few years because of advances in vitrectomy, including wide-field viewing, endolaser treatment, heavy liquids, and bimanual instrumentation to manipulate the retina [112].

Laser and Surgical Interventions for Diabetic Macular Edema

Focal Laser Photocoagulation. There is high quality evidence that focal laser photocoagulation preserves vision in eyes with diabetic macular edema. The ETDRS [91] randomized 1490 eyes with diabetic macular edema to receive focal laser treatment or observation. At 3 years, treatment significantly reduced moderate visual loss as compared with observation [91], with the greatest benefits in eyes with clinically significant diabetic macular edema [113]. However, there remains limited evidence that the type (argon, diode, dye, krypton) or method of laser used influences outcomes [92,114–116].

Adverse effects of focal laser treatment are well documented, and include inadvertent foveal burn, central visual field defect, color vision abnormalities, subretinal fibrosis, and spread of laser scars.

Table 14.5. Randomized Controlled Trials of Surgical Interventions in Proliferative Diabetic Retinopathy and Diabetic Macular Edema

Author	Diagnosis	Intervention	N	Outcome	Comment	Follow up
Proliferative Diabetic Retinopathy						
Diabetic Retinopathy Vitrectomy Study [102,105]	Recent severe diabetic vitreous hemorrhage reducing VA ≤ 5/200 at least 1 month	Early vitrectomy vs. deferral of vitrectomy for 1 year	616 eyes	Early surgery ↑ recovery of VA ≥10/20 (25% vs 15% deferred group) Trend for more frequent loss of LP with early surgery (25% vs 19%) Greatest benefit ↑ VA ≥10/20 in type 1 DM with more severe PDR (36% vs 12% deferred group) and proportion losing LP was similar (28% vs 26%)		4 yrs
Diabetic Retinopathy Vitrectomy Study [102,105]	Advanced PDR with fibrovascular proliferation, and VA ≥10/200	Early vitrectomy vs. conventional management	370 eyes	Early surgery ↑ proportion of eyes with VA≥10/20 (44% vs 28% conventional treatment) No difference in proportion with loss of vision to light perception or less	Most benefit in patients with very advanced PDR. No benefit in group with less severe NV	4 yrs

(*Continued*)

Table 14.5. (Continued)

Author	Diagnosis	Intervention	N	Outcome	Comment	Follow up
Diabetic Macular Edema						
Gillies MC, et al. [106] (2006)	DME and impaired vision that persisted or recurred after laser treatment	Intravitreal triamcinolone acetonide (TA) injections (4 mg) vs subconjunctival saline placebo	43 (69 eyes)	TA ↑BCVA ≥ 5 letters (56% vs. 26%; II = 0.006)	Data for 60 of 69 (87%) eyes of 35 of 41 (85%) patients	2 yr
				TA ↑ Mean VA by 5.7 letters (CI, 1.4–9.9) vs placebo		
				IOP elevation ≥ 5mmHg in 23/34 (68%) vs 3/30 (10%) untreated eyes (P<0.0001)		
				Cataract surgery in 54% vs 0% controls (P<0.0001)		
				2 TA eyes required trabeculectomy		
				1 case of infectious endophthalmitis		
Pearson P, et al. [107]	DME	Sustained release fluocinolone acetonide intravitreal implant (Retisert) vs standard care (randomized 2:1 ratio)	197	Implant ↓ DME (no edema in 58% vs 30% standard care; P<0.001)	↑ IOP in 35%	3 yrs
				Implant ↑ >2 improvement in CMT (45% vs 24%)	28% required a filtering procedure and 5% explanted to manage IOP	
				Trend ↑ VA with implant (VA ↑ ≥3 lines in 28% vs 15%, P<0.05*)		
				Cataract surgery in 95% of phakic implanted eyes		

Study	Indication	Intervention	Number	Outcome	Follow-up	Comments
Yanyali A, et al. [108] (2006)	Bilateral DME unresponsive to grid laser photocoagulation	Vitrectomy with removal of the internal limiting membrane (ILM) randomly in one eye	20 eyes of 10 patients	Surgery ↓ CMT by 165.8 ± 114.8 microns vs 37.8 ± 71.2 microns in untreated eye (P = 0.016) Vitrectomy ↑ VA by ≥2 lines in 4 (40%) vs 1 (10%)*	1 yr	
Thomas et al. [109]	DME (VA≤6/12) unresponsive to laser with no associated traction	Vitrectomy + ILM peel vs further macular laser	40 eyes	Vitrectomy ↓ CMT by 73 microns (20%) vs 29 microns (10.7%) Vitrectomy ↓ mean BCVA by 0.05 logMAR vs ↑ 0.03 logMAR in controls* (not significant)	1 yr	18% loss to FU
Bahadir M, et al. [111]	Diffuse CSME	Vitrectomy + ILM peel (17 eyes) vs vitrectomy without ILM peeling (41 eyes total)	58 eyes of 49 patients	No significant difference between groups in VA outcome VA ↑ in both groups (0.391 ± 0.335 in Vity/ILM and 0.393 ± 0.273 logMAR, P>0.01)	1 yr	Randomization and masking unclear HbA1c and baseline BP not reported

CMT = central macular thickness; DME = diabetic macular edema; VA = visual acuity; ILM = internal limiting membrane; OCT = optical coherence tomography; PPV = pars plana vitrectomy; LP = light perception; IOP = intraocular pressure; FU = follow up; * = not significant; vs. = versus; CSME = clinically significant macular edema; BP = blood pressure; HbA1c = glycosylated hemoglobin.

Surgical Vitrectomy for Diabetic Macular Edema. Vitrectomy may also be useful for treatment of widespread or diffuse diabetic macular edema that is nonresponsive to focal laser photocoagulation [112,117–120]. However, the few clinical trials to date have small sample size and short follow-up, with inconsistent results (Table 14.5). A randomized clinical trial of 28 patients with diffuse diabetic macular edema reported reduced macular thickness and improved visual acuity at 6 months after vitrectomy versus observation [121]. Vitrectomy was superior to focal laser treatment in one randomized clinical trial [122], but not in others [109,110].

Complications of vitrectomy include recurrent vitreous hemorrhage, cataract formation and glaucoma, and retinal tears and detachment. The presence of vitreous or epiretinal traction and macular edema, now readily documented with optical coherence tomography, in association with visual impairment, is currently a frequent indication for vitrectomy.

Intravitreal Corticosteroids. Corticosteroids have potent anti-inflammatory and anti-angiogenesis effects. Intravitreal injection of triamcinolone acetonide (IVTA) [123] has been used for treatment of diabetic macular edema [124–126], with a number of clinical trials demonstrating significant improvements in diabetic macular edema and visual acuity [127–132]. Many of these, however, had small participant numbers and short follow-up. In addition, there are substantial adverse effects, including infection, glaucoma, and cataract formation [106,133–136].

In the largest randomized clinical trial with the longest follow-up yet reported, eyes with persistent diabetic macular edema were randomized to receive 4 mg of IVTA or sham injection (saline injection into subconjunctival space) [106]. After 2 years, 19 of 34 IVTA-treated eyes (56%) had a visual acuity improvement of 5 letters or more compared with 9 of 35 placebo-treated eyes (26%) ($P = 0.007$). Overall, IVTA-treated eyes had twice the chance of improved visual acuity and half the risk of further loss. However, many eyes required repeated injections (mean of 2.2) and there was significant intraocular pressure elevation (≥ 5 mmHg in 68% of treated eyes versus 10% of controls). Cataract surgery was required in 55% of IVTA-treated eyes. Thus, while this study demonstrated significant efficacy of IVTA in persistent diabetic macular edema, larger studies are needed to provide further data on long-term benefits and safety [137].

In addition, the ideal dose of IVTA remains unclear [138]. A phase 2 randomized clinical trial [139] evaluated sub-tenon's injections of triamcinolone either alone or in combination with focal laser photocoagulation in 129 eyes with mild diabetic macular edema and visual acuity (VA) of 20/40 or better. No significant changes in retinal thickening or VA were detected between focal laser, steroid, or combination treatment groups at 34 weeks. The authors concluded a phase III trial to evaluate the benefit of these treatments for mild diabetic macular edema was not warranted.

Intravitreal or retinal implants have also been developed allowing extended drug delivery. A surgically implanted intravitreal fluocinolone acetonide (Retisert, Bausch & Lomb, NY, USA) was evaluated in 97 patients with diabetic macular edema, who were randomized to receive either implant or standard care (laser or observation) [107]. At 3 years, 58% of implant eyes versus 30% of controls had resolution of diabetic macular edema ($P < 0.001$) and associated improvement in visual acuity. However, adverse effects included a substantially higher risk of cataract and glaucoma than that seen in eyes receiving IVTA, with 5% undergoing implant removal to control glaucoma [107]. An injectable biodegradable intravitreal dexamethasone extended-release implant (Posurdex, Allergan, CA, USA) was evaluated in a randomized clinical trial with reported improvements in visual acuity and macular thickness [140]. This study, however, also included eyes with macular edema from other causes (retinal vein occlusion, uveitis and post cataract surgery), and had relatively short follow-up. A larger randomized clinical trial of Posurdex for diabetic macular edema is currently under way.

Intravitreal Anti-vascular Endothelial Growth Factor Agents. Several randomized clinical trials are currently evaluating agents that suppress vascular endothelial growth factor (VEGF) for treatment of diabetic macular edema.

Pegaptanib (Macugen, Pfizer, NY), an aptamer that targets the 165-isoform of VEGF, is licensed for treatment of neovascular age-related macular degeneration. A randomized clinical trial of 172 patients with diabetic macular edema randomized to repeated intravitreal pegaptanib or sham injections showed that treated eyes were more likely to have improvement in visual acuity of ≥10 letters (34% vs. 10%, $P = 0.03$), macular thickness ($P = 0.02$) and need for focal laser treatment ($P = 0.04$) at 36 weeks [141]. Serious infection occurred following 1 of 652 injections (0.15%) and was not associated with severe visual loss [141]. Retrospective data analysis of 16 eyes with proliferative diabetic retinopathy also showed regression of neovascularization [142].

Ranibizumab (Lucentis, Genentech, CA) is an antibody fragment that blocks all isoforms of VEGF. Like pegaptanib, it is also approved for the treatment of neovascular age-related macular degeneration [143,144], and may also be useful for diabetic retinopathy and diabetic macular edema [145]. A phase 2 randomized clinical trial (the RESOLVE study) is currently evaluating ranibizumab in diabetic macular edema.

Bevacizumab (Avastin, Genentech, CA) is the full-length antibody from which ranibizumab is derived. It is approved for the treatment of colorectal cancer and not approved for intraocular use. However, bevacizumab appears to show similar efficacy for treatment of neovascular age-related macular degeneration, and may therefore also be effective for diabetic macular edema and proliferative diabetic retinopathy [146–149]. Bevacizumab has attracted interest because of its low cost, but systemic safety is a concern [150]. A phase 2 randomized clinical trial comparing the effects of focal photocoagulation, two different doses of intravitreal bevacizumab, and combined intravitreal bevacizumab with focal photocoagulation have been published [151]. There are a number of ongoing studies including a randomized clinical trial sponsored by the National Eye Institute comparing the effects of laser treatment, intravitreal ranibizumab, combined intravitreal ranibizumab and laser or sham injection on diabetic macular edema [152] and a study comparing intravitreal ranibizumab with PRP in diabetic retinopathy [153].

SUMMARY OF EVIDENCE

Primary Interventions. This systematic review shows there are high quality data and strong evidence that tight glycemic control reduces the incidence and progression of diabetic retinopathy (Table 14.6). For persons with type 1 diabetes, the DCCT showed that each 10% decrease in HbA1c level (e.g., 9–8%) reduces the risk of diabetic retinopathy by 39%, and this beneficial effect persists long after the period of intensive control. For persons with type 2 diabetes, the UKPDS showed that each 10% decrease in HbA1c level reduces the risk of microvascular events, including diabetic retinopathy, by 25%.

There is also strong evidence that tight blood pressure control in diabetic patients with hypertension is beneficial in reducing visual loss from diabetic retinopathy. The UKPDS showed that each 10 mmHg decrease in systolic blood pressure reduces the risk of microvascular complications by 13%, independent of the effects of glycemic control. There remains uncertainty of the benefit of blood pressure treatment in normotensive diabetic patients.

The benefits of lipid-lowering therapy for diabetic retinopathy prevention remain inconclusive. There is also little evidence that aspirin, other antiplatelet agents and aldose reductase inhibitors confer any benefit in reducing progression of diabetic retinopathy. The role of PKC and growth hormone inhibitors is currently unclear.

Secondary Interventions

Proliferative Diabetic Retinopathy. There are high-quality data and strong evidence that PRP significantly reduces the risk of severe vision loss from proliferative diabetic retinopathy by at least 50%. The benefits are most marked in those with high-risk proliferative diabetic retinopathy in whom PRP should be commenced without delay [84].

Early vitrectomy (between 1 and 6 months after onset) should be considered in patients with type 1 diabetes with persistent vitreous hemorrhage or when hemorrhage prevents other treatment. The benefits of vitrectomy are less clear for those with type 2 diabetes. However, with advances in vitreoretinal surgery, vitrectomy may be indicated earlier in eyes with nonclearing hemorrhage or advanced proliferative diabetic retinopathy.

The effectiveness and safety of several intravitreal anti-VEGF agents for the treatment of proliferative diabetic retinopathy are current being evaluated in clinical trials. Until these results are available, there is currently insufficient evidence recommending their routine use.

Nonproliferative Diabetic Retinopathy. Although there is good evidence that early PRP reduces the risk of severe visual loss in nonproliferative diabetic retinopathy, the absolute benefit of early PRP treatment is small, and the risks of deferred treatment are low. Thus, it is recommended that in mild-to-moderate nonproliferative diabetic retinopathy, systemic factors such as glycemic control and blood pressure should be gradually optimized, and PRP can be deferred provided that follow-up can be maintained.

Table 14.6. Summary of Clinical Recommendations for Primary and Secondary Interventions for Diabetic Retinopathy

Intervention	Recommendation	Evidence*
Glycemic control	Any lowering of HbA1c is advantageous in reducing the development of new and progression of existing DR. In patients with DR, an HbA1c < 7% is ideal	A, I
Blood pressure control	Any lowering of systolic and/or diastolic blood pressure is advantageous in reducing the development and progression of DR. In patients with DR, a systolic BP <130 mmHg is ideal	A, I
Lipid-lowering therapy	Lowering of LDL cholesterol reduces macrovascular complications of diabetes and may be advantageous in DME	A, II
Panretinal laser photocoagulation (PRP)	Prompt PRP is recommended in patients with PDR especially if high-risk features are present. Early PDR with less severe PDR (flat new vessels elsewhere and no high-risk features) and severe NPDR may be observed closely, but treatment is recommended if any difficulty/delay in follow-up is anticipated; there are associated risk factors or signs of progression especially in type 2 diabetics	A, I A, II
Focal laser photocoagulation	Focal laser therapy is recommended in eyes with DME involving the center of the macula and reducing VA. Treatment should be considered to DME threatening the center of the macula, but patients must be warned of potential risks of treatment especially where vision is 6/6 or better. Treatment is ideally guided by a fluorescein angiogram, and is unlikely to be beneficial in the presence of significant macular ischemia.	A, I
Surgical vitrectomy	Early vitrectomy (within 3 months) is recommended in patients with type I diabetes with severe vitreous hemorrhage and significant DR. Vitrectomy should be considered in eyes with severe PDR not responsive to other therapies, especially in the presence of vitreomacular traction.	B, II B, III

(Continued)

Table 14.6. (Continued)

Intervention	Recommendation	Evidence*
Intravitreal steroids	Intravitreal triamcinolone may have a role in diffuse DME that is unresponsive to focal laser treatment. Patients must be warned of the high incidence of secondary intraocular pressure rise, cataract, other potential risks, and the possible need for repeat treatment.	B, II
Intravitreal anti-vascular endothelial growth factor (VEGF) agents	These agents may have a role in reducing PDR and DME, but patients require repeated treatment and the agents have potential adverse effects. There is currently insufficient evidence to recommend their routine use.	B, II/III
Aspirin and other medical treatment	Aspirin does not reduce the risk of developing DR, or increase the incidence of retinal or vitreous hemorrhage.	C, I
	There is currently insufficient evidence to recommend the routine use of PKC inhibitors, GH antagonists and other treatments, but they may have a role in some patients	C, II/III

*Importance of clinical outcome, strength of evidence. **A** = most important or crucial to a good clinical outcome; **B** = moderately important to clinical outcome; **C** = possibly relevant but not critical to clinical outcome; **I** = data providing strong evidence in support of the clinical recommendation; **II** = strong evidence in support of the recommendation but the evidence lacks some qualities, thereby preventing its justifying the recommendation without qualification; **III** = insufficient evidence to provide support for or against recommendation, panel or individual expert opinion.

DR = diabetic retinopathy; DME = diabetic macular edema; CSME = clinically significant macular edema; PRP = panretinal laser photocoagulation; VA = visual acuity; NPDR = nonproliferative diabetic retinopathy; PDR = proliferative diabetic retinopathy; HbA1c = glycosylated hemoglobin.

For patients with severe nonproliferative diabetic retinopathy, the ETDRS and other studies [90] suggest that PRP should be considered, especially in persons with type 2 diabetes. This benefit should be balanced against the small risk of vision loss. Early PRP is recommended in these patients if regular follow-up examination is not feasible, if there is significant media opacity/cataract, which may affect the ability to apply future laser treatment, or if there are concomitant risk factors (e.g., pregnancy) for rapid progression.

Diabetic Macular Edema. There is strong evidence that focal laser photocoagulation reduces the risk of moderate vision loss in diabetic macular edema that poses risk to fixation (or clinically significant diabetic macular edema) by at least 50% and increases the chance of visual improvement. In patients with coexistent proliferative diabetic retinopathy and diabetic macular edema, focal laser treatment prior to or concurrent with PRP is recommended [84].

There is moderate evidence that intravitreal steroids may be useful in eyes with persistent diabetic macular edema and loss of vision despite conventional treatment, including focal laser treatment and attention to systemic risk factors. Patients should be informed of potential adverse effects and the need for reinjection. Further studies are warranted to determine the ideal dose and longer term efficacy and safety.

Intravitreal anti-VEGF agents have shown promising preliminary results, and are currently being evaluated in several clinical trials. Until the results of these trials are available, there is insufficient evidence recommending their routine use.

There is weak evidence that vitrectomy may be beneficial in some patients with diabetic macular edema, particularly in eyes with associated vitreo-macular traction, but well conducted studies with longer follow up are needed.

CONCLUSION

Diabetic retinopathy remains the leading cause of preventable blindness in working adults in the United States and other countries. There are proven effective primary and secondary interventions to limit visual loss. Data from a number of well-conducted RCTs demonstrate that improved control of blood glucose and hypertension and possibly serum lipids can significantly slow the onset and reduce the progression of diabetic retinopathy. Close follow-up and treatment with laser photocoagulation and vitrectomy surgery can prevent moderate and severe visual loss. Newer pharmacological agents, surgical techniques, and the use of intravitreal agents including steroids and anti-VEGF agents are promising adjuncts, which may further improve outcomes. However, the indications, efficacy, and safety of newer medical and surgical treatments require further evaluation.

REFERENCES

1. Diabetes Atlas 2005; Available at http://www.eatlas.idf.org. (Accessed May 2006).
2. Centres for Disease Control and Prevention. National diabetes fact sheet: general information and national estimates on diabetes in the United States, 2005. Atlanta, GA: U.S.

Department of Health and Human Services, Centers for Disease Control and Prevention; 2005.

3. Klein R, Klein BE, Moss SE, Cruickshanks KJ. The Wisconsin Epidemiologic Study of Diabetic Retinopathy: XVII. The 14-year incidence and progression of diabetic retinopathy and associated risk factors in type 1 diabetes. *Ophthalmology.* 1998;105:1801–1815.

4. Wong TY, Klein R, Islam FM, et al. Diabetic retinopathy in a multi-ethnic cohort in the United States. *Am J Ophthalmol.* 2006;141:446–455.

5. Verhagen AP, de Vet HC, de Bie RA, et al. The Delphi list: a criteria list for quality assessment of randomized clinical trials for conducting systematic reviews developed by Delphi consensus. *J Clin Epidemiol.* 1998;51:1235–1241.

6. Minckler. Evidence-based ophthalmology series and content based continuing medical education for the journal. *Ophthalmology.* 2000;107:9–10.

7. Early Treatment Diabetic Retinopathy Study Research Group. Classification of diabetic retinopathy from fluorescein angiograms. ETDRS report number 11. *Ophthalmology.* 1991;98:807–822.

8. Early Treatment Diabetic Retinopathy Study Research Group. Grading diabetic retinopathy from stereoscopic color fundus photographs--an extension of the modified Airlie House classification. ETDRS report number 10. *Ophthalmology.* 1991;98:786–806.

9. Aldington SJ, Kohner EM, Meuer S, Klein R, Sjølie AK. Methodology for retinal photography and assessment of diabetic retinopathy: the EURODIAB IDDM complications study. *Diabetologia.* 1995;38:437–444.

10. Diabetes Control and Complications Trial Research Group. Progression of retinopathy with intensive versus conventional treatment in the Diabetes Control and Complications Trial. *Ophthalmology.* 1995;102:647–661.

11. The Diabetes Control and Complications Trial/Epidemiology of Diabetes Interventions and Complications Research Group. Retinopathy and nephropathy in patients with type 1 diabetes four years after a trial of intensive therapy. *N Engl J Med.* 2000;342:381–389.

12. UK Prospective Diabetes Study Group. Tight blood pressure control and risk of macrovascular and microvascular complications in type 2 diabetes: UKPDS 38. *BMJ* 1998;317:703–713.

13. Klein R, Palta M, Allen C, Shen G, Han DP, D'Alessio DJ. Incidence of retinopathy and associated risk factors from time of diagnosis of insulin-dependent diabetes. *Arch Ophthalmol.* 1997;115:351–356.

14. Olsen BS, Sjølie A, Hougaard P, et al. A 6-year nationwide cohort study of glycaemic control in young people with type 1 diabetes. Risk markers for the development of retinopathy, nephropathy and neuropathy. Danish Study Group of Diabetes in Childhood. *J Diabetes Complications.* 2000;14:295–300.

15. The Diabetes Control and Complications Trial Research Group. The effect of intensive treatment of diabetes on the development and progression of long-term complications in insulin-dependent diabetes mellitus. *N Engl J Med.* 1993;329:977–986.

16. The Diabetes Control and Complications Trial Research Group. The relationship of glycemic exposure (HbA1c) to the risk of development and progression of retinopathy in the diabetes control and complications trial. *Diabetes.* 1995;44:968–983.

17. Diabetes Control and Complications Trial/Epidemiology of Diabetes Interventions and Complications Research Group. Effect of intensive therapy on the microvascular complications of type 1 diabetes mellitus. *JAMA.* 2002;287:2563–2569.

18. UK Prospective Diabetes Study (UKPDS) Group. Intensive blood-glucose control with sulphonylureas or insulin compared with conventional treatment and

risk of complications in patients with type 2 diabetes (UKPDS 33). *Lancet.* 1998;352:837–853.

19. Kohner EM, Stratton IM, Aldington SJ, Holman RR, Matthews DR, UK Prospective Diabetes Study (IKPDS) Group. Relationship between the severity of retinopathy and progression to photocoagulation in patients with Type 2 diabetes mellitus in the UKPDS (UKPDS 52). *Diabet Med.* 2001;18:178–184.

20. Shichiri M, Kishikawa H, Ohkubo Y, Wake N. Long-term results of the Kumamoto Study on optimal diabetes control in type 2 diabetic patients. *Diabetes Care.* 2000;23(Suppl 2):B21–B29.

21. Wang PH, Lau J, Chalmers TC. Meta-analysis of effects of intensive blood-glucose control on late complications of type I diabetes. *Lancet.* 1993;341:1306–1309.

22. Wang PH, Lau J, Chalmers TC. Metaanalysis of the effects of intensive glycemic control on late complications of type I diabetes mellitus. *Online J Curr Clin Trials.* 1993;Doc No 60:[5023 words; 37 paragraphs].

23. Lauritzen T, Frost-Larsen K, Larsen HW, Deckert T. Two-year experience with continuous subcutaneous insulin infusion in relation to retinopathy and neuropathy. *Diabetes.* 1985;34(Suppl 3):74–79.

24. The Kroc Collaborative Study Group. Blood glucose control and the evolution of diabetic retinopathy and albuminuria. A preliminary multicenter trial. *N Engl J Med.* 1984;311:365–372.

25. The Kroc Collaborative Study Group. Diabetic retinopathy after two years of intensified insulin treatment. Follow-up of the Kroc Collaborative Study. *JAMA.* 1988;260:37–41.

26. Beck-Nielsen H, Olesen T, Mogensen CE, et al. Effect of near normoglycemia for 5 years on progression of early diabetic retinopathy and renal involvement. *Diabetes Res.* 1990;15:185–190.

27. Olsen T, Richelsen B, Ehlers N, Beck-Nielsen H. Diabetic retinopathy after 3 years' treatment with continuous subcutaneous insulin infusion (CSII). *Acta Ophthalmol (Copenh).* 1987;65:185–189.

28. Reichard P, Berglund B, Britz A, Cars I, Nilsson BY, Rosenqvist U. Intensified conventional insulin treatment retards the microvascular complications of insulin-dependent diabetes mellitus (IDDM): the Stockholm Diabetes Intervention Study (SDIS) after 5 years. *J Intern Med.* 1991;230:101–108.

29. Dahl-Jørgensen K, Brinchmann-Hansen O, Hanssen KF, et al. Effect of near normoglycaemia for two years on progression of early diabetic retinopathy, nephropathy, and neuropathy: the Oslo study. *Br Med J (Clin Res Ed).* 1986;293:1195–1199.

30. Dahl-Jørgensen K, Brinchmann-Hansen O, Hanssen KF, Sandvik L, Aagenaes O. Rapid tightening of blood glucose control leads to transient deterioration of retinopathy in insulin dependent diabetes mellitus: the Oslo study. *Br Med J (Clin Res Ed).* 1985;290:811–815.

31. Brinchmann-Hansen O, Dahl-Jørgensen K, Sandvik L, Hanssen KF. Blood glucose concentrations and progression of diabetic retinopathy: the seven year results of the Oslo study. *BMJ.* 1992;304:19–22.

32. Stratton IM, Kohner EM, Aldington SJ, et al. UKPDS 50: risk factors for incidence and progression of retinopathy in Type II diabetes over 6 years from diagnosis. *Diabetologia.* 2001;44:156–163.

33. Ohkubo Y, Kishikawa H, Araki E, et al. Intensive insulin therapy prevents the progression of diabetic microvascular complications in Japanese patients with non-insulin-dependent diabetes mellitus: a randomized prospective 6-year study. *Diabetes Res Clin Pract.* 1995;28:103–117.

34. Reichard P, Nilsson BY, Rosenqvist U. The effect of long-term intensified insulin treatment on the development of microvascular complications of diabetes mellitus. *N Engl J Med*. 1993;329:304–309.

35. Reichard P, Pihl M, Rosenqvist U, Sule J. Complications in IDDM are caused by elevated blood glucose level: the Stockholm Diabetes Intervention Study (SDIS) at 10-year follow up. *Diabetologia*. 1996;39:1483–1488.

36. The Diabetes Control and Complications Trial Research Group. Early worsening of diabetic retinopathy in the Diabetes Control and Complications Trial. *Arch Ophthalmol*. 1998;116:874–886.

37. Egger M, Davey Smith G, Stettler C, Diem P. Risk of adverse effects of intensified treatment in insulin-dependent diabetes mellitus: a meta-analysis. *Diabet Med*. 1997;14:919–928.

38. van Leiden HA, Dekker JM, Moll AC, et al. Blood pressure, lipids, and obesity are associated with retinopathy: the hoorn study. *Diabetes Care*. 2002;25:1320–1325.

39. Wong TY, Mitchell P. The eye in hypertension. *Lancet*. 2007;369:614.

40. Klein R, Klein BE, Moss SE, Davis MD, DeMets DL. Is blood pressure a predictor of the incidence or progression of diabetic retinopathy? *Arch Intern Med*. 1989;149:2427–2432.

41. Klein R, Moss SE, Klein BE, Davis MD, DeMets DL. The Wisconsin Epidemiologic Study of Diabetic Retinopathy. XI. The incidence of macular edema. *Ophthalmology*. 1989;96:1501–1510.

42. Matthews DR, Stratton IM, Aldington SJ, Holman RR, Kohner EM, UK Prospective Diabetes Study Group. Risks of progression of retinopathy and vision loss related to tight blood pressure control in type 2 diabetes mellitus: UKPDS 69. *Arch Ophthalmol*. 2004;122:1631–1640.

43. Estacio RO, Jeffers BW, Gifford N, Schrier RW. Effect of blood pressure control on diabetic microvascular complications in patients with hypertension and type 2 diabetes. *Diabetes Care*. 2000;23(Suppl 2):B54–B64.

44. Schrier RW, Estacio RO, Esler A, Mehler P. Effects of aggressive blood pressure control in normotensive type 2 diabetic patients on albuminuria, retinopathy and strokes. *Kidney Int*. 2002;61:1086–1097.

45. Chaturvedi N, Sjolie AK, Stephenson JM, et al. Effect of lisinopril on progression of retinopathy in normotensive people with type 1 diabetes. The EUCLID Study Group. EURODIAB Controlled Trial of Lisinopril in Insulin-Dependent Diabetes Mellitus. *Lancet*. 1998;351:28–31.

46. Patel A, ADVANCE Collaborative Group, MacMahon S, et al. Effects of a fixed combination of perindopril and indapamide on macrovascular and microvascular outcomes in patients with type 2 diabetes mellitus (the ADVANCE trial): a randomised controlled trial. *Lancet*. 2007;370:829–840.

47. Schrier RW, Estacio RO, Jeffers B. Appropriate Blood Pressure Control in NIDDM (ABCD) Trial. *Diabetologia*. 1996;39:1646–1654.

48. Larsen M, Hommel E, Parving HH, Lund-Andersen H. Protective effect of captopril on the blood-retina barrier in normotensive insulin-dependent diabetic patients with nephropathy and background retinopathy. *Graefes Arch Clin Exp Ophthalmol*. 1990;228:505–509.

49. ADVANCE Collaborative Group. ADVANCE—Action in Diabetes and Vascular Disease: patient recruitment and characteristics of the study population at baseline. *Diabet Med*. 2005;22:882–888.

50. Knudsen ST, Bek T, Poulsen PL, Hove MN, Rehling M, Mogensen CE. Effects of losartan on diabetic maculopathy in type 2 diabetic patients: a randomized, double-masked study. *J Intern Med*. 2003;254:147–158.

51. Sjolie AK, Klein R, Porta M, Orchard T, Fuller J, Parving HH, et al. Effect of candesartan on progression and regression of retinopathy in type 2 diabetes (DIRECT-Protect 2): a randomised placebo-controlled trial. *Lancet*. 2008;372:1385–1393.

52. Chaturvedi N, Porta M, Klein R, Orchard T, Fuller J, Parving HH, et al. Effect of candesartan on prevention (DIRECT-Prevent 1) and progression (DIRECT-Protect 1) of retinopathy in type 1 diabetes: randomised, placebo-controlled trials. *Lancet* 2008;372:1394–1402.

53. Chew EY, Ambrosius WT, Howard LT, et al. Rationale, design, and methods of the Action to Control Cardiovascular Risk in Diabetes Eye Study (ACCORD-EYE). *Am J Cardiol*. 2007;99:103i–111i.

54. Klein R, Sharrett AR, Klein BE, et al. The association of atherosclerosis, vascular risk factors, and retinopathy in adults with diabetes: the atherosclerosis risk in communities study. *Ophthalmology*. 2002;109:1225–1234.

55. Chew EY, Klein ML, Ferris FL, et al. Association of elevated serum lipid levels with retinal hard exudate in diabetic retinopathy. Early Treatment Diabetic Retinopathy Study (ETDRS) Report 22. *Arch Ophthalmol*. 1996;114:1079–1084.

56. Sen K, Misra A, Kumar A, Pandey RM. Simvastatin retards progression of retinopathy in diabetic patients with hypercholesterolemia. *Diabetes Res Clin Pract*. 2002;56:1–11.

57. Cullen JF, Town SM, Campbell CJ. Double-blind trial of Atromid-S in exudative diabetic retinopathy. *Trans Ophthalmol Soc UK*. 1974;94:554–562.

58. Keech A, Simes RJ, Barter P, et al. Effects of long-term fenofibrate therapy on cardiovascular events in 9795 people with type 2 diabetes mellitus (the FIELD study): randomised controlled trial. *Lancet*. 2005;366:1849–1861.

59. Early Treatment Diabetic Retinopathy Study Research Group. Effects of aspirin treatment on diabetic retinopathy. ETDRS report number 8. *Ophthalmology* 1991;98:757–765.

60. Chew EY, Klein ML, Murphy RP, Remaley NA, Ferris FL. Effects of aspirin on vitreous/preretinal hemorrhage in patients with diabetes mellitus. Early Treatment Diabetic Retinopathy Study report no. 20. *Arch Ophthalmol*. 1995;113:52–55.

61. The DAMAD Study Group. Effect of aspirin alone and aspirin plus dipyridamole in early diabetic retinopathy. A multicenter randomized controlled clinical trial. *Diabetes*. 1989;38:491–498.

62. The TIMAD Study Group. Ticlopidine treatment reduces the progression of nonproliferative diabetic retinopathy. *Arch Ophthalmol*. 1990;108:1577–1583.

63. The PKC-DRS Study Group. The effect of ruboxistaurin on visual loss in patients with moderately severe to very severe nonproliferative diabetic retinopathy: initial results of the Protein Kinase C beta Inhibitor Diabetic Retinopathy Study (PKC-DRS) multicenter randomized clinical trial. *Diabetes*. 2005;54:2188–2197.

64. PKC-DMES Study Group. Effect of ruboxistaurin in patients with diabetic macular edema: thirty-six month results of the randomized PKC-DMES clinical trial. *Arch Ophthalmol*. 2007;124:318–324.

65. Sorbinil Retinopathy Trial Research Group. A randomized trial of sorbinil, an aldose reductase inhibitor, in diabetic retinopathy. *Arch Ophthalmol*. 1990;108:1234–1244.

66. Gardner TW, Sander B, Larsen ML, et al. An extension of the Early Treatment Diabetic Retinopathy Study (ETDRS) system for grading of diabetic macular edema in the Astemizole Retinopathy Trial. *Curr Eye Res.* 2006;31:535–547.

67. Grant MB, Mames RN, Fitzgerald C, et al. The efficacy of octreotide in the therapy of severe nonproliferative and early proliferative diabetic retinopathy: a randomized controlled study. *Diabetes Care.* 2000;23:504–509.

68. Thomason MJ, Colhoun HM, Livingstone SJ, et al. Baseline characteristics in the Collaborative A to Rvastatin Diabetes Study (CARDS) in patients with Type 2 diabetes. *Diabet Med.* 2004;21:901–905.

69. Colhoun HM, Betteridge DJ, Durrington PN, et al. Primary prevention of cardiovascular disease with atorvastatin in type 2 diabetes in the Collaborative Atorvastatin Diabetes Study (CARDS): multicentre randomised placebo-controlled trial. *Lancet.* 2004;364:685–696.

70. Knopp RH, d'Emden M, Smilde JG, Pocock SJ. Efficacy and safety of atorvastatin in the prevention of cardiovascular end points in subjects with type 2 diabetes: the Atorvastatin Study for Prevention of Coronary Heart Disease Endpoints in non-insulin-dependent diabetes mellitus (ASPEN). *Diabetes Care.* 2006;29:1478–1485.

71. PKC-DRS2 Group, Aiello LP, Davis MD, et al. Effect of ruboxistaurin on visual loss in patients with diabetic retinopathy. *Ophthalmology.* 2006;113:2221–2230.

72. Aiello LP, Davis MD, Milton RC, et al. Protein kinase C inhibitor trials: diabetic retinopathy & diabetic macular edema: University of Wisconsin - Madison; 2005. Available at: http://eyephoto.ophth.wisc.edu/PresentationsPublications/PKCInhibitorTrials.pdf (accessed 2006 Apr 4).

73. Ray BS, Pazianos AG, Greenberg E, Peretz WL, McLean JM. Pituitary ablation for diabetic retinopathy. I. Results of hypophysectomy. (A ten-year evaluation). *JAMA.* 1968;203:79–84.

74. Hardy J, Ciric IS. Selective anterior hypophysectomy in the treatment of diabetic retinopathy. A transsphenoidal microsurgical technique. *JAMA.* 1968;203:73–78.

75. Sönksen PH, Russell-Jones D, Jones RH. Growth hormone and diabetes mellitus. A review of sixty-three years of medical research and a glimpse into the future? *Horm Res.* 1993;40:68–79.

76. Kirkegaard C, Nørgaard K, Snorgaard O, Bek T, Larsen M, Lund-Andersen H. Effect of one year continuous subcutaneous infusion of a somatostatin analogue, octreotide, on early retinopathy, metabolic control and thyroid function in Type I (insulin-dependent) diabetes mellitus. *Acta Endocrinol (Copenh).* 1990;122:766–772.

77. Available at; http://clinicaltrials.gov/ct/show/NCT00248157. (Accessed October 2006.)

78. Available at; http://clinicaltrials.gov/ct/show/NCT00248131. (Accessed October 2006.)

79. Mohamed Q, Wong TY. Emerging drugs for diabetic retinopathy. *Expert Opin Emerg Drugs.* December 2008;13(4):675–694.

80. The Diabetic Retinopathy Study Research Group. Photocoagulation treatment of proliferative diabetic retinopathy: the second report of diabetic retinopathy study findings. *Ophthalmology.* 1978;85:82–106.

81. The Diabetic Retinopathy Study Research Group. Photocoagulation treatment of proliferative diabetic retinopathy. Clinical application of Diabetic Retinopathy Study (DRS) findings, DRS Report Number 8. *Ophthalmology.* 1981;88:583–600.

82. Early Treatment Diabetic Retinopathy Study Research Group. Early Treatment Diabetic Retinopathy Study design and baseline patient characteristics. ETDRS report number 7. *Ophthalmology.* 1991;98:741–756.

83. Rohan TE, Frost CD, Wald NJ. Prevention of blindness by screening for diabetic retinopathy: a quantitative assessment. *BMJ*. 1989;299:1198–1201.

84. Early Treatment Diabetic Retinopathy Study Research Group. Early photocoagulation for diabetic retinopathy. ETDRS report number 9. *Ophthalmology*. 1991;98: 766–785.

85. Flynn HW, Chew EY, Simons BD, Barton FB, Remaley NA, Ferris FL. Pars plana vitrectomy in the Early Treatment Diabetic Retinopathy Study. ETDRS report number 17. The Early Treatment Diabetic Retinopathy Study Research Group. *Ophthalmology*. 1992;99:1351–1357.

86. British Multicentre Study Group. Photocoagulation for proliferative diabetic retinopathy: a randomised controlled clinical trial using the xenon-arc. *Diabetologia*. 1984;26:109–115.

87. British Multicentre Study Group. Photocoagulation for diabetic maculopathy. A randomized controlled clinical trial using the xenon arc. *Diabetes*. 1983;32: 1010–1016.

88. Hercules BL, Gayed II, Lucas SB, Jeacock J. Peripheral retinal ablation in the treatment of proliferative diabetic retinopathy: a three-year interim report of a randomised, controlled study using the argon laser. *Br J Ophthalmol*. 1977;61:555–563.

89. Patz A, Schatz H, Berkow JW, Gittelsohn AM, Ticho U. Macular edema--an overlooked complication of diabetic retinopathy. *Trans Am Acad Ophthalmol Otolaryngol*. 1973;77:OP34–OP42.

90. Lövestam-Adrian M, Agardh CD, Torffvit O, Agardh E. Type 1 diabetes patients with severe non-proliferative retinopathy may benefit from panretinal photocoagulation. *Acta Ophthalmol Scand*. 2003;81:221–225.

91. Early Treatment Diabetic Retinopathy Study research group. Photocoagulation for diabetic macular edema. Early Treatment Diabetic Retinopathy Study report number 1. *Arch Ophthalmol*. 1985;103:1796–1806.

92. Diabetic Retinopathy Clinical Research Network. Comparison of the modified Early Treatment Diabetic Retinopathy Study and mild macular grid laser photocoagulation strategies for diabetic macular edema. *Arch Ophthalmol*. 2007;125:469–480.

93. Blankenship GW. Diabetic macular edema and argon laser photocoagulation: a prospective randomized study. *Ophthalmology*. 1979;86:69–78.

94. Olk RJ. Modified grid argon (blue-green) laser photocoagulation for diffuse diabetic macular edema. *Ophthalmology*. 1986;93:938–950.

95. Photocoagulation in treatment of diabetic maculopathy. Interim report of a multicentre controlled study. *Lancet*. 1975;2:1110–1113.

96. Ladas ID, Theodossiadis GP. Long-term effectiveness of modified grid laser photocoagulation for diffuse diabetic macular edema. *Acta Ophthalmol (Copenh)*. 1993;71:393–397.

97. Pahor D. Visual field loss after argon laser panretinal photocoagulation in diabetic retinopathy: full- versus mild-scatter coagulation. *Int Ophthalmol*. 1998;22:313–319.

98. Buckley SA, Jenkins L, Benjamin L. Fields, DVLC and panretinal photocoagulation. *Eye*. 1992;6(Pt 6):623–625.

99. Fong DS, Girach A, Boney A. Visual side effects of successful scatter laser photocoagulation surgery for proliferative diabetic retinopathy: a literature review. *Retina*. 2007;27:816–824.

100. Early Treatment Diabetic Retinopathy Study Research Group. Focal photocoagulation treatment of diabetic macular edema. Relationship of treatment effect to fluorescein angiographic and other retinal characteristics at baseline: ETDRS report no. 19. *Arch Ophthalmol*. 1995;113:1144–1155.

101. Ho T, Smiddy WE, Flynn HW Jr. Vitrectomy in the management of diabetic eye disease. *Surv Ophthalmol.* 1992;37:190–202.
102. The Diabetic Retinopathy Vitrectomy Study Research Group. Early vitrectomy for severe vitreous hemorrhage in diabetic retinopathy. Two-year results of a randomized trial. Diabetic Retinopathy Vitrectomy Study report 2. *Arch Ophthalmol.* 1985;103:1644–1652.
103. The Diabetic Retinopathy Vitrectomy Study Research Group. Early vitrectomy for severe proliferative diabetic retinopathy in eyes with useful vision. Results of a randomized trial—Diabetic Retinopathy Vitrectomy Study Report 3. *Ophthalmology.* 1988;95:1307–1320.
104. The Diabetic Retinopathy Vitrectomy Study Research Group. Early vitrectomy for severe proliferative diabetic retinopathy in eyes with useful vision. Clinical application of results of a randomized trial—Diabetic Retinopathy Vitrectomy Study Report 4. *Ophthalmology.* 1988;95:1321–1334.
105. Early vitrectomy for severe vitreous hemorrhage in diabetic retinopathy. Four-year results of a randomized trial: Diabetic Retinopathy Vitrectomy Study Report 5. *Arch Ophthalmol.* 1990;108:958–964.
106. Gillies MC, Sutter FK, Simpson JM, Larsson J, Ali H, Zhu M. Intravitreal triamcinolone for refractory diabetic macular edema: two-year results of a double-masked, placebo-controlled, randomized clinical trial. *Ophthalmology.* 2006;113:1533–1538.
107. Pearson, Levy, Comstock, Fluocinolone Acetonide Implant study group. Fluocinolone acetonide intravitreal implant to treat diabetic macular edema: 3-year results of a multi-center clinical trial. *Invest Ophthalmol Vis Sci.* 2006;E-Abstract 5442.
108. Yanyali A, Horozoglu F, Celik E, Ercalik Y, Nohutcu AF. Pars plana vitrectomy and removal of the internal limiting membrane in diabetic macular edema unresponsive to grid laser photocoagulation. *Eur J Ophthalmol.* 2006;16:573–581.
109. Thomas D, Bunce C, Moorman C, Laidlaw DA. A randomised controlled feasibility trial of vitrectomy versus laser for diabetic macular oedema. *Br J Ophthalmol.* 2005;89:81–86.
110. Dhingra N, Sahni J, Shipley J, et al. Vitrectomy and Internal Limiting Membrane (ILM) removal for diabetic macular edema in eyes with absent vitreo-macular traction fails to improve visual acuity: results of a 12 months prospective randomized controlled clinical trial. *Invest Ophthalmol Vis Sci.* 2005;46:1467.
111. Bahadir M, Ertan A, Mertog˘lu O. Visual acuity comparison of vitrectomy with and without internal limiting membrane removal in the treatment of diabetic macular edema. *Int Ophthalmol.* 2005;26:3–8.
112. Smiddy WE, Flynn HW. Vitrectomy in the management of diabetic retinopathy. *Surv Ophthalmol.* 1999;43:491–507.
113. Early Treatment Diabetic Retinopathy Study Research Group. Treatment techniques and clinical guidelines for photocoagulation of diabetic macular edema. Early Treatment Diabetic Retinopathy Study Report Number 2. *Ophthalmology.* 1987;94:761–774.
114. Akduman L, Olk RJ. Diode laser (810 nm) versus argon green (514 nm) modified grid photocoagulation for diffuse diabetic macular edema. *Ophthalmology.* 1997;104:1433–1441.
115. Canning C, Polkinghorne P, Ariffin A, Gregor Z. Panretinal laser photocoagulation for proliferative diabetic retinopathy: the effect of laser wavelength on macular function. *Br J Ophthalmol.* 1991;75:608–610.

116. Akduman L, Olk RJ. Subthreshold (invisible) modified grid diode laser photoco-agulation in diffuse diabetic macular edema (DDME) *Ophthalmic Surg Lasers*. 1999;30:706–714.

117. La Heij EC, Hendrikse F, Kessels AG, Derhaag PJ. Vitrectomy results in diabetic macular oedema without evident vitreomacular traction. *Graefes Arch Clin Exp Ophthalmol*. 2001;239:264–270.

118. Dillinger P, Mester U. Vitrectomy with removal of the internal limiting mem-brane in chronic diabetic macular oedema. *Graefes Arch Clin Exp Ophthalmol*. 2004;242:630–637.

119. Yang CM. Surgical treatment for severe diabetic macular edema with massive hard exudates. *Retina*. 2000;20:121–125.

120. Kralinger MT, Pedri M, Kralinger F, Troger J, Kieselbach GF. Long-term outcome after vitrectomy for diabetic macular edema. *Ophthalmologica*. 2006;220:147–152.

121. Stolba U, Binder S, Gruber D, Krebs I, Aggermann T, Neumaier B. Vitrectomy for persistent diffuse diabetic macular edema. *Am J Ophthalmol*. 2005;140:295–301.

122. Yanyali A, Nohutcu AF, Horozoglu F, Celik E. Modified grid laser photocoagulation versus pars plana vitrectomy with internal limiting membrane removal in diabetic macular edema. *Am J Ophthalmol*. 2005;139:795–801.

123. Sobrin L, D'Amico DJ. Controversies in intravitreal triamcinolone acetonide use. *Int Ophthalmol Clin*. 2005;45:133–141.

124. Jonas JB, Söfker A. Intraocular injection of crystalline cortisone as adjunctive treat-ment of diabetic macular edema. *Am J Ophthalmol*. 2001;132:425–427.

125. Jonas JB, Kreissig I, Söfker A, Degenring RF. Intravitreal injection of triamcinolone for diffuse diabetic macular edema. *Arch Ophthalmol*. 2003;121:57–61.

126. Martidis A, Duker JS, Greenberg PB, et al. Intravitreal triamcinolone for refractory diabetic macular edema. *Ophthalmology*. 2002;109:920–927.

127. Avitabile T, Longo A, Reibaldi A. Intravitreal triamcinolone compared with mac-ular laser grid photocoagulation for the treatment of cystoid macular edema. *Am J Ophthalmol*. 2005;140:695–702.

128. Kang SW, Sa HS, Cho HY, Kim JI. Macular grid photocoagulation after intravit-real triamcinolone acetonide for diffuse diabetic macular edema. *Arch Ophthalmol*. 2006;124:653–658.

129. Jonas JB, Kamppeter BA, Harder B, Vossmerbaeumer U, Sauder G, Spandau UH. Intravitreal triamcinolone acetonide for diabetic macular edema: a prospective, ran-domized study. *J Ocul Pharmacol Ther*. 2006;22:200–207.

130. Massin P, Audren F, Haouchine B, et al. Intravitreal triamcinolone acetonide for diabetic diffuse macular edema: preliminary results of a prospective controlled trial. *Ophthalmology*. 2004;111:218–224; discussion 224–225.

131. Audren F, Erginay A, Haouchine B, et al. Intravitreal triamcinolone acetonide for diffuse diabetic macular oedema: 6-month results of a prospective controlled trial. *Acta Ophthalmol Scand*. 2006;84:624–630.

132. Audren F, Lecleire-Collet A, Erginay A, et al. Intravitreal triamcinolone acetonide for diffuse diabetic macular edema: phase 2 trial comparing 4 mg vs 2 mg. *Am J Ophthalmol*. 2006;142:794–799.

133. Jonas JB, Kreissig I, Spandau UH, Harder B. Infectious and noninfectious endophthal-mitis after intravitreal high-dosage triamcinolone acetonide. *Am J Ophthalmol*. 2006;141:579–580.

134. Jonas JB, Degenring RF, Kreissig I, Akkoyun I, Kamppeter BA. Intraocular pres-sure elevation after intravitreal triamcinolone acetonide injection. *Ophthalmology*. 2005;112:593–598.

135. Gillies MC, Simpson JM, Billson FA, et al. Safety of an intravitreal injection of triamcinolone: results from a randomized clinical trial. *Arch Ophthalmol.* 2004;122:336–340.

136. Westfall AC, Osborn A, Kuhl D, Benz MS, Mieler WF, Holz ER. Acute endophthalmitis incidence: intravitreal triamcinolone. *Arch Ophthalmol.* 2005;123:1075–1077.

137. Available at; http://www.nei.nih.gov/neitrials/viewStudyWeb.aspx?id=105. (Accessed May 2006.)

138. Spandau UH, Derse M, Schmitz-Valckenber P, Papoulis C, Jonas JB. Dosage dependency of intravitreal triamcinolone acetonide as treatment for diabetic macular oedema. *Br J Ophthalmol.* 2005; 89:8, 999–1003.

139. Diabetic Retinopathy Clinical Research Network, Chew E, Strauber S, et al. Randomized trial of peribulbar triamcinolone acetonide with and without focal photocoagulation for mild diabetic macular edema: a pilot study. *Ophthalmology.* 2007;114:1190–1196.

140. Kuppermann BD, Blumenkranz MS, Haller JA, Williams GA, Posurdex Study Group. An intravitreous dexamethasone bioerodible drug delivery system for the treatment of persistent diabetic macular edema. *Invest Ophthalmol Vis Sci.* 2003;44:E-Abstract 4289.

141. Cunningham ET, Adamis AP, Altaweel M, et al. A phase II randomized double-masked trial of pegaptanib, an anti-vascular endothelial growth factor aptamer, for diabetic macular edema. *Ophthalmology.* 2005;112:1747–1757.

142. Adamis AP, Altaweel M, Bressler NM, et al. Changes in retinal neovascularization after pegaptanib (Macugen) therapy in diabetic individuals. *Ophthalmology.* 2006;113:23–28.

143. Brown DM, Kaiser PK, Michels M, et al. Ranibizumab versus verteporfin for neovascular age-related macular degeneration. *N Engl J Med.* 2006;355:1432–1444.

144. Rosenfeld PJ, Brown DM, Heier JS, et al. Ranibizumab for neovascular age-related macular degeneration. *N Engl J Med.* 2006;355:1419–1431.

145. Chun DW, Heier JS, Topping TM, Duker JS, Bankert JM. A pilot study of multiple intravitreal injections of ranibizumab in patients with center-involving clinically significant diabetic macular edema. *Ophthalmology.* 2006;113:1706–1712.

146. Avery RL. Regression of retinal and iris neovascularization after intravitreal bevacizumab (Avastin) treatment. *Retina.* 2006;26:352–354.

147. Avery RL, Pearlman J, Pieramici DJ, et al. Intravitreal bevacizumab (Avastin) in the treatment of proliferative diabetic retinopathy. *Ophthalmology.* 2006;113:1695. e1–1695.e15.

148. Spaide RF, Fisher YL. Intravitreal bevacizumab (Avastin) treatment of proliferative diabetic retinopathy complicated by vitreous hemorrhage. *Retina.* 2006;26:275–278.

149. Rosenfeld, PJ. Intravitreal avastin: the low cost alternative to Lucentis? *Am J Ophthalmol.* 2006;142(1):141–143.

150. Gillies MC. What we don't know about avastin might hurt us. *Arch Ophthalmol.* October 2006;124(10):1478–1479.

151. Diabetic Retinopathy Clinical Research Network. A phase II randomized clinical trial of intravitreal bevacizumab for diabetic macular edema. *Ophthalmology.* 2007;114:1860–1867.

152. Available at http://www.nei.nih.gov/neitrials/viewStudyWeb.aspx?id=129 (last accessed date February 23, 2009).

153. Available at http://www.clinicaltrials.gov/ct/show/NCT00347698?order=12 (last accessed date February 23, 2009).

15

Cataract Management in Diabetes

MITCHELL S. FINEMAN, MD,
WILLIAM E. BENSON, MD,
AND INGRID U. SCOTT, MD, MPH

CORE MESSAGES

- Patients with diabetes develop cataracts more frequently and at a younger age than patients without diabetes.
- Patients with diabetes are at increased risk of pseudophakic cystoid macular edema.
- Cataract surgery may be associated with postoperative progression of diabetic retinopathy.

*I*ndividuals who have diabetes mellitus not only develop cataracts more frequently than nondiabetic patients but also do so at a younger age [1–6]. They account for about 10% of people with visually significant cataracts and represent about 6% of the population of the United States [7–10]. Cataract is a frequent cause of visual loss in older-onset diabetic patients and is second only to proliferative diabetic retinopathy (PDR) in younger-onset diabetic patients [11]. Although the main indication for cataract surgery in diabetic patients is visual rehabilitation, it is occasionally required when the lens opacity prevents adequate diagnosis or treatment of retinopathy [12].

Diabetic patients have a higher risk of both anterior and posterior segment complications following cataract surgery [13]. One of the most significant anterior segment complications is neovascularization of the iris (NVI), because it usually progresses to neovascular glaucoma [14–18]. Other anterior segment complications include pigment dispersion with precipitates on the surface of the intraocular lens (IOL), fibrinous exudate or membrane in the anterior chamber, and posterior synechiae (Fig. 15.1) [19–21]. The incidence of pseudophakic pupillary block with secondary angle-closure glaucoma [22] and postoperative posterior capsular

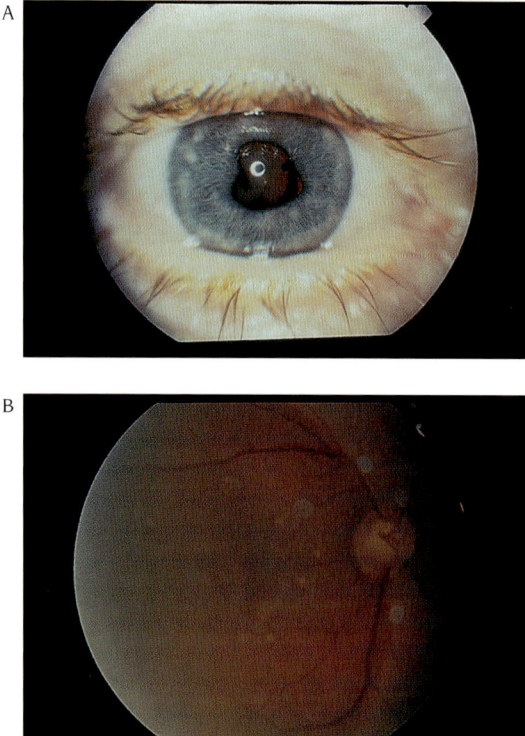

Figure 15.1. (A) Posterior synechiae in an eye of a diabetic patient following extracapsular cataract extraction. (B) Resulting small size of pupil caused poor view of fundus and difficulties with peripheral laser photocoagulation.

opacification (Fig. 15.2) [23,24] is also reported to be greater in diabetic patients. Following cataract surgery in diabetic patients, macular edema, macular ischemia [25–32], PDR [28,33], vitreous hemorrhage [14,33], and tractional retinal detachment [33] may develop or worsen.

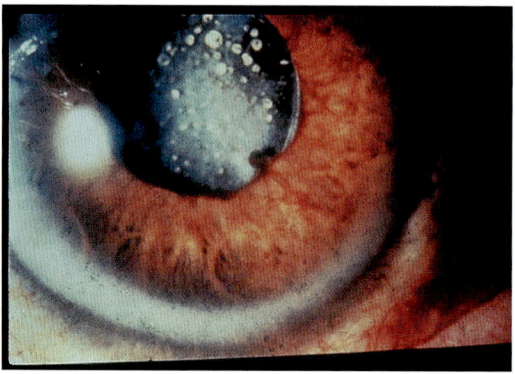

Figure 15.2. Slit-lamp photograph of an eye of a diabetic patient demonstrating severe posterior capsular opacification 2 months following cataract extraction. Posterior synechia is visible between the 4- and 5-o'clock positions.

The best predictor of visual and anatomic outcomes after cataract surgery is the preoperative severity of retinopathy [14,27,28]. Other factors affecting the postoperative visual outcome are the age and gender of the patient [34], insulin treatment [32,35], glycemic control [35,36], prior laser photocoagulation [37], and previous vitrectomy [38].

In this chapter, unless otherwise specified, the term *cataract surgery* means phacoemulsification or extracapsular cataract extraction (ECCE) with placement of a posterior chamber IOL, because these techniques are currently used in nearly all cataract operations performed in the United States.

PREOPERATIVE SEVERITY OF RETINOPATHY

No or Mild Retinopathy. The current results of cataract surgery in diabetic patients with no or minimal retinopathy are comparable to those in nondiabetic persons [28,39–42]. About 85% of eyes can be expected to achieve a postoperative visual acuity of 20/40 or better [43]. However, the risk of angiographic pseudophakic cystoid macular edema (CME) is considerably higher than that in nondiabetic patients, and progression of retinopathy occurs in 15% of eyes within 18 months postoperatively [28].

Nonproliferative Retinopathy. Cataract surgery is often followed by progression of established nonproliferative diabetic retinopathy (NPDR) or by NVI (Fig. 15.3) [27–29,31,32,34,35,41]. In one study, clinically significant macular edema (CSME) developed postoperatively in 50% of eyes that did not have it preoperatively [34]. In some cases, progression of NPDR and CSME caused the postoperative visual acuity to be worse than the preoperative level (Fig. 15.4) [25,27]. Dowler and associates [43] performed a meta-analysis and calculated that 80% of eyes with preoperative NPDR and no macular edema achieve a visual acuity of 20/40 or better following ECCE.

In the Early Treatment Diabetic Retinopathy Study (ETDRS), evaluation of 1-year postoperative visual acuities for all eyes with mild-to-moderate NPDR at the annual visit prior to cataract surgery showed that 53% achieved better than 20/40, 90% better than 20/100, and 10% achieved 5/200 or worse [44]. Severity of retinopathy at the time of lens removal is the most important predictor of poor visual acuity outcome in the study by Dowler and associates [43] and in the ETDRS Report Number 25 [44].

Several investigators have reported that cataract surgery does not lead to progression of preexisting retinopathy [39,45]. Romero-Aroca and associates studied 132 diabetic patients with NPDR who underwent phacoemulsification in one eye; with a mean follow-up interval of 11 months, there was no difference between the operated and fellow eyes in the proportion of eyes with diabetic retinopathy progression [46]. Other investigators have also reported that phacoemulsification with IOL implantation is not associated with diabetic retinopathy progression and that visual improvement is achieved in the majority of patients with NPDR without macular edema; a poorer visual outcome is observed in patients who develop

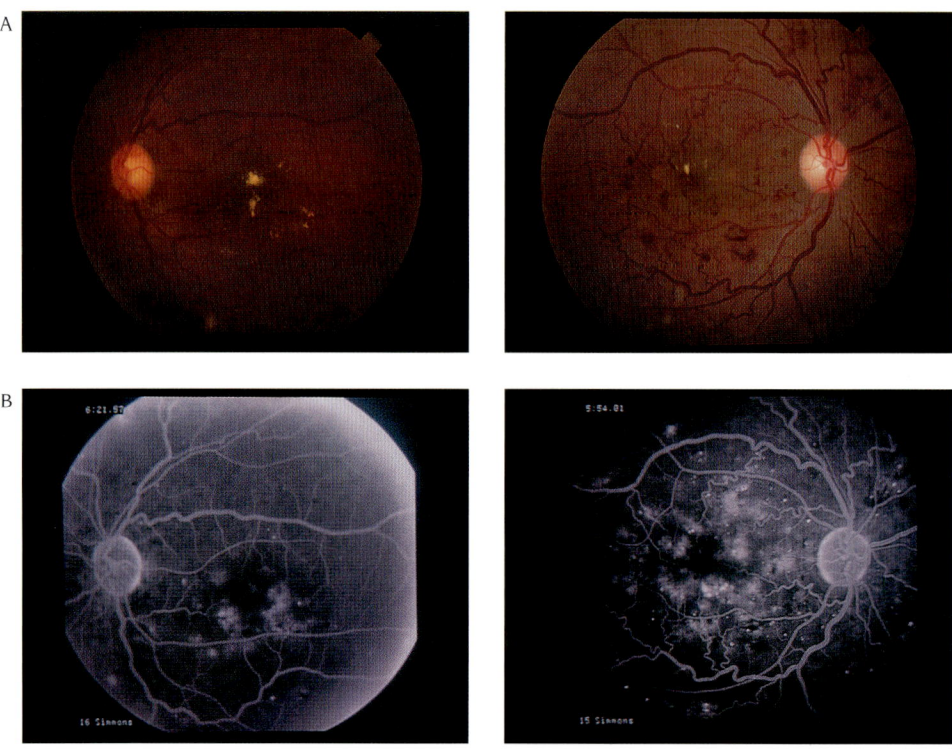

Figure 15.3. (A) Fundus photograph of right and left eyes of a 57-year-old man with nonproliferative diabetic retinopathy (NPDR) who underwent uncomplicated extracapsular cataract extraction with implantation of posterior chamber intraocular lens in right eye 5 months earlier. Retinopathy was symmetric before cataract surgery, but is asymmetric postoperatively. (B) Intravenous fluorescein angiography reveals asymmetry of NPDR, with significantly more microaneurysms and fluorescein leakage in the right eye.

macular edema [47]. Other investigators have reported that although small-incision phacoemulsification improved visual acuity in most diabetic patients, the latter have an overall worse visual outcome than nondiabetic patients; the most important predictors of visual outcome were diabetes and the extent of preoperative diabetic retinopathy [48]. In a prospective, case-controlled study of 50 patients with type 2 diabetes who underwent phacoemulsification in one eye, there was no significant difference in the number of operated and fellow eyes in which the retinopathy progressed postoperatively [49]. Retinopathy progression was associated with a higher mean hemoglobin A1c (HbA1c) level and with insulin treatment. In contrast, in a study of 75 patients who underwent cataract surgery in one eye, the operated eye had more progression of retinopathy than the nonoperated contralateral eye; the presence of preoperative macular edema and poor renal function were associated with retinopathy progression [50].

Nonproliferative Retinopathy with Macular Edema. Eyes with preoperative macular edema have been reported to have a poor visual prognosis, even if they undergo focal macular photocoagulation preoperatively [28,34]. Retinopathy progresses in 30% of eyes, and 50% require supplemental postoperative focal macular

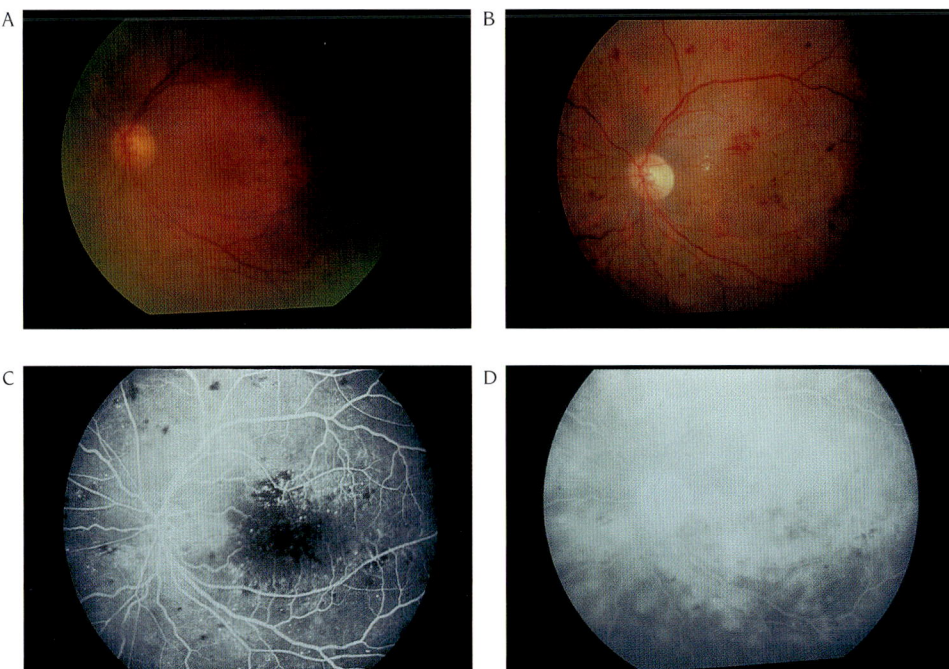

Figure 15.4. (A) Fundus photograph of the left eye of a 65-year-old man with moderate cataract in the clinically significant macular edema setting of mild nonproliferative diabetic retinopathy without clinically significant macular edema. Visual acuity of 20/70 was consistent with density of cataract. (B) About 8 weeks after extracapsular cataract extraction, visual acuity had deteriorated to 20/200 and CSME was present. (C,D) Intravenous fluorescein angiography performed 8 weeks after cataract surgery reveals relatively few microaneurysms in full-venous phase (C) and diffuse leakage of fluorescein in macula in recirculation phase (D). Vision remained poor in this eye due to chronic macular edema despite medical and laser treatment.

photocoagulation for worsening macular edema. Only 50% have a postoperative improvement of visual acuity. A meta-analysis performed by Dowler and associates [43] found that 40% of eyes with preoperative NPDR and maculopathy achieve a visual acuity of 20/40 or better following ECCE. The presence of macular edema prior to cataract surgery worsened by six-fold the odds of obtaining a final visual acuity better than 20/40 [43].

It is the clinical impression of many ophthalmologists that patients with macular edema who are treated with focal laser photocoagulation prior to cataract surgery have less progression than those who are not so treated. However, no controlled series has been published to support this opinion. Moreover, it is unlikely that such a study would ever be undertaken because of concerns about withholding treatment. Even in eyes with previous focal macular photocoagulation, progression of the retinopathy occurs in 30% of eyes; 35% to 50% of eyes require supplemental focal macular photocoagulation for macular edema.

In patients with CSME, focal macular photocoagulation is applied preoperatively or postoperatively to limit the progression of CSME [51]. If CSME is present prior to cataract surgery but cannot be treated with macular laser photocoagulation because the cataract obscures the view, then focal macular photocoagulation in the early postoperative period is usually recommended. More recently, Lam and colleagues reported favorable 6-month outcomes in diabetic patients with cataract and CSME who were treated with combined phacoemulsification and intravitreal traimcinolone acetonide injection [52]. At 6 months, 10 of 17 eyes (58.8%) demonstrated an improvement in Snellen best-corrected visual acuity of 2 or more lines with a mean improvement of 2.4 lines. The peak improvement in best-corrected visual acuity occurred at 4 months.

Proliferative Retinopathy. There are three reasons why PDR is a risk factor for a poor visual acuity outcome:

1. The prevalence of macular edema is related to the overall severity of retinopathy. Macular edema is present in 3% of eyes with mild NPDR, in 38% of eyes with moderate-to-severe NPDR, and in 71% of eyes with PDR [53].
2. Patients with PDR have an increased risk of vitreous hemorrhage and retinal detachment.
3. Patients with PDR have a higher risk of NVI than do patients with NPDR.

When high-risk PDR is present, panretinal laser photocoagulation (PRP) should be performed prior to cataract surgery, when possible. Yellow and red laser wavelengths may penetrate a nuclear sclerotic cataract better than green or blue-green wavelengths. If PRP is not possible and there is no vitreoretinal traction present, standard cataract surgery with IOL placement can be considered and laser treatment can be performed at the time of cataract surgery or shortly thereafter. Alternatively, a combined procedure, including cataract surgery, vitrectomy, and IOL insertion can be considered (see section on combined cataract surgery and vitrectomy).

Intracapsular cataract extraction in the presence of active retinal neovascularization was found to be associated with a significant risk of PDR progression. In one study, 40% of eyes developed neovascular glaucoma within 6 weeks [14]. With current extracapsular and phacoemulsification surgical techniques, this risk is lower. However, neovascular glaucoma has been reported in eyes with an intact posterior capsule [16–18,28] and in eyes that had undergone preoperative PRP [33]. These findings are a reminder that PRP and preservation of the posterior capsule do not guarantee prevention of postoperative NVI.

Eyes that have active PDR have the worst visual prognosis. They have a higher rate of postoperative uveitis and associated fibrin membrane formation. Few can be expected to achieve a final visual acuity of 20/40 or better [54] unless simultaneous vitrectomy and endolaser PRP are performed.

Eyes that have quiescent PDR and undergo cataract surgery have a better visual prognosis compared to eyes with active PDR. Overall, about 50% of eyes that undergo cataract surgery after PRP achieve a visual acuity of 20/40 or better, but 25% have a final visual acuity of 20/200 or worse [43]. The final visual outcome is influenced most by the presence of preoperative macular edema. In the meta-analysis study by Dowler and associates, a postoperative visual acuity of 20/40 or better was achieved in about 60% of eyes with quiescent PDR without macular edema and in about 10% of eyes with quiescent PDR with macular edema [43]. In one study, 33% of eyes required additional PRP in the postoperative period, 10% developed new or recurrent NVI, and 10% underwent a postoperative pars plana vitrectomy [34].

METHOD OF CATARACT SURGERY AND VISUAL ACUITY OUTCOME

Extracapsular Cataract Extraction versus Phacoemulsification. One study found no significant differences in the progression of retinopathy, the types of complications, or in final visual acuity between eyes that underwent ECCE and those that had phacoemulsification [55].

The ETDRS did not distinguish between the two types of cataract surgery in study patients [44]. At 1 year following cataract surgery, visual acuity improvement of two lines from preoperative levels was measured in 64.3% of the operated eyes assigned to early photocoagulation and in 59.3% of eyes assigned to deferral of photocoagulation. In eyes assigned to early photocoagulation, 46% achieved visual acuity better than 20/40, 73% were better than 20/100, and 8% were 5/200 or worse at 1 year after surgery. Visual acuity results for eyes assigned to deferral of laser photocoagulation at 1 year were not as favorable: 36% achieved visual acuity better than 20/40, 55% were better than 20/100, and 17% were 5/200 or worse.

Combined Cataract Surgery and Vitrectomy. A common indication for combined cataract surgery and pars plana vitrectomy in eyes with severe retinopathy is a lens opacity that impairs the surgeon's ability to perform safe vitreoretinal surgery. Although it is possible to perform vitrectomy and cataract surgery as separate procedures, several studies have shown that they can be safely combined (Fig. 15.5) [56–62]. Some surgeons prefer pars plana lensectomy with placement of the IOL in front of the anterior capsule [63,64]. Others prefer ECCE or phacoemulsification with placement of the IOL in the bag or in the sulcus [56,65–71]. All three approaches are effective, and the method chosen usually depends on surgeon's preference and the hardness of the lens [72]. Some surgeons have reported greater improvement in vision, less astigmatism, and fewer postoperative complications in patients undergoing combined phacoemulsification with pars plana vitrectomy compared to ECCE with pars plana vitrectomy [73].

With all these techniques, approximately 80% of eyes have improved postoperative visual acuity. However, because many eyes have severe retinopathy preoperatively, final visual acuity is 20/40 or better in only about 30%. The most common cause for poor final visual acuity is preexisting macular disease [63].

Although the combination of cataract surgery and pars plana vitrectomy has advantages for both the patient and the surgeon, it is not without risks. One study that predated the era of endophotocoagulation reported that the risk of postoperative NVI increased three-fold and the risk of neovascular glaucoma increased

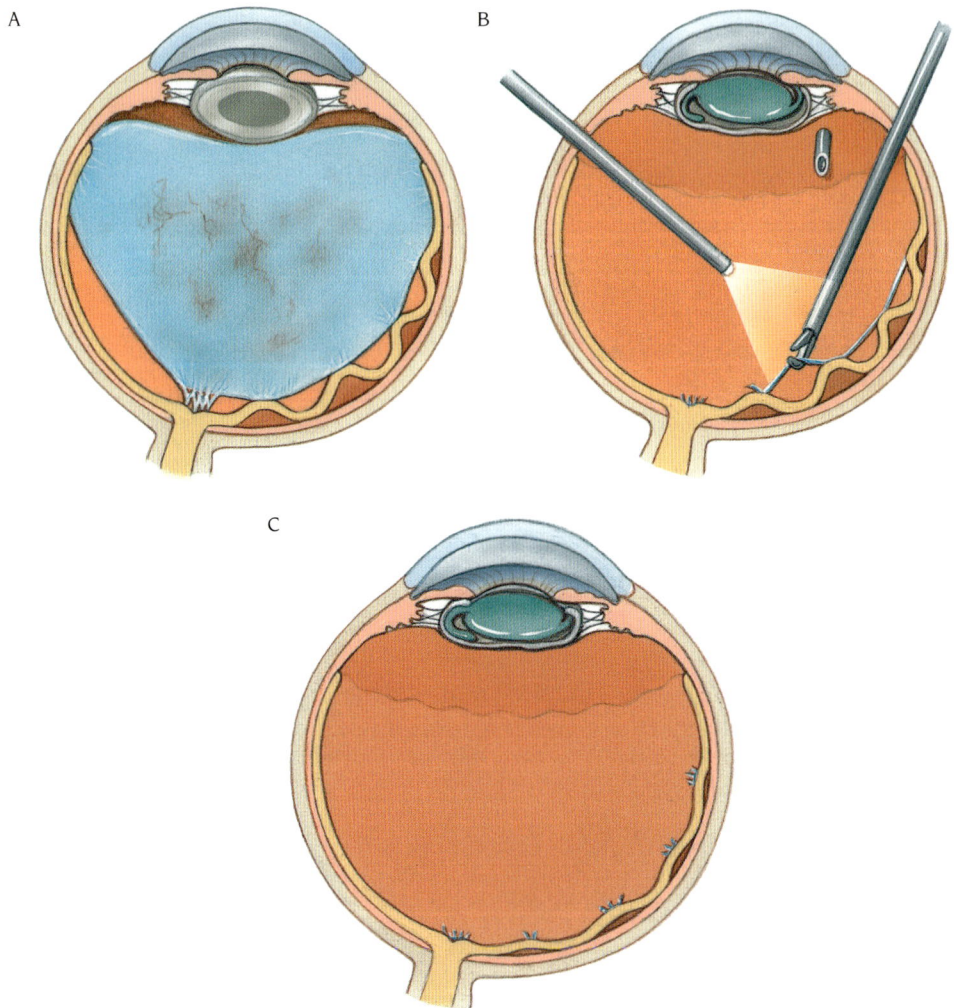

Figure 15.5. (A) Significant lens opacity, which impairs surgical treatment of vitreoretinal disease. (B) After cataract surgery has been performed, standard 3-port pars plana vitrectomy is performed. (C) One operation results in a pseudophakic eye with treated vitreoretinal disease.

four-fold if the lens was removed during vitrectomy and the eye was left aphakic [74]. Severe preoperative retinal neovascularization and the absence of preoperative PRP were also associated with an increased incidence of postoperative NVI. However, Wand and associates did not find an association between postvitrectomy aphakia and the development of neovascular glaucoma in eyes with completed PRP [75]. This study found retinal reattachment and aggressive PRP to be the most important factors in reducing the incidence of postvitrectomy neovascular glaucoma. One minor concern is that the addition of vitrectomy to cataract surgery may result in a small, myopic, postoperative refractive error [76].

FACTORS AFFECTING VISUAL OUTCOME

Age. The patient's age may be a predictor of final visual acuity following cataract surgery with placement of an IOL [34]. Patients aged 63 years or less were more likely to have a final visual acuity of 20/40 or better (58% vs. 38%) and were less likely to have a final visual acuity of 20/200 or less (17% vs. 38%) than older patients. The poor visual acuity outcomes in the older group were caused by progression and persistence of macular edema more often than by complications of PDR. Older patients were twice as likely to receive focal macular photocoagulation (41% vs. 19%), but were less likely to receive scatter PRP (27% vs. 38%) during the course of cataract management.

Gender. One study reported that diabetic women were more likely to have postoperative CSME than were diabetic men [25]. However, other studies failed to show an association between the gender of the patient and visual results following cataract surgery [34].

Previous Vitrectomy. Eyes that required a vitrectomy prior to cataract surgery might be expected to have a poor visual prognosis, because nearly all have had severe retinopathy, the most significant predictor of poor final visual acuity. In addition, phacoemulsification is more difficult after vitrectomy because of reduced vitreous support of the lens and possibly weakened zonules [77–80]. On the other hand, there are reasons why vitrectomy prior to cataract surgery may improve the visual prognosis:

1. The development of endophotocoagulation allows intraoperative PRP before cataract surgery [81–83].
2. Removal of vitreous traction may contribute to the regression of retinal and optic disc neovascularization [84].
3. Separation of the posterior hyaloid from the macula may decrease the severity of the macular edema in some eyes.

Eyes with macular edema are much less likely to have posterior vitreous detachment than are eyes without macular edema [85,86].

About 90% of eyes that have undergone vitrectomy before cataract surgery have an improvement in visual acuity following cataract surgery [34,38,80]. A final visual acuity of 20/40 or better is reported in only 50% of eyes and correlates with the presence of preoperative macular edema [34]. The majority of eyes do not have retinopathy progression, and very few of these eyes require a second pars plana vitrectomy. Therefore, cataract surgery has a high likelihood of visual acuity improvement in patients who have had a successful vitrectomy. However, structural changes in an eye that has undergone vitrectomy should alert the cataract surgeon to possible variations in the intraoperative dynamics of the cataract surgery [77–80]. Retinal ischemia may be an independent factor limiting visual recovery.

ROLE OF POSTERIOR CAPSULOTOMY

Preservation of the posterior lens capsule does not necessarily reduce neovascular complications or slow progression of retinopathy. In eyes with mild-to-moderate NPDR, progression of retinopathy and development of NVI within 1 year of cataract surgery may occur, even though the posterior capsule remains intact [16–18].

The question of whether or not posterior capsulotomy increases the risk of neovascular glaucoma has no clear answer. In a 1985 study, eyes that underwent ECCE with a primary posterior capsulotomy and without placement of an IOL developed neovascular glaucoma more often than eyes with an intact posterior capsule [15]. Another study reported that neovascular glaucoma developed in pseudophakic eyes within 1 month of an Nd:YAG laser posterior capsulotomy [87]. However, other studies have failed to show evidence of an adverse effect from posterior capsulotomy following ECCE with placement of an IOL. It is possible that the presence of a posterior chamber IOL may reduce the rate of NVI by restricting the access of vasoproliferative factors to the anterior chamber [88] and by decreasing the flow of oxygen from the anterior to the posterior segment [89]. In one large series, a posterior capsulotomy did not increase the risk of CSME [34].

TREATMENT OF POSTOPERATIVE MACULAR EDEMA

The evaluation and treatment of macular edema following cataract surgery is difficult, because these eyes may have macular edema and pseudophakic CME (Irvine-Gass syndrome). Although the mechanism of CME following cataract surgery is incompletely understood, fluorophotometry readings suggest a role for breakdown of the blood–retina barrier [90]. In addition, it is known that diabetic eyes may have some breakdown of the blood–retina barrier, even in the absence of retinopathy or previous ocular surgery [91–95]. It is likely that the higher rate of CME seen after cataract surgery in diabetic eyes results from a surgically induced inflammatory insult to an already compromised blood–retina barrier.

The development of CME following ECCE with IOL implantation occurs more frequently in diabetic eyes [96]. Postoperative angiographic or clinical CME develops in 8% of normal eyes, in 32% of diabetic eyes with no retinopathy, and in 81% of eyes with retinopathy. Persistence of the CME at 1 year following cataract surgery is present in 56% of eyes with preoperative retinopathy. Persistent clinical CME (not angiographic CME) at 1 year following cataract surgery is associated with the presence of preoperative retinopathy, progression of retinopathy, and a final visual acuity worse than 20/40. Although angiographic CME following cataract surgery is more common and persists longer in diabetic eyes, in the absence of retinopathy, it does not appear to impact the final visual acuity adversely [97].

Because of many overlapping clinical manifestations of pseudophakic CME and diabetic macular edema, subtle clinical features or fluorescein angiography may help to distinguish between the two [26,29,96]. Topical corticosteroids and nonsteroidal anti-inflammatory agents have been the agents traditionally used to treat

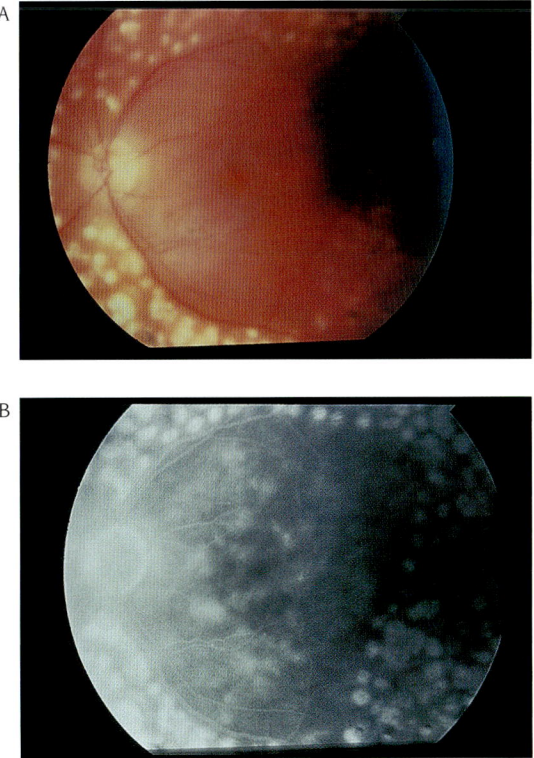

Figure 15.6. (A) Fundus photograph of the left eye of a 62-year-old woman with quiescent proliferative diabetic retinopathy following phacoemulsification cataract extraction with implantation of a posterior chamber intraocular lens. Visual acuity was 20/200. (B) Intravenous fluorescein angiography reveals diffuse leakage of fluorescein in fovea. Note paucity of microaneurysms. About 6 months later, visual acuity had improved to 20/25 without laser treatment.

CME [98,99]. In eyes with macular edema thought to be primarily due to diabetic retinopathy, light laser photocoagulation to visible leaks is usually recommended. To allow the Irvine-Gass component of the edema to regress, the recommendation to delay laser treatment is supported by the observation that some eyes with a significant decrease in visual acuity secondary to macular edema spontaneously improve to 20/40 or better (Fig. 15.6) [34]. One option is to treat with topical medications for 3 to 6 months after cataract surgery before treating with macular laser photocoagulation, to allow time for the CME component to restore. More recently, intravitreal injection(s) of triamcinolone acetonide or an anti-vascular endothelial growth factor (anti-VEGF) agent has been employed as off-label treatments of CME and diabetic macular edema [100–105].

CHOICE OF INTRAOCULAR LENS

The choice of IOL type in a diabetic patient depends on the likelihood that the patient will require macular laser photocoagulation, PRP, or vitreoretinal surgery in the future. It is generally recommended that patients with significant retinopathy have large-diameter (6.5- to 7.0-mm), all-PMMA (polymethylmethacrylate) implants without positioning holes [29,106,107]. A 7-mm IOL provides 36% more optical area than does a 6-mm IOL, enabling the vitreoretinal specialist to view the retinal periphery and provide laser treatment with less difficulty [106]. In addition, other potential problems involving secondary posterior capsulotomy and incarceration of the iris or lens capsule are avoided with the use of these lenses. A large anterior capsulorhexis is also important because a small opening in the anterior lens capsule may negate the advantages of a large IOL.

The shape of the IOL may also be an important factor for those eyes that may ultimately require vitreous substitutes with refractive indexes different from vitreous (that is, air, gas, or silicone). Both planoconvex [106] and convexoconcave [107] posterior chamber IOLs have been recommended for eyes that may require a future vitrectomy. These lens designs minimize refraction consequences caused by changes in the refractive index of the vitreous cavity when the vitreous gel is replaced with gas during vitrectomy [106]. There is considerably less minification during air–fluid exchange, and a standard contact lens, rather than a high-minus lens, can be used to visualize the retina. Further, postoperative slit-lamp photocoagulation is made easier, and there is less refractive error if the eye is filled with silicone oil.

Silicone posterior chamber IOLs are less desirable in diabetic patients for several reasons:

1. Deposition of precipitates on the anterior surface of silicone lenses is much more common than with other lenses [108].
2. During the fluid–air exchange (if vitrectomy is required later), the view of the posterior segment is markedly compromised if the posterior capsule is not intact, because liquid droplets form on the posterior surface of the silicone IOL implant [109]. This may limit achieving vitrectomy objectives.
3. If the vitreous cavity is filled with silicone oil, the oil will adhere to the silicone IOL and may cause reduced visual acuity even when the majority of silicone oil has been removed [110,111].

CONCLUSION

Although the majority of patients with diabetes benefit from cataract surgery, caution must be exercised when considering cataract surgery in patients who have retinopathy. Patients should be informed of the potential postoperative complications, especially progression of preexisting retinopathy. Frequent postoperative evaluations are recommended, with special attention to examining for NVI and macular edema or progression of retinopathy. After removal of the opaque lens, appropriate evaluation and management of active retinopathy with macular focal photocoagulation or PRP should be performed. The visual acuity outcomes and management decisions for diabetic patients with visually significant cataracts are summarized in Figures 15.7 and 15.8.

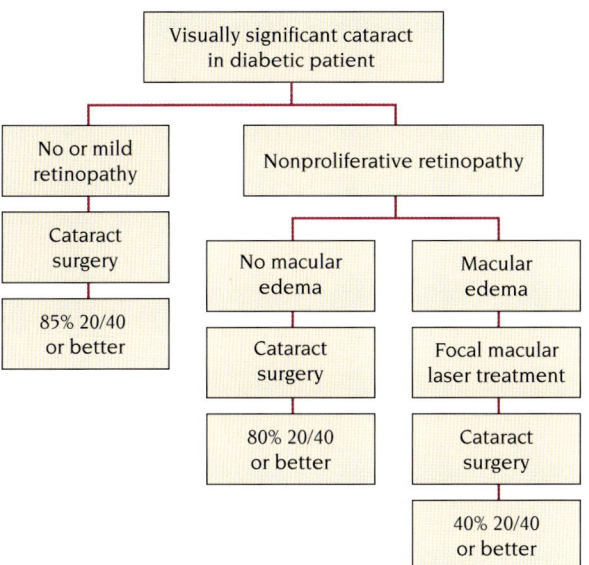

Figure 15.7. Visual acuity outcomes and management decisions for diabetic patients with visually significant cataracts and no or mild retinopathy or nonproliferative diabetic retinopathy with or without macular edema.

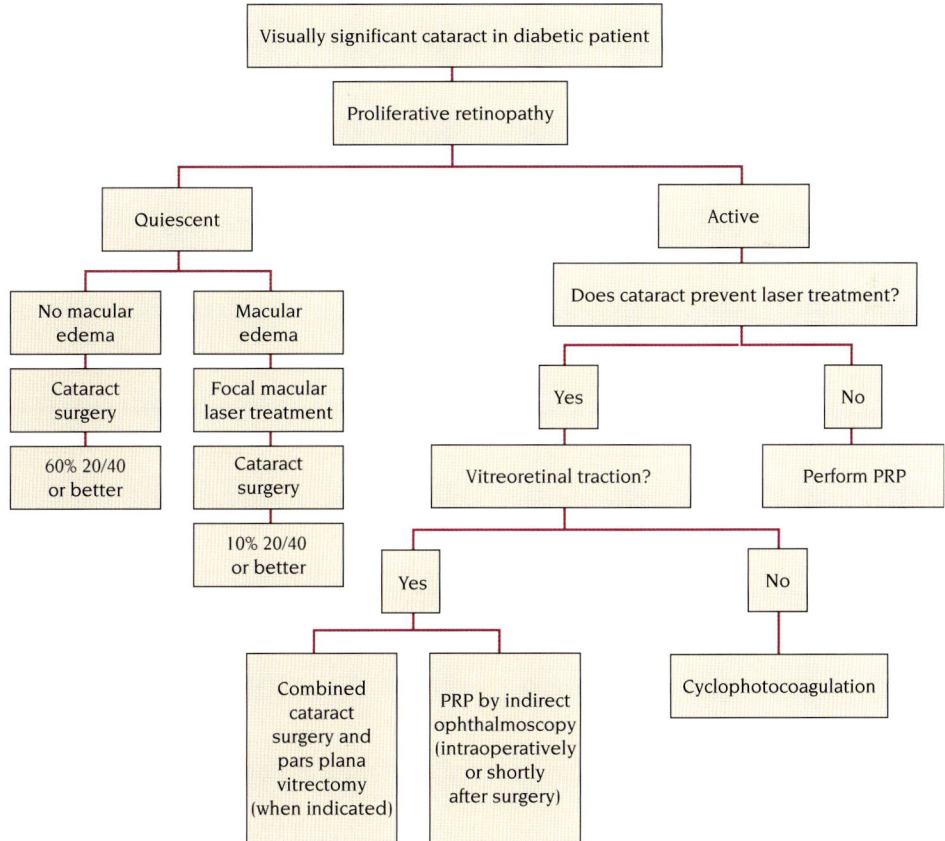

Figure 15.8. Visual acuity outcomes and management decisions for diabetic patients with visually significant cataracts and active or quiescent proliferative diabetic retinopathy with or without macular edema.

REFERENCES

1. Klein BE, Klein R, Moss SE. Incidence of cataract surgery in the Wisconsin Epidemiologic Study of Diabetic Retinopathy. *Am J Ophthalmol.* 1995;119:295–300.
2. Klein BE, Klein R, Moss SE. Prevalence of cataracts in a population-based study of persons with diabetes mellitus. *Ophthalmology.* 1985;92:1191–1196.
3. Bron AJ, Sparrow J, Brown NA, et al. The lens in diabetes. *Eye.* 1993;7:260–275.
4. Mukesh BN, Le A, Dimitrov PN, et al. Development of cataract and associated risk factors: the Visual Impairment Project. *Arch Ophthalmol.* 2006;124:79–85.
5. Saxena S, Mitchell P, Rochtchina E. Five-year incidence of cataract in older persons with diabetes and pre-diabetes. *Ophthalmic Epidemiol.* 2004;11:271–277.
6. Rowe NG, Mitchell PG, Cumming RG, Wans JJ. Diabetes, fasting blood glucose and age-related cataract: the Blue Mountains Eye Study. *Ophthalmic Epidemiol.* 2000;7:103–114.
7. Harding JJ, Egerton M, van Heyningen R, Harding RS. Diabetes, glaucoma, sex, and cataract: analysis of combined data from two case control studies. *Br J Ophthalmol.* 1993;77:2–6.
8. Harris MI, Eastman RC, Cowie CC, et al. Comparison of diabetes diagnostic categories in the U.S. population according to the 1997 American Diabetes Association and 1980–1985 World Health Organization diagnostic criteria. *Diabetes Care.* 1997;20:1859–1862.
9. Harris MI, Robbins DC. Prevalence of adult-onset IDDM in the U.S. population. *Diabetes Care.* 1994;17:1337–1340.
10. Nielsen NV, Vinding T. The prevalence of cataract in insulin-dependent and non–insulin-dependent diabetes mellitus. *Acta Ophthalmol.* 1984;62:595–602.
11. Klein R, Klein BE, Moss SE. Visual impairment in diabetes. *Ophthalmology.* 1984;91:1–9.
12. Edwards MG, Schachat AP, Bressler SB, Bressler NM. Outcome of cataract operations performed to permit diagnosis, to determine eligibility for laser therapy, or to perform laser therapy of retinal disorders. *Am J Ophthalmol.* 1994;118:440–444.
13. Minckler D, Astorino A, Hamilton AM. Cataract surgery in patients with diabetes. *Ophthalmology.* 1998;105:949–950.
14. Aiello LM, Wand M, Liang G. Neovascular glaucoma and vitreous hemorrhage following cataract surgery in patients with diabetes mellitus. *Ophthalmology.* 1983;90:814–820.
15. Poliner LS, Christianson DJ, Escoffery RF, et al. Neovascular glaucoma after intracapsular and extracapsular cataract extraction in diabetic patients. *Am J Ophthalmol.* 1985;100:637–643.
16. Pavese T, Insler MS. Effects of extracapsular cataract extraction with posterior chamber lens implantation on the development of neovascular glaucoma in diabetics. *J Cataract Refract Surg.* 1987;13:197–201.
17. Prasad P, Setna PH, Dunne JA. Accelerated ocular neovascularisation in diabetics following posterior chamber lens implantation. *Br J Ophthalmol.* 1990;74:313–314.
18. Sadiq SA, Chatterjee A, Vernon SA. Progression of diabetic retinopathy and rubeotic glaucoma following cataract surgery. *Eye.* 1995;9:728–738.
19. Suzuki Y, Ohtsuki K, Goto T, Sumiya Y. Comparative study of postoperative complications in primary and secondary implantation of posterior chamber intraocular lens in cataract surgery for diabetic patients. *Nippon Ganka Gakkai Zasshi.* 1992;96:359–363.
20. Krupsky S, Zalish M, Oliver M, Pollack A. Anterior segment complications in diabetic patients following extracapsular cataract extraction and posterior chamber intraocular lens implantation. *Ophthalmic Surg.* 1991;22:526–530.

21. Hykin PG, Gregson RM, Hamilton AM. Extracapsular cataract extraction in diabetics with rubeosis iridis. *Eye*. 1992;6:296–299.
22. Weinreb RN, Wasserstrom JP, Forman JS, Ritch R. Pseudophakic pupillary block with angle-closure glaucoma in diabetic patients. *Am J Ophthalmol*. 1986;102:325–328.
23. Ionides A, Dowler JG, Hykin PG, et al. Posterior capsule opacification following diabetic extracapsular cataract extraction. *Eye*. 1994;8:535–537.
24. Helbig H, Kellner U, Bornfeld N, Foerster MH. Cataract surgery and YAG-laser capsulotomy following vitrectomy for diabetic retinopathy. *Ger J Ophthalmol*. 1996;5:408–414.
25. Jaffe GJ, Burton TC. Progression of nonproliferative diabetic retinopathy following cataract extraction. *Arch Ophthalmol*. 1988;106:745–749.
26. Pollack A, Dotan S, Oliver M. Course of diabetic retinopathy following cataract surgery. *Br J Ophthalmol*. 1991;75:2–8.
27. Pollack A, Dotan S, Oliver M. Progression of diabetic retinopathy after cataract extraction. *Br J Ophthalmol*. 1991;75:547–551.
28. Cunliffe IA, Flanagan DW, George ND, et al. Extracapsular cataract surgery with lens implantation in diabetics with and without proliferative retinopathy. *Br J Ophthalmol*. 1991;75:9–12.
29. Jaffe GJ, Burton TC, Kuhn E, et al. Progression of nonproliferative diabetic retinopathy and visual outcome after extracapsular cataract extraction and intraocular lens implantation. *Am J Ophthalmol*. 1992;114:448–456.
30. Dureau P, Massin P, Chaine G, et al. Extracapsular extraction and posterior chamber implantation in diabetics: prospective study of 198 eyes. *J Fr Ophtalmol*. 1997;20:117–123.
31. Vignanelli M. Progression of diabetic retinopathy following cataract extraction. *Klin Monatsbl Augenheilkd*. 1990;196:334–337.
32. Raniel Y, Teichner Y, Friedman Z. The course of nonproliferative diabetic retinopathy following ECCE with posterior chamber IOL implantation. *Metab Pediatr Syst Ophthalmol*. 1994;17:10–13.
33. Ruiz RS, Saatci OA. Posterior chamber intraocular lens implantation in eyes with inactive and active proliferative diabetic retinopathy. *Am J Ophthalmol*. 1991;111:158–162.
34. Benson WE, Brown GC, Tasman W, et al. Extracapsular cataract extraction with placement of a posterior chamber lens in patients with diabetic retinopathy. *Ophthalmology*. 1993;100:730–738.
35. Henricsson M, Heijl A, Janzon L. Diabetic retinopathy before and after cataract surgery. *Br J Ophthalmol*. 1996;80:789–793.
36. Kodama T, Hayasaka S, Setogawa T. Plasma glucose levels, postoperative complications, and progression of retinopathy in diabetic patients undergoing intraocular lens implantation. *Graefes Arch Klin Exp Ophthalmol*. 1993;231:439–443.
37. Pollack A, Leiba H, Bukelman A, et al. The course of diabetic retinopathy following cataract surgery in eyes previously treated by laser photocoagulation. *Br J Ophthalmol*. 1992;76:228–231.
38. Hutton WL, Pesicka GA, Fuller DG. Cataract extraction in the diabetic eye after vitrectomy. *Am J Ophthalmol*. 1987;104:1–4.
39. Sebestyen JG. Intraocular lenses and diabetes mellitus. *Am J Ophthalmol*. 1986;101:425–428.
40. Straatsma BR, Pettit TH, Wheeler N, Miyamasu W. Diabetes mellitus and intraocular lens implantation. *Ophthalmology*. 1983;90:336–343.
41. Cheng H, Franklin SL. Treatment of cataract in diabetics with and without retinopathy. *Eye*. 1988;2:607–614.

42. Ngui MS, Lim AS, Chong AB. Posterior chamber intraocular lenses in diabetics: review of 63 patients. *Int Ophthalmol.* 1985;8:257–259.
43. Dowler JG, Hykin PG, Lightman SL, Hamilton AM. Visual acuity following extracapsular cataract extraction in diabetes: a meta-analysis. *Eye.* 1995;9:313–317.
44. Early Treatment Diabetic Retinopathy Study Research Group. Results after lens extraction in patients with diabetic retinopathy. ETDRS Report Number 25. *Arch Ophthalmol.* 1999;117:1600–1606.
45. Wagner T, Knaflic D, Rauber M, Mester U. Influence of cataract surgery on the diabetic eye: a prospective study. *Ger J Ophthalmol.* 1996;5:79–83.
46. Romero-Aroca P, Fernandez-Ballart J, Almena-Garcia M, et al. Nonproliferative diabetic retinopathy and macular edema progression after phacoemulsification: prospective study. *J Cataract Refract Surg.* 2006;32:1438–1444.
47. Krepler K, Biowski R, Schrey S, et al. Cataract surgery in patients with diabetic retinopathy: visual outcome, progression of diabetic retinopathy, and incidence of diabetic macular edema. *Graefes Arch Clin Exp Ophthalmol.* 2002;240:735–738.
48. Somaiya MD, Burns JD, Mintz R, et al. Factors affecting visual outcomes after small-incision phacoemulsification in diabetic patients. *J Cataract Refract Surg.* 2002;28:1364–1371.
49. Squirrell D, Bhola R, Bush J, et al. A prospective, case controlled study of the natural history of diabetic retinopathy and maculopathy after uncomplicated phacoemulsification cataract surgery in patients with type 2 diabetes. *Br J Ophthalmol.* 2002;86:565–571.
50. Chung J, Kim MY, Kim HS, et al. Effect of cataract surgery on the progression of diabetic retinopathy. *J Cataract Refract Surg.* 2002;28:626–630.
51. Early Treatment Diabetic Retinopathy Study Research Group. Photocoagulation for diabetic macular edema. ETDRS Report Number 1. *Arch Ophthalmol.* 1985;103:1796–1806.
52. Lam DS, Chan CK, Mohamet S, et al. Phacoemulsification with intravitreal triamcinolone in patients with cataract and coexisting diabetic macular oedmea: a 6-month prospective pilot study. *Eye.* 2005;19:885–890.
53. Klein R, Klein BE, Moss SE, et al. The Wisconsin epidemiologic study of diabetic retinopathy, IV: diabetic macular edema. *Ophthalmology.* 1984;91:1464–1474.
54. Hykin PG, Gregson RM, Stevens JD, Hamilton PA. Extracapsular cataract extraction in proliferative diabetic retinopathy. *Ophthalmology.* 1993;100:394–399.
55. Antcliff RJ, Poulson A, Flanagan DW. Phacoemulsification in diabetics. *Eye.* 1996;10:737–741.
56. Benson WE, Brown GC, Tasman W, McNamara JA. Extracapsular cataract extraction, posterior chamber lens insertion, and pars plana vitrectomy in one operation. *Ophthalmology.* 1990;97:918–921.
57. Senn P, Schipper I, Perren B. Combined pars plana vitrectomy, phacoemulsification, and intraocular lens implantation in the capsular bag: a comparison to vitrectomy and subsequent cataract surgery as a two-step procedure. *Ophthalmic Surg Lasers.* 1995;26:420–428.
58. Diolati S, Senn P, Schmid MK, et al. Combined pars plana vitrectomy and phacoemulsification with intraocular lens implantation in severe proliferative diabetic retinopathy. *Ophthalmic Surg Lasers Imaging.* 2006;37:468–474.
59. Mochizuki Y, Kubota T, Hata Y, et al. Surgical results of combined pars plana vitrectomy, phacoemulsification, and intraocular lens implantation. *Eur J Ophthalmol.* 2006;16:279–286.

60. Lahey JM, Francis RR, Kearney JJ. Combining phacoemulsification with pars plana vitrectomy in patients with proliferative diabetic retinopathy: a series of 223 cases. *Ophthalmology.* July 2003;110(7):1335-1339.

61. Douglas MJ, Scott IU, Flynn HW Jr. Pas plana lensectomy, pars plana vitrectomy, and silicone oil tamponade as initial management of cataract and combined traction/rhegmatogenous retinal detachment involving the macula associated with severe proliferative diabetic retinopathy. *Ophthalmic Surg Lasers Imaging.* 2003;34:270–278.

62. Jun Z, Pavlovic S, Jacobi KW. Results of combined vitreoretinal surgery and phacoemulsification with intraocular lens implantation. *Clin Exp Ophthalmol.* 2001;29: 307–311.

63. Blankenship GW, Flynn HW Jr, Kokame GT. Posterior chamber intraocular lens insertion during pars plana lensectomy and vitrectomy for complications of proliferative diabetic retinopathy. *Am J Ophthalmol.* 1989;108:1–5.

64. Kokame GT, Flynn HW Jr, Blankenship GW. Posterior chamber intraocular lens implantation during diabetic pars plana vitrectomy. *Ophthalmology.* 1989;96:603–610.

65. McElvanney AM, Talbot EM. Posterior chamber lens implantation combined with pars plana vitrectomy. *J Cataract Refract Surg.* 1997;23:106–110.

66. Ullern M, Nicol JL, Ruellan YM, et al. Phacoemulsification by the anterior approach combined with vitreoretinal surgery. *J Fr Ophtalmol.* 1993;16:320–324.

67. Menchini U, Azzolini C, Camesasca FI, Brancato R. Combined vitrectomy, cataract extraction, and posterior chamber intraocular lens implantation in diabetic patients. *Ophthalmic Surg.* 1991;22:69–73.

68. Koenig SB, Mieler WF, Han DP, Abrams GW. Combined phacoemulsification, pars plana vitrectomy, and posterior chamber intraocular lens insertion. *Arch Ophthalmol.* 1992;110:1101–1104.

69. Pagot V, Gazagne C, Galiana A, et al. Extracapsular cataract extraction and implantation in the capsular sac during vitrectomy in diabetics. *J Fr Ophtalmol.* 1991;14:523–528.

70. Mamalis N, Teske MP, Kreisler KR, et al: Phacoemulsification combined with pars plana vitrectomy. *Ophthalmic Surg.* 1991;22:194–198.

71. Mackool RJ. Pars plana vitrectomy and posterior chamber intraocular lens implantation in diabetic patients. *Ophthalmology.* 1989;96:1679–1680.

72. de Ortueta Hilberath D, Losche CC. Choice of surgical technique in the management of cataract combined with vitreous surgery. *Eur J Ophthalmol.* 1997;7:245–250.

73. Hsu SY, Wu WC. Comparison of phacoemulsification and planned extracapsular cataract extraction in combined pars plana vitrectomy and posterior chamber intraocular lens implantation. *Ophthalmic Surg Lasers Imaging.* 2005;36:108–113.

74. Rice TA, Michels RG, Maguire MG, Rice EF. The effect of lensectomy on the incidence of iris neovascularization and neovascular glaucoma after vitrectomy for diabetic retinopathy. *Am J Ophthalmol.* 1983;95:1–11.

75. Wand M, Madigan JC, Gaudio AR, Sorokanich S. Neovascular glaucoma following pars plana vitrectomy for complications of diabetic retinopathy. *Ophthalmic Surg.* 1990;21:113–118.

76. Shioya M, Ogino N, Shinjo U. Change in postoperative refractive error when vitrectomy is added to intraocular lens implantation. *J Cataract Refract Surg.* 1997;23:1217–1220.

77. Sneed S, Parrish RK II, Mandelbaum S, O'Grady G. Technical problems of extracapsular cataract extractions after vitrectomy. *Arch Ophthalmol.* 1986;104:1126–1127.

78. Smiddy WE, Stark WJ, Michels RG, et al. Cataract extraction after vitrectomy. *Ophthalmology.* 1987;94:483–487.

79. Saunders DC, Brown A, Jones NP. Extracapsular cataract extraction after vitrectomy. *J Cataract Refract Surg.* 1996;22:218–221.

80. McDermott ML, Puklin JE, Abrams GW, Eliott D. Phacoemulsification for cataract following pars plana vitrectomy. *Ophthalmic Surg Lasers.* 1997;28:558–564.

81. Charles S. Endophotocoagulation. *Retina.* 1981;1:117–120.

82. Peyman GA, Grisolano JM, Palacio MN. Intraocular photocoagulation with the argon-krypton laser. *Arch Ophthalmol.* 1980;98:2061–2064.

83. Fleischman JA, Swartz M, Dixon JA. Argon laser endophotocoagulation: an intraoperative trans–pars plana technique. *Arch Ophthalmol.* 1981;99:1610–1612.

84. Federman JL, Boyer D, Lanning R, Breit P. An objective analysis of proliferative diabetic retinopathy before and after pars plana vitrectomy. *Ophthalmology.* 1979;86:276–282.

85. Nasrallah FP, Jalkh AE, Van Coppenolle F, et al. The role of the vitreous in diabetic macular edema. *Ophthalmology.* 1988;95:1335–1339.

86. Nasrallah FP, Van de Velde F, Jalkh AE, et al. Importance of the vitreous in young diabetics with macular edema. *Ophthalmology.* 1989;96:1511–1516; discussion 1516–1517.

87. Weinreb RN, Wasserstrom JP, Parker W. Neovascular glaucoma following neodymium-YAG laser posterior capsulotomy. *Arch Ophthalmol.* 1986;104:730–731.

88. Glaser BM. Extracellular modulating factors and the control of intraocular neovascularization. *Arch Ophthalmol.* 1988;106:603–607.

89. Stefansson E, Landers MB III, Wolbarsht ML. Increased retinal oxygen supply following pan-retinal photocoagulation and vitrectomy and lensectomy. *Trans Am Ophthalmol Soc.* 1981;79:307–334.

90. Miyake K. Fluorophotometric evaluation of the blood–ocular barrier function following cataract surgery and intraocular lens implantation. *J Cataract Refract Surg.* 1988;14:560–568.

91. Cunha-Vaz JG. Studies on the pathophysiology of diabetic retinopathy: the blood–retinal barrier in diabetes. *Diabetes.* 1983;32:20–27.

92. Boot JP, van Gerven JM, van Best JA, et al. Blood retinal and blood aqueous barriers in diabetics by fluorophotometry. *Doc Ophthalmol.* 1989;71:19–27.

93. Bordat B, Arnaud C, Guirguis IR, Laudeho A. Fluorophotometric study of lens autofluorescence and the blood–retinal barrier in 56 diabetic patients. *Eur J Ophthalmol.* 1995;5:13–18.

94. Schalnus R, Ohrloff C, Jungmann E, et al. Permeability of the blood–retinal barrier and the blood–aqueous barrier in type I diabetes without diabetic retinopathy: simultaneous evaluation with fluorophotometry. *Ger J Ophthalmol.* 1993;2:202–206.

95. Schalnus R, Ohrloff C. The blood–ocular barrier in type I diabetes without diabetic retinopathy: permeability measurements using fluorophotometry. *Ophthalmic Res.* 1995;27:116–123.

96. Pollack A, Leiba H, Bukelman A, Oliver M. Cystoid macular oedema following cataract extraction in patients with diabetes. *Br J Ophthalmol.* 1992;76:221–224.

97. Menchini U, Bandello F, Brancato R, et al. Cystoid macular oedema after extracapsular cataract extraction and intraocular lens implantation in diabetic patients without retinopathy. *Br J Ophthalmol.* 1993;77:208–211.

98. Jampol LM. Pharmacologic therapy of aphakic and pseudophakic cystoid macular edema: 1985 update. *Ophthalmology.* 1985;92:807–810.

99. Jampol LM. Aphakic cystoid macular edema: a hypothesis. *Arch Ophthalmol.* 1985;103:1134–1135.

100. Haritoglou C, Kook D, Neubauer A, et al. Intravitreal bevacizumab (Avastin) therapy for persistent diffuse diabetic macular edema. *Retina*. 2006;26:999–1005.
101. Audren F, Erginay A, Haouchine B, et al. Intravitreal triamcinolone acetonide for diffuse diabetic macular oedema: 6-month results of a prospective controlled trial. *Acta Ophthalmol Scand*. 2006;84:624–630.
102. Gillies MC, Sutter FK, Simpson JM, et al. Intravitreal triamcinolone for refractory diabetic macular edema: two-year results of a double-masked, placebo-controlled, randomized clinical trial. *Ophthalmology*. 2006;113:1533–1538.
103. Mason JO 3rd, Albert MA Jr, Vail R. Intravitreal bevacizumab (Avastin) for refractory pseudophakic cystoid macular edema. *Retina*. 2006;26:356–357.
104. Scott IU, Flynn HW Jr, Rosenfeld PJ. Intravitreal triamcinolone acetonide for idiopathic cystoid macular edema. *Am J Ophthalmol*. 2003;136:737–739.
105. Cunningham EM Jr, Adamis AP, Altaweel M, et al. A phase II randomized double-masked trial of pegaptanib, an anti-vascular endothelial growth factor aptamer, for diabetic macular edema. *Ophthalmology*. 2005;112:1747–1757.
106. McCuen BW II, Klombers L. The choice of posterior chamber intraocular lens style in patients with diabetic retinopathy. *Arch Ophthalmol*. 1990;108:1376–1377.
107. McCartney DL, Guyton DL. The choice of posterior chamber intraocular lens style in patients with diabetic retinopathy. *Arch Ophthalmol*. 1991;109:615.
108. Apple DJ, Mamalis N, Loftfield K, et al. Complications of intraocular lenses: a historical and histopathological review. *Surv Ophthalmol*. 1984;29:1–54.
109. Eaton AM, Jaffe GJ, McCuen BW II, Mincey GJ. Condensation on the posterior surface of silicone intraocular lenses during fluid–air exchange. *Ophthalmology*. 1995;102:733–736.
110. Apple DJ, Federman JL, Krolicki TJ, et al. Irreversible silicone oil adhesion to silicone intraocular lenses: a clinicopathologic analysis. *Ophthalmology*. 1996;103:1555–1561; discussion 1561–1562.
111. Kusaka S, Kodama T, Ohashi Y. Condensation of silicone oil on the posterior surface of a silicone intraocular lens during vitrectomy. *Am J Ophthalmol*. 1996;121:574–575.

16

Nonretinal Ocular Abnormalities in Diabetes

INGRID U. SCOTT, MD, MPH,
AND HARRY W. FLYNN, JR., MD

CORE MESSAGES

- Corneal abnormalities associated with diabetes include decreased corneal sensitivity, bacterial keratitis, neurotrophic ulcers, persistent epithelial defects, and recurrent epithelial erosions.
- There may be an association between diabetes and primary open-angle glaucoma, angle-closure glaucoma, neovascular glaucoma, and blood-associated glaucoma.
- Lens abnormalities associated with diabetes include refractive changes and cataract.
- Optic nerve abnormalities associated with diabetes include acute optic disc edema, Wolfram syndrome, optic nerve hypoplasia, and optic atrophy.
- Diabetes is associated with cranial nerve III, IV, and IV palsies.
- Diabetes is associated with an increased risk of endophthalmitis and mucormycosis.

Although diabetes-related visual impairment is most commonly due to complications of diabetic retinopathy, many nonretinal ocular abnormalities may contribute to visual loss and must be considered in the management of patients with diabetes.

CORNEAL DISEASES

Diabetic patients may have significantly decreased corneal sensitivity, and the severity of the decreased sensitivity is usually correlated positively with the severity of retinopathy [1–3]. Diabetes has also been reported to be associated with dry eyes, with the severity of dry eyes correlated positively with the severity of diabetic retinopathy [4]. Decreased corneal sensitivity and increased dry eyes may account for the increased incidence of contact lens-associated bacterial corneal ulcers [5] and neurotrophic ulcers [6] in diabetic patients compared with nondiabetic persons (Fig. 16.1).

Intrinsic abnormalities of the epithelial basement membrane complexes [7] and impaired epithelial barrier function [8] predispose to superficial punctuate keratitis, poor epithelial wound healing after trauma, and persistent epithelial defects [6]. The latter are seen frequently in diabetic patients whose corneal epithelium was removed during vitreoretinal surgery (Fig. 16.2) [9].

Diabetic patients are prone to recurrent corneal erosions, especially after photocoagulation and vitrectomy [10]. In a study of 100 vitrectomies performed for advanced diabetic retinopathy with vitreous hemorrhage, persistent epithelial defects or recurrent corneal erosions occurred in 25% of patients [11]. In another study, 55 vitreoretinal surgeons were asked to retrospectively report how many pars plana vitrectomies they performed in 1 year on diabetic eyes and in what percentage of cases the corneal epithelium was debrided [12]. The frequency of epithelial debridement was 17.4%; the use of irrigating contact lenses was associated with a significantly higher rate of debridement compared with the use of sew-on or binocular indirect operating microscope (BIOM) noncontact lenses (23.5% vs. 12.1%, respectively; $P < 0.001$). In another study of patients who underwent pars plana vitrectomy, diabetic patients had more postoperative corneal epithelial defects if hand-held infusion lenses were used (32.1%) than if sew-on lenses (8.8%; $P = 0.011$) or noncontact lenses (0%; $P < 0.001$) were employed [13].

When the epithelium of the diabetic cornea is removed, it often comes off as an intact epithelial sheet, with the basement membrane attached to basal epithelial cells. In the nondiabetic eye, scraping of the epithelium removes only the epithelium and usually leaves the basement membrane intact and adherent to the

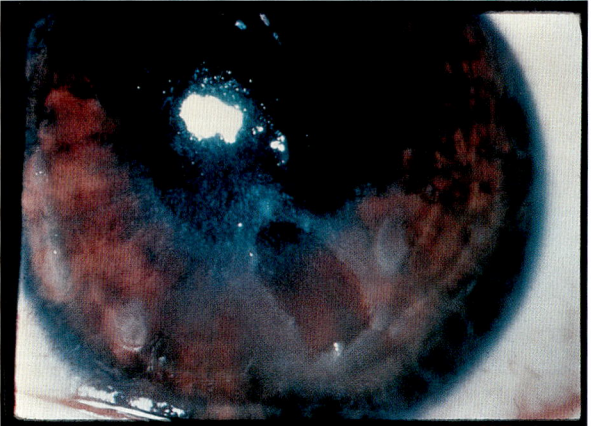

Figure 16.1. Neurotrophic corneal ulcer in a diabetic patient with decreased corneal sensitivity.

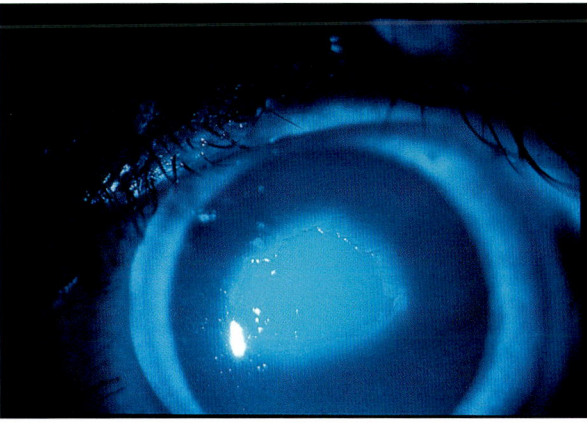

Figure 16.2. Persistent corneal epithelial defect in a diabetic patient after vitreoretinal surgery.

stroma [9,14]. Ultrastructural abnormalities of the diabetic corneal epithelial basement membrane complex mimic findings in epithelial basement membrane dystrophies [15] and include thickening of the multilaminar basement membrane [7], decreased hemidesmosome frequency [16], and decreased penetration of anchoring fibrils [17].

The poor adhesiveness of the diabetic corneal basement membrane may be related to changes in biochemical composition induced by increased sorbitol and fructose produced by the aldose reductase pathway [9]. While topical aldose-reductase inhibitors may promote epithelial regeneration [18–20] and may prevent decreased corneal sensitivity due to diabetes [21] (and oral aldose-reductase inhibitors may improve corneal sensation in diabetic patients) [22], most studies have been performed in rats [18,19,21] and the efficacy of these agents in humans is unproven. In contrast, lubricants, limited epithelial debridement, and bandage contact lenses have proven to be effective in avoiding major ocular surface problems.

GLAUCOMA

Primary Open-Angle Glaucoma. The association between diabetes and primary open-angle glaucoma (POAG) is unclear. Several studies have demonstrated a higher prevalence of elevated mean intraocular pressure (IOP) and POAG among diabetic patients compared with nondiabetic persons [23–25]. Several case-control studies support an association between diabetes and POAG, with the relative odds of having glaucoma among diabetic patients versus controls ranging from 1.6 to 4.7 [26–29]. Other studies, including population-based surveys such as the Baltimore Eye Survey, demonstrated no association between diabetes and POAG [30,31]. Although diabetes was common in participants of the Barbados Eye Survey and participants of the Baltimore Eye Survey, it was unrelated to the prevalence of open-angle glaucoma [31,32]. Similarly, no significant association between diabetes and glaucoma was found in the African Caribbean Eye Survey [33]. In the Beaver Dam Eye Study, older-onset diabetes ($\geq$30 years of age) was associated with a modest increase in the risk of glaucoma [25]. In the Blue Mountains Eye Study, there was a significant association between diabetes (diagnosed from history or from elevated fasting plasma glaucose level) and open-angle glaucoma [34]. The Rotterdam Study also reported a significant association between diabetes and POAG [35]. The Ocular Hypertension Treatment Study (OHTS) found that diabetes mellitus appeared to be protective against the development of POAG in patients with ocular hypertension [36]. However, the diagnosis of diabetes was not confirmed with blood tests and individuals with diabetic retinopathy were excluded from the OHTS, suggesting that an unrepresentative group of patients with diabetes was enrolled in this study. These factors may explain the paradoxical relationship between diabetes and POAG in the OHTS, which contradicts previously published study results.

When patients are treated medically for POAG, it is important to recognize that the potential side effects of beta-adrenergic antagonists include reduced glucose tolerance and masking of hypoglycemic signs. Therefore, this class of antiglaucoma medications should be used cautiously in diabetic patients.

Angle-Closure Glaucoma. Several observations suggest an association between diabetes and angle-closure glaucoma (ACG). One study found that patients with ACG had a higher prevalence of abnormal glucose tolerance test results compared with POAG patients and controls [37]. Patients with ACG also have a high prevalence of non-insulin-dependent diabetes [38]. It has been hypothesized that, in some cases, ACG may be a symptom of diabetes, perhaps due to autonomic dysfunction [39]. Finally, lens swelling related to hyperglycemia may precipitate ACG [40].

Hyperosmotic agents are commonly included in the medical management of acute episodes of elevated IOP. In diabetic patients, isosorbide is preferred to glycerol because isosorbide is not metabolized into sugar, while glycerol is metabolized into sugar and ketone bodies. Glycerol, therefore, can produce hyperglycemia and, rarely, ketoacidosis in diabetic patients.

Neovascular Glaucoma. Despite the widespread use of panretinal photocoagulation (PRP), proliferative diabetic retinopathy (PDR) remains a leading cause of neovascular glaucoma. In a 1973 report of 56 patients with neovascular glaucoma, 43% were attributed to diabetic retinopathy, 37% to central retinal vein occlusion, and the rest to miscellaneous causes [41]. In 1984, Brown and associates reviewed 208 cases of neovascular glaucoma and reported that 36% were caused by central retinal vein occlusion, 32% by diabetic retinopathy, and 13% by carotid occlusive disease [42].

The reported incidence of any neovascularization of the iris (NVI) among diabetic patients ranges from 1% [43] to 17% [44]. In eyes with PDR, the reported incidence in one study was 65% [45]. In the early stages, NVI usually appears as small vascular tufts either at the pupillary margin or in the anterior chamber angle. As these vessels later spread across the iris surface, they are frequently accompanied by fibrous tissue, which contracts and may cause ectropion uveae (Fig. 16.3)

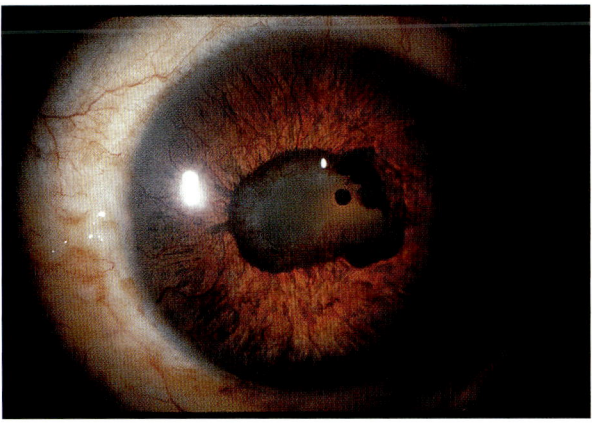

Figure 16.3. Extensive neovascularization of the iris in a patient with proliferative diabetic retinopathy.

and peripheral anterior synechiae. While angle closure can cause severe glaucoma, IOP may be elevated even before any angle is closed, probably because of leakage of protein and cells from the new iris vessels [46].

It is generally well accepted that NVI is associated with retinal hypoxia and PDR [47], and many authors have reported regression of early NVI following PRP [47–49]. In goniophotocoagulation, argon laser treatment is applied directly to new vessels in the anterior chamber angle. Although performed infrequently, goniophotocoagulation has been proposed as a treatment in the early stages of neovascular glaucoma to prevent progressive angle closure, while PRP facilitates regression of the anterior segment neovascularization.

Use of adjunctive 5-fluorouracil or mitomycin C has been shown to increase the success rate of filtering surgery in eyes with neovascular glaucoma [50–53]. Glaucoma drainage devices have gained increasing popularity in recent years to achieve IOP control in various refractory glaucomas, including neovascular glaucoma [54]. A traditional approach to the management of patients with neovascular glaucoma is as follows:

PRP is performed to induce regression of NVI.

Adjunctive anti-vascular endothelial growth factor (anti-VEGF) agents may facilitate regression of NVI.

If IOP is not controlled medically and the eye has visual potential, filtering surgery with an adjunctive antimetabolite or implantation of a glaucoma drainage device is performed. Adjunctive anti-VEGF agents at the time of surgery may also be employed.

If IOP is not controlled medically and the eye has limited visual potential, a cyclodestructive procedure may be considered.

For eyes with NVI and opaque media, an alternative approach is combined pars plana vitrectomy, lensectomy with or without intraocular lens implantation, and implantation of a glaucoma drainage device [54].

Medical management of IOP elevation in neovascular glaucoma principally involves aqueous suppressants, such as alpha-2-agonists, beta-blockers, and topical and oral carbonic anhydrase inhibitors. Miotics are not beneficial when the anterior chamber angle is closed and are avoided, as they can exacerbate intraocular inflammation and may hamper access to the posterior segment. Topical corticosteroids are often useful in treating intraocular inflammation and pain.

Blood-associated Glaucoma. Glaucoma associated with degenerated intraocular blood is not unique to diabetic patients. Ghost-cell glaucoma may occur after vitreous hemorrhage of any cause in an eye with a communication between the vitreous and the anterior segment through a disrupted anterior hyaloid face. Ghost-cell glaucoma was originally observed after early attempts at vitrectomy, when only a core vitrectomy was performed. Blood products in the peripheral vitreous leach out, and degenerated erythrocytes (ghost cells) travel around lens zonules and into the anterior chamber, obstructing the trabecular meshwork and causing elevated IOP within days to weeks postvitrectomy [55].

Slit-lamp examination usually permits differentiation of white inflammatory cells associated with anterior uveitis from khaki-colored ghost cells. In severe cases, it is important to distinguish the white color of a hypopyon due to uveitis or endophthalmitis from the khaki-colored pseudohypopyon characteristic of ghost-cell glaucoma. In questionable cases, anterior chamber aspiration, combined with phase-contrast microscopy, may be performed. In ghost-cell glaucoma, degenerated erythrocytes with precipitated hemoglobin (Heinz bodies) adherent to the inner walls of the cells may be evident [56].

Medical treatment focuses on agents that decrease aqueous production—for example, alpha-2 agonists, beta-adrenergic blocking agents, and carbonic anhydrase inhibitors. Because the trabecular meshwork is obstructed by ghost cells, miotics may be unsuccessful in increasing aqueous outflow. In severe cases or if medical therapy is unsuccessful or not tolerated, surgical management may be limited to anterior chamber washout or may include a pars plana vitrectomy.

Hemolytic glaucoma results when macrophages ingest contents of red blood cells and then accumulate in the trabecular meshwork, where they obstruct aqueous outflow [57]. Examination reveals red-tinted blood cells floating in the aqueous, and the anterior chamber angle is usually open, with the trabecular meshwork covered with reddish brown pigment [58]. As the condition is typically self-limited, it is generally managed medically. Occasionally, anterior chamber lavage is required [58].

First described in 1960, hemosiderotic glaucoma is thought to result from obstruction of the aqueous outflow channels by iron deposition, with subsequent degeneration and inflammatory changes [59]. Hemosiderotic glaucoma is reported to have a later onset than that of ghost-cell glaucoma (patients with hemosiderotic glaucoma typically present with elevated IOP years after the initial intraocular hemorrhage), and ghost cells are not present [60].

Because treatment is similar to that of ghost-cell glaucoma, these two entities (hemolytic glaucoma and hemosiderotic glaucoma) may represent part of the broad spectrum of blood-associated glaucoma.

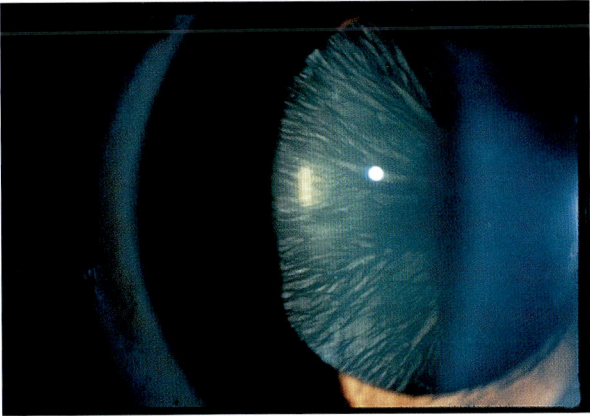

Figure 16.4. "Snowflake" cataract in a patient with type 1 diabetes.

LENS ABNORMALITIES

Refractive Error. Reversible swelling in lenses of diabetic patients causes "fluctuating myopia," which may be a presenting sign of diabetes. It is thought that accumulation of the sugar alcohol sorbitol, an end product of glucose reduction by aldose reductase, exerts an osmotic effect in lens cells [61]. A transient hyperopic shift typically occurs in hyperglycemic patients after such patients improve control of their plasma glucose levels [62]. Because lens shape, and thus refractive error, may fluctuate with blood glucose levels, it is best to prescribe glasses when the blood glucose level is relatively stable. Prior to prescribing glasses in patients with labile blood glucose levels, the clinician may need to evaluate the refractive error on several visits to confirm a stable refractive error.

Cataract. The risk of cataract formation is approximately 2 to 4 times higher in diabetic patients than in nondiabetic persons [63–66]. The risk of cataract increases with duration of diabetes and with poor metabolic control [62,67]. Cataract in diabetic patients usually does not differ morphologically from age-related cataract, but may occur 20 to 30 years earlier than in nondiabetic persons. In young diabetic patients, a rare "snowflake" cataract may develop, with superficial vacuoles and white snowflake opacities (Fig. 16.4) in the subcapsular region, and rapidly progress to a mature cataract.

OPTIC NERVE ABNORMALITIES

Acute Optic Disc Edema. Acute optic disc edema associated with diabetes, or diabetic papillopathy, usually occurs in the second to fourth decades of life and generally shows no correlation with the severity of diabetic retinopathy. It is typically associated with mild loss of vision (≥20/50) [68,69], and the visual field may be normal or may show defects, such as an increased blind spot, arcuate scotoma, or altitudinal scotoma. Fluorescein angiography usually demonstrates diffuse leakage at the disc. The condition presents bilaterally in approximately 50% of cases [70], while in other cases, the second eye may be affected as late as 3 years after initial presentation [69]. The visual prognosis is usually good [71], with nearly all younger patients recovering to a visual acuity of ≥20/30 (Fig. 16.5). Visual field defects infrequently persist [69,72]. While the optic disc appearance usually returns to normal, occasionally, diffuse or segmental atrophy may result (Fig. 16.6).

In diabetic papillopathy, diffuse disc swelling may mimic papilledema of raised intracranial pressure [73]. However, careful visual field testing may demonstrate an arcuate or altitudinal defect, which would be unusual in papilledema. To avoid unnecessary PRP, it is important to differentiate the prominent telangiectasia of disc vessels often seen in diabetic papillopathy from neovascularization of the disc.

Diabetic papillopathy differs from anterior ischemic optic neuropathy (AION). Typical AION is generally seen in middle-aged to elderly frequently

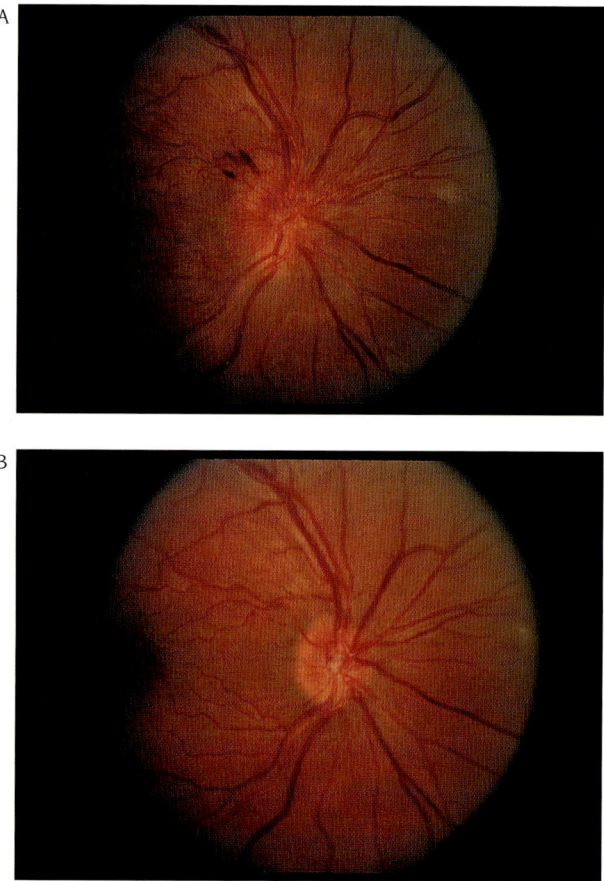

Figure 16.5. Diabetic papillopathy with good visual prognosis. (A) Disc edema, telangiectasia and splinter hemorrhages in a 20-year-old patient. Visual acuity is 20/30[-2]. (B) About 7 months later, disc edema has resolved and there is gliosis on the disc. Visual acuity is 20/25.

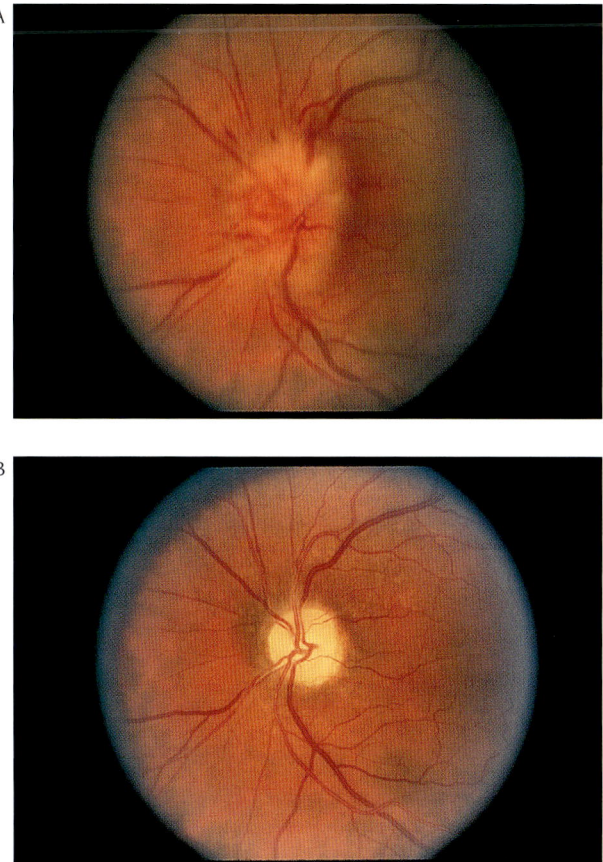

Figure 16.6. Diabetic papillopathy with eventual optic atrophy. (A) Disc edema, hemorrhages, and cotton-wool spots in a 52-year-old patient with a 6-year history of diabetes. Visual acuity is 20/25. (B) About 3 years later, diffuse optic atrophy is present. Visual acuity is 20/100.

hypertensive persons with or without diabetes, and is characterized by acute unilateral moderate-to-marked loss of vision, swelling of the optic disc with variable nerve fiber layer hemorrhages, segmental areas of nonperfusion on fluorescein angiography, poor prognosis for visual recovery, and late optic disc pallor [74].

Wolfram Syndrome. Wolfram syndrome refers to type 1 diabetes mellitus and progressive optic atrophy. The clinical spectrum includes multiple other neurologic and systemic abnormalities, such as neurosensory hearing loss, neurogenic bladder, diabetes insipidus, nystagmus, anosmia, and gonadal dysfunction [75]. The inheritance is autosomal recessive or sporadic. The syndrome has been reported to be associated with mutations of the *WFS1* gene that encodes wolframin, a putative transmembrane glycoprotein of the endoplasmic reticulum [76]. In a series of nine patients reported by Lessell and Rosman, diabetes was diagnosed between the ages of 2 and 11 years, and progressive loss of vision to ≤20/200 occurred within several years [75].

Optic Nerve Hypoplasia. Optic nerve hypoplasia is a congenital anomaly associated with a decreased complement of axons in the optic nerve but relatively normal vessels [77]. Examination may reveal a double-ring sign caused by concentric chorioretinal pigment changes. Optic nerve hypoplasia occurs most often in children born to mothers exposed to anticonvulsants, quinine, excessive alcohol, or lysergic acid diethylamide (LSD) and in children born to mothers with diabetes, but may also be seen in children with congenital intracranial tumors or basal encephaloceles [77,78]. The optic nerve hypoplasia seen in children of diabetic mothers is often superior and segmental, with a corresponding inferior semialtitudinal visual field defect; central acuity is usually normal.

Optic Atrophy. Optic atrophy in diabetic patients may be due to such causes as prior diabetic papillitis or nonarteritic anterior ischemic optic neuropathy. Further, at least two mild forms of optic atrophy are due to diabetic retinopathy [77]:

1. Multiple nerve fiber layer infarcts, which accumulate over time, may cause temporal or diffuse optic atrophy.
2. PRP destroys many retinal ganglion cells.

CRANIAL NERVE ABNORMALITIES

Diabetic patients may have an isolated cranial nerve (III, IV, or VI) palsy due to focal small-vessel occlusion with ischemic demyelination. The differential diagnosis includes microvascular infarction, vasculitic infarction, a compressive lesion, trauma, inflammation, and, in young patients, ophthalmoplegic migraine. Trauma is a frequent cause of nerve IV palsy. A nerve VI palsy may be nonlocalizing and may be a sign of increased intracranial pressure [79]. The risk of a compressive lesion is higher for an isolated nerve III palsy, but is almost always accompanied by pupillary dilation. If nerve III is involved because of microvascular infarction, the pupil is almost always spared (Fig. 16.7). When present, pupillary involvement

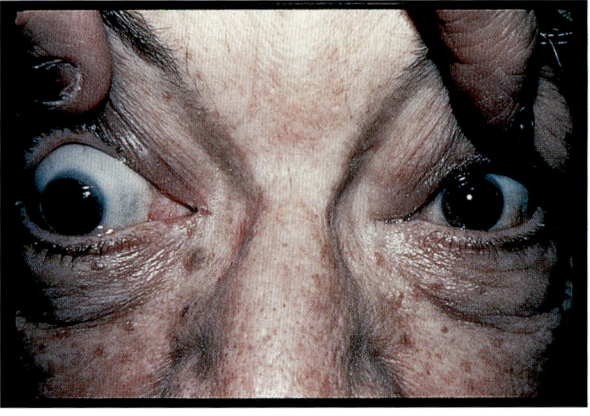

Figure 16.7. Right cranial nerve III palsy in a 71-year-old patient with type 2 diabetes.

generally consists of anisocoria of ≤1 mm rather than a fully dilated unreactive pupil [80], and internal ophthalmoplegia is incomplete [81]. Despite what is often reported, cranial nerve palsies caused by microvascular disease may present with orbital pain in up to 20% of cases [79], and pain may precede the palsy by a few days.

Workup for causes other than microvascular disease is indicated if examination reveals involvement of more than one cranial nerve, other neurologic signs, progressive deterioration, or lack of complete recovery within 3 months. Patients younger than 45 years with an isolated cranial nerve palsy usually do not have a microvascular infarct even if they have long-standing diabetes [77]. Recurrences are not rare and may involve the same or another cranial nerve on either side.

INFECTIOUS DISEASES

Endophthalmitis. Several studies suggest that patients with diabetes may have an increased risk of developing postoperative endophthalmitis (Fig. 16.8) compared to nondiabetic persons [82–85]. In one study of the 5-year incidence rates of endophthalmitis following intraocular surgery, a statistically significant increased incidence of endophthalmitis occurred in diabetic patients (0.163%) compared with nondiabetic patients (0.055%) who underwent extracapsular cataract extraction with or without intraocular lens implantation [82]. In a case-control study of endophthalmitis following secondary intraocular lens implantation, 50% of patients had a history of diabetes compared with 5.9% of control patients [84]. In a report of 162 consecutive patients treated for acute postoperative endophthalmitis, 21% had diabetes [83].

The increased risk of postoperative endophthalmitis among diabetic patients is not surprising, because patients with diabetes have been demonstrated to have impaired cellular and humoral immune responses, as well as altered phagocytic capabilities [86]. Further, it is well known that diabetic patients are more likely than nondiabetic patients to experience delayed wound healing [87]. Thus, diabetic patients may be predisposed to wound breakdown or persistent wound defects or both, which, in turn, may increase their risk of developing endophthalmitis. Finally, vitrectomy for complications of PDR often requires longer surgical time and more instrument changes passing through the pars plana sclerotomies compared with vitrectomy for other diseases.

The Endophthalmitis Vitrectomy Study reported that only 39% of diabetic patients compared with 55% of nondiabetic patients achieved a final visual acuity of 20/40 or better [88]. Both diabetic and nondiabetic patients who presented with vision of only light perception had better visual acuity results with immediate vitrectomy. For those who presented with better than light perception vision, diabetic patients achieved a final visual acuity of 20/40 or better more often with vitrectomy (57%) than with vitreous tap/biopsy (40%), but (perhaps due to small numbers) this difference was not statistically significant. Patients without diabetes did equally well with vitrectomy or vitreous tap/biopsy. In the diabetic group, small numbers did not permit adequate statistical power to test treatment difference.

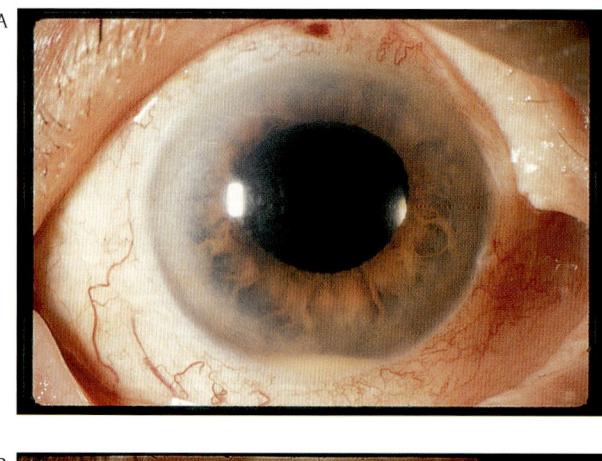

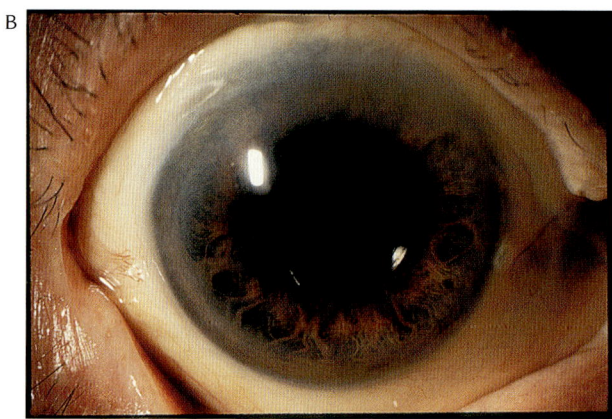

Figure 16.8. (A) *Staphylococcus epidermidis* endophthalmitis in an 86-year-old diabetic man 1 week after small-incision phacoemulsification with posterior chamber intraocular lens implantation. Visual acuity is hand motions at 1 foot. (B) About 5 months later and after pars plana vitrectomy with intraocular antibiotics, visual acuity is 20/40.

Mucormycosis. Mucormycosis is a rare orbital infection that affects diabetic patients, especially those with ketoacidosis. In fact, it is estimated that 50% of mucromycosis cases occur in diabetic patients [89]. The diagnosis should be suspected in any diabetic, immunosuppressed, or debilitated patient who develops facial or orbital pain, diplopia, or other neurologic signs and symptoms, and in diabetic patients with ketoacidosis who remain obtunded after correction of the underlying ketoacidosis.

Orbital mucormycosis usually originates in adjacent sinuses and presents with complete internal and external ophthalmoplegia, decreased vision, proptosis, ptosis, and chemosis. Histopathologic hallmarks of the disease are vascular invasion and tissue necrosis. Clinically, affected areas are characterized by black eschars (Fig. 16.9) and discharge, although this may be a late finding. Mucormycosis is associated with a significant risk of mortality [90,91], which underscores the importance of prompt diagnosis and treatment with tissue debridement and amphotericin B.

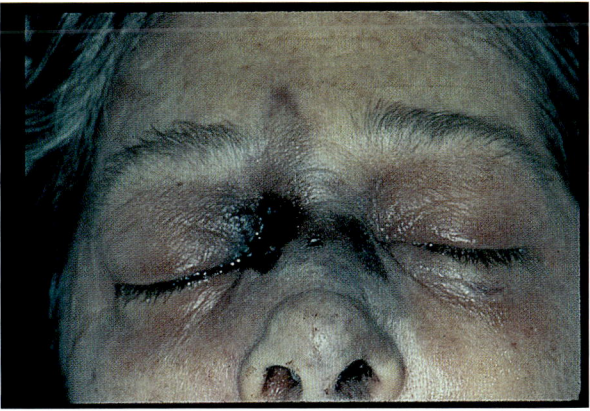

Figure 16.9. Mucormycosis with characteristic black eschar in a patient with uncontrolled diabetes.

CONCLUSION

Diabetes is associated with myriad nonretinal ocular abnormalities. The most common of these include corneal diseases (decreased corneal sensitivity, infectious and neurotrophic ulcers, and epithelial defects and erosions), glaucoma (open-angle, angle-closure, neovascular, and blood-associated), refractive changes, and cataract. Optic and cranial nerve abnormalities are not rare. Endophthalmitis and mucormycosis occur less frequently and are associated with a guarded prognosis, especially if not detected and treated promptly. Care of the diabetic patient usually includes referral to an appropriate primary care physician to ensure optimal metabolic control, with the goal of reducing the rates of ocular and systemic complications from diabetes.

REFERENCES

1. Rogell GD. Corneal hypesthesia and retinopathy in diabetes mellitus. *Ophthalmology.* 1980;87:229–233.
2. Saito J, Enoki M, Hara M, et al. Correlation of corneal sensation, but not of basal or reflex tear secretion, with the stage of diabetic retinopathy. *Cornea.* 2003;22:15–18.
3. Saini JS, Khandalavla B. Corneal epithelial fragility in diabetes mellitus. *Can J Ophthalmol.* 1995;30:142–146.
4. Nepp J, Abela C, Polzer I, Derbolav A, Wedrich A. Is there a correlation between the severity of diabetic retinopathy and keratoconjunctivitis sicca? *Cornea.* 2000;19:487–491.
5. Eichenbaum JW, Feldstein M, Podos SM. Extended-wear soft contact lenses and corneal ulcers. *Br J Ophthalmol.* 1982;66:663–666.
6. Hyndiuk RA, Kazarian EL, Schultz RO, Seideman S. Neurotrophic corneal ulcers in diabetes mellitus. *Arch Ophthalmol.* 1977;95:2193–2196.
7. Kenyon KR. Anatomy and pathology of the ocular surface. *Int Ophthalmol Clin.* 1979;19:3–35.
8. Gekka M, Miyata K, Nagai Y, et al. Corneal epithelial barrier function in diabetic patients. *Cornea.* 2004;23:35–37.

9. Foulks GN, Thoft RA, Perry HD, Tolentino FI. Factors related to corneal epithelial complications after closed vitrectomy in diabetics. *Arch Ophthalmol.* 1979;97: 1076–1078.

10. Arentsen J, Tasman W. Using a bandage contact lens to prevent recurrent corneal erosion during photocoagulation in patients with diabetes. *Am J Ophthalmol.* 1981;92:714–716.

11. Mandelcorn MS, Blankenship G, Machemer R. Pars plana vitrectomy for the manage ment of severe diabetic retinopathy. *Am J Ophthalmol.* 1976;81:561–570.

12. Friberg TR, Ohji M, Scherer JJ, Tano Y. Frequency of epithelial debridement during diabetic vitrectomy. *Am J Ophthalmol.* 2003;135:553–554.

13. Virata SR, Kylstra JA, Singh HT. Corneal epithelial defects following vitrectomy surgery using hand-held, sew-on, and noncontact viewing lenses. *Retina.* 1999;19:287–290.

14. Kenyon KR. Recurrent corneal erosion: pathogenesis and therapy. *Int Ophthalmol Clin.* 1979;19:169–195.

15. Fogle JA, Kenyon KR, Stark WJ, Green WR. Defective epithelial adhesion in anterior corneal dystrophies. *Am J Ophthalmol.* 1975;79:925–940.

16. Tabatabay CA, Bumbacher M, Baumgartner B, Leuenberger PM. Reduced number of hemidesmosomes in the corneal epithelium of diabetics with proliferative vitreoretinopathy. *Graefes Arch Klin Exp Ophthalmol.* 1988;226:389–392.

17. Azar DT, Spurr-Michaud SJ, Tisdale AS, Gipson IK. Decreased penetration of anchoring fibrils into the diabetic stroma: a morphometric analysis. *Arch Ophthalmol.* 1989;107:1520–1523.

18. Datiles MB, Kador PF, Fukui HN, et al. Corneal re-epithelialization in galactosemic rats. *Invest Ophthalmol Vis Sci.* 1983;24:563–569.

19. Matsuda M, Awata T, Ohashi Y, et al. The effects of aldose reductase inhibitor on the corneal endothelial morphology in diabetic rats. *Curr Eye Res.* 1987;6:391–397.

20. Ohashi Y, Matsuda M, Hosotani H, et al. Aldose reductase inhibitor (CT-112) eyedrops for diabetic corneal epitheliopathy. *Am J Ophthalmol.* 1988;105:233–238.

21. Hosotani H, Ohashi Y, Kinoshita S, et al. Effects of topical aldose reductase inhibitor CT-112 on corneal sensitivity of diabetic rats. *Curr Eye Res.* 1996;15:1005–1007.

22. Fujishima H, Shimazaki J, Yagi Y, Tsubota K. Improvement of corneal sensation and tear dynamics in diabetic patients by oral aldose reductase inhibitor, ONO-2235: a preliminary study. *Cornea.* 1996;15:368–375.

23. Leske MC, Podgor MJ. Intraocular pressure, cardiovascular risk variables, and visual field defects. *Am J Epidemiol.* 1983;118:280–287.

24. Klein BE, Klein R, Moss SE. Intraocular pressure in diabetic persons. *Ophthalmology.* 1984;91:1356–1360.

25. Klein BE, Klein R, Jensen SC. Open-angle glaucoma and older-onset diabetes: the Beaver Dam Eye Study. *Ophthalmology.* 1994;101:1173–1177.

26. Morgan RW, Drance SM. Chronic open-angle glaucoma and ocular hypertension: an epidemiological study. *Br J Ophthalmol.* 1975;59:211–215.

27. Reynolds DC. Relative risk factors in chronic open-angle glaucoma: an epidemiological study. *Br J Ophthalmol.* 1975;59:211–215.

28. Wilson MR, Hertzmark E, Walker AM, et al. A case-control study of risk factors in open angle glaucoma. *Arch Ophthalmol.* 1987;105:1066–1071.

29. Katz J, Sommer A. Risk factors for primary open angle glaucoma. *Am J Prev Med.* 1988;4:110–114.

30. Armaly MF, Krueger DE, Maunder L, et al. Biostatistical analysis of the collaborative glaucoma study, I: summary report of the risk factors for glaucomatous visual-field defects. *Arch Ophthalmol.* 1980;98:2163–2171.

31. Tielsch JM, Katz J, Quigley HA, et al. Diabetes, intraocular pressure, and primary open-angle glaucoma in the Baltimore Eye Survey. *Ophthalmology*. 1995;102:48–53.

32. Leske MC, Connell AM, Wu SY, et al. Risk factors for open-angle glaucoma. The Barbados Eye Study. *Arch Ophthalmol*. 1995;113:918–924.

33. Wormald RP, Basauri E, Wright LA, Evans JR. The African Caribbean Eye Survey: risk factors for glaucoma in a sample of African Caribbean people living in London. *Eye*. 1994;8:315–320.

34. Mitchell P, Smith W, Chey T, Healey PR. Open-angle glaucoma and diabetes: the Blue Mountains eye study, Australia. *Ophthalmology*. 1997;104:712–718.

35. Dielemans I, de Jong PT, Stolk R, et al. Primary open-angle glaucoma, intraocular pressure, and diabetes mellitus in the general elderly population. The Rotterdam Study. *Ophthalmology*. 1996;103:1271–1275.

36. Gordon MO, Beiser JA, Brandt JD, et al. The Ocular Hypertension Treatment Study. Baseline factors that predict the onset of primary open-angle glaucoma. *Arch Ophthalmol*. 2002;120:714–720.

37. Mapstone R, Clark CV. Prevalence of type 2 diabetes mellitus in glaucoma. *Br Med J*. 1985;291:93–95.

38. Clark CV, Mapstone R. The prevalence of diabetes mellitus in the family history of patients with primary glaucoma. *Doc Ophthalmol*. 1986;62:161–163.

39. Mapstone R, Clark CV. The prevalence of autonomic neuropathy in glaucoma. *Trans Ophthalmol Soc UK*. 1985;104:265–269.

40. Sorokanich S, Wand M, Nix HR. Angle closure glaucoma and acute hyperglycemia. *Arch Ophthalmol*. 1986;104:1434.

41. Madsen PH. Experiences in surgical treatment of haemorrhagic glaucoma. *Acta Ophthalmol (Copenh)*. 1973;120(suppl):88–91.

42. Brown GC, Magargal LE, Schachat A, Shah H. Neovascular glaucoma: etiologic considerations. *Ophthalmology*. 1984;91:315–320.

43. Armaly MF, Baloglou PJ. Diabetes mellitus and the eye, I: changes in the anterior segment. *Arch Ophthalmol*. 1967;77:485–492.

44. Madsen PH. Haemorrhagic glaucoma: comparative study in diabetic and nondiabetic patients. *Br J Ophthalmol*. 1971;55:444–450.

45. Ohrt V. The frequency of rubeosis iridis in diabetic patients. *Acta Ophthalmol (Copenh)*. 1971;49:301–307.

46. Zirm M. Protein glaucoma—overtaxing of flow mechanisms? Preliminary report. *Ophthalmologica*. 1982;184:155–161.

47. Little HL, Rosenthal AR, Dellaporta A, Jacobson DR. The effect of pan-retinal photocoagulation on rubeosis iridis. *Am J Ophthalmol*. 1976;81:804–809.

48. Laatikainen L. Preliminary report on effect of retinal panphotocoagulation on rubeosis iridis and neovascular glaucoma. *Br J Ophthalmol*. 1977;61:278–284.

49. Pavan PR, Folk JC, Weingeist TA, et al. Diabetic rubeosis and panretinal photocoagulation. *Arch Ophthalmol*. 1983;101:882–884.

50. Heuer DK, Parrish RK II, Gressel MG, et al. 5-Fluorouracil and glaucoma filtering surgery, III: intermediate follow-up of a pilot study. *Ophthalmology*. 1986;93:1537–1546.

51. Rockwood EJ, Parrish RK II, Heuer DK, et al. Glaucoma filtering surgery with 5-fluorouracil. *Ophthalmology*. 1987;94:1071–1078.

52. Kitazawa Y, Kawase K, Matsushita H, Minobe M. Trabeculectomy with mitomycin: a comparative study with fluorouracil. *Arch Ophthalmol*. 1991;109:1693–1698.

53. Skuta GL, Beeson CC, Higginbotham EJ, et al. Intraoperative mitomycin versus postoperative 5-fluorouracil in high-risk glaucoma filtering surgery. *Ophthalmology*. 1992;99:438–444.

54. Lloyd MA, Heuer DK, Baerveldt G, et al. Combined Molteno implantation and pars plana vitrectomy for neovascular glaucomas. *Ophthalmology*. 1991;98:1401–1405.

55. Campbell DG, Simmons RJ, Tolentino FI, McMeel JW. Glaucoma occurring after closed vitrectomy. *Am J Ophthalmol*. 1977;83:63–69.

56. Cameron JD, Havener VR. Histologic confirmation of ghost cell glaucoma by routine light microscopy. *Am J Ophthalmol*. 1983;96:251–252.

57. Fenton RH, Zimmerman LE. Hemolytic glaucoma: an unusual cause of acute open-angle secondary glaucoma. *Arch Ophthalmol*. 1963;70:236–239.

58. Phelps CD, Watzke RC. Hemolytic glaucoma. *Am J Ophthalmol*. 1975;80:690–695.

59. Vannas M, Teir H. Hemosiderosis in eyes with secondary glaucoma after delayed intraocular hemorrhages. *Acta Ophthalmol (Copenh)*. 1960;38:254–267.

60. Campbell DG, Schertzer RM. Ghost cell glaucoma. In: Ritch R, Shields MB, Kurpin T, eds. *The Glaucomas*, 2nd ed. St Louis: CV Mosby Co; 1996:1277–1285.

61. Benson WE, Brown GC, Tasman W. *Diabetes and its Ocular Complications*. Philadelphia: WB Saunders Co; 1988:27–34.

62. Okamoto F, Sone H, Nonoyama T, Hommura S. Refractive changes in diabetic patients during intensive glycaemic control. *Br J Ophthalmol*. 2000;84:1097–1102.

63. Klein BE, Klein R, Moss SE. Prevalence of cataracts in a population-based study of persons with diabetes mellitus. *Ophthalmology*. 1985;92:1191–1196.

64. Hennis A, Wu SY, Nemesure B, et al. Risk factors for incident cortical and posterior subcapsular lens opacities in the Barbados Eye Studies. *Arch Ophthalmol*. 2004;122:525–530.

65. Leske MC, Wu SY, Nemesure B, et al. Risk factors for incident nuclear opacities. *Ophthalmology*. 2002;109:1303–1308.

66. Rowe NG, Mitchell PG, Cumming RG, Wans JJ. Diabetes, fasting blood glucose and age-related cataract: the Blue Mountains Eye Study. *Ophthalmic Epidemiol*. 2000;7:103–114.

67. Schwab IR, Dawson CR, Hoshiwara I, et al. Incidence of cataract extraction in Pima Indians: diabetes as a risk factor. *Arch Ophthalmol*. 1985;103:208–212.

68. Skillern PG, Lockhart G. Optic neuritis and uncontrolled diabetes mellitus in 14 patients. *Ann Intern Med*. 1959;51:468–475.

69. Barr CC, Glaser JS, Blankenship G. Acute disc swelling in juvenile diabetes: clinical profile and natural history of 12 cases. *Arch Ophthalmol*. 1980;98:2185–2192.

70. Bayraktar Z, Alacali N, Bayraktar S. Diabetic papillopathy in type II diabetic patients. *Retina*. 2002;22:752–758.

71. Regillo CD, Brown GC, Savino PJ, et al. Diabetic papillopathy. Patient characteristics and fundus findings. *Arch Ophthalmol*. 1995;113:889–895.

72. Pavan PR, Aiello LM, Wafai MZ, et al. Optic disc edema in juvenile-onset diabetes. *Arch Ophthalmol*. 1980;98:2193–2195.

73. Lubow M, Makley TA Jr. Pseudopapilledema of juvenile diabetes mellitus. *Arch Ophthalmol*. 1971;85:417–422.

74. Hayreh SS, Zahoruk RM. Anterior ischemic optic neuropathy, VI: in juvenile diabetics. *Ophthalmologica*. 1981;182:13–28.

75. Lessell S, Rosman NP. Juvenile diabetes mellitus and optic atrophy. *Arch Neurol*. 1977;34:759–765.

76. Hofmann S, Philbrook C, Gerbitz KD, Bauer MF. Wolfram syndrome: structural and functional analyses of mutant and wild-type wolframin, the WFS1 gene product. *Hum Mol Genet*. 2003;12:2003–2012.

77. Sadun AA. Neuro-ophthalmic manifestations of diabetes. *Ophthalmology*. 1999;106:1047–1048.

78. Nelson M, Lessell S, Sadun AA. Optic nerve hypoplasia and maternal diabetes mellitus. *Arch Neurol*. 1986;43:20–25.

79. Moster M. Paresis of isolated and multiple cranial nerves and painful ophthalmoplegia. In: Yanoff M, Duker JS, Augsburger JJ, et al., eds. *Ophthalmology*. Philadelphia: CV Mosby Co; 1998:16.1–16.12.

80. Jacobson DM. Pupil involvement in patients with diabetes-associated oculomotor nerve palsy. *Arch Ophthalmol*. 1998;116:723–727.

81. Glaser JS, Siatkowski RM. Infranuclear disorders of eye movement. In: Glaser JS, ed. *Neuro-ophthalmology*, 3rd ed. Philadelphia: Lippincott Williams & Wilkins; 1999:405–460.

82. Kattan HM, Flynn HW Jr, Pflugfelder SC, et al. Nosocomial endophthalmitis survey: current incidence of infection after intraocular surgery. *Ophthalmology*. 1991;98: 227–228.

83. Phillips WB II, Tasman WS. Postoperative endophthalmitis in association with diabetes mellitus. *Ophthalmology*. 1994;101:508–518.

84. Scott IU, Flynn HW Jr, Feuer W. Endophthalmitis after secondary intraocular lens implantation: a case-control study. *Ophthalmology*. 1995;102:1925–1931.

85. Lehmann OJ, Bunce C, Matheson MM, et al. Risk factors for development of post-trabeculectomy endophthalmitis. *Br J Ophthalmol*. 2000;84:1349–1353.

86. Moutschen MP, Scheen AJ, Lefebvre PJ. Impaired immune responses in diabetes mellitus: analysis of the factors and mechanisms involved—relevance to the increased susceptibility of diabetic patients to specific infections. *Diabetes Metab*. 1992;18:187–201.

87. Morain WD, Colen LB. Wound healing in diabetes mellitus. *Clin Plast Surg*. 1990;17:493–501.

88. Doft BH, Wisniewski SR, Kelsey SF, et al. Diabetes and postcataract extraction endophthalmitis. *Curr Opin Ophthalmol*. 2002;13:147–151.

89. Behlau I, Baker AS. Fungal infections of the eye. In: Albert DM, Jakobiec FA, eds. *Principles and Practice of Ophthalmology: Clinical Practice*. Philadelphia: WB Saunders Co; 1994:3041–3043.

90. Parfrey NA. Improved diagnosis and prognosis of mucormycosis: a clinicopathologic study of 33 cases. *Medicine*. 1986;65:113–123.

91. Butugan O, Sanchez TG, Goncalez F, et al. Rhinocerebral mucormycosis: predisposing factors, diagnosis, therapy, complications and survival. *Rev Laryngol Otol Rhinol*. 1996;117:53–55.

17

The Effect of Systemic Conditions on Diabetic Retinopathy

EMILY Y. CHEW, MD

CORE MESSAGES

- Diabetic retinopathy is affected by a number of systemic factors and conditions.
- The most important risk factor for the development and progression of diabetic retinopathy remains glucose control in both type 1 and type 2 diabetes. Tight glucose control may decrease the risk of progression by as much as 50% to 75%.
- Hypertension is also an important risk factor for the development and progression of diabetic retinopathy. A modest decrease may retard the progression by as much as 37% and reduce the risk of moderate vision loss by 50%.
- Observational data from several studies suggest that controlling systemic risk factors may decrease the risk of progression to proliferative diabetic retinopathy and the development of clinically significant macular edema.
- Pregnancy may be associated with an accelerated progression of diabetic retinopathy by both the tightening of glycemic control and the effects of pregnancy itself.
- Puberty may be associated with an increased risk of progression of diabetic retinopathy.
- Patients with neuropathy and anemia have an increased risk of diabetic retinopathy.
- Fibrinogen is associated with an increased risk of diabetic retinopathy, indicating that inflammation may play an important role in the pathogenesis of diabetic retinopathy.

Diabetic retinopathy, a leading cause of blindness in the U.S. and in the developed world, can be affected by a number of systemic conditions [1]. These include hyperglycemia, elevated blood pressure, dyslipidemia, and conditions associated with changes in hormones such as pregnancy and puberty. Other microvascular complications of diabetes, neuropathy and nephropathy, may share similar risk factors with diabetic retinopathy and may also be present concurrently with retinopathy. These complications, especially nephropathy, may have an impact on the progression of diabetic retinopathy through secondary effects, such as hypertension. Data to support the changes in retinopathy caused by these systemic changes come from a number of controlled clinical trials as well as epidemiologic studies. This chapter describes some of these important systemic conditions that may influence diabetic retinopathy or that may be associated with the progression of retinopathy.

GLYCEMIC CONTROL

The relationship of glucose control with the complications of diabetes was demonstrated in observational studies [2–6]. The results of these studies showed that increased severity of diabetic retinopathy is associated with increasing hyperglycemia, as measured by glycosylated hemoglobin A1c (HbA1c). Randomized controlled clinical trials of glycemic control were designed to address the role of glucose control in patients with diabetic complications, including diabetic retinopathy. These studies were conducted in separate populations with either type 1 or type 2 diabetes. Such data have provided valuable information regarding the medical management of these patients. Preventive measures of diabetic retinopathy are highly beneficial and may be cost-effective, both to the individual patient and to society.

TYPE 1 DIABETES

In the Diabetes Control and Complications Trial (DCCT), 1441 patients with type 1 diabetes were assigned randomly to either conventional or intensive insulin treatment, and followed for a period of 4 to 9 years [7–11]. The DCCT demonstrated that intensive insulin treatment is associated with a decreased risk of either the development or the progression of diabetic retinopathy in patients with type 1 diabetes. In patients without any visible retinopathy when enrolled in the DCCT, the 3-year risk of developing retinopathy was reduced by 75% in the intensive insulin treatment group compared with the standard treatment group (Fig. 17.1). However, even in the intensively treated group, retinopathy could not be prevented completely over the 9-year course of the study. The benefit of the strict control was also evident in patients with existing retinopathy (50% reduction in the rate of retinopathy progression compared with controls). At 6- and 12-month visits, a small adverse affect of intensive treatment on retinopathy progression was seen, similar to that described in other trials of glucose control (Fig. 17.2) [12]. However, in eyes with little or no retinopathy at the time of initiating intensive glucose control, this

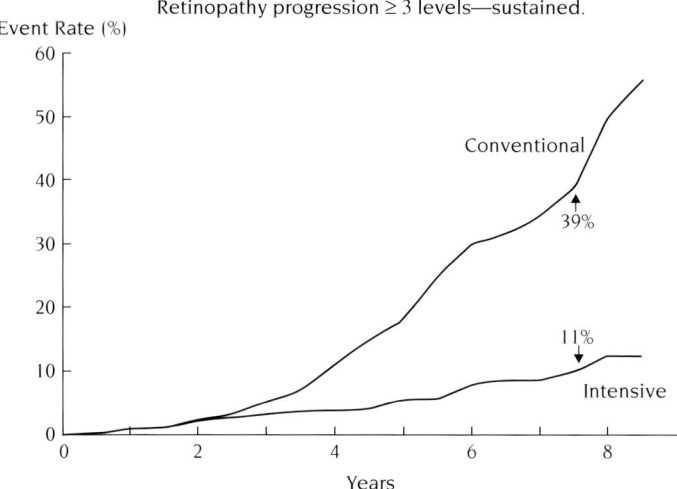

Figure 17.1. Diabetes Control and Complications Trial—primary prevention.

early worsening of retinopathy is unlikely to threaten vision. When the DCCT results were stratified by HbA1c levels, there was a 35% to 40% reduction in the risk of retinopathy progression for every 10% decrease in HbA1c (e.g., from 8% to 7.2%). This represented a five-fold increase in the risk for patients with an HbA1c of approximately 10% versus those with 7%. Furthermore, there was a statistically significant reduction in both diabetic neuropathy and nephropathy with intensive blood glucose control in the DCCT.

The beneficial effects of intensive therapy were evident after 3 years of therapy on all different severities of retinopathy evaluated in the DCCT [13]. Intensive therapy reduced the risk of any retinopathy by 27% ($P = 0.002$). The risk of

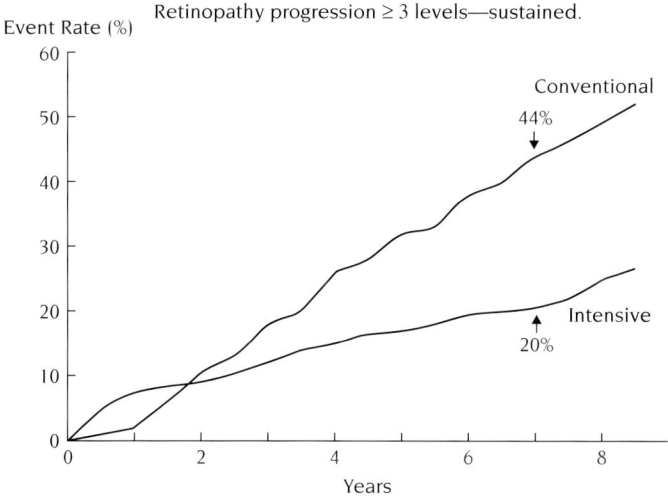

Figure 17.2. Diabetes Control and Complications Trial—secondary intervention.

Table 17.1. Diabetes Control and Complications Trial/Epidemiology of Diabetes Interventions and Complications Study

Intensive treatment of glycemia reduced the risk of progression of diabetic retinopathy by 34% to 76% in persons with type 1 diabetes.
Tight glycemic control was most effective when initiated early in the course of the disease and it had beneficial effect over the entire range of retinopathy and in all patient subgroups
The beneficial effects of tight control lasted for years following the cessation of the randomized trial.

developing retinopathy or progression to clinically significant degrees was reduced by 34% to 76% by intensive treatment of the glycemia. It was most effective when initiated early in the course of the disease and it had beneficial effect over the entire range of retinopathy and in all patient subgroups. This reduction in risk resulted in reduced need for laser treatment and saved sight.

After 6.5 years of follow-up, the DCCT ended, and all patients were encouraged to maintain strict control of blood sugar. These patients are followed in the Epidemiology of Diabetes Interventions and Complications (EDIC) trial, which includes 95% of DCCT subjects, half from each treatment group (Table 17.1). A total of 1294 to 1335 patients have been examined annually in the EDIC. Further progression of diabetic retinopathy during the first 4 years of the EDIC was 66% to 77% less in the former intensive treatment group than in the former conventional treatment group [14]. The benefit persists even at 7 years [15]. This benefit included an effect on severe diabetic retinopathy, including severe nonproliferative diabetic retinopathy, proliferative diabetic retinopathy, clinically significant macular edema, and the need for focal or scatter laser therapy. The decrease in HbA1c from 9% to approximately 8% did not drastically reduce the progression of diabetic retinopathy in the former conventional treatment group, nor did the increase in HbA1c from approximately 7% to 8% drastically accelerate diabetic retinopathy in the former intensive treatment group. Thus, it takes time for improvements in control to negate the long-lasting effects of prior prolonged hyperglycemia, and once the biological effects of prolonged improved control are manifest, the benefits are long lasting. Furthermore, the total glycemic exposure of the patient (i.e., degree and duration) determines the degree of retinopathy observed at any one time.

TYPE 2 DIABETES

The effect of glycemic control on the incidence and progression of diabetic retinopathy is similar in patients with type 2 diabetes, as assessed in observational studies and randomized studies conducted in Japan and the United Kingdom [16–19]. Findings in a study of Japanese patients with type 2 diabetes have shown that multiple insulin-injection treatment reduced the onset of retinopathy from 32% to 8% and reduced a two-step progression retinopathy from 44% to 19% compared with people receiving conventional insulin treatments over 6 years [18]. In the United Kingdom Prospective Diabetes Study (UKPDS), the largest and longest

Table 17.2. **United Kingdom Prospective Diabetes Study**

Tight glycemic control reduced the risk of progression of diabetic retinopathy in patients with type 2 diabetes.

For every percentage point decrease in HbA1c (e.g., 9%–8%), there was a 35% reduction in the risk of microvascular complications.

Results of both the DCCT and UKPDS show that while intensive therapy of glucose does not prevent retinopathy completely, it reduces the risk of the development and progression of diabetic retinopathy. This may be translated clinically to both preservation of vision and reduction in therapy such as laser photocoagulation.

study of 4209 patients with type 2 diabetes followed for 15 years, there was a 25% reduction in the risk of "any diabetes-related microvascular endpoint," including the need for retinal photocoagulation in the intensive treatment group compared to the conventional treatment group (Table 17.2). After 6 years of follow-up, a smaller proportion of patients in the intensive treatment group than in the conventional group had a two-step progression (worsening) in diabetic retinopathy ($P < 0.01$). Epidemiologic analysis of the UKPDS data showed a continuous relationship between the risk of microvascular complications and glycemia, such that for every percentage point decrease in HbA1c (e.g., 9%–8%), there was a 35% reduction in the risk of microvascular complications.

The results of both the DCCT and UKPDS show that while intensive therapy of glucose does not prevent retinopathy completely, it reduces the risk of the development and progression of diabetic retinopathy. This may be translated clinically to both preservation of vision and reduction in therapy such as laser photocoagulation.

HYPERTENSION

The findings of observational studies assessing the importance of blood pressure (BP) in the progression of nonproliferative diabetic retinopathy are inconsistent. However, in the UKPDS, a randomized comparison of more intensive BP control versus less intensive BP control in persons with type 2 diabetes demonstrated that intensive BP control was associated with a decreased risk of retinopathy progression [20]. Of the 1148 hypertensive patients in the UKPDS, 758 were allocated to tight control of BP and 390 to less tight control with a median follow-up of 8.4 years. The target for the intensive treatment was a BP less than 150/85 mmHg versus a less tight BP control goal of less than 180/105 mmHg. The outcome measures included the deterioration of diabetic retinopathy of 2 or more steps along the modified ETDRS final scale, laser photocoagulation, vitreous hemorrhage, and cataract extraction, and analysis of specific retinal lesions (microaneurysms, hard exudates, and cotton-wool spots). Visual acuity was assessed at 3-year intervals.

Tight BP control resulted in a 37% reduction in microvascular diseases, and a reduced risk of retinal photocoagulation, when compared to less tight BP control [21]. Retinal hard exudates increased from a prevalence of 11.2% to 18.3% at 7.5 years after randomization with fewer lesions found in the tight BP control group

(RR, 0.53; P < .001). Cotton-wool spots increased in both groups but less so in the tight BP control group which had fewer cotton-wool spots at 7.5 years (RR, 0.53; P < 0.001). A two-step or more deterioration on the ETDRS scale was significantly different at 4.5 years with fewer people in the tight BP control group progressing two steps or more (RR, 0.75; P = 0.02). Patients assigned to tight BP control were less likely to undergo photocoagulation (RR, 0.65; P = 0.03). This difference was mainly in photocoagulation for diabetic macular edema (RR, 0.58; P = 0.02). There was a 50% reduction in the risk of moderate vision loss as well as with decrease in blindness or vision of 20/200 or worse. The decreased vision of 20/200 or worse in one eye was found in 18/758 for the tight BP control group compared with 12/390 for the less tight BP control group. The absolute risks of such poor vision was of the order of 3.1 to 4.1 per 1000 patient-years, respectively (P = 0.046; RR, 0.76; 99% confidence interval [CI], 0.29–1.99).

A previously published study of BP medication in patients with diabetic retinopathy suggested that there might be a specific benefit of angiotensin-converting enzyme (ACE) inhibition and BP reduction, even in "normotensive" persons, on the progression of diabetic retinopathy [22]. The UKPDS included a randomized comparison of beta-blockers and ACE inhibitors in the tight BP control arm of that study. Benefits from tight BP control were present in both the ß-blocker and ACE inhibitor treatment groups, with no statistically significant difference between them. The results of the UKPDS suggest that the treatment effect is more likely to be secondary to BP reduction than to a specific effect of ACE inhibitors [20].

ELEVATED SERUM LIPID LEVELS

The Wisconsin Epidemiologic Study of Diabetic Retinopathy, a population-based study, and the Early Treatment Diabetic Retinopathy Study (ETDRS) found that elevated levels of serum cholesterol were associated with increased severity of retinal hard exudates (Fig. 17.3) [23,24]. A study of diabetic retinopathy in African Americans with type 1 diabetes also showed the association of macular edema and retinal hard exudates with elevated serum lipids [25]. Patients with a total cholesterol/high-density lipoprotein cholesterol (HDL-C) ratio of 4.5 or greater were almost twice as likely to have retinal hard exudates compared to those with a ratio of less than 4.5. Patients with higher quartile of total cholesterol or low-density lipoprotein cholesterol (LDL) levels were five to six times more likely to have retinal hard exudates than those in the lowest quartiles. In the ETDRS, elevated total cholesterol (240 mg/dL or 6.21 mmol/L) was twice as likely to have retinal hard exudates at baseline (odds ratio [OR]: 2.00, 99% CI: 1.35–2.95). Similar results were found when comparing elevated LDL levels (160 mg/dL or 1.14 mmol/L) with the lowest level of LDL (130 mg/dL or 3.37 mmol/L) and the OR was 1.97, 99% CI: 1.3–2.96. Patients with elevated cholesterol and triglyceride levels were 50% more likely to develop retinal hard exudates. Independent of the accompanying macular edema, the severity of retinal hard exudates at baseline was associated with decreased visual acuity in the ETDRS (Fig. 17.4). The severity of retinal hard exudates was also a significant risk factor for moderate visual loss (15 or more

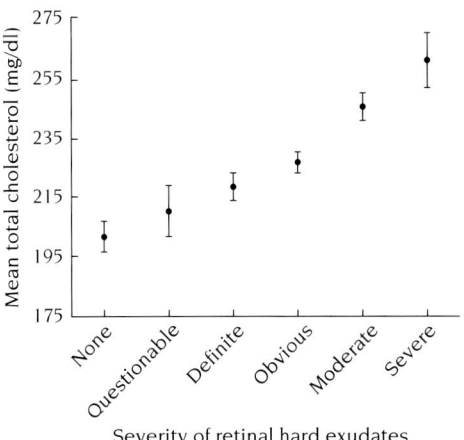

Figure 17.3. Mean total cholesterol by severity of retinal hard exudates at baseline.

letter loss) during the course of the study. Patients with the most severe level of retinal hard exudates had double the risk of experiencing moderate visual loss.

Although the intensive treatment of hyperglycemia substantially reduced the development and progression of diabetic retinopathy in the DCCT/EDIC study, there was no statistically significant effect on macular edema. The investigators evaluated the correlation of serum lipids and the incidence of macular edema and retinal hard exudates in this cohort [26]. Elevated LDL was associated with an increased risk of macular edema. The comparison of the highest quintile vs. the lowest quintile of LDL resulted in a relative risk (RR) of 1.95 (*P* for trend = 0.03). The total-to-HDL cholesterol ratio was also a significant predictor for incident or new cases of clinically significant macular edema with a RR of 3.84 (*P* for

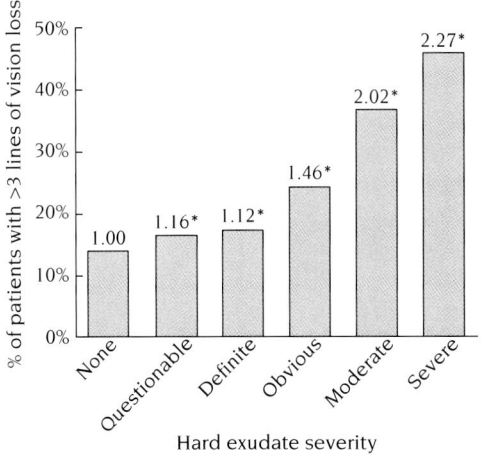

* Odds Ratio Adjusted for:Macular Thickening, HgbA₁C, Age, and Ret. Severity

Figure 17.4. Percent of patients with three or more lines of vision loss (doubling of baseline visual angle) at 5 years.

trend = 0.03). Similar findings were found for association of serum lipids with the development of retinal hard exudates. After adjusting for all known potential risk factors, the following were statistically significant predictors of retinal hard exudates: total cholesterol: RR= 2.37, P for trend = 0.001; LDL cholesterol: 2.77, P for trend = 0.002; total-to-HDL cholesterol ratio: 2.44, P for trend = 0.0004; and triglycerides: 3.20, P for trend = 0.006. These findings were similar to those found in the ETDRS.

In a study of the risk factors associated with the development of subretinal fibrosis in ETDRS patients with diabetic macular edema, the presence of severe hard exudates was the strongest risk factor [27]. Elevated serum triglyceride levels were also associated with a greater risk of developing high-risk proliferative diabetic retinopathy in the ETDRS patients [28]. In a study in Pittsburgh, elevated triglycerides, as well as elevated LDL cholesterol, were found to be associated with proliferative diabetic retinopathy [3].

Although these are all observational findings, the data are compelling to recommend lowering elevated serum lipids in patients with diabetic retinopathy to reduce the risk of vision loss. In addition to reducing the risk of cardiovascular disease, reducing the risk of vision loss should be another motivating factor for patients to lower elevated serum lipids. Currently, the National Heart, Lung, and Blood Institute (NHLBI) of National Institutes of Health (NIH) is addressing this question in the Actions to Control Cardiovascular Risk in Diabetes (ACCORD) Study, a randomized controlled clinical trial of glycemic control, BP control, and management of dyslipidemia in 10,000 subjects with type 2 diabetes. The results from this study will hopefully answer the particular question of possible association of serum cholesterol with progression of diabetic retinopathy and development of diabetic macular edema.

DIABETES AND PREGNANCY

The effects of pregnancy on the development and the rate of progression of underlying diabetic retinopathy have been controversial. Although a number of studies have suggested a worsening of retinopathy during pregnancy [29–32], others have not [33,34]. Diabetic retinopathy can worsen during pregnancy because of the pregnancy itself or the changes in metabolic control, usually a marked improvement in glucose control [29–30].

The DCCT is the largest prospective study to assess the effect of pregnancy on the development and progression of diabetic retinopathy and other microvascular abnormalities [35]. The women in the DCCT were generally younger and had shorter duration of diabetes with fewer or less severe diabetic complications than those reported previously in other studies. Women in the intensive treatment group had HbA1c levels that were near normal for a mean of 3 years prior to conception. When the analyses were stratified by the treatment group, both the intensive and the conventional groups showed a short-term deterioration of retinopathy during pregnancy that persisted through the first year postpartum. In the conventional treatment group, there was a 2.5-fold increase in the risk of retinopathy progression when compared with nonpregnant women. This was statistically significant and not affected by other risk factors. In the intensive treatment group, the adjusted risks were not as great while the risk of retinopathy progression was nominally statistically significant. However, there were fewer events in the early treatment group.

There was a significant trend toward greater worsening of retinopathy with greater reductions in HbA1c. This progression may be similar to that of the early worsening that has been shown to be related to the magnitude of the decrease of HbA1c level with the intensive therapy for glycemic control. However, when the recent changes in retinopathy were compared between the pregnant and nonpregnant women, adjusted for the recent changes in HbA1c, the increased worsening of retinopathy during pregnancy persisted. It would appear that both the effects of pregnancy as well as the effects of intensive therapy are important in the progression (worsening) of retinopathy. The follow-up examinations showed that the effects of pregnancy on retinopathy continued to increase over the first year following delivery of the baby. The cause for this continued effect of accelerated progression following delivery is not known. It is possible that factors other than glucose control may be involved, such as changes in hormones (e.g., growth hormone or cortisol). However, there were no long-term consequences of this worsening of retinopathy as both pregnant and nonpregnant women had similar severity of retinopathy at the end of the study.

Patients with diabetes who are planning to become pregnant are encouraged to achieve glucose control as tight as possible to reduce the risk of malformations and other genetic abnormalities. Patients with diabetes who are planning to become pregnant are encouraged to have their eyes examined prior to conception, to be counseled on the risk of development and/or progression of diabetic retinopathy. During the first trimester, another eye examination should be performed; subsequent follow-up will depend on the level of retinopathy found; and postpartum examination may also be important.

DIABETES AND PUBERTY

The effect of puberty on the progression of diabetic retinopathy has been investigated in a number of epidemiologic studies. Some have found puberty to be not a risk factor for the progression of diabetic retinopathy [36,37], while other investigators have determined puberty to be a significant risk factor [38–40]. Children who were postpubescent had a greater prevalence of retinopathy than those who were not sexually mature. The relative odds of having retinopathy in the postpubescent group compared to prepubescent or pubescent group was 4.8 (95% CI: 1.5–15.3). This study also suggested that minimal retinopathy in children is not rare and that postpubescent children have a greater prevalence of diabetic retinopathy than do prepubescent children with similar duration of diabetes. In the Wisconsin Epidemiologic Study of Diabetic Retinopathy, prepubescent patients had no progression in the 10 year study follow-up [41]. Puberty may increase the risk of progression of diabetic retinopathy.

DIABETIC NEUROPATHY

The risk of proliferative diabetic retinopathy was 5 times more common in patients with diabetic neuropathy compared with those without neuropathy in a cross-sectional analysis of approximately 2500 European patients [42]. In a case-control study of patients with or without proliferative diabetic retinopathy after 15 to 21 years of insulin-dependent diabetes at the Joslin Clinic, the odds of having cardiovascular autonomic neuropathy were about thirty to forty fold greater for those with proliferative diabetic retinopathy than those without [43]. In the ETDRS, the presence of neuropathy increased the risk of development of proliferative diabetic retinopathy by 26 to 32% ($P < 0.0009$) [28].

ANEMIA

In the ETDRS, a progressive increase in the risk of developing high-risk proliferative diabetic retinopathy was associated with decreasing hematocrit [28]. In the lowest category of hematocrit for both men and women, there was a 52% increased risk ($P < 0.0038$). Similar findings were seen in a cross-sectional study of patients in a diabetes clinic in Finland [44].

FIBRINOGEN AND ALBUMIN

In the DCCT, elevated fibrinogen and decreased albumin were associated with increased risk of diabetic retinopathy progression [45]. In the ETDRS, elevated fibrinogen increased the risk of proliferative diabetic retinopathy and this was of borderline statistical significance [28]. Fibrinogen is a marker of inflammation and recent studies have suggested that inflammation may play a critical role in the pathogenesis of diabetic retinopathy [46].

SUMMARY

Following years of debate, randomized, controlled clinical trials of intensive treatment compared with conventional treatment of hyperglycemia demonstrated the important role of glucose control in the development and progression of diabetic retinopathy. In addition to intensive treatment of hyperglycemia, the reduction of elevated blood pressure significantly reduced the risk of progression of diabetic retinopathy and moderate vision loss. The data regarding the association of elevated cholesterol and its components with macular edema, retinal hard exudates, and moderate vision loss are observational but nevertheless compelling. Recommendations to lower elevated cholesterol are important for other macrovascular diseases that are common in the population of persons with diabetes.

States of hormonal changes such as pregnancy and perhaps puberty are associated with progression of retinopathy. Other microvascular complications, neuropathy and nephropathy, are often correlated with retinopathy and may share common risk factors [47]. Another systemic condition that may have an impact on the course of diabetic retinopathy is anemia. There are emerging data to suggest the importance of inflammation in the pathogenesis of diabetic retinopathy and future research in this area will provide important information.

All patients with diabetes should be educated on the importance of tight glycemic control and reduction of elevated blood pressure and of elevated cholesterol levels. These medical measures may prevent the development of, and retard the progression of, diabetic retinopathy. Prevention is preferable to the current treatments, which include laser photocoagulation and other surgical procedures.

REFERENCES

1. The Eye Diseases Prevalence Research Group. Causes and prevalence of visual impairment among adults in the United States. *Arch Ophthalmol.* 2004;122:477–485.
2. Klein R, Klein BEK, Moss SE, Cruickshanks KJ. Relationship of hyperglycemia to the long-term incidence and progression of diabetic retinopathy. *Arch Intern Med.* 1994;154:2169–2178.
3. Lloyd CE, Klein R, Maser RE, Kuller LH, Becker DJ, Orchard TJ. The progression of retinopathy over 2 years: the Pittsburgh Epidemiology of Diabetes Complications (EDC) Study. *J Diab Complic.* 1995;3:140–148.
4. Janka HU, Warram JH, Rand LI, Krolewski AS. Risk factors for progression of background retinopathy in long-standing IDDM. *Diabetes.* 1989;38:460–464.
5. Teuscher A, Schnell H, Wilson PWF. Incidence of diabetic retinopathy and relationship to baseline plasma glucose and blood pressure. *Diabetes Care.* 1988;11:246–251.
6. Krolewski AS, Barzilay J, Warram JH, Martin BC, Pfeifer M, Rand LI. Risk of early-onset proliferative diabetic retinopathy in IDDM is closely related to cardiovascular autonomic neuropathy. *Diabetes.* 1992;41:430–437.
7. The Diabetes Control and Complications Trial Research Group (1993). The effect of intensive treatment of diabetes on the development and progression of long-term complications in insulin-dependent diabetes mellitus. *N Engl J Med.* 1993;329:977–986.
8. The Diabetes Control and Complications Trial Research Group. The effect of intensive diabetes treatment on the progression of diabetic retinopathy in insulin-dependent diabetes mellitus. *Arch Ophthalmol.* 1995;113:36–51.
9. The Diabetes Control and Complications Trial Research Group. The relationship of glycemic exposures (HbA1C) to the risk of development and progression of retinopathy in the Diabetes Control and Complications Trial. *Diabetes.* 1995;44:968–983.
10. The Diabetes Control and Complications Trial Research Group. Perspectives in Diabetes. The absence of a glycemic threshold for the development of long-term complications: the perspective of the Diabetes Control and Complications Trial. *Diabetes.* 1996;45:1289–1289.
11. Reichard P, Nilsson BY, Rosenqvist U. The effect of long-term intensified insulin treatment on the development of microvascular complications of diabetes mellitus. *N Eng J Med.* 1993;329:304–309.
12. The Diabetes Control and Complications Trial Research Group. Early worsening of diabetic retinopathy in the Diabetes Control and Complications Trial. *Arch Ophthalmol.* 1998;116:874–886.
13. The Diabetes Control and Complications Trial Research Group. Progression of retinopathy with intensive versus conventional treatment in the Diabetes Control and Complications Trial. *Ophthalmology.* 1994;103:647–661.

14. The Diabetes Control and Complications Trial/Epidemiology of Diabetes Intervention and Complications Research Group. Retinopathy and nephropathy in patients with type 1 diabetes four years after a trial of intensive therapy. *N Engl J Med*. 2000;342: 381–389.

15. The Diabetes Control and Complications Trial/Epidemiology of Diabetes Intervention and Complications Research Group. Effect of intensive therapy on the microvascular complications of type 1 diabetes mellitus. *JAMA*. 2002;287:2563–2569.

16. Klein R, Klein B, Moss S. Relation of glycemic control to diabetic microvascular complications in diabetes mellitus. *Ann Intern Med*. 1996;124:90–96.

17. Ohkubo Y, Hideke K, Eiichi A, et al. Intensive insulin therapy prevents the progression of diabetic microvascular complications in Japanese patients with non-insulin-dependent diabetes mellitus: a randomized prospective 6-year study. *Diabetes Res Clin Pract*. 1995;28:103–117.

18. UK Prospective Diabetes Study Group. Intensive blood-glucose control with sulphonylureas or insulin compared with conventional treatment and risk of complications in patients with Type 2 diabetes (UKPDS 33). *Lancet*. 1998;352:837–853.

19. UK Prospective Diabetes Study Group. Effect of intensive blood-glucose control with metformin on complications in overweight patients with Type 2 diabetes (UKPDS 34). *Lancet*. 1998;352:854–865.

20. UK Prospective Diabetes Study Group. Tight blood pressure control and risk of macrovascular and microvascular complications in Type 2 diabetes (UKPDS 38). *BMJ*. 1998;317:703–713.

21. Matthews DR, Stratton IM, Aldington SJ, Holman RR, Kohner EM, UK Prospective Diabetes Study Group. Risks of progression of retinopathy and vision loss related to tight blood pressure control in type 2 diabetes mellitus: UIKPDS 69. *Arch Ophthalmol*. 2004;122:1631–1640.

22. Chaturvedi N, Sjolie AK, Stephen JM, et al. Effect of lisinopril on progression of retinopathy in normotensive people with type 1 diabetes. *Lancet*. 1998;351:28–31.

23. Klein BEK, Moss SE, Klein R, Surawicz TS. The Wisconsin Epidemiologic Study of Diabetic Retinopathy, X: relationship of serum cholesterol to retinopathy and hard exudates. *Ophthalmology*. 1991;98:1261–1265.

24. Chew EY, Klein ML, Ferris III FL, et al. Association of elevated serum lipid levels with retinal hard exudates in diabetic retinopathy. *Arch Ophthalmol*. 1996;114: 1079–1084.

25. Roy MS, Klein R. Macular edema and retinal hard exudates in African Americans with type 1 diabetes. The New Jersey 725. *Arch Ophthalmol*. 2001;119:251–259.

26. Miljanovic B, Glynn RJ, Nathan Dm, Manson JE, Schaumberg DA. A prospective study of serum lipids and risk of diabetic macular edema in type 1 diabetes. *Diabetes*. 2000;53:2883–2892.

27. Fong DS, Segal PP, Myers F, Ferris FL, Hubbard LD, Davis MD. Subretinal fibrosis in diabetic macular edema, ETDRS Report No. 23. *Arch Ophthalmol*. 1997;115:873–877.

28. Davis MD, Fisher MR, Gangnon RE, et al. Risk factors for high-risk proliferative diabetic retinopathy and severe visual loss: Early Treatment Diabetic Retinopathy Study Report #18. *Invest Opthalmol Vis Sci*. 1998;39:233–252.

29. Phelps RL, Sakol P, Metzger BE. Jampol LM, Freinkel N. Changes in diabetic retinopathy during pregnancy: correlation with regulation of hyperglycemia. *Arch Ophthalmol*. 1986;104:1806–1810.

30. Klein BE, Moss SE, Klein R. Effect of pregnancy on progression of diabetic retinopathy. *Diabetes Care*. 1990;13:34–40.

31. Chew EY, Mills JL, Metzger BE, et al. Metabolic control and progression of retinopathy. The Diabetes in Early Pregnancy Study. National Institute of Child Health and Human Development Diabetes in Early Pregnancy Study. *Diabetes Care.* 1995;18:631–637.

32. Axer-Stegel R, Hod M, Fin k-Cohen A, et al. Diabetic retinopathy during pregnancy. *Ophthalmology.* 1996;103:1815–1819.

33. Lovestam-Adrian M, Agardh C-D, Aberg A, Agardh E. Pre-eclampsia is a potent risk factor for deterioration of retinopathy during pregnancy in type 1 diabetic patients. *Diabet Med.* 1997;14:1059–1065.

34. Lapolla A, Cardone C, Negrin P, et al. Pregnancy does not induce or worsen retinal or peripheral nerve dysfunction in insulin-dependent diabetic women. *J Diabetes Complications.* 1998;12:74–80.

35. The Diabetes Control and Complications Trial Research Group. Effect of pregnancy on microvascular complications in the Diabetes Control and Complications Trial. *Diabetes Care.* 2000;23:1084–1091.

36. Bognetti E, Calori G, Meschi F, Macellaro P, Bonfanti R, Chiumello G. Prevalence and correlations of early microvascular complications in young type I diabetic patients: role of puberty. *J Pediatr Endocrinol Metab.* 1997;10:587–592.

37. Donaghue KC, Fung AT, Hing S, et al. The effect of prepubertal diabetes duration on diabetes. Microvascular complications in early and late adolescence. *Diabetes Care.* 1997;20:77–80.

38. Porta M, Sjoelie AK, Chaturvedi N, et al. Risk factors for progression to proliferative diabetic retinopathy in the EURODIAB Prospective Complications Study. *Diabetologia.* 2001;44(12):2203–2209.

39. R Klein BE, Moss SE, Klein R. Is menarche associated with diabetic retinopathy? *Diabetes Care.* 1990;13:1034–1038.

40. Murphy RP, Nanda M, Plotnick L, Enger C, Vitale S, Patz A. The relationship of puberty to diabetic retinopathy. *Arch Ophthalmol.* 1990;108:215–218.

41. Klein R, Klein BE, Moss SE, Cruickshanks KJ. The Wisconsin Epidemiologic Study of diabetic retinopathy. XIV. Ten-year incidence and progression of diabetic retinopathy. *Arch Ophthalmol.* 1994;112:1217–1228.

42. Tesfaye S, Stevens LK, Stephenson JM, et al. Prevalence of diabetic peripheral neuropathy and its relation to glycaemic control and potential risk factors: the EURODIAB IDDM Complications Study. *Diabetologia.* 1995102:647–661.

43. Krolewski AS, Warram JH, Rand LJ, Christlieb AR, Busick EJ, Kahn CR. Risk of proliferative diabetic retinopathy in juvenile-onset type 1 diabetes: a 40 year follow-up study. *Diabetes Care.* 1986;9(5):443–552.

44. Qiao Q, Keinänen-Kiukaanniemi S, Läärä E. The relationship between hemoglobin levels and diabetic retinopathy. *J Clin Epidemiol.* 1997;50:153–158.

45. McMillan DE, Malone JI, Rand LJ, Steffes MW. Hemorheological plasma proteins predicts future retinopathy and nephropathy in the DCCT. *Diabetologia.* 1986;29:23–29.

46. Miyamoto K. Khorsrof S, Bursell SE, et al. Prevention of leukostasis and vascular leakage in streptozotocin-induced diabetic retinopathy via intercellular adhesion molecule-1 inhibition. *Proc Natl Aca Sci USA.* 1999;96:10836–10841.

47. Cusick M, Meleth AD, Agron E, et al. Associations of mortality and diabetes complications in patients with type 1 and type 2 diabetes: Early Treatment Diabetic Retinopathy Study Report no. 27. *Diabetes Care.* 2005;28:617–625.

18

Medical Management of the Diabetic Patient

JAY S. SKYLER, MD

CORE MESSAGES

- Randomized controlled clinical trials have demonstrated the benefit in patients with diabetes of meticulous glycemic control, stringent blood pressure control, and aggressive control of elevated serum lipids.
- Patients with diabetes should be screened regularly for early signs of diabetic retinopathy, diabetic nephropathy, diabetic neuropathy, and cardiovascular disease.

The major toll of diabetes mellitus, in terms of morbidity, mortality, and economic burden, is a consequence of the devastating chronic complications of the disease. Therefore, medical management of the diabetic patient has as one of its major goals the reduction of risk of chronic complications, including diabetic retinopathy. Controlled clinical trials have demonstrated that aggressive glycemic control reduces the risk and slows the progression of microvascular complications—including retinopathy, nephropathy, and neuropathy. As a consequence, current recommendations for glycemic control are to aim for glycated hemoglobin (A1c) to be <7% (normal range ~4.0%–6.0%), with fasting and pre-prandial capillary plasma glucose of 90 to 130 mg/dL (5.0–7.2 mmol/L), and peak postprandial capillary plasma glucose of <180 mg/dL (<10.0 mmol/L), with recognition that more stringent goals may further reduce the risk of complications [1]. It has also been demonstrated by controlled clinical trials that aggressive blood pressure control reduces the risk of both microvascular and macrovascular complications, such that current recommendations for glycemic control are to aim for blood pressure to be <130/80 mmHg in adults with diabetes [1]. Controlled clinical trials have demonstrated that the risk of macrovascular complications (including coronary artery disease, cerebral vascular disease, and peripheral vascular disease) can be reduced by careful control of plasma lipids, with current targets in people with diabetes being low density lipoprotein-cholesterol (LDL-C) of <100 mg/ dL (<2.6 mmol/L), high density lipoprotein-cholesterol (HDL-C) of >40 mg/dL (>1.1 mmol/L), and triglycerides <150 mg/dL (<1.7 mmol/L) [1], although it has been suggested that for individuals with diabetes and known coronary artery disease the targets be even more stringent, that is, an LDL-C target of <70 mg/dL (<1.8 mmol/L) [1,2]. Further, if drug-treated patients do not reach targets on maximal tolerated statin therapy, a reduction in LDL cholesterol of 30% to 40% from baseline is an alternative therapeutic goal [1]. This chapter reviews the treatment strategies and available modalities to achieve these goals.

GLYCEMIC CONTROL

Evidence. The evidence of the role of treatment of hyperglycemia and its impact on diabetic microvascular disease is unambiguous. Analyses from epidemiologic studies demonstrate a significant relationship between prevailing level of glycemia and microvascular disease, particularly retinopathy [3]. More importantly, randomized controlled clinical trials have demonstrated a beneficial effect on microvascular disease of lowering glycemia to a level close to normal. The Diabetes Control and Complications Trial (DCCT) showed that improved glycemic control, attained through intensive insulin therapy, can delay the onset and slow the progression of retinopathy, nephropathy, and neuropathy in patients with type 1 diabetes mellitus [4]. The DCCT may be the most important clinical study ever conducted in the field of diabetes, as its results were so dramatic that they effectively ended the debate as to whether glycemic control influences the development of diabetic complications. Importantly, too, in the DCCT, there was no "glycemic threshold"; rather, there was a continuous relationship between glycemic exposure and risk of complications [5,6]. Further, the Epidemiology of Diabetes Interventions and Complications (EDIC) follow-up study of the DCCT cohort showed the perhaps somewhat surprising result that the beneficial effects of improved glycemic control are sustained even after there is some slippage in the degree of control attained, and that the adverse effects of hyperglycemia continue even when there is subsequent improvement in glycemic control [7]. Indeed, in the EDIC extension, after a follow-up period of up to 20 years after enrollment on DCCT, there was even a reduction in macrovascular disease events—including death from coronary artery disease [8]. These observations suggest either that there is some sort of "metabolic memory" or that once the processes leading to microvascular complications are initiated, they are self-perpetuating. The lesson is that patients should strive for the best possible control as early as possible in the course of the disease, ideally from the time of diagnosis of their diabetes.

Other trials have confirmed the relationship between glycemic control and diabetic complications in both type 1 diabetes [9,10] and type 2 diabetes [11–13]. The United Kingdom Prospective Diabetes Study (UKPDS) was the largest of these in type 2 diabetes [12,13]. Epidemiologic analysis of all UKPDS subjects also demonstrated that there was a continuous relationship between glycemic exposure and risk of complications [14]. Moreover, as in the DCCT-EDIC study [8], long-term follow-up of the UKPDS cohort also demonstrated a "legacy effect" of earlier gly-cemic control, resulting in sustained benefit on microvascular complications, and the emergence of a statistically significant benefit on macrovascular complications and on death [15]. In contrast, three recent studies (ACCORD, ADVANCE, and VADT) with much shorter duration of follow-up failed to demonstrate a bene-ficial effect of glycemic control on macrovascular disease [16–18]. In addition, ACCORD, which sought a glycemic target of A1c < 6%, had an increased death rate in the intensive treatment group [16]. As a consequence of these studies and concerns raised about them, the American Diabetes Association, the American College of Cardiology, and the American Heart Association combined to review the data and present a statement about the studies and their implications on clinical practice [19]. That statement specifically noted that "the lack of significant reduc-tion in CVD events with intensive glycemic control in ACCORD, ADVANCE, and VADT should not lead clinicians to abandon the general target of an A1c of <7.0% and thereby discount the benefit of good control on serious and debilitating micro-vascular complications" [19]. It also noted that "subset analyses of ACCORD, ADVANCE, and VADT suggest the hypothesis that patients with shorter duration of type 2 diabetes and without established atherosclerosis might reap cardiovascu-lar benefit from intensive glycemic control" [19], which is consistent with the ben-eficial effects of early glycemic control in DCCT-EDIC [8] and UKPDS [15].

Management—Background. The vast majority of cases of diabetes fall into the two main categories: type 1 diabetes and type 2 diabetes. Type 1 diabetes is usually due to an immune-mediated destruction of pancreatic insulin-producing islet β-cells with consequent insulin deficiency and the need to replace insulin [20]. Although usually having an abrupt clinical onset, the disease process unfolds slowly, with progressive loss of β-cells over time. Type 1 diabetes presents as a consequence of significant loss of β-cell mass and/or function and invariably requires therapeutic replacement of insulin.

Type 2 diabetes, the more common type, is usually due to resistance to insulin action in the setting of inadequate compensatory insulin secretory response [21,22]. This is depicted in Figure 18.1. Insulin resistance is actually quite common, as it arises as a consequence of obesity, a sedentary lifestyle, and aging (Fig. 18.2), with resulting hyperglycemia and diabetes, blood pressure elevation, and dyslipidemia. In fact, collectively these abnormalities—which often occur together—have been des-ignated the "metabolic syndrome" (or more properly the "dysmetabolic syndrome"). Type 2 diabetes does not emerge in all persons with insulin resistance, but rather only in those with a genetic defect in insulin secretory capacity such that pancreatic insulin secretion fails to compensate for the insulin resistance (Fig. 18.1). Initially, the insulin secretory abnormality is manifest by a loss of "first phase" insulin secre-tion after a glucose challenge, resulting in excessive postprandial hyperglycemia. Ultimately, however, in type 2 diabetes, there is a progressive loss of pancreatic islet β-cells, resulting in insulin deficiency and the need to replace insulin [23].

The basis of the abnormalities in carbohydrate, fat, and protein metabolism in diabetes primarily is deficient action of insulin on target tissues, resulting from inadequate insulin secretion and/or diminished tissue responses to insulin at one or more points in the complex pathways of hormone action. Actually, it is a bit more

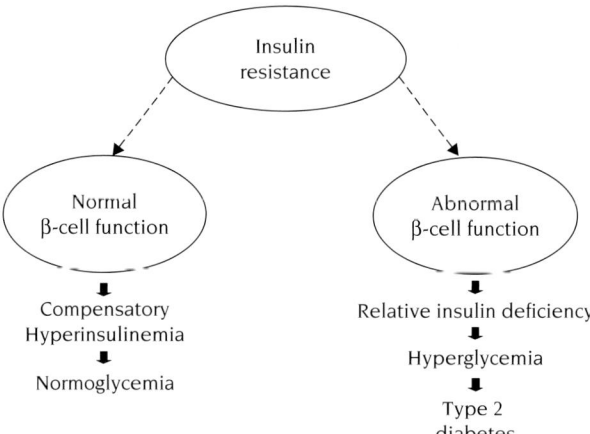

Figure 18.1. Schematic depiction of the dual defect that is necessary for type 2 diabetes to be manifest: insulin resistance in the setting of impaired β-cell function inadequate to compensate for the insulin resistance.

complex than that, with other hormones playing an important contributory role in glucose homeostasis. Glucagon, a hormone produced by the pancreatic islet α-cells that is normally secreted in response to protein and also to hypoglycemia, stimulates glucose production and release by the liver. In contrast, insulin modulates glucose production and release by the liver, to prevent it from becoming excessive. Thus, hepatic glucose production is regulated by a balance between stimulation by glucagon and inhibition by insulin (Fig. 18.3).

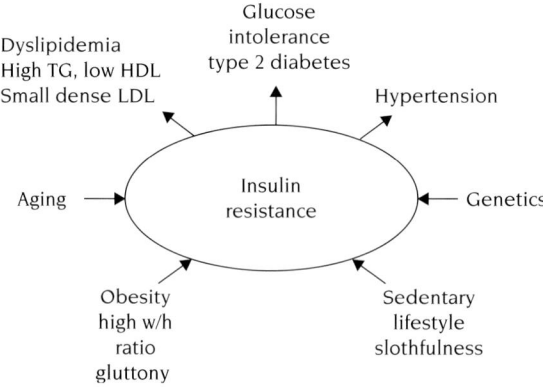

Figure 18.2. Causes and consequences of insulin resistance. Insulin resistance arises from obesity (particularly central obesity), a sedentary lifestyle, aging (perhaps related to progressive loss of muscle mass or sarcopenia), and may have a genetic proclivity to occurrence in some individuals. Potential consequences of insulin resistance include hyperglycemia and type 2 diabetes, blood pressure elevation (potentially leading to hypertension in those with a genetic risk of essential hypertension), and a dyslipidemia characterized by elevated triglycerides, low high density lipoprotein-cholesterol, and small dense low density lipoprotein-cholesterol (an atherogenic lipid pattern).

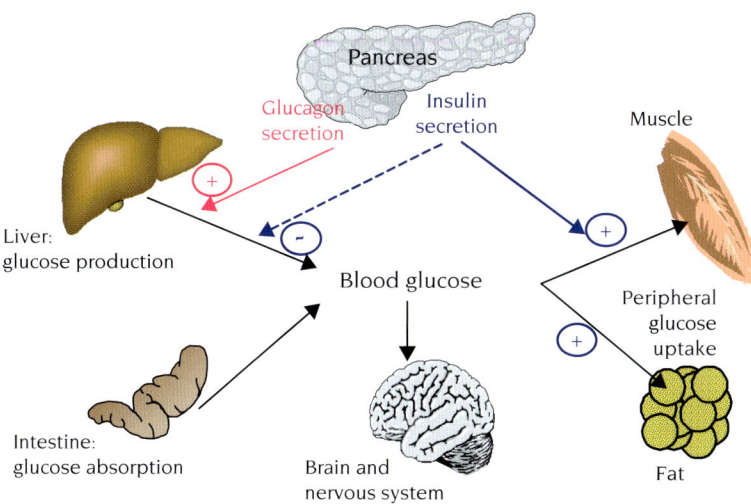

Figure 18.3. Scheme of regulation of blood glucose. Glucose input is from food intake via the gastrointestinal tract, or during the basal state from hepatic glucose production, which is modulated (inhibited) by basal insulin secretion and stimulated by glucagon. The brain and nervous tissue use glucose independent of insulin, while insulin stimulates glucose uptake and utilization by peripheral tissues (here represented by muscle and adipose tissue).

One can conceptually divide the day into two basic time periods—the basal or fasting state (overnight and between meals) and the prandial state (after consuming meals). Hyperglycemia occurs in the basal or fasting state because of increased hepatic glucose production, which is a consequence of both an insulin secretory abnormality (lack of first phase insulin secretion) and hepatic resistance to insulin, the net result being inadequate modulation by insulin of the hepatic glucose production [21,22]. Hepatic glucose production is stimulated by increased glucagon secretion, which coupled with decreased insulin secretion results in a decrease of the insulin/glucagon ratio, important in regulating hepatic glucose production [24]. In contrast, hyperglycemia in the prandial state arises because of (1) increased absorption of glucose from the gastrointestinal tract; (2) continued hepatic glucose production, due to lack of adequate prompt insulin availability to modulate glucose production; and (3) decreased ability to dispose of the consumed glucose load, due to inadequate insulin secretion to compensate for resistance to insulin action in tissues where glucose is disposed—principally muscle and adipose tissue [21,22]. Figure 18.3 depicts the scheme of regulation of blood glucose and provides a number of potential targets for therapeutically regulating blood glucose.

Management—Strategy. Contemporary diabetes management is based on the concept of "targeted glycemic control." Therapy, based on glycemic goals, utilizes progressive step-wise additions of whatever treatment modality is necessary to achieve glycemic goals [25]. Lifestyle modification—including medical nutritional therapy and promotion of physical activity—is the cornerstone of treatment of diabetes and is needed for all patients, as is basic education on diabetes.

Type 1 Diabetes. Modern management of type 1 diabetes focuses on replication of normal insulin secretion [26–29]. Also called "flexible diabetes therapy," this strategy calls for insulin delivery that comprises a basal and a prandial component, frequent home self-monitoring of blood glucose, a flexible dietary plan that accommodates most foods but with specific guidelines on how to alter therapy (such as insulin dose) based on carbohydrate intake. Most importantly, patients require the self-management skills to correct alterations in metabolic control at the time of such occurrences. This could include a change in insulin dose for premeal hyperglycemia, treatment of hypoglycemia, or addition of carbohydrate at bedtime to compensate for exercise earlier in the day. In addition, patients should understand basic principles of diabetes management during illness—"sick day guidelines." All too often, patients with type 1 diabetes either fail to administer enough insulin during a viral gastroenteritis or fail to measure urinary ketones during illness. As a consequence, life-threatening ketoacidosis may develop.

Flexible diabetes therapy is accomplished, as in the DCCT, with insulin administered either by continuous subcutaneous insulin infusion (CSII) with an insulin pump or by multiple daily insulin injections (MDI); frequent self-monitoring of blood glucose (SMBG); and meticulous attention to balancing insulin dose, food intake, and energy expenditure [26–29]. If, as stated above, one conceptually divides the day into the basal or fasting state and the prandial state, then the insulin program follows logically—a basal insulin (or basal rate in an insulin pump) to work throughout the day, and prandial insulin (or bolus activation of an insulin pump) for each meal. If one fails to achieve near-normal glycemic control (and near-normal A1c), preprandial injections of pramlintide may be added to the treatment program [30,31]. Pramlintide is an analog of the hormone amylin, which is secreted together with insulin from the pancreatic islet β-cell, and allows correction of concomitant amylin deficiency [32]. Studies have demonstrated that the addition of pramlintide to insulin results in better postprandial glycemic control and improved A1c without weight gain [30–32].

Type 2 Diabetes. In type 2 diabetes, when lifestyle modification alone does not result in normalization or near-normalization of metabolic abnormalities, pharmacologic therapy is required. Before 1995 in the United States, only insulin and sulfonylureas were available for the treatment of diabetes. Among patients with type 2 diabetes, more than 50% of patients were treated with oral monotherapy, 40% of patients were treated with insulin therapy, and a small percentage of patients were using sulfonylureas in combination with insulin. Since 1995, there has been an explosion of introductions of new classes of pharmacologic agents [33–37]. Currently available antidiabetic agents are listed in Tables 18.1 and 18.2, with Table 18.2 summarizing insulin preparations, including insulin analogues.

The classes of pharmacologic agents currently available include insulins and insulin analogues [38–40], sulfonylureas [41], glinides [41], biguanides [42–44], glitazones (thiazolidinediones) [45,46], α-glucosidase inhibitors [47], amylin agonists [31,32], incretin mimetics [37,48,49], incretin enhancers (DPP-4 inhibitors) [37], and bile acid sequestrants [50–52]. Combination products have been introduced as well.

Table 18.1. Anti-diabetic Agents Available in the United States

Generic Name	Brand Name
Sulfonylureas	
Tolbutamide	Orinase—now generic
Chlorpropamide	Diabinese—now generic
Tolazamide	Tolinase—now generic
Acetohexamide	Dymelor—now generic
Glipizide	Glucotrol—now generic
Glipizide-GITS	Glucotrol-XL—now generic
Glyburide	Diabeta, Micronase—now generic
Glyburide-(Micronized)	Glynase—now generic
Glimiperide	Amaryl—now generic
Glinides (Meglitinides)	
Repaglinide	Prandin
Nateglinide	Starlix
Biguanides	
Metformin	Glucophage—now generic
Metformin-XR	Glucophage-XR, Glumetza, Fortamet, and generic
PPARγ-Activators (Glitazones)	
Rosiglitazone	Avandia
Pioglitazone	Actos
Alpha-Glucosidase Inhibitors	
Acarbose	Precose
Miglitol	Glyset
Amylin Analogues	
Pramlintide	Symlin
Incretin Mimetics	
Exenatide	Byetta
Incretin Enhancers (DPP-4 Inhibitors)	
Sitagliptin	Januvia
Bile Acid Sequestrants	
Colesevelam	Welchol
Combination Therapies	
Glyburide-Metformin	Glucovance
Glipizide-Metformin	Metaglip

(Continued)

Table 18.1. (Continued)

Generic Name	Brand Name
Rosiglitazone-Glimiperide	Avandaryl
Pioglitazone-Metformin	ActoPlus Met
Pioglitazone-Glimiperide	Duetact
Sitagliptin-Metformin	Janumet

Table 18.2. Insulin Preparations Available in the United States

Generic Name	Brand Name
Short-Acting Preparations	
Regular human insulin	Humulin-R, Novolin-R
Insulin lispro	Humalog
Insulin aspart	Novolog
Insulin glulisine	Apidra
Intermediate-Acting Preparations	
NPH human insulin	Humulin-N, Novolin-N
Long Acting Preparations	
Insulin glargine	Lantus
Insulin detemir	Levemir
Premixed Preparations	
70% NPH/30% Regular	Humulin 70/30, Novolin 70/30
50% NPH/50% Regular	Humulin 50/50
75% Intermediate/25% Lispro	Humalog Mix 75/25
50% Intermediate/50% Lispro	Humalog Mix 50/50
70% Intermediate/30% Aspart	Novolog Mix 70/30

The new insulin analogs [40] include both rapid-acting insulin analogs (insulin lispro, insulin aspart, and insulin glulisine), which are designed to replace regular (soluble) insulin for prandial glycemic control, and relatively peakless long-acting insulin analogs (insulin glargine and insulin detemir), which are designed to replace NPH (isophane), lente, and ultralente insulin for basal glycemic control. Indeed, lente and ultralente insulin are no longer sold in the United States.

The newer insulin secretagogues [41] include both long-acting sulfonylureas (glimiperide, glipizide-GITS) designed for once or twice daily use, and the very short acting glinides (repaglinide, natiglinide) designed for prandial use. There are two classes of insulin sensitizers—the biguanides (metformin) [42–44], which act principally by restraining hepatic glucose production, and the glitazones (rosiglitazone, pioglitazone, and the now defunct troglitazone) [45,46], which act through activation of the nuclear transcription factor PPARγ and which have effects on glucose metabolism that results in increased glucose utilization. Also available are the α-glucosidase inhibitors (acarbose, miglitol) [47] that retard glucose absorption from the gastrointestinal tract. Recently available is an amylin analog (pramlintide) [31,32] whose antidiabetic effects arise from interactions via cognate receptors located in the central nervous system resulting in postprandial glucagon suppression, modulation of nutrient absorption rate, and reduction of food intake. Also recently introduced is the first of the incretin mimetics (exenatide) [37,48,49], which exerts at least some of its pharmacologic actions as an agonist at the glucagon-like peptide-1 (GLP-1) receptor, with several consequent actions, including glucose-dependent insulinotropic effects (and the potential to preserve or improve β-cell function), correction of excessive glucagon secretion, reduction of food intake, and modulation of nutrient absorption. Another recent class to be introduced is the incretin enhancers—or dipeptidyl peptidase-4 (DPP-4) inhibitors—which prevent inactivation of the incretins GLP-1 and GIP (glucose-dependent insulinotropic peptide), two key glucoregulatory hormones [37]. In addition, the bile acid sequestrant colesevelam, already used for lipid reduction, has been shown to have beneficial effects on glycemic control as well, by limiting glucose absorption [50–52].

Thus, each of the classes of drugs has effects on one or more of the major pathways of glucose regulation depicted in Figure 18.3. The major pathways impacted by each class are summarized in Table 18.3, while the major limitations of each

Table 18.3. Principal Glucose-lowering Actions of Currently Available Classes of Agents for Treatment of Diabetes Mellitus

	Correct Insulin Deficiency	Stimulate Insulin Secretion	Decrease Hepatic Glucose Production	Increase Muscle Glucose Utilization	Retard Carbohydrate Absorption
Insulin or insulin analogs	X				
Sulfonylureas		X			
Glinides		X			
Biguanides			X	(X)	
PPARγ activators			(X)	X	
α-Glucosidase inhibitors					X
Amylin analogs			X		X
Incretin mimetics		X	X		X
Incretin enhancers		X	X		
Bile acid sequestrants					X

X indicates minimal effect.

Table 18.4. Principal Limiting Factors in the Use of Currently Available Classes of Agents for Treatment of Diabetes Mellitus

	Hypoglycemia	Weight Gain	Other
Insulin or insulin analogs	√	√	Injections
Sulfonylureas	√	√	
Glinides	√	√	
Biguanides	No	No	Lactate production; GI side effects
PPARγ activators	No	√√	Fluid retention
α-glucosidase inhibitors	No	No	GI side effects
Amylin analogs	No	Weight loss	Injections; GI side effects
Incretin mimetics	No	Weight loss	Injections; GI side effects
Incretin enhancers	No	No	Modest GI side effects
Bile acid sequestrants	No	No	GI side effects

class are summarized in Table 18.4. The availability of agents with differing and complementary mechanisms of action allows them to be used in various combinations, thus increasing the likelihood that satisfactory glycemic control can be achieved in any given patient. Some debate exists over what sequence agents should be added, although most authorities start with metformin, as recommended in current guidelines [53]. The concept of "targeted glycemic control" calls for progressive step-wise additions in order to achieve near-normal glycemic goals.

BLOOD PRESSURE CONTROL

Evidence. Many randomized controlled clinical trials have addressed the influence of blood pressure control in diabetes. The Hypertension in Diabetes Study (HDS) was embedded in the UKPDS by using a factorial design [54,55]. There were substantial risk reductions for "any diabetes-related endpoint," diabetes-related death, heart failure, stroke, and microvascular disease (deterioration of retinopathy or of visual acuity). An "epidemiological" assessment of HDS demonstrated that the lower the systolic blood pressure, the lower the risk, and suggested a systolic blood pressure target of ≤130 mmHg [56].

The Hypertension Optimal Treatment (HOT) Study was a randomized trial involving 18,790 hypertensive patients (including 1501 patients with diabetes at baseline) with diastolic blood pressure of 100 to 115 mmHg [57]. They were randomly assigned to three different target diastolic blood pressure groups: ≤90, ≤85, and ≤80 mmHg. Felodipine was given as baseline therapy with the addition of other agents, according to a five-step regimen. In the patients with diabetes in HOT, with the lowest target blood pressure (≤80 mmHg), there was a decline in the rate of major cardiovascular events, cardiovascular mortality, and total mortality. In the group randomized to ≤80 mmHg, the risk of major cardiovascular events was halved in comparison with that of the target group ≤90 mmHg. These results suggest a diastolic blood pressure target of ≤80 mmHg in people with diabetes [57]. As a consequence of the above studies, current treatment recommendations for hypertension in patients with diabetes are to target a blood pressure of ≤130/80 mmHg [58–61]. Yet, the recently reported Comparison of Amlodipine vs Enalapril to Limit Occurrences of Thrombosis (CAMELOT) study in patients with coronary artery disease (CAD) but normal blood pressure found beneficial results of treatment in patients with a baseline blood pressure that averaged 129/78 mmHg [62]. Benefit was particularly seen in terms of atherosclerosis progression as measured by intravascular ultrasound [62]. This prompted an editorialist to suggest that the optimal target level of systolic blood pressure "is clearly lower than 140 mmHg and perhaps in the 120 mmHg range" [63].

The Systolic Hypertension in the Elderly Program (SHEP) and Systolic Hypertension in Europe (Syst-Eur) trials demonstrated that diabetic patients with isolated systolic hypertension benefited from treatment [64,65]. The Heart Outcomes Prevention Evaluation (HOPE) study demonstrated beneficial effects of intervention with an angiotensin-converting enzyme (ACE) inhibitor in diabetic patients with cardiovascular risk [66]. The Losartan Intervention for Endpoint reduction in hypertension study (LIFE) also showed a reduction in cardiovascular morbidity and mortality with an angiotensin receptor blocker (ARB) [67]. ARBs were also shown to be of benefit in diabetic patients with nephropathy, both early and late [68–70]. Yet, several other studies have found little or no difference amongst the various antihypertensive classes or agents [71–73], suggesting that it is blood pressure per se that is the critical issue [74]. However, most of these studies did not focus on diabetes per se. As a consequence, it is reasonable to continue to recommend that either an ACE inhibitor or an ARB be used in patients with diabetes.

Current Recommendations. There are consistent and substantial beneficial effects of improved blood pressure control in diabetic patients, impacting on various diabetic complications. In patients with diabetes, current blood pressure recommendations of the American Diabetes Association appear in its Position Statement on Treatment of Hypertension in Diabetes [58], which is based on a Technical Review on the same subject [59]. Similar recommendations are contained in the "Seventh Report of the Joint National Committee on Detection, Evaluation, and Treatment of High Blood Pressure" [60] and in the Guidelines developed by the European Society of Hypertension and European Society of Cardiology [61].

The primary goal of therapy for (nonpregnant) adults (>18 years of age) with diabetes is to decrease blood pressure to, and maintain it, at <130 mmHg systolic and <80 mmHg diastolic. In children, blood pressure should be decreased to the corresponding age-adjusted 90th percentile values. It should be noted, however, that in the general population, the risks for end-organ damage appear to be lowest when the systolic blood pressure is <120 mmHg and the diastolic blood pressure is <70 mmHg. For patients with an isolated systolic hypertension of >180 mmHg, the initial goal of treatment is to reduce the systolic blood pressure to <160 mmHg. For those with systolic blood pressure of 160 to 179 mmHg, the goal is a reduction of 20 mmHg. If these goals are achieved and well tolerated, further lowering to <140 mmHg may be appropriate.

Many experts are concerned about the selection of antihypertensive agents in individuals with diabetes. In clinical trials, the best demonstration of benefit to diabetic patients has been with ACE inhibitors or ARBs, particularly in terms of renal function and cardiovascular disease. It has been demonstrated that even in normotensive individuals with diabetes, ACE inhibitors have beneficial effects in kidney function.

CONTROL OF DYSLIPIDEMIA

Evidence. Several randomized controlled clinical trials have addressed the influence of lipid lowering with statin therapy in diabetes.

The Scandinavian Simvastatin Survival Study (4S) was a randomized trial involving patients with known coronary heart disease (CHD) manifested by angina pectoris or previous myocardial infarction who had total cholesterol levels of 5.5 to 8.0 mmol/L (213–310 mg/dL) while on a lipid-lowering diet [75]. The study included 202 diabetic patients. However, a post hoc subgroup analysis comparing the diabetic and nondiabetic patients demonstrated that in the diabetic patients, treatment with simvastatin reduced total mortality, major cardiovascular events, and any atherosclerotic event [76]. A further analysis suggested that both patients with diabetes and those with impaired fasting glucose benefited [77].

The Cholesterol and Recurrent Events (CARE) trial was a randomized trial involving patients with previous myocardial infarction who had plasma total cholesterol levels below 6.2 mmol/L (240 mg/dL) [78]. The study included 586 patients with clinical diagnoses of diabetes and 342 patients with impaired fasting glucose (IFG) at entry [79]. Treatment with pravastatin reduced the likelihood of a fatal coronary event or a nonfatal myocardial infarction. Post hoc analysis comparing the diabetic and nondiabetic patients showed that diabetic patients suffered more recurrent coronary events and a similar relative risk reduction as nondiabetic patients [79].

The Heart Protection Study (HPS) was a randomized trial involving patients with coronary disease, other occlusive arterial disease, or diabetes who had total cholesterol concentrations of at least 3.5 mmol/L (135 mg/dL) [80]. The study included 5963 diabetic patients [81]. Among the diabetic patients, treatment with simvastatin reduced major coronary events, strokes, and revascularizations. Beneficial effects were seen amongst diabetic participants who did not have any diagnosed occlusive arterial disease at entry, and amongst diabetic participants whose pretreatment LDL cholesterol concentration was <3.0 mmol/L (116 mg/dL).

The Collaborative Atorvastatin Diabetes Study (CARDS) was a randomized trial involving patients with type 2 diabetes without raised cholesterol levels and without prior clinical history of coronary, cerebrovascular, or peripheral vascular disease [82]. The study included 2838 diabetic patients. Treatment with low-dose atorvastatin reduced major coronary events, strokes, and revascularizations.

The Anglo-Scandinavian Cardiac Outcomes Trial-Lipid Lowering Arm (ASCOT-LLA) was a randomized trial involving hypertensive patients with at least three other cardiovascular risk factors but with total cholesterol concentrations <6.5 mmol/L (252 mg/dL) [83]. The study included 2532 diabetic patients. Treatment with low-dose atorvastatin reduced total cardiovascular events, total coronary events, and strokes.

The Pravastatin or Atorvastatin Evaluation and Infection Therapy-Thrombolysis in Myocardial Infarction (PROVE-IT) trial was a randomized trial involving people who had been hospitalized for an acute coronary syndrome within the preceding 10 days and it compared pravastatin standard therapy with atorvastatin high-dose intensive therapy [84]. The study included 734 diabetic patients. Intensive therapy showed a greater reduction in total cardiovascular events, total coronary events, and strokes.

Collectively, these studies unambiguously demonstrate the beneficial effects of lipid-lowering therapy with statins in people with diabetes. The benefits are seen across the spectrum of baseline level of cholesterol, and whether or not there are other cardiovascular risk factors.

Current Recommendations. The National Cholesterol Education Program Expert Panel on Detection, Evaluation, and Treatment of High Blood Cholesterol in Adults (Adult Treatment Panel III) identified diabetes as a high-risk condition [85,86]. More recently, these recommendations have been updated, taking into account the recent studies cited here [2]. The recommendations of the American Diabetes Association are similar and appear in their Position Statement on Treatment of Dyslipidemia in Diabetes [87], and were recently updated [1]. The designation of diabetes as a high-risk condition is based on evidence that the majority of patients with diabetes in higher-risk populations have a relatively high 10-year risk for developing cardiovascular disease (CVD). Thus, patients with the combination of diabetes and CVD deserve intensive lipid-lowering therapy. In high-risk persons, the recommended goal is low-density lipoprotein cholesterol (LDL-C) <100 mg/dL (2.6 mmol/L), but when risk is very high, an LDL-C goal of <70 mg/dL (1.8 mmol/L) is a therapeutic option, that is, a reasonable clinical strategy, on the basis of available clinical trial evidence. For patients with diabetes plus CVD, it is reasonable to attempt to achieve a very low LDL-C level, <70 mg/dL (1.8 mmol/L). On the basis of HPS, the presence of this combination appears to support initiation of statin therapy regardless of baseline LDL-C levels. This therapeutic option extends also to patients at very high risk who have a baseline LDL-C <100 mg/dL (<2.6 mmol/L).

Lipid-associated risk for CVD events is graded and continuous. Target LDL-C levels for adults with diabetes are <100 mg/dL (2.6 mmol/L); target HDL-C levels are >40 mg/dL (1.02 mmol/L); and target triglyceride levels are <150 mg/dL (1.7 mmol/L). In women, who tend to have higher HDL-C levels than men, an HDL-C goal of 10 mg/dL higher may be appropriate. Moreover, when a diabetic patient, particularly one with high risk, has high triglycerides or low HDL-C, consideration can be given to combining a fibrate or nicotinic acid along with an LDL-lowering drug.

The current ADA recommendations are that statin therapy should be added to lifestyle therapy, regardless of baseline lipid levels, for diabetic patients either

(a) with overt cardiovascular disease (CVD), or (b) without CVD who are over the age of 40 and have one or more other CVD risk factors [1]. These recommendations state further that for lower-risk patients (i.e., without overt CVD and under the age of 40), statin therapy should be considered if LDL cholesterol remains above 100 mg/dL (2.6 mmol/L) or in those with multiple CVD risk factors [1]. This assumes that in individuals without overt CVD, the primary goal is an LDL cholesterol <100 mg/dL (2.6 mmol/L), and in individuals with overt CVD, a lower LDL cholesterol goal of <70 mg/dL (1.8 mmol/L) using a high dose of a statin. Moreover, that if drug-treated patients do not reach targets on maximal tolerated statin therapy, a reduction in LDL cholesterol of 30% to 40% from baseline is an alternative therapeutic goal.

ANTI-PLATELET (ASPIRIN) THERAPY

Current Recommendations. The current ADA recommendation is to use aspirin therapy (75–162 mg/day) as a primary prevention strategy in those with type 1 or type 2 diabetes at increased CVD risk, including those over 40 years old or younger if there are additional risk factors (family history of CVD, hypertension, smoking, dyslipidemia, or albuminuria) [1].

CONCLUDING REMARKS

Randomized controlled clinical trials have established the benefit in patients with diabetes of meticulous glycemic control, stringent blood pressure control, and aggressive control of elevated lipids. Contemporary treatment of diabetes must pay attention to each of these three areas—blood glucose, blood pressure, and blood lipids—and to anti-platelet therapy, all in an effort to reduce the risk of cardiovascular disease and other diabetic complications. In addition, patients with diabetes must be screened regularly for early signs of diabetic retinopathy, diabetic nephropathy, diabetic neuropathy (especially that affecting the feet), and cardiovascular disease. A combination approach that stresses all of these variables has proven to be beneficial [88–91]. Improving interventions provide patients the hope that careful attention to preventive therapies will result in a markedly reduced burden of the potentially devastating complications of diabetes.

REFERENCES

1. American Diabetes Association. Standards of Medical Care in Diabetes. *Diabetes Care.* 2009;32(Suppl. 1):S13–S61.
2. Grundy SM, Cleeman JI, Merz CN, et al. Implications of recent clinical trials for the National Cholesterol Education Program Adult Treatment Panel III guidelines. *Circulation.* 2004;110:227–239.
3. Klein R. Hyperglycemia and microvascular and macrovascular disease in diabetes. *Diabetes Care.* 1995;18:258–268.
4. Diabetes Control and Complications Trial Research Group. The effect of intensive treatment of diabetes on the development and progression of long-term complications in insulin-dependent diabetes mellitus. *N Engl J Med.* 1993;329:683–689.

5. The Diabetes Control and Complications Trial Research Group. The relationship of glycemic exposure (HbA1c) to the risk of development and progression of retinopathy in the diabetes control and complications trial. *Diabetes*. 1995;44:968–983.

6. DCCT Research Group. The absence of a glycemic threshold for the development of long-term complications: the perspective of the Diabetes Control and Complications Trial. *Diabetes*. 1996;45:1285–1298.

7. The Diabetes Control and Complications Trial/Epidemiology of Diabetes Interventions and Complications Research Group. Retinopathy and nephropathy in patients with type 1 diabetes four years after a trial of intensive therapy. *N Engl J Med*. 2000;342:381–389.

8. The Diabetes Control and Complications Trial/Epidemiology of Diabetes Interventions and Complications (DCCT/EDIC) Study Research Group. Intensive diabetes treatment and cardiovascular disease in patients with type 1 diabetes. *N Engl J Med*. 2005;353:2643–2653.

9. Reichard P, Nilsson BY, Rosenqvist U. The effect of long-term intensified insulin treatment on the development of microvascular complications of diabetes mellitus. *N Engl J Med*. 1993;329:304–309.

10. Wang PH, Lau J, Chalmers TC. Meta-analysis of effects of intensive blood glucose control on late complications on type I diabetes. *Lancet*. 1993;341:1306–1309.

11. Ohkubo Y, Kishikawa H, Araki E, et al. Intensive insulin therapy prevents the progression of diabetic microvascular complications in Japanese patients with non-insulin-dependent diabetes mellitus: a randomized prospective 6-year study. *Diabetes Res Clin Pract*. 1995;28:103–117.

12. UK Prospective Diabetes Study Group. Intensive blood-glucose control with sulphonylureas or insulin compared with conventional treatment and risk of complications in patients with type 2 diabetes (UKPDS 33). *Lancet*. 1998;352:837–853.

13. UK Prospective Diabetes Study Group. Effect of intensive blood-glucose control with metformin on complications in overweight patients with type 2 diabetes (UKPDS 34). *Lancet*. 1998;352:854–865.

14. Stratton IM, Adler AI, Neil HA, et al. Association of glycaemia with macrovascular and microvascular complications of type 2 diabetes (UKPDS 35): prospective observational study. *BMJ*. 2000;321:405–412.

15. Holman RR, Paul SK, Bethel MA, Matthews DR, Neil HAW. 10-year follow-up of intensive glucose control in type 2 diabetes. *N Engl J Med*. 2008;359:1577–1589.

16. Action to Control Cardiovascular Risk in Diabetes Study Group, Gerstein HC, Miller ME, et al. Effects of intensive glucose lowering in type 2 diabetes. *N Engl J Med*. 2008;358:2545–2559.

17. ADVANCE Collaborative Group, Patel A, MacMahon S, et al. Intensive blood glucose control and vascular outcomes in patients with type 2 diabetes. *N Engl J Med*. 2008;358:2560–2572.

18. Duckworth W, Abraira C, Moritz T, et al. Intensive glucose control and complications in American veterans with type 2 diabetes. *N Engl J Med*. 2009;360:129–139.

19. Skyler JS, Bergenstal R, Bonow RO, et al. Intensive glycemic control and the prevention of cardiovascular events: implications of the ACCORD, ADVANCE, and VADT diabetes trials. A Position Statement of the American Diabetes Association and A Scientific Statement of the American College of Cardiology Foundation and the American Heart Association. *Diabetes Care*. 2009;32:187–192, *Circulation*. 2009;119;351–357; *J Am Col Cardiol*. 2009;53:298–304.

20. Atkinson MA, Eisenbarth GS. Type 1 diabetes: new perspectives on disease pathogenesis and treatment. *Lancet*. 2001;358:221–229.

21. Gerich JE. Contributions of insulin-resistance and insulin-secretory defects to the pathogenesis of type 2 diabetes mellitus. *Mayo Clin Proc.* 2003;78:447–456.
22. Kahn SE. The relative contributions of insulin resistance and beta-cell dysfunction to the pathophysiology of Type 2 diabetes. *Diabetologia.* 2003;46:3–19.
23. Butler A, Janson J, Bonner-Weir S, Ritzel R, Rizza RA, Butler PC. β-Cell deficit and increased β-cell apoptosis in humans with type 2 diabetes. *Diabetes.* 2003;52: 102–110.
24. Mitrakou A, Kelley D, Mokan M, et al. Role of reduced suppression of glucose production and diminished early insulin release in impaired glucose tolerance. *N Engl J Med.* 1992;326:22–29.
25. Skyler JS. Diabetes mellitus: pathogenesis and treatment strategies. *J Med Chem.* 2004;47:4113–4117.
26. DCCT Research Group. Implementation of treatment protocols in the Diabetes Control and Complications Trial. *Diabetes Care.* 1995;18:361–376.
27. Schade DS, Santiago JV, Skyler JS, Rizza R: *Intensive Insulin Therapy.* Princeton, N.J.: Excerpta Medica; 1983.
28. Hirsch IB. Intensive treatment of type 1 diabetes. *Med Clin North Am.* 1998;82:689–719.
29. Bolli GB. Physiological insulin replacement in type 1 diabetes mellitus. *Exp Clin Endocrinol Diabetes.* 2001;109(Suppl. 2):S317–S332.
30. Whitehouse F, Kruger DF, Fineman M, et al. A randomized study and open-label extension evaluating the long-term efficacy of pramlintide as an adjunct to insulin therapy in type 1 diabetes. *Diabetes Care.* 2002;25(4):724–730.
31. Edelman S, Garg S, Frias J, et al. A double-blind, placebo-controlled trial assessing pramlintide treatment in the setting of intensive insulin therapy in type 1 diabetes. *Diabetes Care.* 2006;29:2189–2195.
32. Kruger DF, Gloster MA. Pramlintide for the treatment of insulin-requiring diabetes mellitus: rationale and review of clinical data. *Drugs.* 2004;64:1419–1432.
33. Feinglos MN, Bethel MA. Treatment of type 2 diabetes mellitus. *Med Clin North Am.* 1998;82:757–790.
34. DeFronzo RA. Pharmacologic therapy for type 2 diabetes mellitus. *Ann Intern Med.* 1999;131:281–303.
35. Inzucchi SE. Oral antihyperglycemic therapy for type 2 diabetes: scientific review. *JAMA.* 2002;287:360–372.
36. Lebovitz HE. Oral antidiabetic agents: 2004. *Medical Clinics of North America* 2004;88:847–863.
37. Drucker DJ, Nauck MA. The incretin system: glucagon-like peptide-1 receptor agonists and dipeptidyl peptidase-4 inhibitors in type 2 diabetes. *Lancet.* 2006;368: 1696–1705.
38. DeWitt DE, Hirsch IB. Outpatient insulin therapy in type 1 and type 2 diabetes mellitus: scientific review. *JAMA.* 2003;289:2254–2264.
39. DeWitt DE, Dugdale DC. Using new insulin strategies in the outpatient treatment of diabetes: clinical applications. *JAMA.* 2003;289:2265–2269.
40. Hirsch IB. Insulin analogues. *N Engl J Med.* 2005;352:174–183.
41. Lebovitz HE. Insulin secretagogues: old and new. *Diabetes Rev.* 1999;7:139–153.
42. Cusi K, DeFronzo RA. Metformin: a review of its metabolic effects. *Diabetes Rev.* 1998;6:89–131.
43. Kirpichnikov D, McFarlane SI, Sowers JR. Metformin: an update. *Ann Intern Med.* 2002;137:25–33.

44. Hundal RS, Inzucchi SE. Metformin: new understandings, new uses. *Drugs.* 2003;63: 1879–1894.

45. Diamant M, Heine RJ. Thiazolidinediones in type 2 diabetes mellitus: current clinical evidence. *Drugs.* 2003;63:1373–1405.

46. Yki-Jarvinen H. Thiazolidinediones. *N Engl J Med.* 2004;351:1106–1118.

47. Lebovitz HE. α-Glucosidase inhibitors as agents in the treatment of diabetes. *Diabetes Rev.* 1998;6:132–145.

48. Nauck MA, Meier JJ. Glucagon-like peptide 1 and its derivatives in the treatment of diabetes. *Regul Pept.* 2005;128:135–148.

49. Joy SV, Rodgers PT, Scates AC. Incretin mimetics as emerging treatments for type 2 diabetes. *Ann Pharmacother.* 2005;39:110–118.

50. Fonseca VA, Rosenstock J, Wang AC, Truitt KE, Jones MR. Colesevelam HCl improves glycemic control and reduces LDL cholesterol in patients with inadequately controlled type 2 diabetes on sulfonylurea-based therapy. *Diabetes Care.* 2008;31: 1479–1484.

51. Goldberg RB, Fonseca VA, Truitt KE, Jones MR. Efficacy and safety of colesevelam in patients with type 2 diabetes mellitus and inadequate glycemic control receiving insulin-based therapy. *Arch Intern Med.* 2008;168:1531–1540.

52. Bays HE, Goldberg RB, Truitt KE, Jones MR. Colesevelam hydrochloride therapy in patients with type 2 diabetes mellitus treated with metformin: glucose and lipid effects. *Arch Intern Med.* 2008;168:1975–1983.

53. Nathan DM, Buse JB, Davidson MB, et al. Medical management of hyperglycemia in type 2 diabetes: a consensus algorithm for the initiation and adjustment of therapy: a consensus statement of the American Diabetes Association and the European Association for the Study of Diabetes. *Diabetes Care.* 2009;32:193–203; *Diabetologia.* 2009;52:17–30.

54. UK Prospective Diabetes Study Group. Tight blood pressure control and risk of macrovascular and microvascular complications in type 2 diabetes: UKPDS 38. *BMJ.* 1998;317:703–713.

55. UK Prospective Diabetes Study Group. Efficacy of atenolol and captopril in reducing risk of macrovascular and microvascular complications in type 2 diabetes: UKPDS 39. *BMJ.* 1998;317:713–720.

56. Adler AI, Stratton IM, Neil AW, et al. Association of systolic blood pressure with macrovascular and microvascular complications of type 2 diabetes (UKPDS 36): prospective observational study. *BMJ.* 2000;321:412–419.

57. Hansson L, Zanchetti A, Carruthers SG, et al. Effects of intensive blood-pressure lowering and low-dose aspirin in patients with hypertension: principal results of the Hypertension Optimal Treatment (HOT) randomised trial. *Lancet.* 1998;351: 1755–1762.

58. American Diabetes Association Position Statement. Hypertension management in adults with diabetes. *Diabetes Care.* 2004;27(Suppl. 1):S65–S67.

59. Arauz-Pacheco C, Parrott MA, Raskin P. The treatment of hypertension in adult patients with diabetes (Technical Review). *Diabetes Care.* 2002;25:134–147.

60. Chobanian AV, Bakris GL, Black HR, et al. The Seventh Report of the Joint National Committee on Prevention, Detection, Evaluation, and Treatment of High Blood Pressure: the JNC 7 report. *JAMA.* 2003;289:2560–2572.

61. ESH/ESC Hypertension Guidelines Committee. 2003 European Society of Hypertension–European Society of Cardiology guidelines for the management of arterial Hypertension. *J Hypertens.* 2003;21:1011–1053.

62. Nissen SE, Tuzcu EM, Libby P, et al. Effect of antihypertensive agents on cardiovascular events in patients with coronary disease and normal blood pressure the CAMELOT study: a randomized controlled trial. *JAMA*. 2004;292:2217–2226.
63. Pepine CJ. What is the optimal blood pressure and drug therapy for patients with coronary artery disease? *JAMA*. 2004;292:2271–2273.
64. Tuomilehto J, Rastenyte D, Birkenhager WH, et al. Effects of calcium-channel blockade in older patients with diabetes and systolic hypertension. *N Engl J Med*. 1999;340:677–684.
65. Curb JD, Pressel SL, Cutler JA, et al. Effect of diuretic based antihypertensive treatment on cardiovascular disease risk in older diabetic patients with isolated systolic hypertension. Systolic Hypertension in the Elderly Program Cooperative Research Group. *JAMA*. 1996;276:1886–1892. [Erratum, *JAMA*. 1997;277:1356].
66. Heart Outcomes Prevention Evaluation (HOPE) Study Investigators. Effects of ramipril on cardiovascular and microvascular outcomes in people with diabetes mellitus: results of the HOPE study and MICRO-HOPE substudy. *Lancet*. 2000;355:253–259.
67. Lindholm LH, Ibsen H, Dahlöf B, et al. Cardiovascular morbidity and mortality in patients with diabetes in the Losartan Intervention For Endpoint reduction in hypertension study (LIFE): a randomised trial against atenolol. *Lancet*. 2002;359:1004–1010.
68. Parving H-H, Lehnert H, Brocher-Mortensen J, et al. The effect of irbesartan on the development of diabetic nephropathy in patients with type 2 diabetes. *N Engl J Med*. 2001;345:870–878.
69. Brenner BM, Cooper ME, de Zeeuw D, et al. Effects of losartan on renal and cardiovascular outcomes in patients with type 2 diabetes and nephropathy. *N Engl J Med*. 2001; 345:861–869.
70. Lewis EJ, Hunsicker LG, Clarke WR, et al. Renoprotective effect of the angiotensin-receptor antagonist irbesartan in patients with nephropathy due to type 2 diabetes. *N Engl J Med*. 2001;345:851–860.
71. The ALLHAT Officers and Coordinators for the ALLHAT Collaborative Research Group. Major outcomes in high-risk hypertensive patients randomized to angiotensin-converting enzyme inhibitor or calcium channel blocker vs diuretic: the Antihypertensive and Lipid-Lowering Treatment to Prevent Heart Attack Trial (ALLHAT). *JAMA*. 2002;288:2981–2997.
72. Pepine CJ, Handberg EM, Cooper-DeHoff RM, et al. A calcium antagonist vs a non-calcium antagonist hypertension treatment strategy for patients with coronary artery disease. *JAMA*. 2003;290:2805–2816.
73. Bakris GL, Fonseca V, Katholi RE, et al. Metabolic effects of carvedilol vs metoprolol in patients with type 2 diabetes mellitus and hypertension: a randomized controlled trial. *JAMA*. 2004;292:2227–2236.
74. Alderman MH. The Return on INVEST. *JAMA*. 2003;290:2859–2861.
75. Scandinavian Simvastatin Survival Study Group. Randomised trial of cholesterol lowering in 4444 patients with coronary heart disease: the Scandinavian Simvastatin Survival Study (4S). *Lancet*. 1994;344:1383–1389.
76. Pyrälä K, Pedersen TR, Kjekshus J, Faergeman O, Olsson AG, Thorgeirsson G. Cholesterol lowering with simvastatin improves prognosis of diabetic patients with coronary heart disease. A subgroup analysis of the Scandinavian Simvastatin Survival Study (4S). *Diabetes Care*. 1997;20:614–620.
77. Haffner SM, Alexander CM, Cook TJ, et al. Reduced coronary events in simvastatin-treated patients with coronary heart disease and diabetes or impaired fasting glucose levels: subgroup analyses in the Scandinavian Simvastatin Survival Study. *Arch Intern Med*. 1999;159:2661–2667.

78. Sacks FM, Pfeffer MA, Moye LA, et al. The effect of pravastatin on coronary events after myocardial infarction in patients with average cholesterol levels. *N Engl J Med.* 1996;335:1001–1009.

79. Goldberg RB, Mellies MJ, Sacks FM, et al. Cardiovascular events and their reduction with pravastatin in diabetic and glucoseintolerant myocardial infarction survivors with average cholesterol levels: subgroup analyses in the cholesterol and recurrent events (CARE) trial. The Care Investigators. *Circulation.* 1998;98:2513–2519.

80. Heart Protection Study Collaborative Group. MRC/BHF Heart Protection Study of cholesterol lowering with simvastatin in 20,536 high-risk individuals: a randomised placebo-controlled trial. *Lancet.* 2002;360:7–22.

81. Heart Protection Study Collaborative Group. MRC/BHF Heart Protection Study of cholesterol-lowering with simvastatin in 5963 people with diabetes: a randomised placebocontrolled trial. *Lancet.* 2003;361:2005–2016.

82. Colhoun HM, Betteridge DJ, Durrington PN, et al. Primary prevention of cardiovascular disease with atorvastatin in type 2 diabetes in the Collaborative Atorvastatin Diabetes Study (CARDS): multicentre randomized placebo controlled trial. *Lancet.* 2004;364:685–696.

83. Sever PS, Dahlof B, Poulter NR, et al. Prevention of coronary and stroke events with atorvastatin in hypertensive patients who have average or lower-than-average cholesterol concentrations, in the Anglo-Scandinavian Cardiac Outcomes Trial-Lipid Lowering Arm (ASCOT-LLA): a multicentre randomised controlled trial. *Lancet.* 2003;361:1149–1158.

84. Cannon CP, Braunwald E, McCabe CH, et al. Intensive versus moderate lipid lowering with statins after acute coronary syndromes. *N Engl J Med.* 2004;350:1495–1504.

85. Expert Panel on Detection, Evaluation, and Treatment of High Blood Cholesterol in Adults. Executive Summary of the Third Report of the National Cholesterol Education Program (NCEP) Expert Panel on Detection, Evaluation, and Treatment of High Blood Cholesterol in Adults (Adult Treatment Panel III). *JAMA.* 2001;285:2486–2497.

86. National Cholesterol Education Program Expert Panel on Detection, Evaluation, and Treatment of High Blood Cholesterol in Adults (Adult Treatment Panel III). Third Report of the National Cholesterol Education Program (NCEP) Expert Panel on Detection, Evaluation, and Treatment of High Blood Cholesterol in Adults (Adult Treatment Panel III) Final Report. *Circulation.* 2002;106:3145–3421.

87. American Diabetes Association Position Statement. Dyslipidemia management in adults with diabetes. *Diabetes Care.* 2004;27(Suppl. 1):S68–S71.

88. Gæde P, Vedel P, Parving HH, Pedersen O. Intensified multifactorial intervention in patients with type 2 diabetes mellitus and microalbuminuria: the Steno type 2 randomised study. *Lancet.* 1999;353:617–622.

89. Gæde P, Vedel P, Larsen N, Jensen GVH, Parving HH, Pedersen O. Multifactorial intervention and cardiovascular disease in patients with type 2 diabetes. *N Engl J Med.* 2003;348:383–393.

90. Gæde P, Pedersen O. Intensive integrated therapy of type 2 diabetes—implications for long-term prognosis. *Diabetes.* 2004;53(Suppl. 3):S39–S47.

91. Gaede P, Lund-Andersen H, Parving H-H, Pedersen O. Effect of a multifactorial intervention on mortality in type 2 diabetes. *N Engl J Med.* 2008;358:580–591.

19

Telemedicine for Diabetic Retinopathy

HELEN K. LI, MD,
AND MATTHEW T.S. TENNANT, MD, FRCSC

CORE MESSAGES

- Screening for diabetic retinopathy is cost effective and reduces the risk of blindness. Telemedicine evaluation of diabetic retinopathy is an opportunity to improve detection of diabetic retinopathy.
- The American Telemedicine Association's *Telehealth Practice Recommendations for Diabetic Retinopathy* provides recommendations for designing and implementing a diabetic retinopathy ocular telehealth program.
- Telemedicine systems are available in a variety of configurations including mydriatic and nonmydriatic fundus cameras and other imaging devices.
- The Early Treatment Diabetic Retinopathy Study (ETDRS) standard seven-field, 30-degree stereoscopic slide film photographs of the retina protocol serve as the reference standard for identifying diabetic retinopathy.
- Telemedicine evaluation of diabetic retinopathy does not replace a comprehensive eye examination.

Diabetes has become epidemic in many communities around the world [1,2]. Increasing numbers of people with diabetes have led to increases in diabetic retinopathy. Fortunately, much of the vision loss from diabetic retinopathy can be reduced or prevented through early identification and treatment [3,4]. Diabetic retinopathy screening programs have proven to be cost effective in reducing the rate of vision loss within a community [5,6]. Unfortunately, many people with diabetes do not have access to eye care or do not receive timely evaluation for diabetic retinopathy. Telemedicine for these people offers the promise of a healthier future.

OVERVIEW

Telemedicine is the delivery of health services and information through integrated networks of computer and telecommunications technology. It offers the possibility of increased access to health care, particularly specialty care, when and where it is most needed. Telemedicine may also reduce escalating medical costs by substituting effective, but less expensive, alternatives to traditional health care delivery systems [7].

Diabetic retinopathy is well suited for assessment by telemedicine. Slide film photography has been used in large, multicenter diabetic retinopathy clinical trials for remote evaluation since 1970. The progression of disease between treatment and observation groups has been compared successfully through photography [8]. Digital photography significantly advances health care delivery options. Digital images can be transmitted electronically from remote locations directly to specialists for evaluation. Digital photographs can also be reviewed immediately onsite because they do not require the processing time normally associated with film photography.

The integration of computers and telecommunications into the care of diabetic retinopathy is an opportunity to make dramatic inroads into this serious public health problem. Telemedicine can extend health care resources to underserved areas, increasing the number of diabetic patients assessed for retinopathy. Telemedicine can also improve screening rates by making evaluation more convenient for patients, even in areas where specialty care is available. Patient visits to specialists could be streamlined by telemedicine directing only those with retinopathy or in need of treatment to traditional evaluation.

DIABETIC RETINOPATHY TELEMEDICINE PROGRAMS

Worldwide use of telemedicine to identify diabetic retinopathy is growing in response to the increasing prevalence of diabetes and the decreasing cost of teletechnology. In Australia, high rates of diabetes in indigenous populations have led to the development of innovative telemedicine projects. Various systems are in place to screen for diabetic retinopathy in people of aboriginal ancestry living in rural communities. Programs use nonmydriatic retinal cameras linked to digital backs. People from the community are often trained and credentialed as photographers, providing the additional benefit of local employment and education [9]. Once identified, patients with diabetic retinopathy are referred to an ophthalmologist for assessment [10–12]. At the Lions Eye Institute in Perth, researchers are working on the development of a portable handheld camera that could be used to screen for diabetic retinopathy and other eye diseases [13].

The creation of a teleophthalmology reimbursement code in some Canadian provinces has led to the development of a web-based, stereoscopic telemedicine system (Fig. 19.1). Funding for the Web server's development and maintenance is generated by telemedicine patient evaluations. Costs for remote mobile camera units including personnel are covered by the federal and provincial governments.

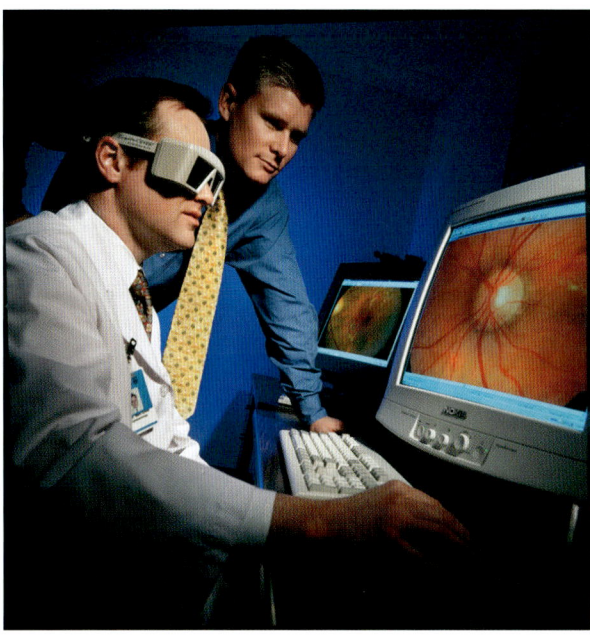

Figure 19.1. Photograph showing the use of LCD shutter goggles for stereo viewing of retinal images at the University of Alberta Tele-Ophthalmology Reading Center. (Source: Courtesy of Richard Siemens with permission from the University of Alberta Folio, 28 April 2000; Vol. 37, Number 16.)

In Alberta, two mobile retinal units with mydriatic cameras travel to 44 First Nations (North American Indian) communities to identify sight-threatening levels of diabetic retinopathy and other eye diseases. Additional testing includes urinalysis, and hemoglobin A1c and cholesterol levels. Nutritional and diabetic counseling is also provided. Visual acuity and intraocular pressures are measured and seven-field, 30-degree digital retina images captured through dilated pupils. Nonsimultaneous stereoscopic pairs of photographs of the disc and macula only are captured, eliminating the need for extra skills to stereo image the peripheral retina. The photography protocol maximizes the benefit of stereopsis for identifying macular edema and neovascularization of the disc. The protocol also minimizes the duration of photography sessions. Once photographs are captured, images and patient information are uploaded to the Web server as encrypted files to be graded by a retinal specialist. Files are protected by two-factor authentication and passwords as images are graded by ophthalmologists with a computer-assisted ETDRS algorithm. Only patients with clinically significant macular edema (CSME) and/or proliferative diabetic retinopathy (PDR) are referred for treatment [14,15]. Once treated, patients are followed over distance by teleophthalmology. Other Canadian telemedicine programs screen for diabetic retinopathy using nonmydriatic digital retinal cameras [16–18].

Some health care organizations contract diabetic retinopathy telemedicine services to commercial enterprises. The Inoveon Corporation of Oklahoma City,

Oklahoma, developed a telemedicine system in the United States to detect diabetic retinopathy based on the ETDRS photography protocol. Stereoscopic, seven-field digital photography of the retina is taken through dilated pupils [19]. Images are ETDRS graded by trained readers through a private intranet. The Joslin Diabetes Center's Joslin Vision Network (JVN) is a telemedicine program that images diabetic retinas without pupillary dilation [20]. Once captured, three 45-degree retina fields are sent through a private intranet to the JVN reading center for grading (Fig. 19.2). The system is being used in a number of locations throughout the United States by the Department of Defense, Indian Health Service and Veterans Administration. EyeTel Imaging, Inc., offers their DigiScope diabetic retinopathy screening system to primary care physicians. Red-free fundus images are reviewed at the EyeTel-Wilmer Reading Center and reports sent back within 48 hours to the primary physician [21].

Mass screening telemedicine programs in other countries are also underway to identify diabetic retinopathy. A Helsingborg, Sweden, telemedicine program screens for diabetic retinopathy and approximately 75% of the diabetic population has already been assessed through retinal photography. The program has recently migrated from slide film to digital imaging following a validation study [22,23]. In Great Britain, telemedicine screening projects rely on nonmydriatic digital retinal cameras [24]. In Gloucestershire, England, a mobile digital retinal camera unit travels to the offices of 85 family doctors. Patients with diabetes undergo pupillary dilation followed by retinal photography. A minimum of four images (768 × 568 pixel resolution) per patient are sent electronically to an ophthalmologist for reading [25]. Diabetic retinopathy telescreening services supported by the EU-Commission were established in five European countries (Czech Republic, Denmark, Germany, Ireland and UK) [26]. Sixteen screening centers in the

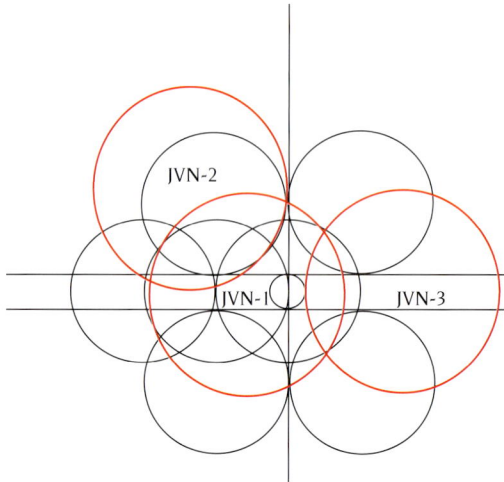

Figure 19.2. Joslin Vision Network's three 45-degree fields overlaid on Early Treatment Diabetic Retinopathy Study seven standard fields.

Ile-de-France region were linked in a telemedical network to facilitate access to annual diabetic retinal evaluation [27].

CLINICAL RESEARCH

Telemedicine technology is also proving to be a useful tool in clinical diabetic retinopathy research. For example, the Diabetic Retinopathy Clinical Research Network (DRCR.net), established in 2003 and sponsored by the National Eye Institute, deployed electronic visual acuity testers (EVA) and wireless tablet personal computers to facilitate electronic collection and web submission of clinical data. Patients view a computer monitor controlled by a study coordinator equipped with an EVA personal digital assistant (PDA) that automatically calculates a visual acuity score [28].

VALIDATION STUDIES

More than a decade of epidemiology data [29] has been derived by following patients with the ETDRS photographic and classification protocols: seven-field, 30-degree, stereoscopic, 35 mm slides (Fig. 19.3). This is currently the most comprehensive method for classifying levels of diabetic retinopathy [30,31]. Because no similar standard yet exists for digital media, ETDRS is commonly used as a reference standard for validating diagnostic accuracy of new telemedicine systems.

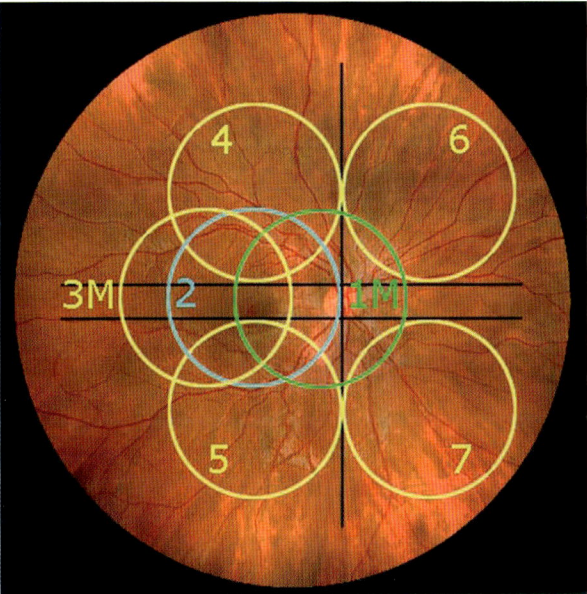

Figure 19.3. Early Treatment Diabetic Retinopathy Study seven standard fields, courtesy of Wisconsin Fundus Photograph Reading Center.

Table 19.1. Comparison of Sample Teleophthalmology Imaging Systems

Authors	Fundus Camera	Resolution	Dilation	# of Fields	Display	# of Diabetic Patients	Results
Fransen et al. [19]	Mydriatic Zeiss FF450 with Kodak DCS520 digital back	1152 × 1152 24-bit color No compression	Yes	7 × 30° Stereo	StereoGraphics Corp. LCD with shuttering glasses	290	6.6% eyes ur gradeable. Sensitivity = 98% and specificity = 89% for identifying *threshold* disease (severe NPDR, questionable or definite CSME or ungradeable image).
Rudinsky et al. [34]*	Mydriatic Zeiss FF450 with Kodak DCS560 digital back	3040 × 2008 24-bit color No compression	Yes	7 × 30° Only fields 1 and 2 are stereo	StereoGraphics Corp. LCD (1024 × 768) with shuttering glasses	105	0% ungradeable. Sensitivity = 91% and specificity = 92% for identifying CSME.
Bursell et al. [20]	Nonmydriatic Topcon TRC-NW5S linked to Sony 970-MD color video camera	640 × 480 24-bit color 10:1 JPEG compression	No	3 × 45° Stereo	StereoGraphics Corp. LCD (1280 × 1024) with shuttering glasses	54	12% ungradeable. *Proliferative DR* Sensitivity = 89% and specificity = 97% *Mild/Moderate NPDR* Sensitivity = 86% and specificity = 76% *Severe/Very Severe NPDR* Sensitivity = 57% and specificity = 99% CSME Sensitivity = 27% and specificity = 98%

Massin et al. [32]	Nonmydriatic Topcon TRC-NW6S linked to Sony DXC-950P video back	800 × 600 24-bit No compression	No	5 × 45° Not stereo	21-inch monitor (1280 × 1024)	74	11% ungradeable. *Moderate/Severe* NPDR Sensitivity = 92% and specificity = 85% was the lowest among three graders. Sensitivity and specificity was not reported for other levels.
Lin et al. [33]	Nonmydriatic Canon CR5–45NM	640 × 480 8-bit No compression	No	1 × 45° Not stereo		197	8% ungradeable. Sensitivity = 78% and specificity = 86% for binary Kaiser referral categories (no referral if less than mild NPDR).

*Rudnisky's study compared to contact lens biomicroscopy instead of 35 mm.

DR = diabetic retinopathy; NPDR = nonproliferative diabetic retinopathy; PDR = proliferative diabetic retinopathy; CSME = clinically significant macula edema.

1. Fransen enrolled patients consecutively: 27 eyes had PDR; 65 eyes had macular edema.

2. Rudnisky enrolled patients consecutively: 42 patients had CSME in at least one eye.

3. Brusell enrolled patients with an identified range of retinopathy level; 8 eyes had CSME; 9 eyes had PDR.

4. Massin used hard exudates within one disc diameter of the fovea as a surrogate marker of macular edema; 12 patients had CSME; 0 had PDR.

5. Lin found all patients with macular edema screened positive for referral due to retinopathy findings including microaneurysms and hemorrhages in photographs; the number of patients with macular edema was not reported.

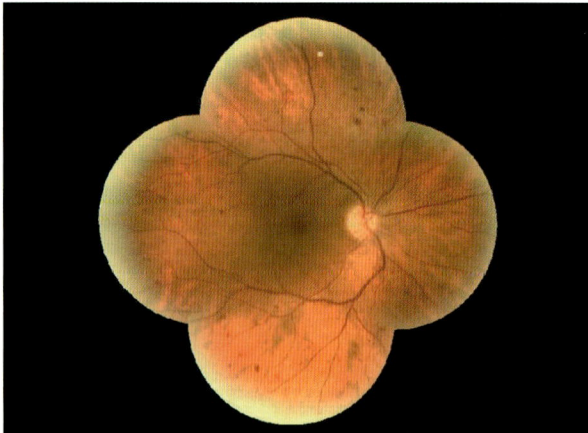

Figure 19.4. Mosaic image from five 45-degree fields taken with Topcon TRC-NW6S using IMAGEnet 2000 software.

Table 19.1 summarizes features of mydriatic and nonmydriatic retinal camera telemedicine systems from studies with published validation results. Fransen et al. [19], Bursell et al. [20], Massin et al. [32] and Lin et al. [33] compared systems to ETDRS (Figs. 19.4 and 19.5). Rudnisky et al. [34] compared digital stereoscopic photography to contact lens biomicroscopy (CLBM) for identification of CSME because other investigators had shown CLBM may be more sensitive [35]. Fransen and Rudnisky show the possibility of using stereoscopic digital systems with *mydriatic* cameras to identify diabetic retinopathy with sight-threatening stages of disease. The other studies demonstrate the possibility of diabetic retinopathy programs deploying *nonmydriatic* cameras to take single or multiple images through undilated pupils. Bursell's study used stereo images but Massin and Lin did not.

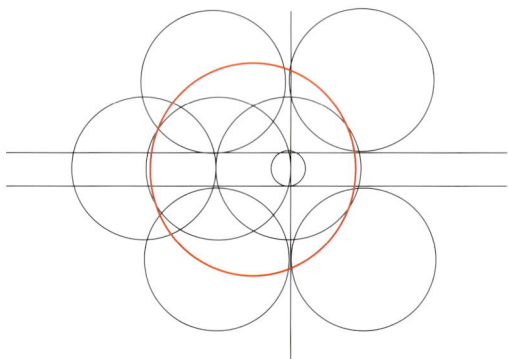

Figure 19.5. Lin's single 45-degree field overlaid on Early Treatment Diabetic Retinopathy Study seven standard fields.

NONMYDRIATIC RETINAL CAMERA TELEMEDICINE SYSTEMS

Nonmydriatic cameras take advantage of infrared technology, allowing retinal images to be photographed through undilated pupils. The Department of Ophthalmology and Visual Sciences at The University of Texas Medical Branch (UTMB) in Galveston, Texas was an early pioneer in the use of telemedicine to evaluate patients with diabetic retinopathy using nonmydriatic cameras. Imaging operator ease-of-use is an important factor when deploying a telemedicine system. Several features available exclusively on nonmydriatic cameras facilitate retinal photography. Nonmydriatic cameras focus and align under infrared conditions instead of the visible light used in mydriatic cameras. Infrared light is much more comfortable for patients than visible light. With a mydriatic camera, operators use a viewfinder to focus and align, requiring considerable skill and experience. Some nonmydriatic cameras such as the Topcon TRC-NW6S offer on-screen guides that help even inexperienced photographers take excellent photographs (Fig. 19.6A and 19.6B). The Topcon TRC-NW6S also has nine internal fixation positions in six patterns. When taking fields peripheral to the central field, fixed internal targets allow operators to easily achieve consistent field definition.

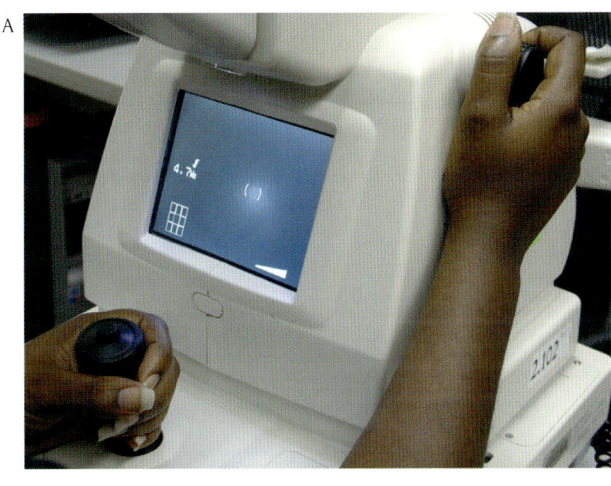

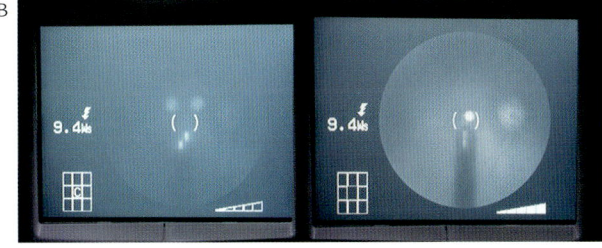

Figure 19.6. Topcon TRC-NW6S on-screen guides. (A) Operating the joystick, the camera is moved to bring two round spots together inside a bracket to achieve alignment. (B) Operating the focusing knob, the two slit lines are brought together for focus.

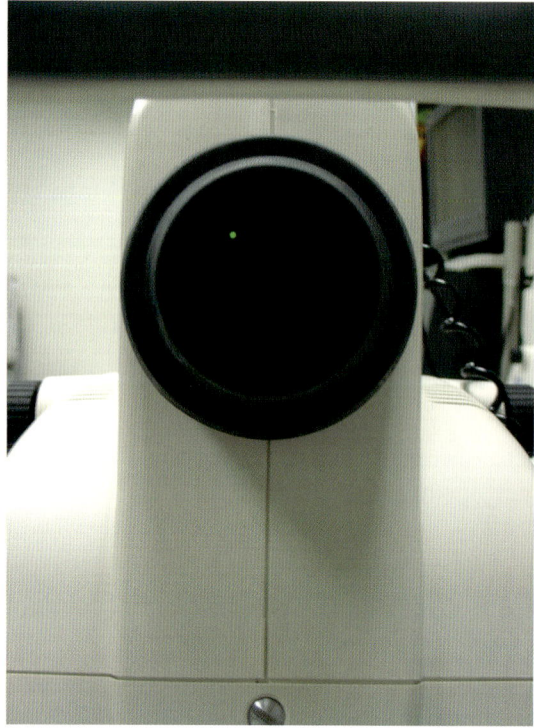

Figure 19.7. Topcon TRC-NW6S internal fixation target. The patient follows the green light as the operator moves the fixation target from one position to the next.

Internal targets are also easier for patients to see and follow than external targets (Fig. 19.7).

Topcon's IMAGEnet 2000 software constructs a large mosaic from nine digital photographs covering about the same posterior pole retina size as the ETDRS seven fields (Fig. 19.8). Many diabetic patients at UTMB's Starks Diabetes Center (located on the other side of campus from the department of ophthalmology) benefited from retinal evaluations at Starks. Images taken through small pupils are often too dark or have low contrast. Consequently, image quality suffers as a number of flash photographs are acquired in rapid succession through undilated pupils. For this reason, pupils were pharmacologically dilated. Nine photographs were taken per eye. Comparison of 141 eyes' wide-angle digital imagery to standard ETDRS seven-field stereo 35-degree slides using the ETDRS nine-step scale protocol found 88% ± 1 step agreement [36].

Other manufacturers such as Canon, Kowa, Nidek and Zeiss also make nonmydriatic cameras, many with similar features to Topcon. Kowa's nonmydriatic camera uses three internal fixation positions: central, nasal, and temporal. Some nonmydriatic systems can be outfitted with seven internal targets fixated at similar field definitions as ETDRS fields. This should allow grading retinopathy levels that exactly follow ETDRS protocols.

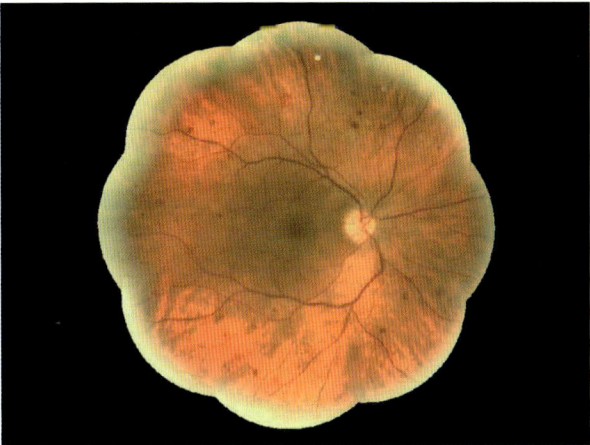

Figure 19.8. Mosaic image from nine photographs taken with a Topcon TRC-NW6S through a dilated pupil using IMAGEnet 2000 software.

OTHER CAMERAS AND IMAGING TOOLS

The Panoramic 200 (Optos Inc. Marlborough, MA,) is a scanning laser ophthalmoscope able to capture a 120-degree digital image (2000 × 2000 pixel resolution) and has been shown to identify diabetic retinopathy (Fig. 19.9) [37].

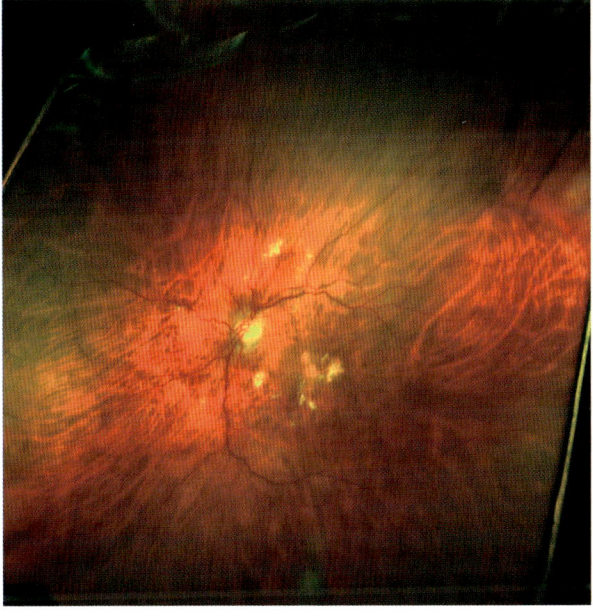

Figure 19.9. Panoramic 200 scanning laser ophthalmoscope wide-angle image.

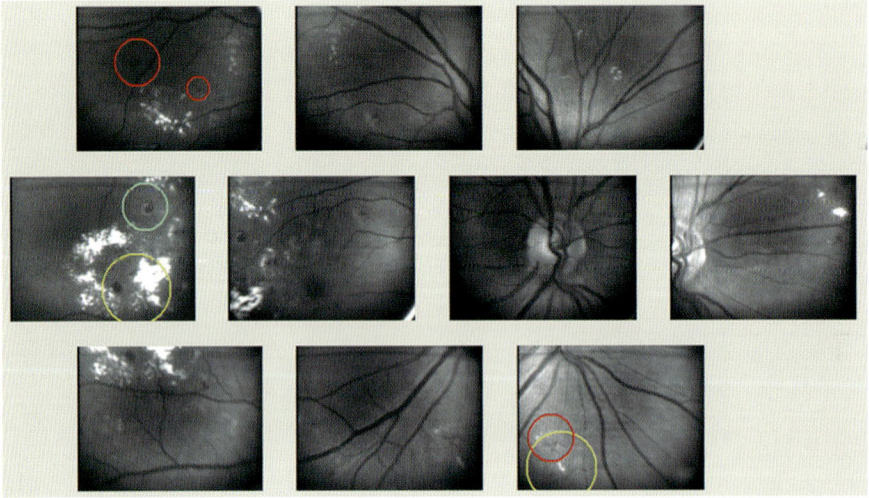

Figure 19.10. DigiScope images. (Source: Image courtesy of Ingrid Zimmer-Galler, MD.)

The DigiScope (EyeTel-Imaging Centerville, VA) captures multiple retinal fields with a black-and-white digital video camera, revealing about a 50-degree field to screen for diabetic retinopathy (Fig. 19.10) [38].

ARIS (Automated Retinal Imaging System) was introduced in 2004 by Visual Pathways Incorporated. The system utilizes automatic alignment and eye tracking to automatically acquire constant-base stereo images in multiple wavelengths, including near infrared, red and green (Fig. 19.11). Computer voice prompts assist the patient in looking in the appropriate direction. Prompts are available in different languages.

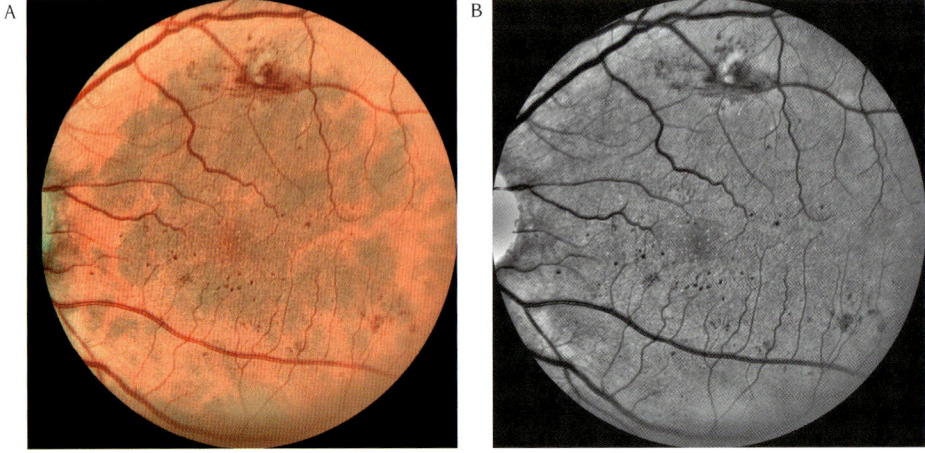

Figure 19.11. ARIS™ (Automated Retinal Imaging System) images. (A) One member of a combined color stereo pair. (B) One member of a red-free stereo pair. (Source: Image courtesy of Visual Pathways Incorporated.)

Brown and associates [39] compared the sensitivity of optical coherence tomography (OCT) to CLBM in the identification of macular edema from diabetic retinopathy. Ninety-five patients (172 eyes) were enrolled consecutively. Excellent agreement was found between the two methods when foveal thickness was within normal limits (<200 microns) or moderately increased (>300 microns). Agreement was poor when retinal thickness was minimal (201–300 microns), suggesting that OCT is more sensitive than clinical examination at identifying mild macular edema. Sanchez-Tocino and associates [40] found that OCT was able to identify early macular edema prior to the development of CSME. OCT might be a useful supplementary tool in a telemedicine program for evaluating macular edema.

Neubauer and colleagues [41] compared routine ophthalmologic examinations to tele-screening images captured with a retinal thickness analyzer (RTA) in 31 consecutive eyes with diabetic retinopathy. The RTA images were graded by three independent and masked graders. RTA images were found to be sensitive (mean = 93%) in the identification of macular edema but less specific (58–96%) than clinical examination. Although the results of this study show promise in the identification of macular edema, further validation is needed if a RTA is to be used as part of a telemedicine system.

PRACTICE RECOMMENDATIONS

The American Telemedicine Association (ATA), the ATA Ocular Telehealth Special Interest Group, and the United States National Institute of Standards and Technology Working Group met in 2003 to discuss current diabetic retinopathy telehealth clinical and administrative issues. Their work culminated with the publication of *Telehealth Practice Recommendations for Diabetic Retinopathy* [42]. The document provides recommendations for designing and implementing a diabetic retinopathy ocular telehealth program. Because of the diverse nature of health care at diabetic patient points of care, the *Recommendations* advise telemedicine programs to clearly define goals. Available resources may vary from one setting to another. Building a telemedicine program should match economics, human resources, and telecommunication infrastructures with community needs.

The *Recommendations* also advocate that every telemedicine program validate and define performance. It is recommended that programs compare kappa values for agreement of diagnosis, false positive and false negative readings, positive predictive value, negative predictive value, sensitivity and specificity of diagnosing levels of retinopathy and macular edema to ETDRS film photography. The *Recommendations* describe four categories of validation ranging from Category 1 (distinguishing between no or minimal DR and more than minimal DR) to Category 4 (distinguishing retinopathy levels equivalent to or exceeding ETDRS) (Table 19.2). The performance of a telemedicine program should be assessed as an integrated system, from image capture to image review—not as a series of individual processes or components. For example, the performance of two teleophthalmology systems based on identical fundus cameras equipped with identical 1280×1024 pixel resolution digital backs may not be the same if one system uses a 800×600 pixel video monitor for review while the other uses a 1280×1024 monitor.

Table 19.2. American Telemedicine Association's Recommended Validation Categories

ETDRS	1	2*	3*	4*
Level 10	No or Minimal DR	No or non-sight-threatening DR	No or questionable DR	Matches or exceeds ETDRS performance
Level 14/15	No or Minimal DR	No or non-sight-threatening DR	No or questionable DR	Matches or exceeds ETDRS performance
Level 20	Mild DR or worse	No or non-sight-threatening DR	Mild DR	Matches or exceeds ETDRS performance
Level 35	Mild DR or worse	No or non-sight-threatening DR	Mild DR	Matches or exceeds ETDRS performance
Level 43	Mild DR or worse	No or non-sight-threatening DR	Moderate DR	Matches or exceeds ETDRS performance
Level 47	Mild DR or worse	No or non-sight-threatening DR	Moderate DR	Matches or exceeds ETDRS performance
Level 53	Mild DR or worse	Sight-threatening DR	Severe DR	Matches or exceeds ETDRS performance
Level 61	Mild DR or worse	Sight-threatening DR	Proliferative DR	Matches or exceeds ETDRS performance
Level 65	Mild DR or worse	Sight-threatening DR	Proliferative DR	Matches or exceeds ETDRS performance
Level 71	Mild DR or worse	Sight-threatening DR	Proliferative DR	Matches or exceeds ETDRS performance
Level 90	Cannot grade	Cannot grade	Cannot grade	

* category able to detect clinically significant macula edema.
ETDRS = Early Treatment Diabetic Retinopathy Study; DR = diabetic retinopathy

The *Telehealth Practice Recommendations for Diabetic Retinopathy* also specifies qualifications and responsibilities for personnel and recommends that programs include quality assurance policies and procedures to monitor system performance. The *Recommendations* acknowledge that diabetic patients be aware that teleophthalmology examination of the retina, while substituting for a traditional face-to-face dilated retinal evaluation, is not a replacement for a comprehensive eye examination. The document notes, A comprehensive eye examination by a qualified provider continues to be essential.... A licensed eye care provider with expertise in evaluation and management of diabetic retinopathy should oversee image evaluation and ultimately be responsible for diagnoses.

CONSIDERATIONS IN IMPLEMENTING A TELEMEDICINE PROGRAM

Resources that societies have or are willing to devote to medical care vary by community and by country. Implementing a telemedicine system may be hindered by legal issues, limited acceptance of telemedicine by local health care professionals and payers, lack of funding for new technology and equipment, limited training of associated health care personnel, physician remuneration, computer network charges and maintenance, and other factors. The cost of implementing a telemedicine program to detect retinopathy should consider all resources needed to build and run the program, including resources to manage diabetic retinopathy once identified.

A number of factors should be considered when initially planning a diabetic retinopathy telemedicine program. Among these are [43]:

- The number of diabetic patients in the population being considered for the program
- The percentage of patients evaluated for retinopathy without teleophthalmology
- The percentage of patients who would be evaluated if teleophthalmology was implemented

Careful consideration of technology should precede implementation of any telemedicine system. Technological considerations include:

- System compliance with relevant health information guidelines and requirements such as HIPPA (Health Insurance Portability and Accountability Act)
- Archiving health information and images
- Expected lifespan of the archival media
- DICOM (Digital Imaging and Communications in Medicine) compliance
- HL7 (Health Level 7) compliance
- Network and/or Web access security such as two-factor authentication, encryption and/or passwords

Once a diabetic retinopathy telemedicine system is up and running, general factors to consider in administering and sustaining the program include:

- Patient convenience
- Appropriate referral of patients evaluated by telemedicine
- Assessment quality
- Quality control

Not all diabetic retinopathy telemedicine systems require sensitivity in detecting all levels of retinopathy. Sensitivity requirements can vary depending on resources available to clinicians and patients. For example, a diabetic patient living in a remote location without access to eye care may need a highly sensitive evaluation to screen for retinopathy requiring treatment. This telemedicine system should be able to identify levels of retinopathy including severe nonproliferative, proliferative, and clinically significant macular edema stages. In addition, the system should be sensitive and specific enough to allow follow-up after treatment. In an urban environment, where distance to specialist care is not a barrier, a community may be better served by a system with only enough sensitivity to identify patients without diabetic retinopathy. Each program should define goals and set clinically acceptable operating points.

Networked telemedicine systems offer potential advantages over stand-alone systems. New software can be downloaded and installed and network servers updated. Web, intranets, and private networks allow use of inexpensive, browser-compliant computers to access telemedicine systems instead of expensive, dedicated workstations. Hardware independence also allows various cameras, operating systems, and other technologies to coexist, providing maximum flexibility to customize systems to local needs. Web-based systems allow instant and simultaneous access to registered users almost anywhere in the world. The development of DICOM standards for ophthalmology will facilitate the transfer of electronic information between different medical devices and components while maintaining data integrity [44].

EMERGING TECHNOLOGY

The use of digital imaging and the growing availability of clinical information in digital form are spurring the development of computer-aided detection and diagnosis for various medical conditions. Potential advantages of automated image analysis and detection include increased efficiency, improved consistency and reliability of interpretation, enhanced accuracy and objective quantification of pathology, and reduction of inter-observer variability [45]. Mammography computer-aided diagnosis (CAD) received FDA approval in 2002 [46]. Studies have shown a 19% increase in cancer detection using CAD [47]. Computer-aided diagnosis for multi-detector computed tomography (MDCT) of pulmonary nodules received approval in July, 2004 [48]. CAD is also being developed in other areas of radiology including detection of polyps in virtual colonoscopy scans, pulmonary nodules and other lung interstitial diseases on chest radiographs, brain lesions on CT and MRI brain scans, and prostate lesions.

Diabetic retinopathy's distinct characteristics can be used by computer algorithms to detect and analyze disease. Microaneurysms' circular features or the high intensity and edge sharpness of hard exudates are relatively easy for computers to identify. Hard exudates in the macula and their proximity to the central macula serve as surrogate markers for macular edema. Microaneurysm quantity is a surrogate measure of diabetic retinopathy severity [49,50]. For these reasons, microaneurysms and hard exudates are logical diabetic retinal lesions for automatic analysis investigation. Neovascularization, unfortunately, is not. Because neovascularization is less frequent, appears in various forms, and has borders that are often indistinct, neovascularization is harder to detect automatically.

Hipewell investigated automated detection of microaneurysms in digital red-free photographs as a diabetic retinopathy screening tool. The study of 925 subjects achieved a sensitivity of 85% and specificity of 76% in the detection of subjects with retinopathy. Two EURODIAB 50-degree fields per eye were analyzed per subject using 1024×1024 pixel, 8-bit images [51].

Another group investigated automated detection of red lesions (microaneurysm and retinal hemorrhage) in photos [52]. This 2003 study analyzed 35 mm slides, 60-degree images digitized at 1350 dpi and 12 bits per color channel. The 137-patient photograph study correctly identified 90% of patients with retinopathy and 81% without retinopathy. By adjusting visibility threshold, their algorithm adapts to different screening priorities: high-sensitivity identification for diabetic retinopathy or high-specificity identification for absence of retinopathy [53]. White lesion detection algorithms for hard exudates have also been studied. [54,55]

A recent intelligent image analysis study to detect retinopathy by looking for exudates, hemorrhages and/or microaneurysms showed 84% sensitivity and 64%

specificity [56]. Another study found 90.5% sensitivity and 67.4% specificity in the detection of technical failures or diabetic retinopathy [57].

Another promising image analysis approach applied to the automated diagnosis of diabetic retinopathy is content-based image retrieval. Investigators have used pictorial content to retrieve related images from large database collections to predict disease presence and severity [58].

In general, automated detection processes include:

Image Processing
1. Pre-processing of images to enhance contrast
2. Identification of optic disc, retinal vessels, and fovea
3. Identification of bright pathology lesions (hard exudates) and dark pathology lesions (hemorrhages/microaneurysms)
4. Extraction of pathology features via size, shape, hue, and intensity

Classification
1. Identification of each lesion as a true lesion or noise (using an *artificial neural network*)
2. Identification of each image and patient as without retinopathy or with retinopathy according to the presence or absence of lesions (based on *mathematical rules*)

Although no automated detection of diabetic retinopathy program is yet approved by the FDA, substantial progress is being made. It is likely that using computers to semi-automatically distinguish images with pathology will eventually become an integral part of evaluating diabetic retinopathy.

Investigations of other computer-assisted tools are also underway. Image enhancement algorithms to maximize suboptimal contrast from uneven illumination or retinal pigmentation variation among individuals are being developed. These algorithms are designed to maximize image quality, decreasing the number of unreadable images. Computer tools for annotating and quantifying pathology are also increasingly available. Digital images embedded with metadata such as patient information, eye/retina characteristics, and digital image specifications offer new possibilities in specialist monitoring and managing diabetic retinopathy through telemedicine.

IMAGINING THE FUTURE

Today's telemedicine technological requirements are being developed and limitations studied through investigative applications and validation research. New standards and protocols for telemedicine technology will accelerate the future use of telemedicine, as will scientific evidence supporting clinical and cost effectiveness.

Diabetic retinopathy is a leading cause of blindness worldwide. Telemedicine offers new methods of health care delivery that can facilitate the goal of all diabetic patients having access to eye care. It may also prove to be the most cost-effective and efficacious solution for mass screening people with diabetes. In countries with socialized medicine programs or single health care payers, cost savings associated with telemedicine have allowed the early development and implementation of telemedicine programs. In other countries, the introduction of diabetic retinopathy telemedicine fee codes or other remuneration for physicians should provide further incentives for expansion.

Within the next 10 years, we expect diabetic retinopathy telemedicine systems to be in place throughout the United States and most of the developed world. Systems will utilize multi-field, digital retinal photography, with or without pupil dilation. Images will be graded utilizing ETDRS, modified ETDRS, or entirely new standards specific to digital imagery.

Technology, of course, does not stand still. Within 20 years, we expect systems will detect diabetic retinopathy more accurately than current seven-field, stereoscopic, film photography. Telemedicine technology will be portable, inexpensive, accurate, and widely available. It will rely on computer algorithms to detect and identify treatable diabetic retinopathy. And if a cure for diabetes is found, telemedicine may play the pivotal role in eliminating the last vestiges of this blinding disease.

SUMMARY FOR THE CLINICIAN

- Telemedicine is being integrated into many aspects of health care
- Telemedicine for diabetic retinopathy protocols and equipment may vary, but all are targeted to early identification of the disease
- An eye care specialist continues to be responsible for diabetic retinopathy identified through telemedicine

Telemedicine Pros
- Patient convenience
- Extends health care resources and specialists
- Potential increase in quality consistency
- Potential increase in patient referral efficiency

Telemedicine Cons
- Not a substitute for comprehensive eye examination
- Technology investment required
- Specialized training and/or new support personnel required
- New compliance protocols associated with computer systems sharing patient information

REFERENCES

1. Bonow RO, Gheorghiade M. The diabetes epidemic: a national and global crisis. *Am J Med.* 2004;116(Suppl 5A):2S–10S.
2. Wild S, Roglic G, Green A, Sicree R, King H. Global prevalence of diabetes: estimates for the year 2000 and projections for 2030. *Diabetes Care.* 2004;27:1047–1053.
3. The Diabetic Retinopathy Study Research Group. Four risk factors for severe visual loss in diabetic retinopathy. The third report from the Diabetic Retinopathy Study. *Arch Ophthalmol.* 1979;97:654–655.

4. Early Treatment Diabetic Retinopathy Study Research Group. Photocoagulation for diabetic macular edema. Early Treatment Diabetic Retinopathy Study report number 1. *Arch Ophthalmol*. 1985;103:1796–1806.

5. Javitt JC, Aiello LP. Cost-effectiveness of detecting and treating diabetic retinopathy. *Ann Intern Med*. 1996;124:164–169.

6. Lairson DR, Pugh JA, Kapadia AS, Lorimor RJ, Jacobson J, Velez R. Cost-effectiveness of alternative methods for diabetic retinopathy screening. *Diabetes Care*. 1992;15:1369–1377.

7. Bashshur RL, Mandil SH, Shannon GW. Telemedicine/telehealth: an international perspective. Executive summary. *Telemed J E Health*. 2002;8:95–107.

8. The Diabetic Retinopathy Study Research Group. Preliminary report on effects of photocoagulation therapy. *Am J Ophthalmol*. 1976;81:383–396.

9. Save Sight Institute Telemedicine. Available at: http://www.eye.usyd.edu.au/service/telemedicine.html. 2004. Accessed March 18, 2009.

10. Harper CA, Livingston PM, Wood C, et al. Screening for diabetic retinopathy using a non-mydriatic retinal camera in rural Victoria. *Aust N Z J Ophthalmol*. 1998;26:117–121.

11. Lee SJ, McCarty CA, Taylor HR, Keeffe JE. Costs of mobile screening for diabetic retinopathy: a practical framework for rural populations. *Aust J Rural Health*. 2001;9:186–192.

12. Mak DB, Plant AJ, McAllister I. Screening for diabetic retinopathy in remote Australia: a program description and evaluation of a devolved model. *Aust J Rural Health*. 2003;11:224–230.

13. Constable IJ, Yogesan K, Eikelboom R, Barry C, Cuypers M. Fred Hollows lecture: digital screening for eye disease. *Clin Experiment Ophthalmol*. 2000;28:129–132.

14. Tennant MT, Greve MD, Rudnisky CJ, Hillson TR, Hinz BJ. Identification of diabetic retinopathy by stereoscopic digital imaging via teleophthalmology: a comparison to slide film. *Can J Ophthalmol*. 2001;36:187–196.

15. Tennant MT, Rudnisky CJ, Hinz BJ, MacDonald IM, Greve MD. Tele-ophthalmology via stereoscopic digital imaging: a pilot project. *Diabetes Technol Ther*. 2000;2:583–587.

16. Boucher MC, Gresset JA, Angioi K, Olivier S. Effectiveness and safety of screening for diabetic retinopathy with two nonmydriatic digital images compared with the seven standard stereoscopic photographic fields. *Can J Ophthalmol*. 2003;38:557–568.

17. Maberley D, Cruess AF, Barile G, Slakter J. Digital photographic screening for diabetic retinopathy in the James Bay Cree. *Ophthalmic Epidemiol*. 2002;9:169–178.

18. Maberley D, Walker H, Koushik A, Cruess A. Screening for diabetic retinopathy in James Bay, Ontario: a cost-effectiveness analysis. *CMAJ*. 2003;168:160–164.

19. Fransen SR, Leonard-Martin TC, Feuer WJ, Hildebrand PL. Clinical evaluation of patients with diabetic retinopathy: accuracy of the Inoveon diabetic retinopathy-3DT system. *Ophthalmology*. 2002;109:595–601.

20. Bursell SE, Cavallerano JD, Cavallerano AA, et al. Stereo nonmydriatic digital-video color retinal imaging compared with Early Treatment Diabetic Retinopathy Study seven standard field 35-mm stereo color photos for determining level of diabetic retinopathy. *Ophthalmology*. 2001;108:572–585.

21. Zimmer-Galler I, Zeimer R. Results of implementation of the DigiScope for diabetic retinopathy assessment in the primary care environment. *Telemed J E Health*. 2006;12:89–98.

22. Henricsson M, Karlsson C, Ekholm L, et al. Colour slides or digital photography in diabetes screening—a comparison. *Acta Ophthalmol Scand.* 2000;78:164–168.

23. Henricsson M, Nystrom L, Blohme G, et al. The incidence of retinopathy 10 years after diagnosis in young adult people with diabetes: results from the nationwide population-based Diabetes Incidence Study in Sweden (DISS). *Diabetes Care.* 2003;26:349–354.

24. Younis N, Broadbent DM, James M, Harding SP, Vora JP. Current status of screening for diabetic retinopathy in the UK. *Diabet Med.* 2002;19(Suppl 4):44–49.

25. Gloucestershire Diabetic Eye Screening Project (Diabetic Eye Screening). Available at: http://www.tcis.port.ac.uk/jsp/search/activity.jsp?project=861. Accessed March 18, 2009.

26. Schneider S, Aldington SJ, Kohner EM, et al. Quality assurance for diabetic retinopathy telescreening. *Diabet Med.* 2005;22:794–802.

27. Massin P, Chabouis A, Erginay A, et al. OPHDIAT: a telemedical network screening system for diabetic retinopathy in the Ile-de-France. *Diabetes Metab.* 2008;34:227–234.

28. Beck RW, Moke PS, Turpin AH, et al. A computerized method of visual acuity testing: adaptation of the early treatment of diabetic retinopathy study testing protocol. *Am J Ophthalmol.* 2003;135:194–205.

29. Klein R, Klein BE, Moss SE, Cruickshanks KJ. The Wisconsin Epidemiologic Study of Diabetic Retinopathy: XVII. The 14-year incidence and progression of diabetic retinopathy and associated risk factors in type 1 diabetes. *Ophthalmology.* 1998;105:1801–1815.

30. Diabetic Retinopathy Study. Report Number 6. Design, methods, and baseline results. Report Number 7. A modification of the Airlie House classification of diabetic retinopathy. *Invest Ophthalmol Vis Sci.* 1981;21:1–226.

31. Early Treatment Diabetic Retinopathy Study Research Group. Grading diabetic retinopathy from stereoscopic color fundus photographs—an extension of the modified Airlie House classification. ETDRS report number 10. *Ophthalmology.* 1991;98:786–806.

32. Massin P, Erginay A, Ben Mehidi A, et al. Evaluation of a new non-mydriatic digital camera for detection of diabetic retinopathy. *Diabet Med.* 2003;20:635–641.

33. Lin DY, Blumenkranz MS, Brothers RJ, Grosvenor DM. The sensitivity and specificity of single-field nonmydriatic monochromatic digital fundus photography with remote image interpretation for diabetic retinopathy screening: a comparison with ophthalmoscopy and standardized mydriatic color photography. *Am J Ophthalmol.* 2002;134:204–213.

34. Rudnisky CJ, Hinz BJ, Tennant MT, de Leon AR, Greve MD. High-resolution stereoscopic digital fundus photography versus contact lens biomicroscopy for the detection of clinically significant macular edema. *Ophthalmology.* 2002;109:267–274.

35. Kinyoun J, Barton F, Fisher M, Hubbard L, Aiello L, Ferris F, 3rd. Detection of diabetic macular edema. Ophthalmoscopy versus photography—Early Treatment Diabetic Retinopathy Study Report Number 5. The ETDRS Research Group. *Ophthalmology.* 1989;96:746–750; discussion 750–751.

36. Harding TM, Florez-Arango JF, Hubbard LD, et al. Mosaic of wide-angle digital color images vs. ETDRS stereo 7-field images for grading diabetic retinopathy severity. (Abstract). *Invest Ophthalmol Vis Sci.* 2008;49:2737.

37. Friberg TR, Pandya A, Eller AW. Non-mydriatic panoramic fundus imaging using a non-contact scanning laser-based system. *Ophthalmic Surg Lasers Imaging.* 2003;34:488–497.

38. Zeimer R, Zou S, Meeder T, Quinn K, Vitale S. A fundus camera dedicated to the screening of diabetic retinopathy in the primary-care physician's office. *Invest Ophthalmol Vis Sci.* 2002;43:1581–1587.

39. Brown JC, Solomon SD, Bressler SB, Schachat AP, DiBernardo C, Bressler NM. Detection of diabetic foveal edema: contact lens biomicroscopy compared with optical coherence tomography. *Arch Ophthalmol.* 2004;122:330–335.

40. Sanchez-Tocino H, Alvarez-Vidal A, Maldonado MJ, Moreno-Montanes J, Garcia-Layana A. Retinal thickness study with optical coherence tomography in patients with diabetes. *Invest Ophthalmol Vis Sci.* 2002;43:1588–1594.

41. Neubauer AS, Welge-Lussen UC, Thiel MJ, et al. Tele-screening for diabetic retinopathy with the retinal thickness analyzer. *Diabetes Care.* 2003;26:2890–2897.

42. The American Telemedicine Association, Ocular Telehealth Special Interest Group, and the National Institute of Standards and Technology Working Group. Telehealth practice recommendations of diabetic retinopathy. *Telemed J E Health.* 2004;10:469–482.

43. Aoki N, Dunn K, Fukui T, Beck JR, Schull WJ, Li HK. Cost-effectiveness analysis of telemedicine to evaluate diabetic retinopathy in a prison population. *Diabetes Care.* 2004;27:1095–1101.

44. Kuzmak PM, Dayhoff RE. The use of digital imaging and communications in medicine (DICOM) in the integration of imaging into the electronic patient record at the Department of Veterans Affairs. *J Digit Imaging.* 2000;13:133–137.

45. Sharp PF, Olson J, Strachan F, et al. The value of digital imaging in diabetic retinopathy. *Health Technol Assess.* 2003;7:1–119.

46. 2001 mammography and CAD survey. *Radiol Manage.* 2001;23:56.

47. Freer TW, Ulissey MJ. Screening mammography with computer-aided detection: prospective study of 12,860 patients in a community breast center. *Radiology.* 2001;220:781–786.

48. FDA approves software system to help detect lung nodules. Available at: http://www.fda.gov/bbs/topics/answers/2004/ANS01300.html. Accessed March 18. 2009.

49. Kohner EM, Sleightholm M. Does microaneurysm count reflect severity of early diabetic retinopathy? *Ophthalmology.* 1986;93:586–589.

50. Klein R, Meuer SM, Moss SE, Klein BE. Retinal microaneurysm counts and 10-year progression of diabetic retinopathy. *Arch Ophthalmol.* 1995;113:1386–1391.

51. Hipwell JH, Strachan F, Olson JA, McHardy KC, Sharp PF, Forrester JV. Automated detection of microaneurysms in digital red-free photographs: a diabetic retinopathy screening tool. *Diabet Med.* 2000;17:588–594.

52. Larsen M, Godt J, Larsen N, et al. Automated detection of fundus photographic red lesions in diabetic retinopathy. *Invest Ophthalmol Vis Sci.* 2003;44:761–766.

53. Larsen N, Godt J, Grunkin M, Lund-Andersen H, Larsen M. Automated detection of diabetic retinopathy in a fundus photographic screening population. *Invest Ophthalmol Vis Sci.* 2003;44:767–771.

54. Niemeijer M, van Ginneken B, Russell SR, et al. Automated detection and differentiation of drusen, exudates, and cotton-wool spots in digital color fundus photographs for diabetic retinopathy diagnosis. *Invest Ophthalmol Vis Sci.* 2007;48:2260–2267.

55. Sopharak A, Uyyanonvara B, Barman, S et al. Automatic detection of diabetic retinopathy exudates from non-dilated retinal images using mathematical morphology methods. *Comput Med Imaging Graph.* 2008;32:720–727.

56. Abràmoff MD, Niemeijer M, Suttorp-Schulten MS, et al. Evaluation of a system for automatic detection of diabetic retinopathy from color fundus photographs in a large population of patients with diabetes. *Diabetes Care.* 2008;31:193–198.

57. Philip S, Fleming AD, Goatman KA, et al. The efficacy of automated disease/no disease grading for diabetic retinopathy in a systematic screening programme. *Br J Ophthalmol.* 2007;91:1512–1517.

58. Chaum E, Karnowski TP, Govindasamy VP, et al. Automated diagnosis of retinopathy by content-based image retrieval. *Retina.* 2008;28:1463–1477.

20

Future Therapies: Rationale for and Status of Antiangiogenic and Antipermeability Interventions

NIGEL H. TIMOTHY, MD,

JENNIFER K. SUN, MD,

JERRY CAVALLERANO, OD, PhD,

THOMAS W. GARDNER, MD, MS,

AND LLOYD PAUL AIELLO, MD, PhD

CORE MESSAGES

- There have been several recent advances in the development and clinical testing of antiangiogenic and antipermeability agents for treatment of diabetic retinopathy.
- Unresolved challenges include method of drug delivery, duration of action, and potential toxicity.

*E*ven though diabetic retinopathy remains the leading cause of new-onset blindness among working-age Americans [1,2], dramatic advances have been achieved over the preceding three decades in our understanding of the natural history of the disease, and in the development and validation of therapeutic modalities. Current therapeutic approaches permit remarkable reductions in diabetes-associated visual loss if timely and appropriate ocular care is provided to all patients with diabetes [3]. Nevertheless, laser photocoagulation, the mainstay of current therapy, is an inherently destructive procedure that obliterates areas of retina in an effort to preserve vision. Thus, the treatment itself can be associated with significant side effects and visual loss can progress despite timely and appropriate therapy.

Recent diverse investigations into the many models, mechanisms, and mediators of diabetic retinopathy have clearly supported the potential of novel therapies targeted specifically against key molecular steps in the development of diabetic complications. These rationally designed therapies have the theoretical potential to provide equivalent or improved efficacy, but without the side effects inherent with current treatment modalities. Numerous recent advances in this rapidly evolving field have led to nondestructive and even orally administered interventional approaches for which clinical trial data are now available or will be forthcoming shortly. In the past seven years, some of these approaches have already been evaluated success-fully in initial clinical investigations while others are currently in phase II and III multicenter randomized clinical trials. This chapter describes the rationale behind these modalities, the available supporting experimental data and the developmental status of these strategies, and speculates on their future clinical implications.

HISTORICAL PERSPECTIVES

Diabetic retinopathy is a complex, multifactorial process that occurs as a result of the similarly complex systemic disease diabetes mellitus. Numerous mechanisms explaining the clinical manifestations of diabetic retinopathy have been inves-tigated, including evaluation of the polyol pathway [4], advanced glycation end products [5], oxidative stress [6], protein kinase C signaling [7], cell–matrix and cell–cell interactions [8], retinal blood flow abnormalities [9], and the role of pro-tein factors with angiogenic, inflammatory, and vasopermeability characteristics. A comprehensive discussion of each of these areas is beyond the scope of this chap-ter, although inhibition of any of these pathways might at least partially ameliorate the ocular complications of diabetes.

Diabetic retinopathy is the prototypical example of a group of disorders known as ischemic retinopathies that are characterized by areas of poor retinal perfu-sion and the development of intraocular angiogenesis and retinal edema. Recent

Table 20.1. Disorders Associated with Intraocular Neovascularization

Retinal Neovascularization	*Choroidal Neovascularization*
Diabetic Mellitus	Age-related Macular Degeneration (wet)
Retinopathy of Prematurity	Ocular Histoplasmosis Syndrome
Retinal Vein Occlusion	Myopic Degeneration
Retinal Arteriolar Occlusion	Angioid Streaks
Retinal Embolization	Best's Disease
Sickle Cell Disease	Serpiginous Chorioretinopathy
Radiation Retinopathy	Choroidal Melanoma
Chronic Retinal Detachment	Choroidal Nevus
Eales' Disease	Others
Ocular Ischemic Syndrome	
Familial Exudative Vitreoretinopathy	
Hyperviscosity Syndromes	
Sarcoidosis	
Retinal Vasculitis	
Pars Planitis	
Incontinentia Pigmenti	
Familial Telangiectasia	
Retinitis Pigmentosa	
Others	

investigations have expanded our understanding of the angiogenic factors and molecular mechanisms that mediate vessel growth and excessive retinal permeability. As a result, numerous targets for the pharmacologic inhibition of diabetic retinopathy have become apparent. Agents directed against some of these targets have already been evaluated in controlled clinical trials, and many are now being investigated in late preclinical and phase I to III clinical trials. The development of growth factor inhibitors serves as a useful paradigm for the discussion of future therapies for diabetic retinopathy and is the principle focus of this chapter.

Table 20.1 presents a partial list of the ischemic retinopathies and several other disorders associated with intraocular neovascularization. These conditions share numerous clinical features (Fig. 20.1).

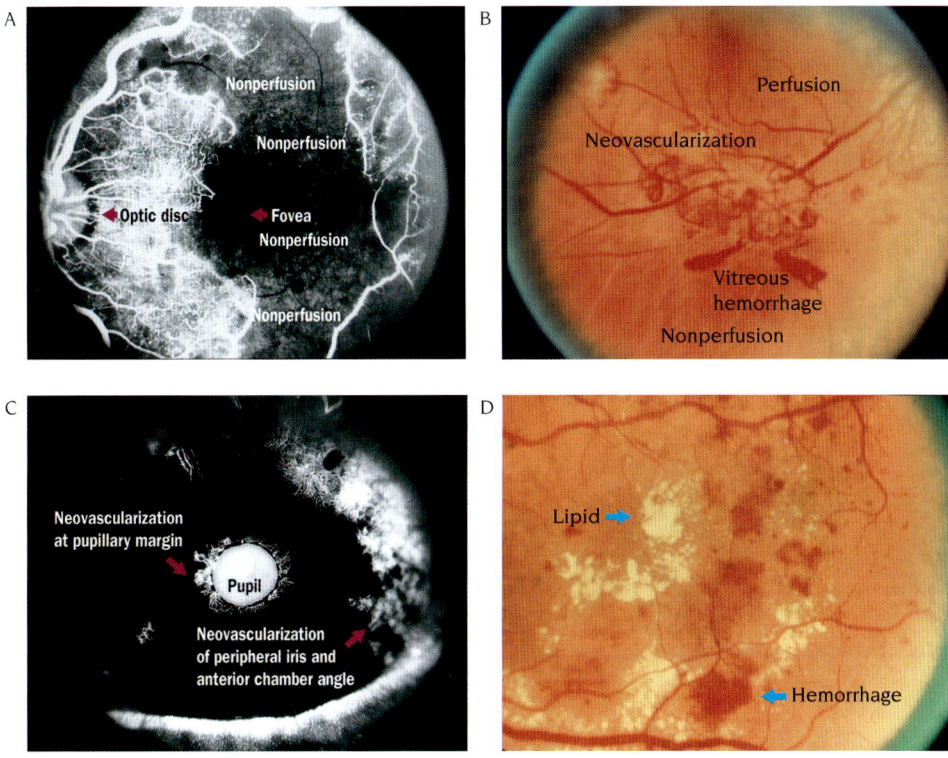

Figure 20.1. Clinical features shared by diabetic retinopathy and other ischemic retinopathies. The ischemic retinopathies share numerous clinical features. Neovascularization is often preceded by the development of areas of nonperfusion as demonstrated by the fluorescein angiogram of a patient with diabetes in (A). Retinal neovascularization often occurs at the border of perfused and nonperfused zones (B). These vessels are fragile and often bleed resulting in vitreous hemorrhage. Neovascularization can also occur at distant sites in the retina or anteriorly at the pupillary margin and the anterior chamber angle. (C) is an iris angiogram of a diabetic patient with iris neovascularization at both the pupillary margin and the anterior chamber angle. The retinal vessels often exhibit increased vascular permeability with transudation of serum components and deposition of lipid (D). (Source: A, C and D courtesy Wilmer Ophthalmological Institute, also Eye Complications of Diabetes for the Atlas of Clinical Endocrinology, volume 2, entitled Diabetes, edited by C. Ronald Kahn, M.D. Panel B is Early Treatment Diabetic Retinopathy Study standard photograph 7 from the modified Airlie House symposium [167].)

Neovascularization is often preceded by, and spatially associated with, retinal capillary nonperfusion (Fig. 20.1A) [10,11]. Retinal neovascularization commonly arises at the border of perfused and nonperfused zones and is universally associated with increased vessel permeability (Fig. 20.1B and 20.1D) [12,13]. The extent of capillary nonperfusion is correlated with the risk of neovascularization [14], and the risk of iris neovascularization (Fig. 20.1C) is increased following cataract surgery in patients with diabetic retinopathy, presumably due to removal of the lens and its barrier function [15]. Nearly six decades ago, it was recognized that the clinical attributes shared by intraocular neovascular disorders suggested a common mechanism for the development of the neovascular and permeability complications in conditions such as diabetic retinopathy [16].

THE GROWTH FACTOR HYPOTHESIS OF NEOVASCULARIZATION

On the basis of these observations, Dr. I.C. Michaelson proposed the growth factor hypothesis of intraocular neovascularization in 1948 [16]. This theory was later refined by his student Ashton and others [16,17]. In essence, the hypothesis states that ischemia of the retina induces a factor or factors capable of stimulating the growth of new vessels (Fig. 20.2). These factors must meet several criteria in order to account completely for the classic clinical observations (Table 20.2). The factors should be freely diffusible within the eye to account for neovascularization of retinal tissue both adjacent to, and distant from, areas of nonperfusion, including neovascularization of the iris and anterior chamber angle. The factors should also be endothelial mitogens capable of inducing proliferation of

Table 20.2. Expected Attributes of a Major Growth Factor Mediator of Neovascularization in Diabetic Retinopathy

Attribute:	Rationale:
• Induced by ischemia	• Accounts for association of neovascularization with areas of retinal ischemia
• Produced by retinal cells	• Accounts for factor production from ischemic area
• Secreted and diffusible	• Accounts for both local factor effect and effects distant to areas of retinal ischemia
• Stimulates endothelial cell growth	• Accounts for endothelial cell growth during vasculogenesis
• Specific receptors on endothelial cells	• Accounts for mechanism by which factors can induce action in the endothelial cells
• Elevated with or before onset of neovascularization	• Necessary if factor is actually inducing the neovascularization
• Diminished with treated or quiescent neovascularization	• Expected if reduction of growth factor stimulus is responsible for neovascular regression
• Intraocular concentration is greater posteriorly than anteriorly within the eye	• Accounts for clearance of retinal-produced factor by diffusion down concentration gradient and removal through trabecular meshwork. Also accounts for neovascularization at the iris and anterior chamber angle

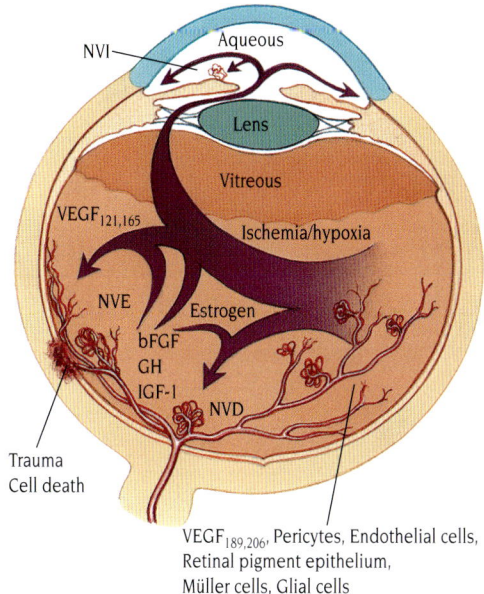

Figure 20.2. Schematic representation of the growth factor hypothesis of neovascularization. Growth factors such as Vascular endothelial growth factor (VEGF) produced by numerous retinal cells act locally within the retina or are free to diffuse through the vitreous down concentration gradients represented by the arrow width in the figure. The larger VEGF isoforms (VEGF$_{189,206}$) tend to be nondiffusible and act locally, while the shorter isoforms (VEGF$_{121,165}$) are freely diffusible within the eye. Because of their potential for diffusion, the growth factors can therefore elicit neovascularization at distant sites in the retina or on the iris and within the anterior chamber angle, where they are eventually cleared through the trabecular meshwork. Other factors such as basic fibroblast growth factor (bFGF), growth hormone (GH) and insulin like growth factor 1 (IGF-1) probably act as synergistic or mediating factors, respectively. Basic FGF release is increased by trauma and cell death. (Source: Adapted from Aiello [55], with permission.)

new vessels, their expression should be induced by retinal hypoxia, and retinal endothelial cells should possess receptors for these molecules to permit cellular responses. Intraocular concentrations that progressively decline more anteriorly within the eye would account for diffusion of a retinal-produced factor towards the trabecular meshwork for clearance and for neovascularization arising at the iris and anterior chamber angle. Finally, concentrations of a postulated contributory growth factor would be expected to increase during or just prior to periods of active intraocular neovascularization and to diminish when neovascularization becomes quiescent due to either natural progression of the disease or successful therapy.

The process of growth factor stimulation of intraocular neovascularization can be broken down into a series of stages presented schematically in Figure 20.3. Diabetes mellitus induces vascular damage to the retina through a variety of mechanisms resulting in vascular nonperfusion and retinal ischemia (Fig. 20.3A). These changes stimulate expression and secretion of the growth factors from a variety of retinal cells (Fig. 20.3B). The growth factors diffuse within the retina

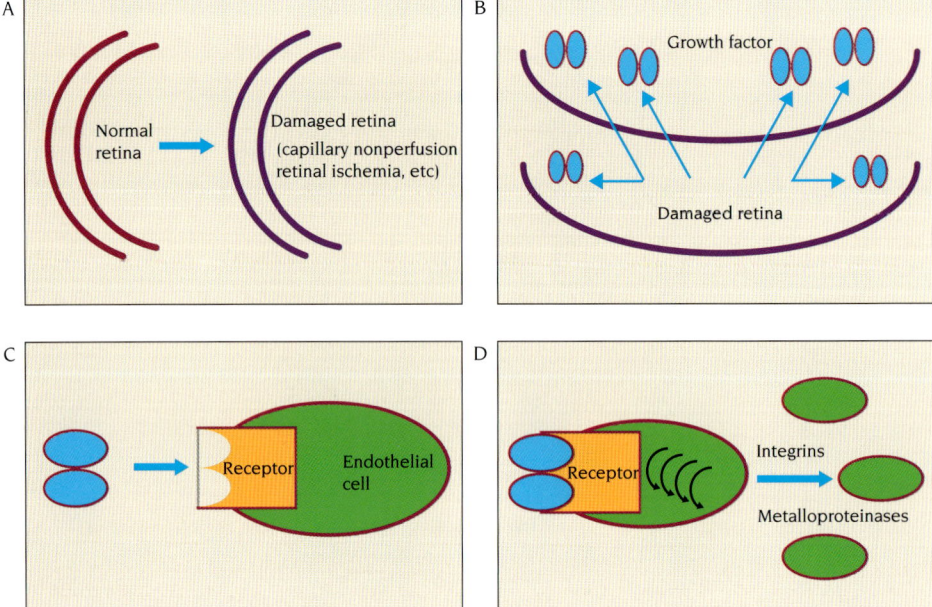

Figure 20.3. Schematic representation of the basic stages of growth factor induction of intraocular neovascularization. (A) Diabetes results in retinal damage by a diverse array of mechanisms, eventually leading to capillary nonperfusion and retinal ischemia. (B) The damaged retina induces the production of growth factors (light blue) such as Vascular endothelial growth factor (VEGF, partially as a result of) retinal ischemia. The factors are free to act within the retina or to diffuse into the vitreous. (C) The growth factors bind to high affinity receptors (orange) on retinal endothelial cells (green). (D) The receptor binding induces a series of intracellular reactions (black arrows), producing an intracellular signal transduction cascade, that ultimately results in endothelial cell proliferation via a complex mechanism. This cascade likely involves numerous mediators such as the integrins and metalloproteases. (Source: Adapted from Aiello [53], with permission.)

and eye, eventually binding to high-affinity receptors on retinal endothelial cells (Fig. 20.3C). Receptor binding induces a series of intracellular biochemical reactions that transmit the signals for cell replication and increased permeability (Fig. 20.3D). Each of these steps is a potential target site for a therapeutic intervention. Once the intracellular signal is transmitted, the regulation of cell proliferation involves numerous other molecules such as the integrins [8,18], angiostatin [19], endostatin [20], and metalloendoproteases [21–23], all of which may be exploited as targets in the development of therapeutic modalities for diabetic retinopathy.

CANDIDATE MEDIATORS OF INTRAOCULAR NEOVASCULARIZATION IN DIABETIC RETINOPATHY

Numerous growth factors have been evaluated as possible mediators of intraocular neovascularization. Some of those that have received the most extensive investigation with regard to diabetic retinopathy are listed in Table 20.3. These include basic fibroblast growth factor (bFGF), growth hormone (GH), insulin-like growth

Table 20.3. Candidate Mediators of Diabetic Retinopathy

Growth Factor or Mediating Molecule	Principal Effect on Angiogenesis in Diabetic Retinopathy		
	Primary	Permissive	Synergistic[*]
Growth Hormone	Unlikely	Probable	Unlikely
IGF-1	Unlikely	Probable	Unlikely
Basic FGF	Unlikely	Probable	Probable
VEGF	Probable	Unknown	Probable
HGF	Possible	Unknown	Unknown
Integrins	Possible	Probable	Unlikely
Angiostatin, Endostatin	Unlikely	Possible Inhibitor	Unlikely
Erythropoietin	Probable	Unknown	Probable
PEDF	Unlikely	Probable inhibitor	Unlikely
Angiopoietin-1[**]	Unlikely	Probable inhibitor	Unknown
Angiopoietin-2[††]	Unlikely	Possible	Possible
Tumor necrosis factor-alpha[‡‡]	Unlikely	Possible	Unknown
Matrix metalloproteinases[‡‡,***]	Possible	Possible	Unknown
Hypoxia inducible factor[††]	Possible	Probable	Unknown

[*]Synergistic with regard to the action of other growth factors. Therapies combining inhibitors of multiple factors would be expected to have increased effectiveness over single agents in most cases.

Watanabe D, Suzuma K, Matsui S, et al. Erythropoietin as a retinal angiogenic factor in proliferative diabetic retinopathy. N Engl J Med. 2005;353:782–792.

‡Zhang SX, Wang JJ, Gao G, Parke K, Ma JX. Pigment epithelium-derived factor downregulates vascular endothelial growth factor (VEGF) expression and inhibits VEGF–VEGF receptor 2 binding in diabetic retinopathy. J Mol Endocrinol. August 2006;37(1):1–12.

**Tsujikawa A, Qin W, QaumT, et al. Suppression of diabetic retinopathy with angiopoietin-1. Am J Pathol. 2002;160:1683–1693.

††Oh H, Takagi H, Suzuma K, Otani A, Matsumura M, Honda Y. Hypoxia and vascular endothelial growth factor selectively up-regulate angiopoietin-2 in bovine microvascular endothelial cells. J Biol Chem. 1999;274:15732–15739.

‡‡Majka S, McGuire PG, Das A. Regulation of matrix metalloproteinase expression by tumor necrosis factor in a murine model of retinal neovascularization. Invest Ophthalmol Vis Sci. January 2002;43(1):260–266.

***Ottino P, Finley J, Rojo E, et al. Hypoxia activates matrix metalloproteinase expression and the VEGF system in monkey choroid-retinal endothelial cells: involvement of cytosolic phospholipase A2 activity. Mol Vis. May 17, 2004;10:341–350.

††Arjamaa O, Nikinmaa M. Oxygen-dependent diseases in the retina: role of hypoxia-inducible factors. Exp Eye Res. September 2006;83(3):473–483.

factor 1 (IGF-1), and vascular endothelial growth factor (VEGF). There are three main actions by which growth factors could influence the development of diabetic retinopathy: (1) as a primary stimulator of angiogenesis, (2) as permissive agents allowing other primary stimulators to induce neovascularization but not primarily stimulating the neovascularization themselves, and/or (3) in a synergistic fashion to increase the angiogenic ability of other factors. The current understanding of the relative role of each growth factor is indicated in Table 20.3.

Basic fibroblast growth factor (bFGF) is tightly associated with the extracellular matrix [24,25] and induces endothelial cell proliferation, migration, and vasculogenesis; however, bFGF is not secreted from cells by classical mechanisms [26–28]. Basic FGF has been demonstrated in the retina [29] but no causal relationship with neovascularization has been identified [30]. Studies using transgenic mice have demonstrated that bFGF is neither necessary nor sufficient to induce retinal neovascularization [31]; however, bFGF is synergistic in its mitogenic activity with VEGF [32–34] and probably acts primarily as a potentiating factor in diabetic retinopathy.

Growth hormone (GH) and its biological mediator *insulin-like growth factor 1* (IGF-1 [35] have been studied for many years as possible mediators of diabetic retinopathy [36,37], leading to a brief period during which hypophysectomy was employed as a treatment for diabetic retinopathy [38]. Although GH/IGF-1 reduction was modestly correlated with regression of proliferative diabetic retinopathy, this treatment was also associated with extensive morbidity in diabetic patients and was abandoned with the advent of laser photocoagulation. Studies using an inhibitor of GH secretion and transgenic mice expressing a GH antagonist suggest that GH plays a permissive role in ischemia-induced retinopathy rather than acting as the principal stimulating factor [39].

As a result of these data, somatostatin analogs that are GH release inhibitors have been investigated in human clinical studies for their potential ability to ameliorate diabetic retinopathy. Initial results from a small case series were encouraging with proliferative disease stabilizing or regressing in all patients [40]. In another study of 46 eyes in which the somatostatin analogue octreotride was used to treat patients with severe nonproliferative diabetic retinopathy (NPDR) and early proliferative diabetic retinopathy (PDR), the incidence of disease progression was decreased from 42% to 27%. In addition, only one of the octreotride treated patients required scatter (panretinal) photocoagulation compared to nine of the control patients [41]. Boehm et al. further noted that octreotride significantly reduced the risk of vitreous hemorrhage in 19 patients with severe PDR [42]. However, in a study of 25 patients with PDR who were administered a growth hormone receptor antagonist for a period of 12 weeks, retinopathy progressed in nine (36%) patients and was unchanged in 16 (64%) [43]. On the basis of two phase III multicenter clinical trials that failed to demonstrate significant efficacy of intramuscular injection of octreotride to treat PDR, further development of this compound for diabetic retinopathy was terminated [44,45].

Hepatocyte growth factor (HGF), a protein with mitogenic and motogenic effects on many nonocular cells, is elevated in the vitreous of patients with PDR [46]. Concentrations of HGF are highest in patients with active PDR and are reduced when proliferation is quiescent. The extent of HGF's role in mediating PDR remains unknown. *Angiostatin* [19] and *endostatin* [20] are endogenous inhibitors of angiogenesis known to be involved in tumor suppression. Their significance in diabetic retinopathy is also currently unknown.

The role of *vascular endothelial growth factor* (VEGF) in the eye has been evaluated extensively for nearly 15 years. Considerable evidence now suggests that VEGF mediates a significant portion of the retinal neovascularization and excessive vascular permeability associated with PDR. VEGF appears involved in the development of macular edema as well, although it may not be the sole mediator of this condition. VEGF may also play a role in the development and progression of NPDR as discussed below.

VEGF is a highly conserved protein with potent vasopermeability [47] and angiogenic activities [48,49]. Five different forms of VEGF exist in the human [50]. The smaller two isoforms ($VEGF_{121,165}$) are freely diffusible, whereas the larger molecules ($VEGF_{189,206}$) are nondiffusible because they are bound to cell surfaces and basement membranes (Fig. 20.2). The general functions of VEGF in ocular disease have been reviewed extensively [51–54] and will not be described in detail here; however, it is important to note that VEGF possesses all of the attributes predicted for a major mediator of neovascularization in diabetic retinopathy as detailed in Table 20.2. VEGF is an endothelial cell mitogen [55], whose expression is increased up to thiry-fold by hypoxia in various cultured ocular cells [56]. At least two types of high-affinity VEGF receptors exist [55,57,58], and numerous retinal cells express VEGF including pigment epithelial cells [53], pericytes, endothelial cells, glial cells, Müller cells, and ganglion cells [56,59]. Thus, the actions of VEGF within the eye are highly consistent with the classic paradigm for growth factor mediation of diabetic retinopathy.

CLINICAL ASSOCIATIONS OF VEGF IN PROLIFERATIVE DIABETIC RETINOPATHY

The in vivo evidence associating VEGF with retinal and iris neovascularization in PDR is extensive. Ischemia-induced retinal neovascularization that histologically resembles diabetic retinopathy is observed in neonatal rats [60], cats [61], and mice (Fig. 20.4A and 20.4B) [62,63]. Similar iris neovascularization is observed in the primate [64]. VEGF expression is correlated temporally with neovascularization in these models, increasing just prior to the onset of neovascularization (Fig. 20.4C and 20.4D) [60,61,63–66] and slowly declining as neovascularization regresses.

VEGF concentrations are elevated in the vitreous of patients with PDR as compared with vitreous from those with nonproliferative disease or quiescent proliferative disease or from nondiabetic patients without neovascularization as shown in Figure 20.5 [67–69]. Intravitreal VEGF concentrations are also correlated with diabetic macular edema [70,71] and are elevated when neovascularization is present owing to other ischemic retinal disorders such as central retinal vein occlusion. Neovascular membranes obtained from patients with PDR demonstrate near-universal VEGF expression (Fig. 20.6) [72–78].

VEGF INDUCTION OF DIABETES-LIKE RETINAL PATHOLOGY

VEGF in Proliferative Diabetic Retinopathy. Several findings support the conclusion that VEGF can induce intraocular neovascularization resembling that of PDR. Growth of retinal microvascular endothelial cells in culture is increased by

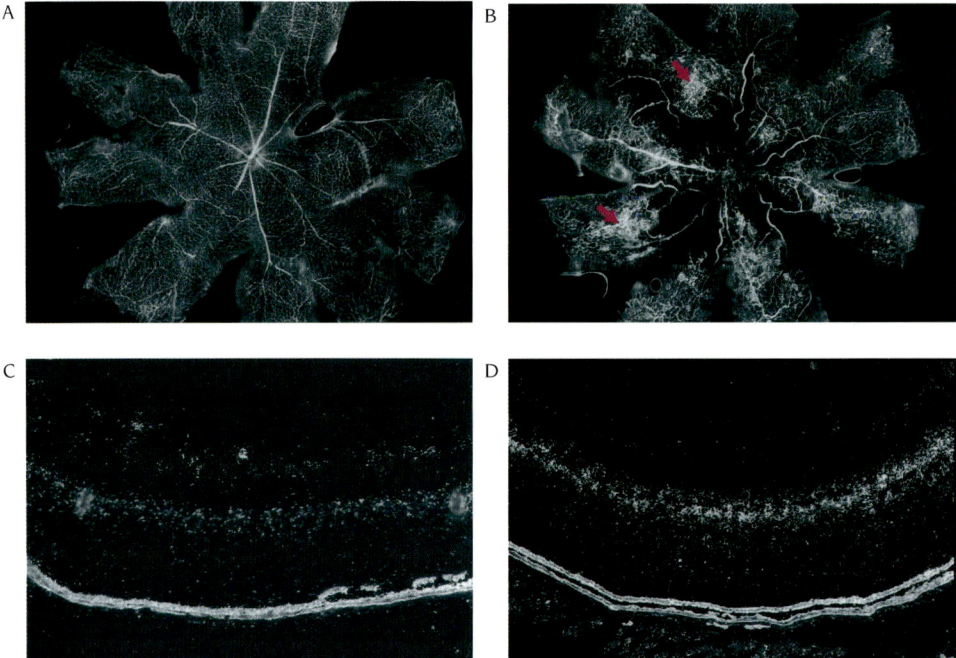

Figure 20.4. Correlation of Vascular endothelial growth factor (VEGF) expression and ischemic retinal neovascularization in the mouse. When neonatal mice are exposed to alterations in oxygen concentration for several days, the normal vascularization pattern of the retina (A) is altered resulting in areas of nonperfusion (B, dark central areas) and retinal neovascularization (arrows) that closely resemble those observed in diabetic retinopathy. The production of VEGF is low under normal conditions (C) and markedly increased just prior to the onset of retinal neovascularization (D). (A and B) are retinal flat mounts from neonatal mice whose vasculature has been perfused with a fluorescein-conjugated dextran for visualization purposes. (C and D) are cross sectional *in situ* hybridization photomicrographs showing location of VEGF production. (Source: Adapted from Pierce et al. [65], with permission.)

concentrations of VEGF well below those found in eyes with active PDR (Fig. 20.7) [55]. Repetitive intravitreal injections of recombinant human VEGF are sufficient to produce iris neovascularization in a nonhuman primate leading to ectropion uveae and neovascular glaucoma (Fig. 20.8) [79]. Similarly, transgenic mice that overexpress VEGF in the photoreceptors develop extensive intraretinal neovascularization as confirmed by light, confocal and standard fluorescent microscopy (Fig. 20.9) [80,81]. Interestingly, the vessels originate from the retinal vasculature and grow toward the VEGF-producing photoreceptor layer, a morphology that is inverted compared to that observed in diabetic retinopathy.

Although increased permeability can occur in the absence of neovascularization as is often observed with diabetic macular edema (Fig. 20.1D), a universal characteristic of retinal proliferation is a corresponding increase in vascular permeability. VEGF is a very effective inducer of permeability, being 50,000 times more potent in the dermal microvasculature than is histamine in this regard [82]. In the eye, extravasated albumin and VEGF immunoreactivity co-localize [83,84]. Repeated injections of high concentrations of VEGF result in leakage of fluorescein dye from

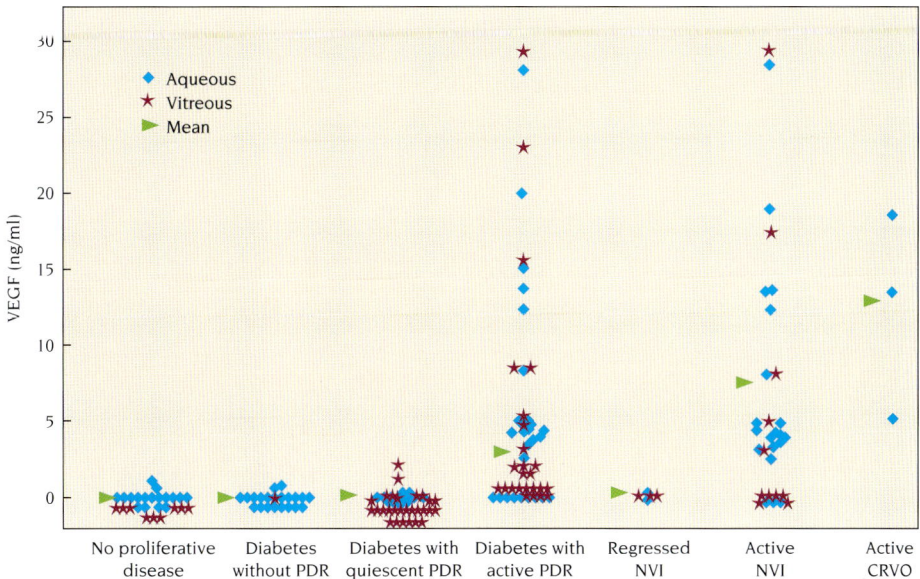

Figure 20.5. Intraocular Vascular endothelial growth factor (VEGF) concentrations are elevated in active proliferative diabetic retinopathy. Aqueous (yellow), vitreous (red) and mean (green) VEGF concentrations are indicated for patients with the particular clinical findings noted under each group of values. Values of 0 or below denote concentrations below the detection limit of the assay (50 pg/mL). NV, neovascularization; CRVO, central retinal vein occlusion (Source: From Aiello et al. [67], with permission.)

the retinal vessels [85]. Use of vitreous fluorophotometry and albumin-sized fluorescein-conjugated dextrans has demonstrated that physiologic concentrations of VEGF administered intravitreally induce a rapid three- to five-fold increase in retinal vascular permeability in rats (Fig. 20.10) [86]. Data suggest that VEGF may exert its effects of retinal vascular permeability by altering tight junction proteins such as occludin and adherens junction proteins such as VE-cadherin [87,88].

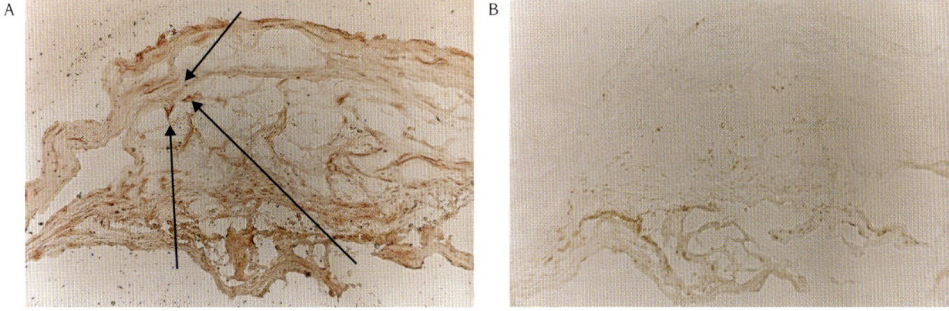

Figure 20.6. Neovascular membranes from patients with proliferative diabetic retinopathy express high levels of Vascular endothelial growth factor (VEGF). Immunohistochemical localization of VEGF protein in membranes derived from patients with proliferative diabetic retinopathy show markedly increased VEGF expression (A, arrows). Negative control staining of an adjacent serial section showed minimal nonspecific staining (B). (Source: Adapted from Frank et al. [75], with permission.).

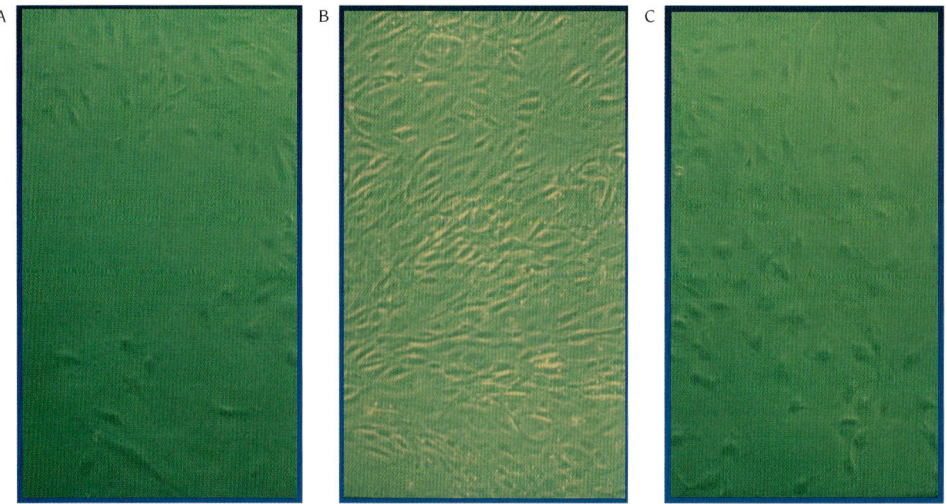

Figure 20.7. Vascular endothelial growth factor (VEGF) stimulates retinal endothelial cell growth. Photographs show retinal microvascular endothelial cells in culture 4 days after plating each group at the same density. Cell number in the presence of physiologic concentration of VEGF (VEGF) is markedly higher than in control cells (no VEGF). Cells grown in the presence of VEGF but with the addition of the PKCβ isoform-selective inhibitor LY333531 proliferated at approximately the same rate as the control cells [54].

VEGF in Nonproliferative Diabetic Retinopathy. Although the role of VEGF in NPDR is less firmly established than it is in proliferative disease, recent findings suggest that it may be an important factor in the development of earlier stages of diabetic retinopathy. One study observing VEGF expression in normal and diabetic human retinas did not detect any difference in VEGF mRNA or protein [89]; however, this study evaluated postmortem eyes where effects of hypoxia and time until

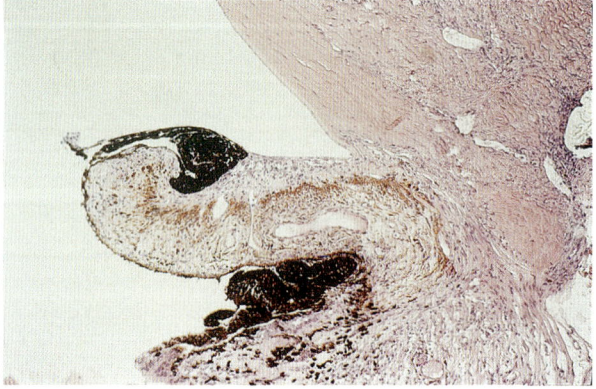

Figure 20.8. Intravitreal Vascular endothelial growth factor (VEGF) injections induce iris neovascularization and neovascular glaucoma. Repetitive intravitreal injections of high concentration of VEGF resulted in iris neovascularization, ectropion uveae, and trabecular meshwork scarring, findings similar to those of neovascular glaucoma from advanced proliferative diabetic retinopathy. (Source: Adapted from Tolentino et al. [79], with permission.)

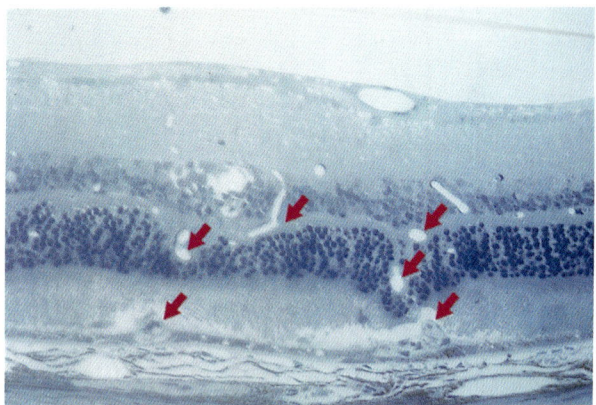

Figure 20.9. Transgenic expression of Vascular endothelial growth factor (VEGF) in the photoreceptors produces intraretinal neovascularization. Transgenic mice over-expressing VEGF in the photoreceptors demonstrated marked intraretinal neovascularization (arrows) that appeared to be proliferating toward the site of VEGF expression in the outer retina. (Source: Adapted from Okamoto et al. [81], with permission.)

tissue isolation can have significant effects. In contrast, an immunohistochemical evaluation of postmortem human eyes with NPDR, but without extensive retinal nonperfusion, demonstrated increased VEGF expression as compared with nondiabetic controls (Fig. 20.11) [90,91]. Repeated injections of high concentrations of VEGF into the normal nonhuman primate eye produce retinal changes resembling NPDR including vascular tortuosity, capillary abnormalities resembling microaneurysms, and leakage of fluorescein (Fig. 20.12) [85]. Intravitreal injections of physiologic concentrations of VEGF in rats alter retinal blood flow and venous caliber in the same manner as observed in diabetic patients with increasingly severe diabetic retinopathy [92]. Furthermore, diabetes accentuates the retina's response to VEGF as compared with nondiabetic animals. As shown in Figure 20.13, these data suggest that, even early in the course of diabetes, the retina may have both increased expression as well as an accentuated response to VEGF. Such expression and response could theoretically result in a positive feedback loop that might eventually induce enough retinal ischemia and VEGF expression to stimulate intraocular neovascularization. This hypothesis raises the intriguing possibility that inhibitors of VEGF action might prove beneficial not only for the neovascular and permeability complications of diabetes, but also as a prevention of retinopathy progression in the nonproliferative stages.

VEGF AS CAUSAL MEDIATOR OF ISCHEMIA-INDUCED RETINAL NEOVASCULARIZATION

Direct evidence that VEGF expression is necessary for ischemia-induced retinal and iris neovascularization in animals has been obtained using multiple different agents that inhibit VEGF. These originally included VEGF receptor chimeric proteins [93], neutralizing antibodies [94], and antisense phosphorothioate

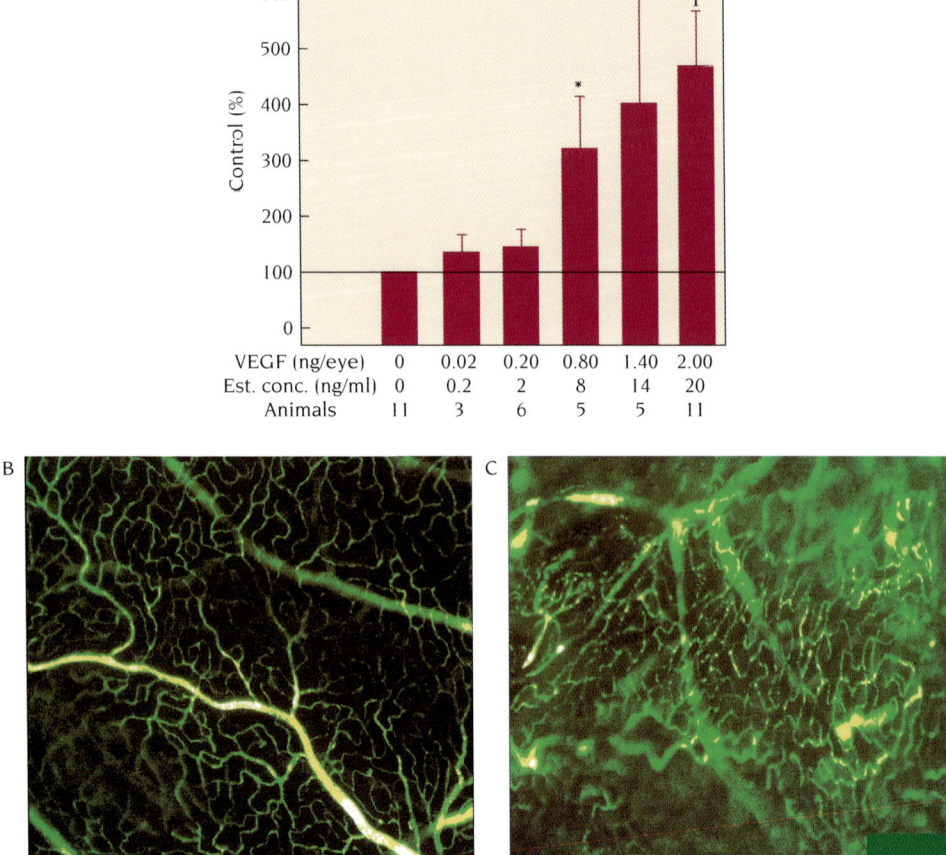

Figure 20.10. Vascular endothelial growth factor (VEGF) induces retinal vascular permeability. The ability of intravitreal injections of VEGF to induce retinal vascular permeability in rats was evaluated utilizing vitreous fluorophotometry (A). A dose-dependent five-fold increase in retinal vascular permeability was evident with physiologic concentrations of VEGF that were consistent with those observed in patients with active proliferative diabetic retinopathy (Fig. 20.5). The retinal vasculature was also perfused with a fluorescein-conjugated dextran approximately the size of albumin that is retained within the lumen of normal vessels. The normal retinal vessel architecture of an animal that received a control intravitreal injection is shown in (B). Note that the fluorescence is primarily retained within the vasculature. However, as shown in (C), intravitreal VEGF injection induced a readily apparent increase in vessel permeability to the fluorescent compound. (Source: Adapted from Aiello et al. [86], with permission.)

oligodeoxynucleotides [95]. These VEGF inhibitors suppressed ischemia-induced intraocular neovascularization by up to 77% in up to 100% of animals studied. The average magnitude of inhibition was approximately 50%. Similar results were obtained for iris neovascularization in primates [94] (Fig. 20.14A and 20.14B) and retinal neovascularization in mice (Fig. 20.14B and 20.14C) [93]. No toxicity

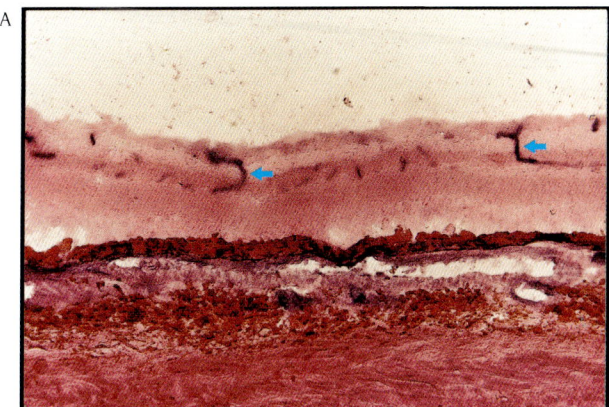

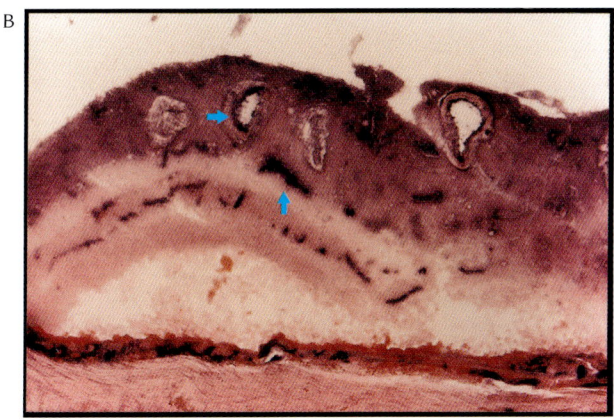

Figure 20.11. Vascular endothelial growth factor (VEGF) expression is increased in patients with nonproliferative diabetic retinopathy and minimal retinal ischemia. Immunohistochemical evaluation of VEGF protein was performed in patients with nonproliferative diabetic retinopathy without extensive areas of retinal nonprofusion. Increased VEGF expression (arrows) was observed in the periphery (A) and the macula (B). (Source: Adapted from Amin et al. [91], with permission.)

was evident by light microscopic evaluation in these relatively short duration studies. As discussed earlier, VEGF over-expression in the photoreceptors of a transgenic mouse was sufficient to produce extensive retinal neovascularization (Fig. 20.9) [80,81]. These data demonstrate that, although the neovascular response is undoubtedly modulated by a wide variety of factors, VEGF appears necessary and sufficient to induce retinal and iris angiogenesis, particularly as a sequelae of the retinal ischemia characteristic of diabetic retinopathy. In addition, these findings strongly suggest that any agent that blocks VEGF action may result in a significant, although perhaps not a complete, reduction in intraocular neovascularization. However, early clinical studies as discussed below show remarkable sensitivity of PDR to anti-VEGF molecules with near-total resolution of neovascularization within 1 week of treatment [96–98]. In contrast, clinical impression is that the response of macular edema to anti-VEGF treatment may not be as sensitive or as complete.

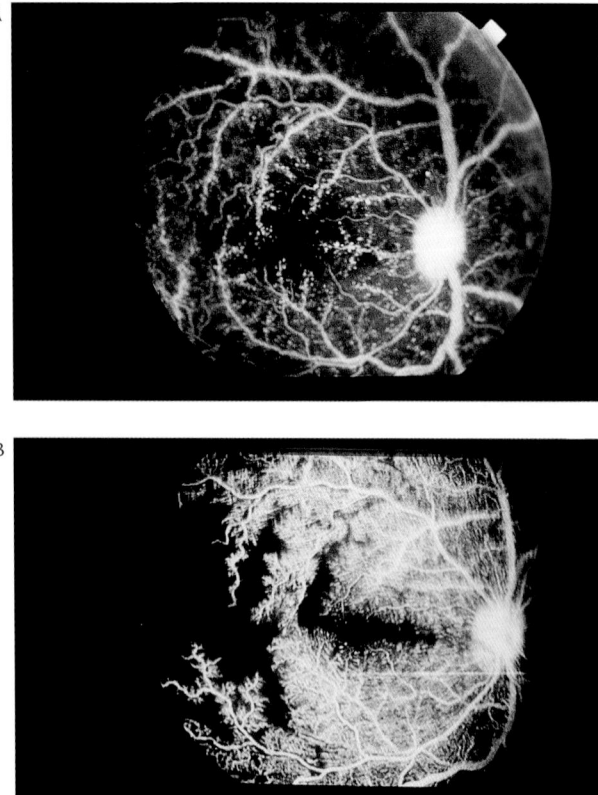

Figure 20.12. Intravitreal injection of Vascular endothelial growth factor (VEGF) into the nonhuman primate induces retinal changes resembling nonproliferative diabetic retinopathy. Repetitive intravitreal injections of VEGF into the normal primate eye resulted in vascular tortuosity and capillary abnormalities resembling microaneurysms (A). Increased VEGF dose resulted in capillary nonperfusion and retinal vascular leakage of fluorescein (B). (Source: Adapted from Tolentino et al. [85], with permission.)

BASIC MECHANISMS AND TARGETS IN DIABETIC RETINOPATHY

The detailed biochemical mechanisms that underlie the intracellular processes permitting VEGF expression and signaling are becoming better understood. One important area, from a potential therapeutic standpoint, is the mechanism by which hypoxia increases VEGF expression. The endogenous nucleoside adenosine appears to serve an important role in this regard (Fig. 20.15) [99–103]. As demonstrated in Figure 20.15, hypoxia increases adenosine concentrations several-fold [99,101,102] by inhibiting an enzyme (adenosine kinase) that usually converts adenosine to adenosine monophospate (AMP) [104]. In retinal endothelial cells, the specific adenosine receptors that mediate the induction of VEGF expression are known. In addition, several of the molecules involved in the intracellular signaling of the adenosine stimulus have been identified and include adenyl cyclase and protein kinase A [103]. Adenosine receptors also work in concert with the VEGF receptor to increase endothelial cell migration and vessel formation [102].

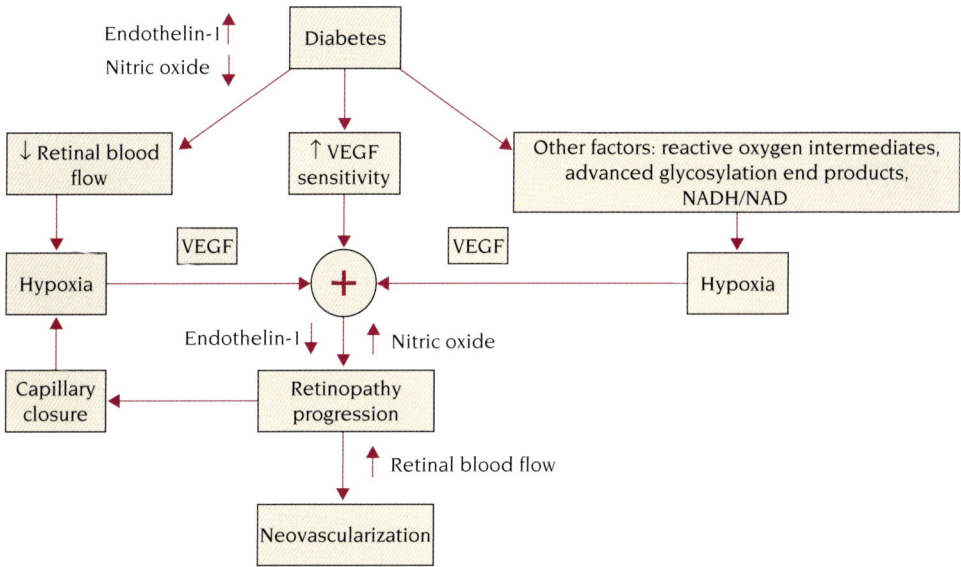

Figure 20.13. Theoretical mechanism by which Vascular endothelial growth factor (VEGF) may mediate the progression of nonproliferative diabetic retinopathy. In early diabetes, molecules such as ET-1 and NO reduce retinal blood flow. This combined with oxidative stress may produce an initial hypoxic stimulus for VEGF expression. The diabetic state further enhances retinal VEGF sensitivity, inducing the vascular abnormalities characteristic of nonproliferative diabetic retinopathy. A positive feedback loop occurs as the development of ischemic areas creates localized hypoxia and further stimulates VEGF production. The down-regulation of ET-1 and nitric oxide by VEGF further increases retinal blood flow as retinopathy advances. Once vascular damage results in extensive retinal ischemia, VEGF concentrations become high enough to induce intraocular neovascularization. ET-1, endothelin 1; NO, nitric oxide; RBF, retinal blood flow. (Source: Adapted from Clermont et al. [92], with permission.)

Thus, inhibition of adenosine or its receptors would be expected to suppress VEGF expression under hypoxic conditions and decrease subsequent vasculogenesis. Inhibitors of adenosine receptors do indeed have this action in cell culture suggesting that they might prove useful in the treatment of diabetic retinopathy [100–103]; however, more study is required to determine the actual clinical applicability of these agents.

Basic FGF (bFGF) was studied extensively as a probable mediator of angiogenesis in diabetic retinopathy until the transgenic mouse data discussed earlier made it unlikely that the induction of neovascularization is its primary role [31]. It should be noted, however, that the mitogenic actions of bFGF and VEGF are potently synergistic both in vivo [32] and in vitro [33,34]. The mechanism of this synergy has been partially elucidated. As shown in Figure 20.16, bFGF increases VEGF [105,106] and VEGF receptor 2 expression (kinase domain receptor [KDR], VEGFR2) [107]. VEGF activity is closely correlated with cellular KDR expression. Even under conditions where KDR expression is low and VEGF's stimulatory activity is minimal, bFGF dramatically increases KDR expression subsequently

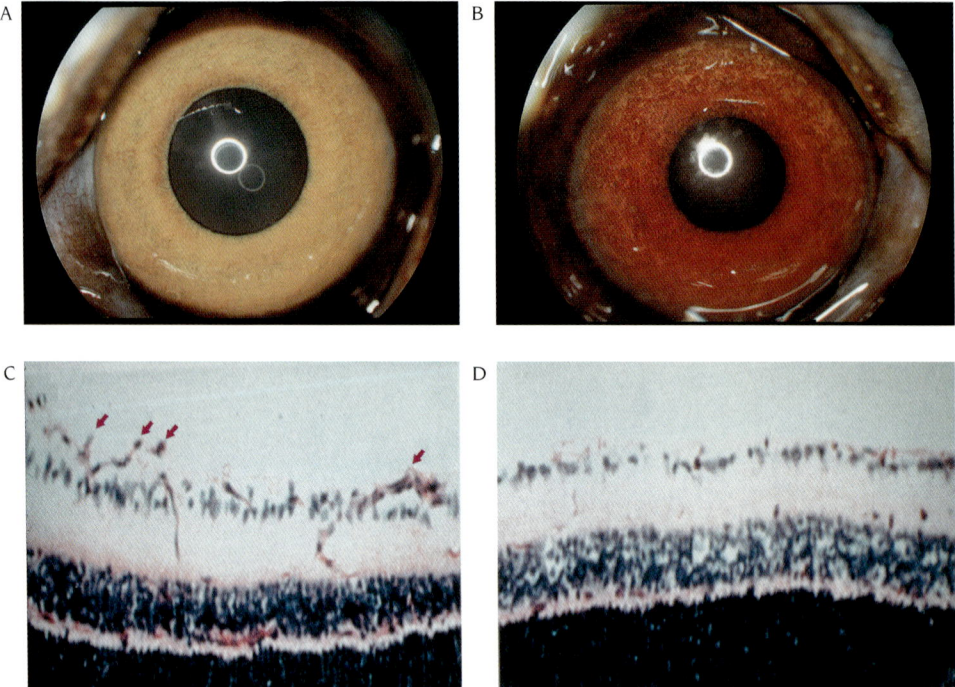

Figure 20.14. Inhibition of Vascular endothelial growth factor (VEGF) suppresses retinal ischemia-induced iris and retinal neovascularization. Retinal ischemia in the primate characteristically produces iris neovascularization while similar ischemia in the neonatal mouse produces retinal neovascularization. VEGF neutralizing antibodies injected into the vitreous of primates with retinal ischemia produced by laser-induced retinal vein occlusion resulted in marked suppression of the iris neovascularization (A, normal yellow iris color) that is normally observed in eyes not receiving the inhibitor (B, abnormal red iris color). Similarly, a VEGF chimeric receptor protein, which binds to VEGF and inhibits its action, was injected intravitreally into neonatal mice with retinal ischemia. These animals universally develop retinal neovascularization in the absence of VEGF inhibition (C, arrows). However, intravitreal injection of the VEGF receptor chimeric protein reduced retinal neovascularization as shown here in the contralateral eye of the same animal (D). (Source: A and B adapted from Adamis et al. [94], C and D adapted from Aiello et al. [93]; with permission.)

allowing VEGF to efficiently induce both mitogenesis and further KDR expression. Basic FGF's induction of VEGF receptor expression requires activation of PKC and MAP kinase. VEGF also increases both thrombin [108] and plasminogen activator expression [109], which can release bioactive bFGF from the extracellular matrix and further potentiate the response [110]. These data demonstrate that the VEGF receptor KDR is a critical regulating component of the VEGF pathway and suggest that compounds that inhibit its function or reduce its expression are likely to be effective inhibitors of neovascularization associated with diabetes. Indeed, this approach has already been proven successful in animals by suppressing angiogenesis, endothelial cell proliferation, tumor growth, tumor metastasis and cancer-associated mortality [95,111–117].

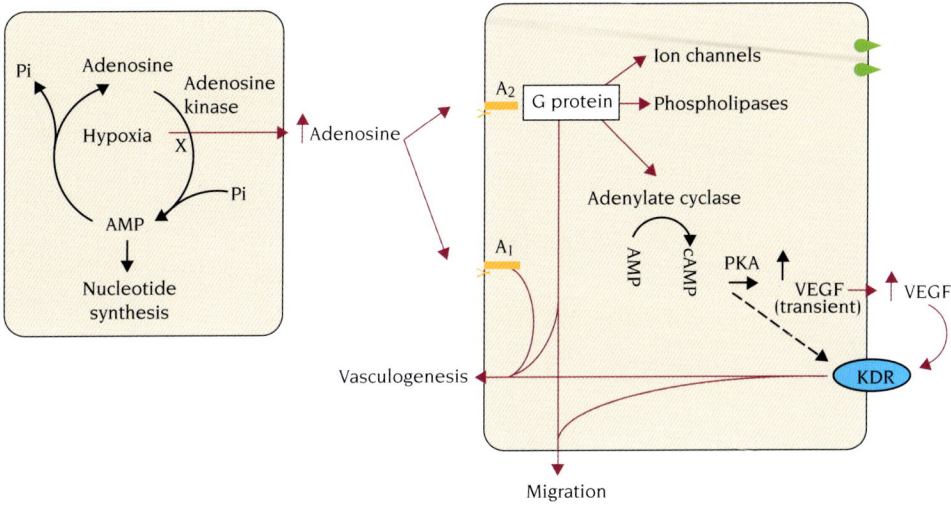

Figure 20.15. Role of adenosine in the hypoxic induction of Vascular endothelial growth factor (VEGF) expression in retinal cells. Hypoxia reduces activity of adenosine kinase (A. Kinase) resulting in increased release of adenosine that primarily binds to the A_2 receptor, activating adenylate cyclase through a G protein-coupled mechanism. The resulting increase in intracellular cAMP activates protein kinase A (PKA), ultimately resulting in increased expression of VEGF through as-yet unidentified mechanisms. Adenosine A_2 receptor activation also induces a transient decrease in VEGF receptor expression (KDR). Combined activation of both the adenosine A_2 receptor and KDR synergistically increased cell migration while contributions of both adenosine receptors and KDR result in a synergistic increase in vasculogenesis. Pi represents inorganic phosphate. (Source: Modified from Aiello LP, Hata Y. Molecular Mechanisms of Growth Factor Action in Diabetic Retinopathy. In *Current Opinion Endocrinology and Diabetes*. 1999; 6:146–156 and Aiello [53]; with permission.)

THE ROLE OF PKC IN DIABETIC RETINOPATHY

The hyperglycemia of diabetes mellitus results in numerous metabolic changes including increases in oxidative stress, polyol pathway flux, advanced glycation end products, and diacylglycerol. Although each of these alterations can elicit numerous biological effects, one of their shared outcomes is an activation of the enzyme protein kinase C (PKC) (Fig. 20.17). PKC is present in many body tissues and exists as numerous related, but structurally different, isoforms [7]. Different isoforms predominate in different body tissues and respond differently to various cytokines. In diabetes, PKC activation is observed in the tissues in which complications are most prevalent, including the retina, peripheral nerves, kidneys, and heart.

Within the eye, the β isoform of PKC is of particular interest. As discussed above, the hyperglycemia of diabetes is thought to induce considerable vascular dysfunction leading to retinal hypoxia and increased VEGF expression that subsequently mediates both intraocular neovascularization and increased vasopermeability (Fig. 20.18). Early in the course of diabetes, PKC-β is activated in the retina by the hyperglycemia-induced *de novo* synthesis of diacylglycerol, the physiologic activator of PKC [118]. This PKC activation appears to account for several biochemical

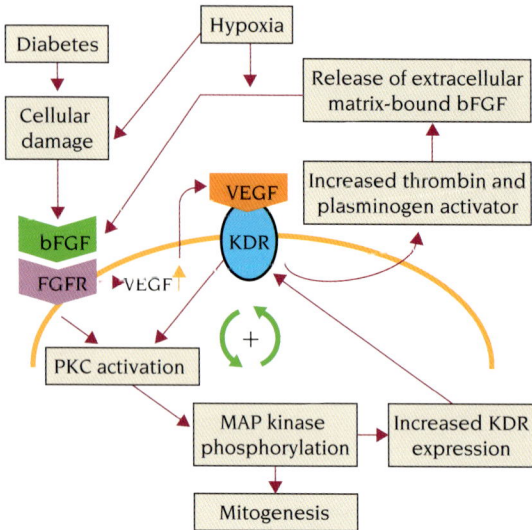

Figure 20.16. Possible mechanisms mediating the synergistic activities of Vascular endothelial growth factor (VEGF) and basic Fibroblast growth factor (bFGF). Both diabetes and hypoxia can result in cellular damage, which releases intracellular bFGF allowing binding to its receptors on the cell surface with subsequent activation of protein kinase C (PKC) and MAP kinase. MAP kinase activation results in mitogenesis and also increases VEGF receptor kinase domain receptor (KDR) expression. Under conditions where VEGF receptor KDR is limiting, VEGF may have little mitogenic effect. However, bFGF stimulation under these conditions increases KDR expression, subsequently permitting VEGF action. VEGF also activates the PKC and MAP kinase pathway, resulting in mitogenesis. In addition, VEGF increases thrombin and plasminogen activator, which release extracellular matrix-bound bFGF, further potentiating the response. (Source: From Aiello LP, Hata Y. Molecular Mechanisms of Growth Factor Action in Diabetic Retinopathy. In Current Opinion Endocrinology and Diabetes. 1999; 6:146–156.)

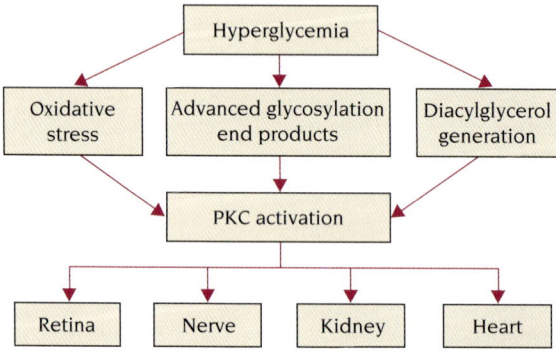

Figure 20.17. Diabetes-induced activation of protein kinase C (PKC). Hyperglycemia increases oxidative stress, diacylglycerol, and advanced glycosylation end product formation. All of these actions can ultimately result in PKC activation in the tissues primarily affected by diabetes: retina, nerve, kidney, and heart.

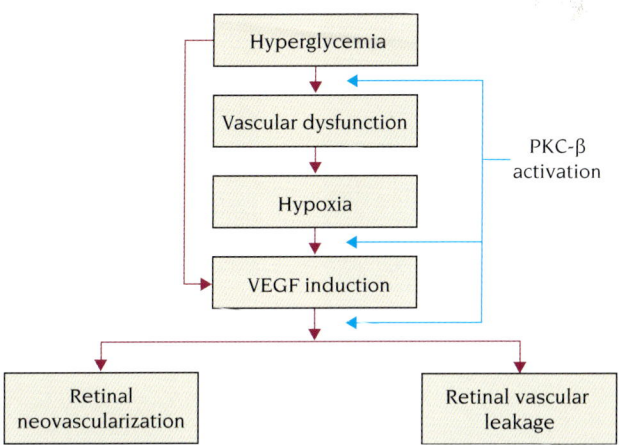

Figure 20.18. The role Protein kinase (PKC)-β in diabetic retinal complications. The hyperglycemia of diabetes induces vascular dysfunction leading to hypoxia and induction of Vascular endothelial growth factor (VEGF) expression. It is thought that VEGF mediates much of the retinal neovascularization and retinal vascular leakage characteristic of diabetic retinopathy. The activation of PKC occurs at multiple steps as indicated in the figure. Thus, inhibition of PKCβ would be expected to reduce hyperglycemia-induced retinal complications by acting at numerous locations along this pathway.

abnormalities associated with the diabetic state, presumably leading to progression of diabetic retinopathy.

PKC activation is a step in the hypoxic and hyperglycemic stimulation of VEGF expression [119,120] and in VEGF enhancement of endothelial cell survival [121]. Physiologic concentrations of VEGF induce rapid, dose-dependent increases in retinal PKC activity with translocation from the cytosolic (inactive) to the membranous (active) fraction [122]. In cell culture, VEGF-induced retinal endothelial cell growth is inhibited using the PKC-β inhibitor, ruboxistaurin (Fig. 20.7). Furthermore, oral ingestion of ruboxistaurin in pigs with laser-induced occlusion of the retinal veins suppresses the development of subsequent retinal neovascularization [123].

PKC-β activation is also required for VEGF to induce its permeability effects and to some degree its proliferative effects as well [78,111,112]. Both physiologic concentrations of VEGF and direct activation of PKC result in a rapid three- to five-fold increase in retinal vascular permeability in rats (Fig. 20.8) [86]. In this model, intravitreal and orally administered PKC-β inhibitor dramatically suppressed VEGF-induced permeability (Fig. 20.19A and 20.19B).

VEGF Inhibitors in Diabetic Retinopathy. As VEGF appears to be a primary mediator of several abnormalities in diabetes, clinical trials are currently evaluating VEGF inhibitors for treatment of diabetic retinal disease. Pegaptanib (Macugen, Eyetech Pharmaceuticals) is an aptamer with high affinity for only the VEGF$_{165}$ isoform and is FDA approved for the treatment of neovascular age-related macular degeneration (AMD) [124]. Recently, a Phase II trial of pegaptanib intravitreally injected every 6 weeks was completed [125]. Best-corrected visual acuity (VA), central retinal thickness as assessed by optical coherence tomography (OCT), and need for additional therapy with photocoagulation between weeks 12 and 36 were primary endpoints

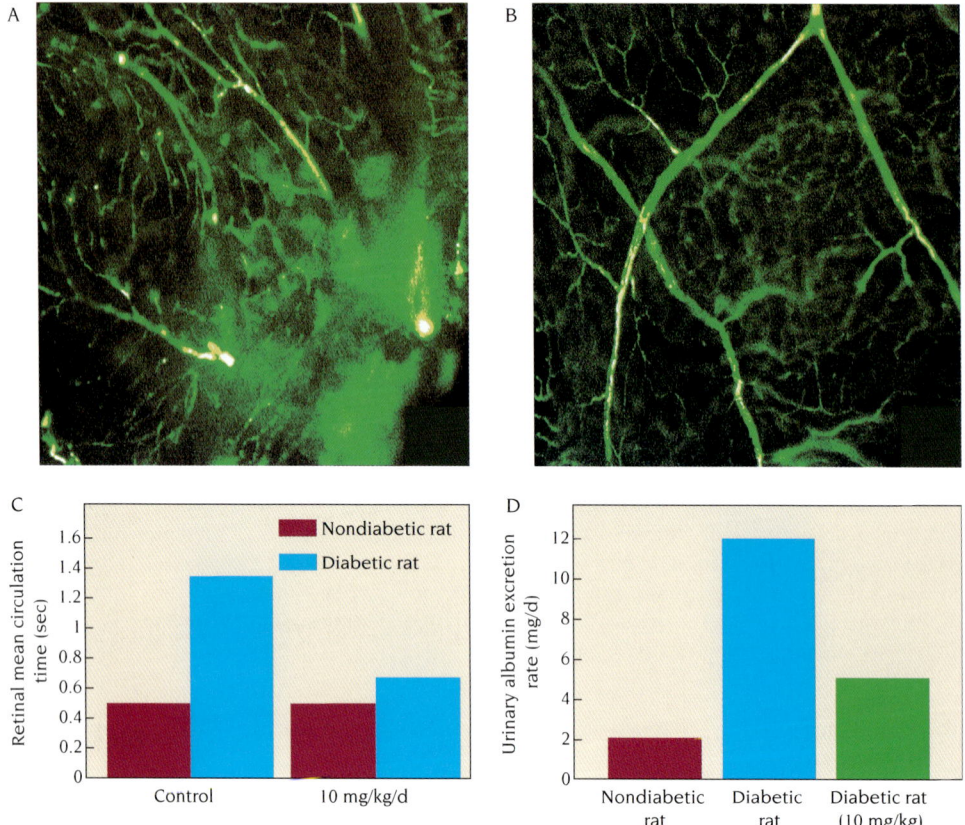

Figure 20.19. Protein kinase (PKC)-β inhibitor ruboxistaurin inhibits Vascular endothelial growth factor (VEGF)-induced retinal vascular permeability and ameliorates diabetes-induced retinal blood flow and renal abnormalities. Intravitreal injection of VEGF increases retinal vascular permeability in rats (see Fig. 20.8). Fluorescein-conjugated dextran of approximately the molecular weight of albumin becomes permeable through the retinal vasculature after the addition of physiologic concentrations of VEGF (A; see also Fig. 20.8C). However, when rats are fed a diet containing the PKCβ selective inhibitor ruboxistaurin for one week prior to evaluation, the ability of VEGF to induce retinal vascular permeability is markedly reduced (B). Orally administered ruboxistaurin was evaluated in diabetic and nondiabetic rats for its effect on typical diabetes-induced abnormalities including changes in retinal blood flow (C) and urine albumin excretion rate (D). Mean retinal blood circulation time is abnormally increased in control diabetic rats. However, in diabetic rats fed with a chow containing 10 mg/kg per day of ruboxistaurin, the diabetes-induced change in retinal circulation time was ameliorated. Similarly, diabetic rats have increased urinary albumin excretion rate. However, one week of oral treatment with ruboxistaurin significantly normalized this abnormality. (Source: A and B adapted from Aiello et al. [86]; with permission. C and D adapted from Ishii et al. [135]; with permission.)

in this cohort of patients with clinically significant diabetic macular edema at baseline. In the 172 patients who participated in the study, median visual acuity was better at week 36 after treatment with 0.3 mg pegaptanib (20/50), than it was with sham injection (20/63, $P = 0.04$). A larger proportion of patients receiving pegaptanib improved visual acuity by 10 or more letters on the Early Treatment Diabetic Retinopathy Study (ETDRS) vision chart (34% vs. 10%, $P = 0.003$, Fig. 20.20A). Mean central retinal thickness on OCT was reduced in the pegaptanib group by

68 microns on average compared with a 4-micron increase in retinal thickness in the sham-treated group ($P = 0.02$). Larger proportions of those receiving 0.3 mg had an absolute decrease of 100 microns or more (42% vs. 16%, $P = 0.02$). Patients receiving pegaptanib were also almost half as likely to receive photocoagulation than those in the placebo group (25% vs. 48%, $P = 0.04$). Interestingly, 8 of 13 (62%) subjects with retinal neovascularization at baseline who were treated with pegaptanib showed regression of neovascularization by week 36 as compared with none of the four patients with retinal neovascularization at baseline in the sham group [126]. These findings suggest a possible direct effect of pegaptanib upon retinal neovascularization in patients with diabetes mellitus. Phase III trials with pegaptanib for diabetic macular edema are currently underway.

Ranibizumab (Lucentis, Genentech) is a recombinant humanized antibody fragment injected intravitreally every 4 weeks that binds all isoforms of VEGF-A and is FDA approved for the treatment of neovascular AMD [127]. Studies evaluating ranibizumab for diabetic macular edema (DME) are currently ongoing. Chun et al reported 10 eyes in 10 patients who received 0.3 or 0.5 mg of ranibizumab for treatment of DME involving the center of the macula [128]. A total of three ranibizumab treatments were administered, 1 month apart over a period of 2 months. At 3 months, five patients had visual improvement of ≥10 ETDRS letters while four patients improved ≥15 letters (Fig. 20.20C). This effect decreased after 6 months. There was improvement in OCT central subfield thickness in both treatment arms, which was statistically significant for the 0.5 mg group and maintained through 6 months follow-up.

Another study evaluated 10 patients with chronic DME in a nonrandomized manner who received intravitreal injections of 0.5 mg of ranibizumab at baseline and at 1, 2, 4, and 6 months. After 7 months (1 month after the fifth injection), the mean foveal thickness was reduced by 246 microns ($P = 0.005$), the macular volume was reduced by 1.75 mm³ ($P = 0.009$) and mean visual acuity was improved from 20/63 to 20/40 ($P = 0.005$). In both studies, the injections were well tolerated with no ocular or systemic adverse events [129]. Phase III trials evaluating ranibizumab for diabetic macular edema are currently underway. Intravitreal administration of the full-length recombinant humanized monoclonal anti-VEGF antibody bevacizumab (Avastin, Genentech, Inc.) for treatment of PDR and iris neovascularization has also been investigated [130]. In small published case series, rapid regression of PDR and iris neovascularization along with resolution of vitreous hemorrhage was demonstrated [96,97]. A recently published prospective study evaluating 32 patients demonstrated at least partial regression of neovascularization by clinical exam and reduced leakage on fluorescein angiography in all patients within one week of bevacizumab injection (Fig. 20.20B). Complete regression occurred in 73%. Leakage from iris neovascularization resolved completely in 82% of eyes. In all but one patient, these findings were maintained at 11 weeks' follow-up [98]. Preoperative intravitreal bevacizumab therapy may also facilitate pars plana vitrectomy for diabetic tractional retinal detachment by reducing intraoperative intraocular bleeding [131].

Intravitreal injection of 1.25 or 2.5 mg bevacizumab is also being evaluated in a phase II trial in combination with and without macular laser photocoagulation as treatment for diabetic macular edema. Pending these results, further long-term

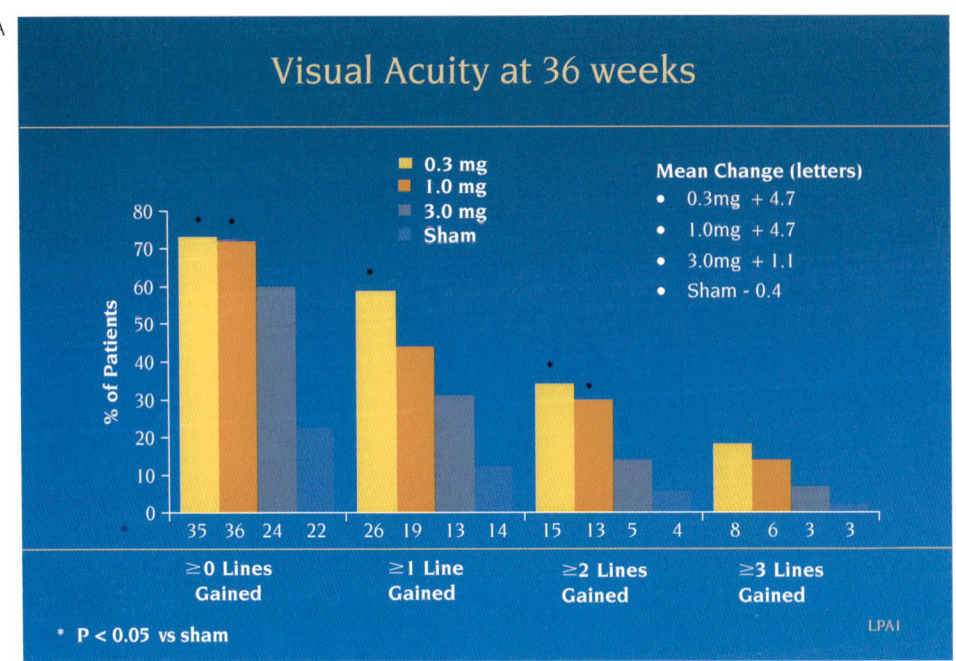

Visual Acuity at 36 weeks

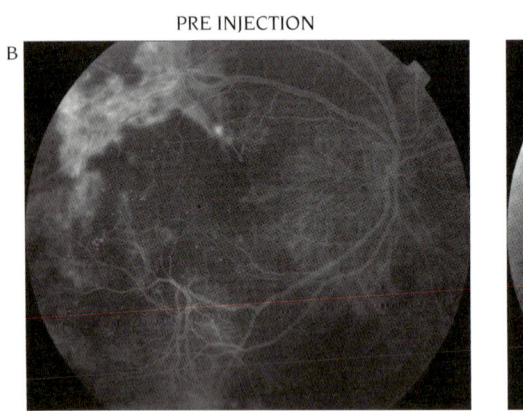
PRE INJECTION

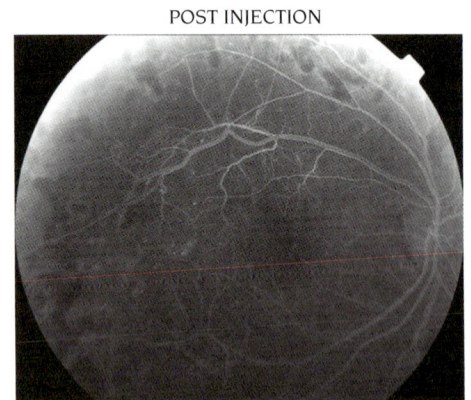
POST INJECTION

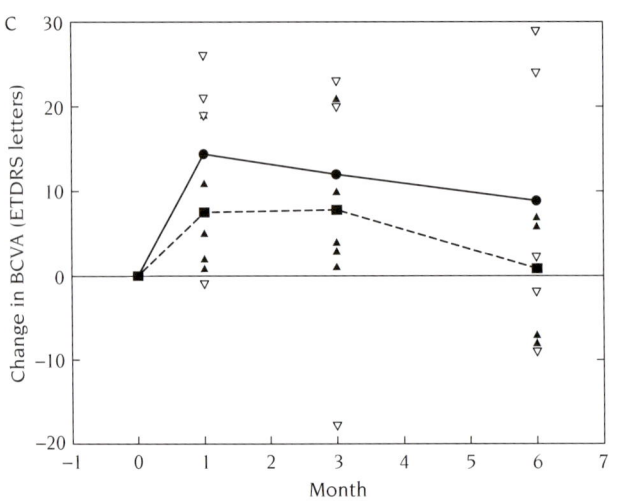

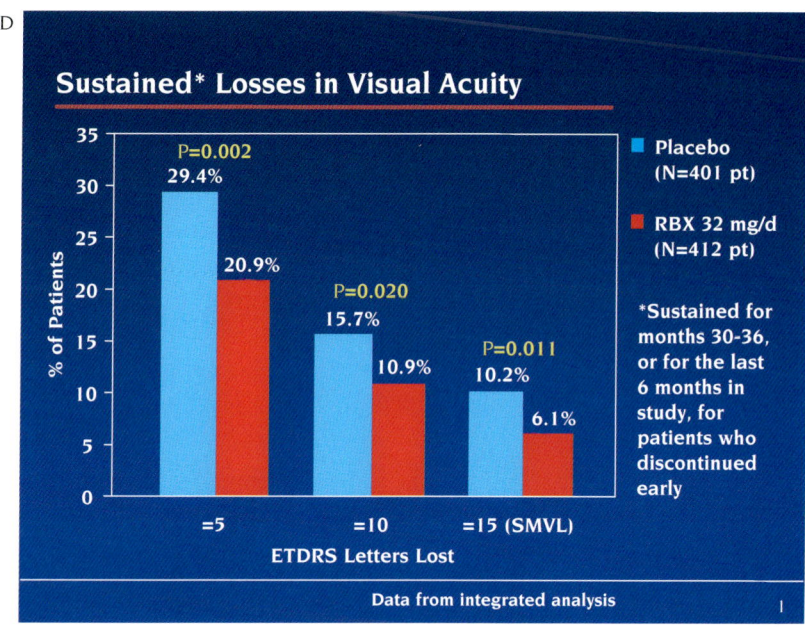

Figure 20.20. Clinical effects of novel therapies for diabetic retinopathy and macular edema. Clinical trials in patients with diabetic macular edema have been performed using the intravitreally administered Vascular endothelial growth factor (VEGF)-inhibitors pegaptanib, bevacizumab, and ranibizumab as well as the orally-administered protein kinase C (PKC) β selective inhibitor ruboxistaurin. A 39-center, phase II, randomized, sham-controlled, double-masked, parallel, dose-ranging study evaluated intravitreal injection of pegaptanib for diabetic macular edema (DME). Injections were performed every six weeks up to and including week 12 (3 injections) without additional laser, after which time, further injections were at the discretion of the treating ophthalmologist. Retinal edema was decreased by pegaptanib therapy and, as shown in (A), visual acuity was improved. (B) A prospective study evaluating intravitreal bevacizumab in 32 patients with DME demonstrated at least partial regression of neovascularization by clinical exam and reduced leakage on fluorescein angiography in all patients within 1 week of bevacizumab injection. Complete regression occurred in 73% and leakage from iris neovascularization completely resolved in 82% of eyes. (B) demonstrates the marked regression in retinal neovascularization observed within 1 week of intravitreal bevacizumab injection. (Source: With permission from Robert L. Avery, MD.) (C) Intravitreal ranibizumab was studied in a single-center, open-label, dose-escalating pilot study of 10 eyes of 10 patients with DME involving the center of the macula with a resulting mean decrease in retinal thickening and 50% of patients gaining 10 or more letters after 3 months. (D) A 3-year phase III trial of the PKC β selective inhibitor ruboxistaurin in patients with moderately severe to very severe nonproliferative diabetic retinopathy at baseline demonstrated a 40% reduction in sustained moderate visual loss (D), 30% reduction in the need for initial focal/grid photocoagulation, less progression of macular edema to within 100 microns of the center of the macula and more than twice as many patients experiencing a 15 or more letter improvement in vision. (Source: A adapted from the Macugen Diabetic Retinopathy Study Group [125], B adapted with permission from Avery et al. [98], C adapted from Chun et al. [128], and D adapted from The PKC-DRS2 Research Group [131].)

randomized prospective studies will be needed to fully evaluate the role of bevaci-zumab in the treatment of diabetic eye disease.

Another VEGF inhibitor under investigation as treatment for diabetic ocular disease is VEGF trap (VEGF Trap-Eye, Regeneron Pharmaceuticals, Inc.), a soluble protein that fuses the binding domains of VEGF receptors 1 and 2 with the Fc por-tion of immunoglobulin G. This recombinant molecule binds all VEGF isoforms with exceptionally high affinity [132]. VEGF trap has been shown to significantly reduce vascular permeability in a mouse model of VEGF-induced breakdown of the blood–retinal barrier [133]. Results are pending from a phase I study exam-ining the effect of VEGF trap on diabetic macular edema as assessed by central retinal thickness and visual acuity measurements. VEGF trap is an inhibitor that binds VEGF (as are bevacizumab, ranibizumab, and pegaptanib) and, therefore, it is likely that VEGF trap may have inhibitory effects on PDR and iris neovascu-larization in addition to effects on DME. Both systemic and intravitreally admin-istered VEGF trap prevent the development of choroidal angiogenesis in a mouse model of laser-induced choroidal neovascularization. VEGF trap is currently being evaluated in phase II clinical trials in patients with choroidal neovascular mem-branes associated with age-related macular degeneration.

PKC INHIBITORS IN DIABETIC RETINOPATHY

PKC-β activation is induced by hyperglycemia through several mechanisms and in part mediates the development of vascular dysfunction, VEGF expression, and VEGF signal transduction. Thus, inhibition of PKC-β might be expected to ame-liorate diabetes-induced vascular complications by several mechanisms. The syn-thesis of a PKC-β isoform-selective inhibitor (ruboxistaurin) has provided diverse data to substantiate this hypothesis [134]. Orally ingested ruboxistaurin amelio-rates diabetes-induced abnormalities of retinal blood flow, glomerular filtration rate, and albumin excretion rate in animals (Fig. 20.19C and D) [135]. These data supported the evaluation of orally administered ruboxistaurin in clinical trials as a potential noninvasive and nondestructive inhibitor of the progression of diabetic retinopathy and diabetic macular edema [136].

Data from two three-year phase III trials of ruboxistaurin in patients with moderate to severe NPDR have been reported [131,137]. Results were very sim-ilar in both trials. In the larger PKC-DRS2 study, 685 patients with moderate to severe NPDR (ETDRS retinopathy level > 47A and < 53E), and no prior scatter (panretinal) photocoagulation in at least one eye were evaluated after receiving oral ruboxistaurin (32 mg/day) over a period of 36 months [131]. Sustained mod-erate visual loss (SMVL: 15-letter or more decrease in ETDRS visual acuity score maintained for the last 6 months of study participation) occurred in 5.5% of ruboxistaurin-treated patients and 9.1% of placebo-treated patients (40% risk reduction, $P = 0.034$, Fig. 20.20D). In individual eyes, ruboxistaurin reduced SMVL by 45% ($P = 0.011$). Mean visual acuity was better in the ruboxistau-rin-treated patients from 12 months onward. In ruboxistaurin-treated patients, visual improvement of 15 or more letters was more frequent (4.9% vs. 2.4%) and

15 or more letter loss was less frequent (6.7% vs. 9.9%) than in placebo-treated patients. When clinically significant macular edema was >100 microns from the center of the macula at baseline, ruboxistaurin treatment was associated with less frequent progression of edema to within 100 microns (68% vs. 50%). Initial laser treatment for macular edema was 26% less frequent in eyes of ruboxistaurin-treated patients. In patients who did require focal/grid laser for diabetic macular edema during the course of the study, patients receiving ruboxistaurin had less SMVL than did patients who had received laser but were receiving placebo (P = 0.032). Ruboxistaurin therapy was very well tolerated and has had an excellent safety profile to date [138]. No effect was observed on progression of NPDR severity. Thus, oral ruboxistaurin reduced vision loss, macular edema progression, and need for laser treatment, while increasing the chance of visual improvement in patients with moderate to severe NPDR. The compound has received an Approvable rating by the FDA under the trade name Arxxant (Eli Lilly). Several additional studies are underway and at least one more phase 3 trial would be required for FDA marketing approval.

Corticosteroids. As discussed above, VEGF and inflammation pathways are involved in the pathogenesis of diabetic retinopathy and macular edema. Corticosteroids, which have known anti-inflammatory properties, have also been shown to inhibit the VEGF gene expression [139]. In vitro studies have shown that the pro-inflammatory molecules platelet derived growth factor (PDGF) and platelet activating factor (PAF) induce expression of VEGF in human vascular cell lines and that administration of corticosteroids can abolish this effect in a dose dependent manner [140]. Corticosteroids are thought to inhibit macrophages that release angiogenic growth factors [141,142] and have been shown to inhibit angiogenesis through the breakdown of capillary basement membrane extracellular matrix proteins, particularly laminin and fibronectin via inhibition of bFGF-induced activation of MMP-2 [143].

In a porcine model of branch retinal vein occlusion (BRVO), intravitreal triamcinolone (TA) inhibits optic disc neovascularization [144]. In a rat model of retinopathy of prematurity, the angiostatic steroid anecortave acetate decreased neovascularization by increasing mRNA expression of the antiangiogenic molecule plasminogen activator inhibitor (PAI)-1 [145]. In a human study of 12 patients with PDR and iris neovascularization who underwent pars plana vitrectomy with perioperative injection of intravitreal steroid, regression of iris neovascularization was noted in all eyes over a mean follow-up period of 1.1 months [146]. In another case series of 14 patients with iris neovascularization, all of whom received a 20-mg intravitreal injection of TA, iris neovascularization regressed by an average of 50% with average intraocular pressure (IOP) reduction from 33.4 to 20.7 mmHg after three months of follow up [147]. Although these data suggest that corticosteroids may have beneficial effects on proliferative diabetic retinopathy, these actions appear less potent than those observed on macular edema.

Corticosteroids have been studied extensively for the treatment of diabetic macular edema. Intravitreal triamcinolone (Kenalog 40, Bristol-Myers-Squibb, Princeton, NJ) has been the most commonly investigated formulation. Although

Kenalog is FDA approved for nonophthalmic indications and is readily available and widely utilized by ophthalmologists, it should be noted that this drug is not FDA approved for intravitreal injection to treat diabetic macular edema or any other interocular complication, and it contains potentially retina-toxic compounds in the vehicle including polysorbate-80 and benzyl alcohol [148]. The 4 mg (0.1 cc) dose is the most widely used as it represents a readily injectable volume with reported clinical benefits. However, compelling scientific evidence as to the optimal dose is lacking and other concentrations have been employed [149].

Martides et al. described a case series of 16 eyes with clinically significant macular edema (CSME) that were treated with 4 mg of intravitreal TA and followed for up to 6 months. These authors noted a mean reduction in foveal thickness of 55% in the 14 eyes evaluated at 1 month (533 microns to 242 microns); however, in 8 eyes that were followed for 6 months, foveal thickness had increased to 335 microns. Visual acuity improved by 2.4 lines at 1 month, but this improvement decreased to 1.3 lines at 6 months [150]. Jonas et al. noted visual acuity improvement from 20/165 to 20/105 with reduced leakage on fluorescein angiogram in 26 eyes with at least a one-year history of macular edema that were treated with intravitreal TA (25 mg), and followed for an average of 6.6 months [146]. In contrast, there was no visual improvement in any of the control patients who were treated with focal/grid photocoagulation. In a group of 12 patients with bilateral diffuse CSME who were treated with 4 mg of intravitreal TA in one eye, with the other eye serving as the control, visual acuity improved by at least two lines in five of the 12 steroid-treated eyes and did not improve in any of the control eyes [151].

Recently, 2-year safety and efficacy outcomes have been reported from a prospective, double-masked, placebo-controlled, randomized clinical trial of intravitreal TA injections (4 mg in 0.1cc) in eyes with diabetic macular edema and impaired vision that persisted or recurred after laser treatment [152]. Sixty-nine eyes of 43 patients were evaluated and 34 eyes were randomized to receive TA and 35 placebo. Two-year data were reported for 60 of 69 (87%) eyes of 35 of 41 (85%) patients with 9 eyes of 6 patients being lost to follow-up (6 placebo, 3 TA). Eyes randomized to placebo received a subconjunctival injection of saline. Improvement of 5 or more letters best-corrected visual acuity occurred in 19 of 34 (56%) eyes treated with intravitreal TA, compared with 9 of 35 (26%) eyes treated with placebo ($P = 0.006$). The mean improvement in visual acuity was 5.7 letters (95% confidence interval, 1.4–9.9) more in the intravitreal TA-treated eyes than in those treated with the placebo. An increase of IOP of ≥5 mmHg was observed in 23 of 34 (68%) TA-treated versus 3 of 30 (10%) untreated eyes ($P < 0.0001$). Glaucoma medication was required in 15 of 34 (44%) treated versus 1 of 30 (3%) untreated eyes ($P = 0.0002$). Cataract surgery was performed in 15 of 28 (54%) treated versus 0 of 21 (0%) untreated eyes ($P < 0.0001$). Two eyes in the intravitreal TA-treated group required trabeculectomy. There was one case of infectious endophthalmitis in the treatment group.

These results suggest that intravitreal TA may improve vision and reduce macular thickness in eyes with refractory diabetic macular edema. With repeated treatment, these effects can be evident for up to 2 years. Progression of cataract, elevation of IOP, need for trabeculectomy, and endophthalmitis were treatment risks that need be weighed against the observed efficacy and the occasional spontaneous improvement over years that still occurred in some eyes that are apparently severely affected by diabetic macular edema.

Most recently, results from a multicenter, randomized clinical trial by the Diabetic Retinopathy Clinical Research Network (DRCR.net) were reported evaluating the potential benefit in 840 study eyes of 693 patients with diabetic macular edema of intravitreal injection using a preservative-free and pH-balanced TA preparation specially formulated for intraocular injection (Allergan). ETDRS laser photocoagulation was used as the control arm. Although at 4 months mean visual acuity was better in the 4 mg TA-treated group than the other two groups, beginning at 16 months and extending out to 2 years, eyes treated with focal/grid photocoagulation had better mean visual acuity and less macular thickening than eyes treated with steroid. Furthermore, there were four-fold fewer adverse events in terms of IOP rise and cataract development necessitating surgery in the laser group as compared with the two steroid-treated groups [153]. Additional phase III trials utilizing sustained-release dexamethasone (Retisert, Bausch & Lomb) and fluocinolone acetonide (Medidur, Alimera Sciences) implants for diabetic macular edema are also underway.

In addition to the evidence that laser photocoagulation treatment results in better visual acuity and anatomic outcomes over the long term as compared with intravitreal steroid treatment, enthusiasm for use of intravitreal steroids is further tempered by known side effects. Complications include high prevalence of cataract, elevated IOP (in some instances severe enough to require trabeculectomy), and endophthalmitis. In a comprehensive review of the published risks of intravitreal injection through 2004, sustained IOP elevation was reported in 38.3% (100/261) of cases of TA injection. All of these cases were managed successfully with topical IOP-reducing medication over a period of several months [154]. Jonas et al. reported an increase in IOP greater than 21 mmHg in 9 of 26 eyes after a single intravitreal injection of 25 mg of triamcinolone. All of these cases of high IOP were controlled successfully with topical medications without evidence of glaucomatous optic nerve damage [146]. The phase III DRCR trial comparing intraviteal TA to laser photocoagulation treatment revealed that IOP increased by 10 mmHg or more in 4%, 16% and 33% of eyes in the laser group, 1 mg TA group, and 4 mg TA groups, respectively [153].

Endophthalmitis, including cases referred to as pseudo or sterile endophthalmitis, has been reported in 1.4% of eyes undergoing TA injection. Several of these cases may have been secondary to inflammatory reactions due to the steroid vehicle. The prevalence of truly infectious endophthalmitis cases is estimated to be closer to 0.6% (10/1703) [154]. Cataract prevalence was reported as 9.9% (8/81) in phakic eyes after intravitreal steroid injection. Incidence was more common in eyes with longer follow-up and in those that were subjected to repeated intravitreal steroid injections. More recently, rates of cataract extraction in patients receiving multiple doses of 4 mg intravitreal TA over 2 years have been found to be as high as 51% [153].

Periocular corticosteroids have also being investigated for potential therapeutic value in treating diabetic macular edema. Significant previous clinical experience exists for the use of peribulbar/retrobulbar steroid injections in nondiabetic cystoid macular edema due to conditions such as uveitis and following cataract extraction. For diabetic macular edema, one case series of six eyes with persistent diabetic macular edema demonstrated that treatment with 12 mg of posterior subtenon's TA applied after vitrectomy improved visual acuity in three eyes [155].

A phase II pilot study performed by the DRCR.net in 32 centers nationwide has recently reported 34-week follow-up primary endpoint data [156]. In this study, neither anterior (20 mg) nor posterior (40 mg) peribulbar injection of Kenalog, either in combination with laser therapy or alone, was more effective than focal/grid laser. Thus, the DRCR.net is not pursuing further peribulbar steroid injection studies at this time.

CURRENT STATUS OF NOVEL THERAPEUTIC AGENTS IN CLINICAL TRIAL

Advances in the development and clinical testing of antiangiogenic and antipermeability agents continue to accelerate remarkably. Significant mechanistic discoveries, initiation of clinical investigations, and new data from controlled clinical trials are now forthcoming each year. Most large pharmaceutical and biotechnology companies currently have active programs devoted to the identification, development, and testing of novel approaches applicable to diabetic macular edema and/or diabetic retinopathy [157]. Indeed, many agents that are being investigated as potential therapies for various vascular cancers and pathologic permeability have clear implications for the treatment of diabetic eye disease. Soon to be initiated or currently ongoing clinical trials in diabetic retinopathy and macular edema include studies of bevacizumab (phase III); dexamethasone, fluocinolone acetonide, pegaptanib (III); ranibizumab (phase III); ruboxistaurin (phase III); triamcinolone acetonide (including preservative-free preparations in phase III investigation); and VEGF trap among others. A variety of other therapeutic approaches are in early stages of development, including gene therapy, anti-inflammatory agents, receptor tyrosine kinase inhibitors, integrin blockers, advanced glycation end product inhibitors, and vitreoretinal interface disruptors such as microplasmin.

CHALLENGES FOR ANTIANGIOGENIC THERAPY OF DIABETIC RETINOPATHY

Although the data supporting the human use of antiangiogenic and antipermeability agents for the treatment of PDR and macular edema are compelling, there are several as-yet unresolved issues that will be important to clarify if these approaches are to achieve routine and highly effective clinical application. The method of drug delivery and the duration of action will become critical issues. Local delivery would presumably have fewer side effects than systemic administration, but achieving adequate concentrations of these agents at the retina is difficult using a topical or peribulbar approach. Indeed, as discussed above, recent evaluation of peribulbar Kenalog with and without additional laser showed that this approach was not more effective than laser alone [156]. Intravitreal injections allow for delivery of high intraocular concentrations of an agent, but frequent repeated intravitreal injections for the treatment of a life-long chronic disease such as diabetic retinopathy are suboptimal because of physician and patient inconvenience and the cumulative risks of endophthalmitis, retinal detachment, and potential toxicity. This drawback is especially notable for the treatment of diabetic retinopathy in light of the remarkable effectiveness of current laser photocoagulation, a noninvasive and relatively well-tolerated intervention [158,159]. Thus, evolution of therapies with duration of action substantially longer than the 4- to 6-week period required for current anti-VEGF therapies, or clear demonstration that duration of therapy will be self-limited rather than life-long, will be necessary for achieving optimal care.

Regardless of systemic or local therapy, it is not known whether excessive inhibition of VEGF in the adult will lead to side effects resulting from a physiological requirement for basal expression of VEGF in the eye or other tissues. Indeed, VEGF has neuroprotective properties that may be important for normal retinal function [160–162]. Thus, especially with a long duration of treatment, careful titration of the extent of VEGF inhibition might be necessary and the therapeutic window could be smaller than initially assumed. This consideration is of particular concern in the neonatal eye, in which VEGF directs appropriate retinal vascular development [61,66]. Antiangiogenic agents would be expected to cause developmental defects if administered systemically during embryogenesis and, thus, their use during pregnancy is likely to be problematic.

Even if a well-tolerated, easily administered antiagiogenic agent with limited toxicity was available, there are likely to be instances where a normal neovascular response would be desired in the patient, and the angio-suppressive action of retinopathy treatment might be detrimental. Although local drug delivery might obviate a part of this problem, systemic administration could be challenging when extensive wound healing or vascular collateralization is required. In patients with diabetes, this scenario might commonly arise following significant trauma, in the presence of concomitant nonhealing ulcers or following myocardial infarction. Increased systemic levels of VEGF may be beneficial in these cases. Indeed, direct myocardial gene transfer of VEGF in five patients with symptomatic myocardial ischemia resulted in reduced symptoms and improved myocardial perfusion [163]. Antiangiogenic agents that can be rapidly reversed or have short half-lives might permit prompt return of angiogenic capabilities in patients when required.

Results from numerous future clinical trials will be necessary to determine the optimal manner in which these agents will contribute to our therapeutic options for treatment of diabetic retinopathy and macular edema. Various therapeutic scenarios include antiangiogenic monotherapy, antiangiogenic therapy prior to laser, concurrent use with laser, or perhaps application only if laser therapy is ineffective. Mounting evidence suggests that, especially in the case of diabetic macular edema, multiple molecules and various pathways are likely to be involved [164], thus suggesting that combination therapies (as proven effective in cancer and AIDS) may provide a powerful approach to the treatment of diabetic eye disease [165].

SUMMARY

For over six decades, there has been an excellent appreciation of the fundamental processes underlying the ocular complications of diabetes. Only recently, however, has an extraordinary series of scientific advances provided a detailed understanding of the molecular mechanisms involved in the evolution of diabetic retinopathy. These observations have suggested novel interventional approaches that hold promise as potentially efficacious, noninvasive, and nondestructive treatments of both diabetic retinopathy and diabetic macular edema. Several of these novel therapeutic modalities now have data derived from clinical trials, are currently under clinical trial evaluation, or will soon be evaluated in clinical trials. Ultimately, it is the results of these randomized clinical investigations that will help resolve the remaining unanswered clinical issues and determine whether any of these approaches may yet prove to be sufficiently effective and adequately free of side effects to have a substantial impact on the clinical care of diabetic retinal disease. Indeed, antiangiogenic agents are now of proven benefit in the treatment of cancer and AMD [124,127,166]. It is enlightening to remember that more than 20 years before the discovery of insulin, Dr Elliot P. Joslin routinely advised his diabetic patients to "Live, so that you may profit from some new discovery." The scientific progress achieved in the past few years, and the information soon to become available from ongoing clinical trials continue to provide validation of this advice, and a new ophthalmic frontier of pharmacologic therapy will continue to evolve with substantial benefits for our patients with diabetes.

REFERENCES

1. The Eye Disease Prevalence Research Group. The prevalence of diabetic retinopathy among adults in the United States. *Arch Ophthalmol.* 2004;122:552–563.
2. Zhang X, Gregg EW, Cheng YJ, et al. Diabetes mellitus and visual impairment. National Health and Nutrition Examination Survey, 1999–2004. *Arch Ophthalmol.* 2008;126:1421–1427.
3. Ferris FL. How effective are treatments for diabetic retinopathy? *JAMA.* 1993;269:1290–1291.
4. Greene DA, Sima AA, Stevens MJ, et al. Aldose reductase inhibitors: an approach to the treatment of diabetic nerve damage. *Diabetes Metab.Rev.* 1993;9:189–217.
5. Brownlee M. The pathological implications of protein glycation. *Clin Invest Med.* 1995;18:275–281.
6. Baynes JW, Thorpe SR. Role of oxidative stress in diabetic complications. A new perspective on an old paradigm. *Diabetes.* 1999;48:1–9.
7. Koya D, King GL. Protein kinase C activation and the development of diabetic complications. *Diabetes.* 1998;47:859–866.
8. Horton MA. The alpha v beta 3 integrin vitronectin receptor. *Int J Biochem Cell Biol.* 1997;29:721–725.
9. King GL, Shiba T, Oliver J, Inoguchi T, Bursell SE. Cellular and molecular abnormalities in the vascular endothelium of diabetes mellitus. *Annu Rev Med.* 1994;45:179–188.
10. Gartner S, Henkind P. Neovascularization of the iris (rubeosis iridis). *Surv Ophthalmol.* 1978;22:291–312.

11. Henkind P. Ocular neovascularization. The Krill memorial lecture. *Am J Ophthalmol*. 1978;85:287–301.

12. The Early Treatment Diabetic Retinopathy Study Research Group. Fluorescein angiographic risk factors for progression of diabetic retinopathy: ETDRS report number 13. *Ophthalmology*. 1991;98:834–840.

13. The Early Treatment Diabetic Retinopathy Study Research Group. Classification of diabetic retinopathy from fluorescein angiograms: ETDRS report number 11. *Ophthalmology*. 1991;98:807–822.

14. Anonymous. Argon laser scatter photocoagulation for prevention of neovascularization and vitreous hemorrhage in branch vein occlusion. A randomized clinical trial. Branch Vein Occlusion Study Group. *Arch Ophthalmol*. 1986;104:34–41.

15. Aiello LM, Wand M, Liang G. Neovascular glaucoma and vitreous hemorrhage following cataract surgery in patients with diabetes mellitus. *Ophthalmology*. 1983;90:814–820.

16. Michaelson IC. The mode of development of the vascular system of the retina, with some observations on its significance for certain retinal diseases. *Trans Ophthalmol Soc UK*. 1948;68:137–180.

17. Ashton N. Retinal neovascularization in health and disease. *Am J Ophthalmol*. 1957;44:7–24.

18. Friedlander M, Theesfeld CL, Sugita M, et al. Involvement of integrins alpha v beta 3 and alpha v beta 5 in ocular neovascular diseases. *Proc Natl Acad Sci USA*. 1996;93:9764–9769.

19. O'Reilly MS, Holmgren L, Shing Y, et al. Angiostatin: a novel angiogenesis inhibitor that mediates the suppression of metastases by a Lewis lung carcinoma [see comments]. *Cell*. 1994;79:315–328.

20. O'Reilly MS, Boehm T, Shing Y, et al. Endostatin: an endogenous inhibitor of angiogenesis and tumor growth. *Cell*. 1997;88:277–285.

21. Grant MB, Caballero S, Tarnuzzer RW, et al. Matrix metalloproteinase expression in human retinal microvascular cells. *Diabetes*. 1998;47:1311–1317.

22. De La Paz MA, Itoh Y, Toth CA, Nagase H. Matrix metalloproteinases and their inhibitors in human vitreous. *Invest Ophthalmol Vis Sci*. 1998;39:1256–1260.

23. Brown D, Hamdi H, Bahri S, Kenney MC. Characterization of an endogenous metalloproteinase in human vitreous. *Curr Eye Res*. 1994;13:639–647.

24. Burgess WH, Maciag T. The heparin-binding (fibroblast) growth factor family of proteins. *Annu Rev Biochem*. 1989;58:575–606.

25. Vlodavsky I, Folkman J, Sullivan R, et al. Endothelial cell-derived basic fibroblast growth factor: synthesis and deposition into subendothelial extracellular matrix. *Proc Natl Acad Sci USA*. 1987;84:2292–2296.

26. Abraham JA, Mergia A, Whang JL, et al. Nucleotide sequence of a bovine clone encoding the angiogenic protein, basic fibroblast growth factor. *Science*. 1986;233:545–548.

27. Kandel J, Bossy-Wetzel E, Radvanyi F, Klagsbrun M, Folkman J, Hanahan D. Neovascularization is associated with a switch to the export of bFGF in the multistep development of fibrosarcoma. *Cell*. 1991;66:1095–1104.

28. McNeil PL, Muthukrishnan L, Warder E, D'Amore PA. Growth factors are released by mechanically wounded endothelial cells. *J Cell Biol*. 1989;109:811–822.

29. Gao H, Hollyfield JG. Basic fibroblast growth factor (bFGF) immunolocalization in the rodent outer retina demonstrated with an anti-rodent bFGF antibody. *Brain Res*. 1992;585:355–360.

30. Sivalingam A, Kenney J, Brown GC, Benson WE, Donoso L. Basic fibroblast growth factor levels in the vitreous of patients with proliferative diabetic retinopathy. *Arch Ophthalmol.* 1990;108:869–872.

31. Ozaki H, Okamoto N, Ortega S, et al. Basic fibroblast growth factor is neither necessary nor sufficient for the development of retinal neovascularization [see comments]. *Am J Pathol.* 1998;153:757–765.

32. Asahara T, Bauters C, Zheng LP, et al. Synergistic effect of vascular endothelial growth factor and basic fibroblast growth factor on angiogenesis in vivo. *Circulation.* 1995;92:II365–II371.

33. Goto F, Goto K, Weindel K, Folkman J. Synergistic effects of vascular endothelial growth factor and basic fibroblast growth factor on the proliferation and cord formation of bovine capillary endothelial cells within collagen gels [see comments]. *Lab Invest.* 1993;69:508–517.

34. Pepper MS, Ferrara N, Orci L, Montesano R. Potent synergism between vascular endothelial growth factor and basic fibroblast growth factor in the induction of angiogenesis in vitro. *Biochem Biophys Res Commun.* 1992;189:824–831.

35. LeRoith D, Roberts CT. Insulin-like growth factors. *Ann N Y Acad Sci.* 1993;692:1–9.

36. Poulsen J. Diabetes and anterior pituitary insufficiency. Final course and postmortem study of a diabetic patient with Sheehan's syndrome. *Diabetes.* 1966;15:73–77.

37. Poulsen JE. The Houssay phenomenon in man. Recovery from retinopathy in a case of diabetes with Simmonds' disease. *Diabetes.* 1953;2:7–12.

38. Sharp P, Fallon T, Brazier O, Sandler L, Joplin G., Kohner E. Long-term follow-up of patients who underwent Yttrium-90 pituitary implantation for treatment of proliferative diabetic retinopathy. *Diabetologia.* 1987;30:199–207.

39. Smith LE, Kopchick JJ, Chen W, et al. Essential role of growth hormone in ischemia-induced retinal neovascularization. *Science.* 1997;276:1706–1709.

40. Mallet B, Vialettes B, Haroche S, et al. Stabilization of severe proliferative diabetic retinopathy by long-term treatment with SMS 201-995. *Diabetes Metab.* 1992;18:438–444.

41. Grant MB, Mames RN, Fitzgerald C, et al. The efficacy of octreotide in the therapy of severe nonproliferative and early proliferative diabetic retinopathy: a randomized controlled study. *Diabetes Care.* 2000;23:504–509.

42. Boehm BO, Lang GK, Jehle PM, et al. Octreotide reduces vitreous hemorrhage and loss of visual acuity risk in patients with high-risk proliferative diabetic retinopathy. *Horm Metab Res.* 2001;33:300–306.

43. Growth Hormone Antagonist for Proliferative Diabetic Retinopathy Study Group. The effect of a growth hormone receptor antagonist drug on proliferative diabetic retinopathy. *Ophthalmology.* 2001;108:2266–2272.

44. Novartis media release, http://cws.huginonline.com/N/134323/PR/200604/1046164_5.html. Last accessed February 25, 2009.

45. Grant MB, Caballero S Jr. The potential role of octreotide in the treatment of diabetic retinopathy. *Treat Endocrinol.* 2005;4(4):199–203.

46. Katsura Y, Okano T, Noritake M, et al. Hepatocyte growth factor in vitreous fluid of patients with proliferative diabetic retinopathy and other retinal disorders. *Diabetes Care.* 1998;21:1759–1763.

47. Senger DR, Galli SJ, Dvorak AM, Perruzzi CA, Harvey VS, Dvorak HF. Tumor cells secrete a vascular permeability factor that promotes accumulation of ascites fluid. *Science.* 1983;219:983–985.

48. Keck PJ, Hauser SD, Krivi G, et al. Vascular permeability factor, an endothelial cell mitogen related to PDGF. *Science.* 1989;246:1309–1312.

49. Leung DW, Cachianes G, Kuang WJ, Goeddel DV, Ferrara N. Vascular endothelial growth factor is a secreted angiogenic mitogen. *Science*. 1989;246:1306–1309.

50. Ferrara N, Houck KA, Jakeman LB, Winer J, Leung DW. The vascular endothelial growth factor family of polypeptides. *J Cell Biochem*. 1991;47:211–218.

51. Williams B. Vascular permeability/vascular endothelial growth factors: a potential role in the pathogenesis and treatment of vascular diseases. *Vasc Med*. 1996;1:251–258.

52. Miller JW, Adamis AP, Aiello LP. Vascular endothelial growth factor in ocular neovascularization and proliferative diabetic retinopathy. *Diabetes Metab Rev*. 1997; 13:37–50.

53. Aiello LP. Clinical implications of vascular growth factors in proliferative retinopathies. *Curr Opin Ophthalmol*. 1997;8:19–31.

54. Aiello LP. Vascular endothelial growth factor. 20th-century mechanisms, 21st-century therapies. *Invest Ophthalmol Vis Sci*. 1997;38:1647–1652.

55. Thieme H, Aiello LP, Takagi H, Ferrara N, King GL. Comparative analysis of vascular endothelial growth factor receptors on retinal and aortic vascular endothelial cells. *Diabetes*. 1995; 44:98–103.

56. Aiello LP, Northrup JM, Keyt BA, Takagi H, Iwamoto MA. Hypoxic regulation of vascular endothelial growth factor in retinal cells. *Arch Ophthalmol*. 1995;113: 1538–1544.

57. De Vries C, Escobedo JA, Ueno H, Houck K, Ferrara N, Williams LT. The fms-like tyrosine kinase, a receptor for vascular endothelial growth factor. *Science*. 1992;255: 989–991.

58. Millauer B, Wizigmann-Voos S, Schnurch H, et al. High affinity VEGF binding and developmental expression suggest Flk-1 as a major regulator of vasculogenesis and angiogenesis. *Cell*. 1993;72:835–846.

59. Simorre-Pinatel V, Guerrin M, Chollet P, et al. Vasculotropin-VEGF stimulates retinal capillary endothelial cells through an autocrine pathway. *Invest Ophthalmol Vis Sci*. 1994;35:3393–3400.

60. Dorey CK, Aouididi S, Reynaud X, Dvorak HF, Brown LF. Correlation of vascular permeability factor/vascular endothelial growth factor with extraretinal neovascularization in the rat [see comments] [published erratum appears in *Arch Ophthalmol*. February 1997;115(2):192]. *Arch Ophthalmol*. 1996;114:1210–1217.

61. Stone J, Chan-Ling T, Pe'er J, Itin A, Gnessin H, Keshet E. Roles of vascular endothelial growth factor and astrocyte degeneration in the genesis of retinopathy of prematurity. *Invest Ophthalmol Vis Sci*. 1996;37:290–299.

62. Smith LE, Wesolowski E, McLellan A, et al. Oxygen-induced retinopathy in the mouse. *Invest Ophthalmol Vis Sci*. 1994;35:101–111.

63. Donahue ML, Phelps DL, Watkins RH, LoMonaco MB, Horowitz S. Retinal vascular endothelial growth factor (VEGF) mRNA expression is altered in relation to neovascularization in oxygen induced retinopathy. *Curr Eye Res*. 1996;15:175–184.

64. Miller JW, Adamis AP, Shima DT, et al. Vascular endothelial growth factor/vascular permeability factor is temporally and spatially correlated with ocular angiogenesis in a primate model. *Am J Pathol*. 1994;145:574–584.

65. Pierce EA, Avery RL, Foley ED, Aiello LP, Smith LE. Vascular endothelial growth factor/vascular permeability factor expression in a mouse model of retinal neovascularization. *Proc Natl Acad Sci USA*. 1995;92:905–909.

66. Pierce EA, Foley ED, Smith LE. Regulation of vascular endothelial growth factor by oxygen in a model of retinopathy of prematurity [see comments] [published erratum appears in *Arch Ophthalmol*. March 1997;115(3):427]. *Arch Ophthalmol*. 1996;114:1219–1228.

67. Aiello LP, Avery RL, Arrigg PG, et al. Vascular endothelial growth factor in ocular fluid of patients with diabetic retinopathy and other retinal disorders [see comments]. N Engl J Med. 1994;331:1480–1487.
68. Adamis AP, Miller JW, Bernal MT, et al. Increased vascular endothelial growth factor levels in the vitreous of eyes with proliferative diabetic retinopathy. Am J Ophthalmol. 1994;118:445–450.
69. Burgos R, Simo R, Audi L, et al. Vitreous levels of vascular endothelial growth factor are not influenced by its serum concentrations in diabetic retinopathy. Diabetologia. 1997;40:1107–1109.
70. Funatsu H, Yamashita H, Nakamura S, et al. Various levels of pigmentepithelium-derived factor and vascular endothelial growth fact are related to diabetic macular edema. Ophthalmology. February 2006;113(2):294–301.
71. Patel JI, Tombran-Tink J, Hykin PG, Gregor ZJ, Cree IA. Vitreous and aqueous concentrations of proangiogenic, antiangiogenic factors and other cytokines in diabetic retinopathy patients with macular edema: implications for structural differences in macular profiles. Exp Eye Res. May 2006;82(5):798–806.
72. Pe'er J, Folberg R, Itin A, Gnessin H, Hemo I, Keshet E. Upregulated expression of vascular endothelial growth factor in proliferative diabetic retinopathy. Br J Ophthalmol. 1996;80:241–245.
73. Armstrong D, Augustin AJ, Spengler R, et al. Detection of vascular endothelial growth factor and tumor necrosis factor alpha in epiretinal membranes of proliferative diabetic retinopathy, proliferative vitreoretinopathy and macular pucker. Ophthalmologica. 1998;212:410–414.
74. Chen YS, Hackett SF, Schoenfeld CL, Vinores MA, Vinores SA, Campochiaro PA. Localisation of vascular endothelial growth factor and its receptors to cells of vascular and avascular epiretinal membranes. Br J Ophthalmol. 1997;81:919–926.
75. Frank RN, Amin RH, Eliott D, Puklin JE, Abrams GW. Basic fibroblast growth factor and vascular endothelial growth factor are present in epiretinal and choroidal neovascular membranes. Am J Ophthalmol. 1996;122:393–403.
76. Malecaze F, Clamens S, Simorre-Pinatel V, et al. Detection of vascular endothelial growth factor messenger RNA and vascular endothelial growth factor-like activity in proliferative diabetic retinopathy. Arch Ophthalmol. 1994;112:1476–1482.
77. Tang S, Le-Ruppert KC, Gabel VP. Proliferation and activation of vascular endothelial cells in epiretinal membranes from patients with proliferative diabetic retinopathy. An immunohistochemistry and clinical study. Ger J Ophthalmol. 1994;3:131–136.
78. Schneeberger SA, Hjelmeland LM, Tucker RP, Morse LS. Vascular endothelial growth factor and fibroblast growth factor 5 are colocalized in vascular and avascular epiretinal membranes. Am J Ophthalmol. 1997;124:447–454.
79. Tolentino MJ, Miller JW, Gragoudas ES, Chatzistefanou K, Ferrara N, Adamis AP. Vascular endothelial growth factor is sufficient to produce iris neovascularization and neovascular glaucoma in a nonhuman primate. Arch Ophthalmol. 1996;114:964–970.
80. Tobe T, Okamoto N, Vinores MA, et al. Evolution of neovascularization in mice with overexpression of vascular endothelial growth factor in photoreceptors. Invest Ophthalmol Vis Sci. 1998;39:180–188.
81. Okamoto N, Tobe T, Hackett SF, et al. Transgenic mice with increased expression of vascular endothelial growth factor in the retina: a new model of intraretinal and subretinal neovascularization [see comments]. Am J Pathol. 1997;151:281–291.

82. Senger DR, Connolly DT, Van de Water L, Feder J, Dvorak HF. Purification and NH2-terminal amino acid sequence of guinea pig tumor-secreted vascular permeability factor. *Cancer Res*. 1990;50:1774–1778.

83. Murata T, Ishibashi T, Khalil A, Hata Y, Yoshikawa H, Inomata H. Vascular endothelial growth factor plays a role in hyperpermeability of diabetic retinal vessels. *Ophthalmic Res*. 1995;27:48–52.

84. Murata T, Nakagawa K, Khalil A, Ishibashi T, Inomata H, Sueishi K. The relation between expression of vascular endothelial growth factor and breakdown of the blood-retinal barrier in diabetic rat retinas. *Lab Invest*. 1996;74:819–825.

85. Tolentino MJ, Miller JW, Gragoudas ES, et al. Intravitreous injections of vascular endothelial growth factor produce retinal ischemia and microangiopathy in an adult primate. *Ophthalmology*. 1996;103:1820–1828.

86. Aiello LP, Bursell SE, Clermont A, et al. Vascular endothelial growth factor-induced retinal permeability is mediated by protein kinase C in vivo and suppressed by an orally effective beta-isoform-selective inhibitor. *Diabetes*. 1997;46:1473–1480.

87. Antonetti DA, Barber AJ, Khin S, Lieth E, Tarbell JM, Gardner TW. Vascular permeability in experimental diabetes is associated with reduced endothelial occludin content: vascular endothelial growth factor decreases occludin in retinal endothelial cells. Penn State Retina Research Group. *Diabetes*. 1998;47:1953–1959.

88. Kevil CG, Payne DK, Mire E, Alexander JS. Vascular permeability factor/vascular endothelial cell growth factor-mediated permeability occurs through disorganization of endothelial junctional proteins. *J Biol Chem*. 1998;273:15099–15103.

89. Gerhardinger C, Brown LF, Roy S, Mizutani M, Zucker CL, Lorenzi M. Expression of vascular endothelial growth factor in the human retina and in nonproliferative diabetic retinopathy. *Am J Pathol*. 1998;152:1453–1462.

90. Boulton M, Foreman D, Williams G, McLeod D. VEGF localisation in diabetic retinopathy. *Br J Ophthalmol*. 1998;82:561–568.

91. Amin RH, Frank RN, Kennedy A, Eliott D, Puklin JE, Abrams GW. Vascular endothelial growth factor is present in glial cells of the retina and optic nerve of human subjects with nonproliferative diabetic retinopathy. *Invest Ophthalmol Vis Sci*. 1997;38:36–47.

92. Clermont AC, Aiello LP, Mori F, Aiello LM, Bursell SE. Vascular endothelial growth factor and severity of nonproliferative diabetic retinopathy mediate retinal hemodynamics in vivo: a potential role for vascular endothelial growth factor in the progression of nonproliferative diabetic retinopathy. *Am J Ophthalmol*. 1997;124:433–446.

93. Aiello LP, Pierce EA, Foley ED, et al. Suppression of retinal neovascularization in vivo by inhibition of vascular endothelial growth factor (VEGF) using soluble VEGF-receptor chimeric proteins. *Proc Natl Acad Sci USA*. 1995;92:10457–10461.

94. Adamis AP, Shima DT, Tolentino MJ, et al. Inhibition of vascular endothelial growth factor prevents retinal ischemia-associated iris neovascularization in a nonhuman primate. *Arch Ophthalmol*. 1996;114:66–71.

95. Robinson GS, Pierce EA, Rook SL, Foley E, Webb R, Smith LE. Oligodeoxynucleotides inhibit retinal neovascularization in a murine model of proliferative retinopathy. *Proc Natl Acad Sci USA*. 1996;93:4851–4856.

96. Oshima Y, Sakaguchi H, Fumi Gomi F, Yasuo T. Regression of iris neovascularization after intravitreal injection of bevacizumab in patients with proliferative diabetic retinopathy. *Am J Ophthalmol*. 2006;142:155–158.

97. Spaide RF, Fisher YL. Intravitreal bevacizumab (Avastin) treatment of proliferative diabetic retinopathy complicated by vitreous hemorrhage. *Retina*. 2006;26:275–278.

98. Avery RL, Joel Pearlman J, Pieramici DJ, et al. Intravitreal bevacizumab (Avastin) in the treatment of proliferative diabetic retinopathy. *Ophthalmology*. 2006;113: 1695–1715.

99. Fischer S, Sharma HS, Karliczek GF, Schaper W. Expression of vascular permeability factor/vascular endothelial growth factor in pig cerebral microvascular endothelial cells and its upregulation by adenosine. *Brain Res Mol Brain Res*. 1995;28: 141–148.

100. Fischer S, Knoll R, Renz D, Karliczek GF, Schaper W. Role of adenosine in the hypoxic induction of vascular endothelial growth factor in porcine brain derived microvascular endothelial cells [In Process Citation]. *Endothelium*. 1997;5:155–165.

101. Hashimoto E, Kage K, Ogita T, Nakaoka T, Matsuoka R, Kira Y. Adenosine as an endogenous mediator of hypoxia for induction of vascular endothelial growth factor mRNA in U-937 cells. *Biochem Biophys Res Commun*. 1994;204:318–324.

102. Lutty GA, Mathews MK, Merges C, McLeod DS. Adenosine stimulates canine retinal microvascular endothelial cell migration and tube formation. *Curr Eye Res*. 1998;17:594–607.

103. Takagi H, King GL, Robinson GS, Ferrara N, Aiello LP. Adenosine mediates hypoxic induction of vascular endothelial growth factor in retinal pericytes and endothelial cells. *Invest Ophthalmol Vis Sci*. 1996;37:2165–2176.

104. Bontemps F, Vincent MF, Van den Berghe G. Mechanisms of elevation of adenosine levels in anoxic hepatocytes. *Biochem J*. 1993;290:671–677.

105. Stavri GT, Zachary IC, Baskerville PA, Martin JF, Erusalimsky JD. Basic fibroblast growth factor upregulates the expression of vascular endothelial growth factor in vascular smooth muscle cells. Synergistic interaction with hypoxia. *Circulation*. 1995;92:11–14.

106. Milanini J, Vinals F, Pouyssegur J, Pages G. p42/p44 MAP kinase module plays a key role in the transcriptional regulation of the vascular endothelial growth factor gene in fibroblasts. *J Biol Chem*. 1998;273:18165–18172.

107. Hata Y, Rook S, Aiello LP. Basic fibroblast growth factor induces expression of VEGF receptor KDR through a protein kinase C and p44/p42 mitogen-activated protein kinase-dependent pathway. *Diabetes*. 1999;48:1145–1155.

108. Zucker S, Mirza H, Conner CE, et al. Vascular endothelial growth factor induces tissue factor and matrix metalloproteinase production in endothelial cells: conversion of prothrombin to thrombin results in progelatinase A activation and cell proliferation. *Int J Cancer*. 1998;75:780–786.

109. Mandriota SJ, Pepper MS. Vascular endothelial growth factor-induced in vitro angiogenesis and plasminogen activator expression are dependent on endogenous basic fibroblast growth factor. *J Cell Sci*. 1997;110:2293–2302.

110. Benezra M, Vlodavsky I, Ishai-Michaeli R, Neufeld G, Bar-Shavit R. Thrombin-induced release of active basic fibroblast growth factor-heparan sulfate complexes from subendothelial extracellular matrix. *Blood*. 1993;81:3324–3331.

111. Witte L, Hicklin DJ, Zhu Z, et al. Monoclonal antibodies targeting the VEGF receptor-2 (Flk1/KDR) as an anti-angiogenic therapeutic strategy. *Cancer Metastasis Rev*. 1998;17:155–161.

112. Zhu Z, Rockwell P, Lu D, et al. Inhibition of vascular endothelial growth factor-induced receptor activation with anti-kinase insert domain-containing receptor single- chain antibodies from a phage display library. *Cancer Res*. 1998;58: 3209–3214.

113. Ruckman J, Green LS, Beeson J, et al. 2'-Fluoropyrimidine RNA-based aptamers to the 165-amino acid form of vascular endothelial growth factor (VEGF165). Inhibition

of receptor binding and VEGF-induced vascular permeability through interactions requiring the exon 7-encoded domain. *J Biol Chem.* 1998;273:20556–20567.

114. Goldman CK, Kendall RL, Cabrera G, et al. Paracrine expression of a native soluble vascular endothelial growth factor receptor inhibits tumor growth, metastasis, and mortality rate. *Proc Natl Acad Sci USA.* 1998;95:8795–8800.

115. Siemeister G, Schirner M, Reusch P, Barleon B, Marme D, Martiny-Baron G. An antagonistic vascular endothelial growth factor (VEGF) variant inhibits VEGF-stimulated receptor autophosphorylation and proliferation of human endothelial cells. *Proc Natl Acad Sci USA.* 1998;95:4625–4629.

116. Kong HL, Hecht D, Song W, et al. Regional suppression of tumor growth by in vivo transfer of a cDNA encoding a secreted form of the extracellular domain of the flt-1 vascular endothelial growth factor receptor. *Hum Gene Ther.* 1998;9: 823–833.

117. Strawn LM, McMahon G, App H, et al. Flk-1 as a target for tumor growth inhibition. *Cancer Res.* 1996;56:3540–3545.

118. Xia P, Inoguchi T, Kern TS, Engerman RL, Oates PJ, King GL. Characterization of the mechanism for the chronic activation of diacylglycerol-protein kinase C pathway in diabetes and hypergalactosemia. *Diabetes.* 1994;43:1122–1129.

119. Mazure NM, Chen EY, Laderoute KR, Giaccia AJ. Induction of vascular endothelial growth factor by hypoxia is modulated by a phosphatidylinositol 3-kinase/Akt signaling pathway in Ha-ras-transformed cells through a hypoxia inducible factor-1 transcriptional element. *Blood.* 1997;90:3322–3331.

120. Williams B, Gallacher B, Patel H, Orme C. Glucose-induced protein kinase C activation regulates vascular permeability factor mRNA expression and peptide production by human vascular smooth muscle cells in vitro. *Diabetes.* 1997;46:1497–1503.

121. Gerber HP, McMurtrey A, Kowalski J, et al. Vascular endothelial growth factor regulates endothelial cell survival through the phosphatidylinositol 3'-kinase/Akt signal transduction pathway. Requirement for Flk-1/KDR activation. *J Biol Chem.* 1998;273:30336–30343.

122. Xia P, Aiello LP, Ishii H, et al. Characterization of vascular endothelial growth factor's effect on the activation of protein kinase C, its isoforms, and endothelial cell growth. *J Clin Invest.* 1996;98:2018–2026.

123. Danis RP, Bingaman DP, Jirousek M, Yang Y. Inhibition of intraocular neovascularization caused by retinal ischemia in pigs by PKCbeta inhibition with LY333531. *Invest Ophthalmol Vis Sci.* 1998;39:171–179.

124. Gragoudas ES, Adamis AP, Cunningham ET Jr, Feinsod M, Guyer DR; VEGF Inhibition Study in Ocular Neovascularization Clinical Trial Group. Pegaptanib for neovascular age-related macular degeneration. *N Engl J Med.* December 30, 2004;351(27):2805–2816.

125. Macugen Diabetic Retinopathy Study Group. A phase II randomized double-masked trial of pegaptanib, an anti-vascular endothelial growth factor aptamer, for diabetic macular edema. *Ophthalmology.* 2005;112:1747–1757.

126. Adamis AP, Altaweel M, Bressler NM, et al. Changes in retinal neovascularization after pegaptanib (Macugen) therapy in diabetic individuals. *Ophthalmology.* January 2006;113(1):23–28.

127. Rosenfeld PJ, Brown DM, Heier JS, et al. Ranibizumab for neovascular age-related macular degeneration. *N Engl J Med.* October 5, 2006;355(14):1419–1431.

128. Chun DW, Heier JS, Topping TM, Duker JS, Bankert JM. A pilot study of multiple intravitreal injections of ranibizumab in patients with center-involving clinically significant diabetic macular edema. *Ophthalmology.* 2006;113:1706–1712.

129. Nguyen QD, Tatlipinar S, Shah SM, et al. Vascular endothelial growth factor is a critical stimulus for diabetic macular edema. *Am J Ophthalmol.* December 2006;14(6):961–969.

130. Scott IU, Edwards AR, Beck RW, the Diabetic Retinopathy Clinical Research Network. A phase II randomized clinical trial of intravitreal bevacizumab for diabetic macular edema. *Ophthalmology.* 2007;114:1860–1867.

131. The PKC-DRS2 Research Group, Aiello LP, Davis MD et al. Effect of ruboxistaurin on visual loss in patients with diabetic retinopathy. *Ophthalmology.* December 2006;113(12);2135–2136;

132. Holash J, Davis S, Papadopoulos N, et al. VEGF-Trap: a VEGF blocker with potent antitumor effects. *Proc Natl Acad Sci USA.* 2002;99:11393–11398.

133. Saishin Y, Saishin Y, Takahashi K, et al. VEGF-TRAP(R1R2) suppresses choroidal neovascularization and VEGF-induced breakdown of the blood-retinal barrier. *J Cell Physiol.* 2003;195:241–248.

134. Jirousek MR, Gillig JR, Gonzalez CM, et al. (S)-13-[(dimethylamino)methyl]-10,11, 14,15-tetrahydro-4,9:16, 21-dimetheno-1H, 13H-dibenzo[e,k]pyrrolo[3,4-h][1,4,13] oxadiazacyclohexadecene-1,3(2H)-d ione (LY333531) and related analogues: isozyme selective inhibitors of protein kinase C beta. *J Med Chem.* 1996;39:2664–2671.

135. Ishii H, Jirousek MR, Koya D, et al. Amelioration of vascular dysfunctions in diabetic rats by an oral PKC beta inhibitor [see comments]. *Science.* 1996;272:728–731.

136. Aiello LP. The potential role of PKC beta in diabetic retinopathy and macular edema. *Surv Ophthalmol.* 2002;47:S263–S269.

137. The PKC-DRS Study Group. The effect of ruboxistaurin on visual loss in patients with moderately severe to very severe nonproliferative diabetic retinopathy: initial results of the Protein Kinase C beta Inhibitor Diabetic Retinopathy Study (PKC-DRS) multicenter randomized clinical trial. *Diabetes.* July 2005;54(7):2188–2197.

138. McGill JB, King GL, Berg PH, et al. Clinical safety of the selective PKC-beta inhibitor, ruboxistaurin. *Expert Opin Drug Saf.* November 2006;5(6):835–845.

139. Nauck M, Karakiulakis G, Perruchoud AP, et al. Corticosteroids inhibit the expression of the vascular endothelial growth factor gene in human vascular smooth muscle cells. *Eur J Pharmacol.* 1998;341:309–315.

140. Nauck M, Roth M, Tamm M, et al. Induction of vascular endothelial growth factor by platelet-activating factor and platelet-derived growth factor is downregulated by corticosteroids. *Am J Respir Cell Mol Biol.* 1997;16:398–406.

141. Challa JK, Gillies MC, Penfold PL, et al. Exudative macular degeneration and intravitreal triamcinolone: 18 month follow up. *Aust N Z J Ophthalmol.* 1998;26: 277–281.

142. Ishibashi T, Miki K, Sorgente N, et al. Effects of intravitreal administration of steroids on experimental subretinal neovascularization in the subhuman primate. *Arch Ophthalmol.* 1985;103:708–711.

143. Wang YS, Friedrichs U, Eichler W, et al. Inhibitory effects of triamcinolone acetonide on bFGF-induced migration and tube formation in choroidal microvascular endothelial cells. *Graefes Arch Clin Exp Ophthalmol.* 2002;240:42–48.

144. Danis RP, Bingaman DP, Yang Y, Ladd B. Inhibition of preretinal and optic nerve head neovascularization in pigs by intravitreal triamcinolone acetonide. *Ophthalmology.* 1996;103:2099–2104.

145. Penn JS, Rajaratnam VS, Collier RJ, Clark AF. The effect of an angiostatic steroid on neovascularization in a rat model of retinopathy of prematurity. *Invest Ophthalmol Vis Sci.* 2001;42:283–290.

146. Jonas JB, Hayler JK, Sofker A, Panda-Jonas S. Intravitreal injection of crystalline cortisone as adjunctive treatment of proliferative diabetic retinopathy. *Am J Ophthalmol.* 2001;131:468–471.

147. Jonas JB, Hayler JK, Sofker A, Panda-Jonas S. Regression of neovascular iris vessels by intravitreal injection of crystalline cortisone. *J Glaucoma.* 2001;10:284–287.

148. Yu SY, Damico FM, Viola F, D'Amico DJ, Young LH. Retinal toxicity of intravitreal triamcinolone acetonide: a morphological study. *Retina.* May–June 2006;26(5):531–536.

149. Jonas JB, Sofker A. Intraocular injection of crystalline cortisone as adjunctive treatment of diabetic macular edema. *Am J Ophthalmol.* 2001;132:425–427.

150. Martidis A, Duker JS, Greenberg PB, et al. Intravitreal triamcinolone for refractory diabetic macular edema. *Ophthalmology.* 2002;109:920–927.

151. Massin P, Audren F, Haouchine B, et al. Intravitreal triamcinolone acetonide for diabetic diffuse macular edema: preliminary results of a prospective controlled trial. *Ophthalmology.* 2004;111:218–224.

152. Gillies MC, Sutter FK, Simpson JM, Larsson J, Ali H, Zhu M. Intravitreal triamcinolone for refractory diabetic macular edema: two-year results of a double-masked, placebo-controlled, randomized clinical trial. *Ophthalmology.* September 2006;113(9):1533–1538.

153. Diabetic Retinopathy Clinical Research Network. A randomized trial comparing intravitreal triamcinolone acetonide and focal/grid photocoagulation for diabetic macular edema. *Ophthalmology.* September 2008;115(9):1447–1459.

154. Jager RD, Aiello LP, Patel SC, Cunningham ET, Jr. Risks of intravitreous injection: a comprehensive review. *Retina.* 2004;24:676–698.

155. Ohguro N, Okada AA, Tano Y. Trans-Tenon's retrobulbar triamcinolone infusion for diffuse diabetic macular edema. *Graefes Arch Clin Exp Ophthalmol.* 2004;242:444–445.

156. Scott M. Freidman. Results of peribulbar Steroids for Diabetic Macular Edema. Retina Subspecialty Day Presentation. American Academy of Ophthalmology Annual Meeting, Las Vegas, NV. Available at http://www.aao.org/annual_meeting/subspecialty/upload/06RET_Schedule_10_23_06.pdf Last accessed February 25, 2009.

157. Casey R, Li WW. Factors controlling ocular angiogenesis. *Am J Ophthalmol.* 1997; 124:521–529.

158. Ferris FL 3rd, Davis MD, Aiello LM. Treatment of diabetic retinopathy. *N Engl J Med.* August 26, 1999;341(9):667–678.

159. Aiello LP, Gardner TW, King GL, et al. Diabetic retinopathy. *Diabetes Care.* January 1998;21(1):143–156.

160. Gora-Kupilas K, Josko J. The neuroprotective function of vascular endothelial growth factor (VEGF). *Folia Neuropathol.* 2005;43(1):31–39.

161. Ostrowski RP, Colohan AR, Zhang JH. Mechanisms of hyperbaric oxygen-induced neuroprotection in a rat model of subarachnoid hemorrhage. *J Cereb Blood Flow Metab.* May 2005;25(5):554–571.

162. Sun FY, Guo X. Molecular and cellular mechanisms of neuroprotection by vascular endothelial growth factor. *J Neurosci Res.* January 1–15, 2005;79(1–2):180–184.

163. Losordo DW, Vale PR, Symes JF, et al. Gene therapy for myocardial angiogenesis: initial clinical results with direct myocardial injection of phVEGF165 as sole therapy for myocardial ischemia [In Process Citation]. *Circulation.* 1998;98: 2800–2804.

164. Watanabe D, Suzuma K, Matsui S, et al. Erythropoietin as a retinal angiogenic factor in proliferative diabetic retinopathy. *N Engl J Med*. August 25, 2005;353(8):782–792.
165. Aiello LP. Angiogenic pathways in diabetic retinopathy. *N Engl J Med*. August 25, 2005;353(8):839–841.
166. Yang JC, Haworth L, Sherry RM, et al. A randomized trial of bevacizumab, an anti-vascular endothelial growth factor antibody, for metastatic renal cancer. *N Engl J Med*. July 31, 2003;349(5):427–434.
167. The Early Treatment Diabetic Retinopathy Study Research Group. Grading diabetic retinopathy from stereoscopic color fundus photographs—an extension of the modified Airlie House classification. ETDRS report number 10. *Ophthalmology*. 1991;98:786–806.

21

Abstracts of Major Collaborative Multicenter Trials for Diabetic Retinopathy

Compiled by
INGRID U. SCOTT, MD, MPH,
NAUMAN A. CHAUDHRY, MD,
AND HARRY W. FLYNN, JR., MD

A-1

DIABETIC RETINOPATHY STUDY (DRS)

1. Diabetic Retinopathy Study Research Group: Preliminary report of effects of photocoagulation therapy. *Am J Ophthalmol.* 1976;81:383–396. Copyright 1976. Reprinted with permission from Elsevier Science.

Summary Analyses of visual acuity and visual field results in the DRS provide evidence that photocoagulation treatment as carried out according to the study protocol (extensive "scatter" photocoagulation and focal treatment of new vessels) is of benefit in preventing severe visual loss, over a 2-year follow-up period, in eyes with proliferative retinopathy. Location of new vessels relative to the disc, severity of new vessels, and the presence of hemorrhage (vitreous or preretinal) all proved to be important prognostic factors. On the basis of these findings, these steps have been taken: All patients in the study have been informed of results to date and given an explanation of their implications. Photocoagulation treatment will be considered for the initially untreated eyes which now or in the future fulfill any one of the following criteria: (1) moderate or severe new vessels on or within 1 disc diameter of the optic disc; (2) mild new vessels on or within 1 disc diameter of the optic disc if fresh hemorrhage is present; and (3) moderate or severe new vessels elsewhere if fresh hemorrhage is present. Follow-up of all patients will continue to allow long-term comparison between the argon and xenon treatment techniques employed. Further analysis of accumulating data will be performed to evaluate more completely the efficacy of photocoagulation therapy.

2. Diabetic Retinopathy Study Research Group: Photocoagulation treatment of proliferative diabetic retinopathy: the second report of Diabetic Retinopathy Study findings. *Ophthalmology* 1978;85;82–106. Courtesy of *Ophthalmology*.

Abstract Data from the DRS show that photocoagulation, as used in the study, reduced the rate of development of severe visual loss and inhibited the progression of retinopathy. These beneficial effects were noted to some degree in all those stages of diabetic retinopathy which were included in the study. Some deleterious effects of treatment were also found, including losses of visual acuity and constriction of peripheral visual field. The risk of these harmful effects was considered acceptable in the eyes with retinopathy in the moderate or severe proliferative stage when the risk of severe visual loss without treatment was great. In early proliferative or severe nonproliferative retinopathy, when the risk of severe visual loss without treatment was less, the risks of harmful treatment effects assumed greater importance. In these earlier stages, DRS findings have not led to a clear choice between prompt treatment and deferral of treatment unless and until progression to a more severe stage occurs. The purpose of this interim report is to present the data on which these conclusions are based. More detailed reports of the study findings will appear in the future.

3. Diabetic Retinopathy Study Research Group: Four risk factors for severe visual loss in diabetic retinopathy: the third report from the Diabetic Retinopathy Study. *Arch Ophthalmol.* 1979;97:654–655. Copyright 1979, American Medical Association. Reprinted with permission.

Abstract The DRS Research Group has so far identified four retinopathy factors that increase the 2-year risk of developing severe visual loss. The risk grows as the number of risk factors increases. Eyes with three or more risk factors (eyes with "high-risk characteristics") are at a much higher risk than eyes with two or fewer factors. The DRS protocol was changed in 1976 to require consideration of treatment for these "high-risk" eyes.

4. Diabetic Retinopathy Study Research Group: Photocoagulation treatment of proliferative diabetic retinopathy: a short report of long range results. DRS Report Number 4. In: *Proceedings of the 10th Congress of the International Diabetes Federation.* Amsterdam: Excerpta Medica;1980. Reprinted with permission of Elsevier.

Summary The 4-year follow-up information presented in this report confirms our previous general conclusion that photocoagulation treatment, as used in the DRS, reduces the risk of severe visual loss by more than 50% and extends this conclusion to the mildest stages of retinopathy included in the study. The reduction of the rate of severe visual loss remains somewhat greater in the xenon treatment group than in the argon group, but its magnitude is not sufficient to outweigh the more frequent occurrence of harmful side effects of the DRS xenon technique. Study findings continue to support prompt treatment when proliferative retinopathy is moderately severe. Persistent decreases in visual acuity resulted from study treatment techniques with sufficient frequency to suggest caution in applying them to eyes with mild proliferative or severe nonproliferative retinopathy. For eyes in these stages of retinopathy,

DRS findings do not provide a clear choice between prompt treatment and deferral of treatment unless and until progression to a more severe stage occurs.

5. Diabetic Retinopathy Study Research Group: Photocoagulation treatment of proliferative diabetic retinopathy: relationship of adverse treatment effects to retinopathy severity. DRS Report Number 5. *Dev Ophthalmol.* 1981;21:248–261. Reprinted with permission of Karger Medical and Scientific Publishers.

Summary Xenon arc photocoagulation, as carried out in the DRS, is attended by an increased risk of severe macular damage secondary to vitreoretinal traction. This risk is of particular importance in eyes with severe fibrous proliferation and/or localized traction retinal detachment. Little evidence was found of such an effect following argon laser photocoagulation, although some, mostly less serious, visual acuity decreases were attributable to this treatment as well. After 4 years of follow-up, the beneficial effect of xenon photocoagulation in reducing the risk of severe visual loss outweighed its harmful effect, even in eyes with severe fibrous proliferation and/or traction retinal detachment. A beneficial effect of approximately equal magnitude was present in the argon group.

6. Diabetic Retinopathy Study Research Group: Design, methods, and baseline results. DRS Report Number 6. *Invest Ophthalmol Vis Sci.* 1981;21:149–209. Copyright 1981, Association for Research in Vision and Ophthalmology. Reprinted with permission.

Summary The DRS is a collaborative clinical trial supported by the NEI. The main objectives of the DRS were the following three questions: (1) Does photocoagulation help prevent severe visual loss from proliferative diabetic retinopathy: (2) Is there a difference with respect to efficacy and safety between two treatment techniques: (a) extensive scatter treatment with the argon laser plus focal treatment of surface new vessels, elevated new vessels, and new vessels on or near the disc; or (b) extensive scatter treatment with the xenon arc plus focal treatment of surface new vessels? (3) Are there some stages of retinopathy in which treatment is helpful but others in which it is of no value or harmful? Fifteen clinical centers participated in the DRS. Patient recruitment started in April 1972, and the last patient was treated in September 1975; a total of 1758 patients were enrolled. Patients enrolled in the study had one eye randomly assigned to prompt photocoagulation with either argon or xenon and the other eye to no treatment. The primary response variable was visual acuity, but visual fields and changes in the retina and vitreous were also considered in the evaluation of treatment. All completed study forms and fundus photograph readings were sent to the Coordinating Center for editing, analysis, and storage. The DRS data were reviewed by the Data Monitoring Committee for evidence of adverse and beneficial treatment effects. The following are highlights of the characteristics of the patients enrolled in this study: (1) Patients were predominantly white, and there were slightly more men than women. (2) The age distribution of the enrolled patients was bimodal, with peaks at 20 to 29 years and 50 to 59 years of age. (3) Approximately 45% of the patients could be classified as juvenile-onset diabetics. (4) Two thirds of the patients had borderline or definite hypertension, on the basis of supine blood pressure readings at entry. (5) Visual acuity was equal to or better than 20/20 in approximately half of the eyes, and there was approximately the same distribution of visual acuity levels for all four groups of eyes: eyes assigned to argon treatment; eyes assigned to xenon treatment; and the fellow eyes of patients in each of these groups. (6) Over 90% of the eyes had intraocular pressure 20 mmHg or less. (7) Fifty percent of the eyes had NVD (neovascularization of the disc), and nearly 75% had NVE (neovascularization elsewhere) as determined by the ophthalmic examination at initial visit. (8) Twenty-five percent had definite macular edema involving the center of the macula with or without cystoid changes as identified by the ophthalmic examination at baseline. On the basis of the baseline variables considered, there was no evidence of lack of comparability of the patients assigned to argon and xenon or lack of comparability of the four groups of eyes at baseline. Two previous reports contained the findings that led to the protocol changes in 1976 and 1977. Additional papers dealing with assessment of treatment effects are being prepared for publication.

7. Diabetic Retinopathy Study Research Group: A modification of the Airlie House classification of diabetic retinopathy. DRS Report Number 7. *Invest Ophthalmol Vis Sci.* 1981;21:210–226. Copyright 1981, Association for Research in Vision and Ophthalmology. Reprinted with permission.

Summary A modification of the Airlie House classification of diabetic retinopathy is described in detail. The classification uses a combination of standard stereo-scopic photographs and written definitions to grade more than 20 lesions on a three- to six-step scale.

8. Diabetic Retinopathy Study Research Group: Photocoagulation treatment of proliferative diabetic retinopathy: clinical application of Diabetic Retinopathy Study (DRS) findings. DRS Report Number 8. *Ophthalmology.* 1981;88:583–600. Courtesy of *Ophthalmology.*

Abstract Additional follow-up confirms previous reports from the DRS that photocoagulation, as used in the study, reduces the risk of severe visual loss by 50% or more. Decreases of visual acuity of one or more lines and constriction of peripheral visual field due to treatment were also observed in some eyes. These harmful effects were more frequent and more severe following the DRS xenon technique. The 2-year risk of severe visual loss without treatment outweighs the risk of harmful treatment effects for two groups of eyes: (1) eyes with new vessels and pre-retinal or vitreous hemorrhages; and (2) eyes with new vessels on or within 1 disc diameter of the optic disc (NVD) (neovascularization of the disc) equaling or exceeding 1/4 to 1/3 disc area in extent, even in the absence of preretinal or vitreous hemorrhage. For eyes with these characteristics, prompt treatment is usually advisable. For eyes with less severe retinopathy, DRS findings do not provide a clear choice between prompt treatment or deferral unless progression to these more severe stages occur.

9. Diabetic Retinopathy Study Research Group: Assessing possible late treatment effects in stopping a clinical trial early: a case study. DRS Report Number 9.

Abstract Suppose a fixed-sample trial in a disease with a long response time shows a statistically significant benefit of the experimental treatment before patients have completed the planned follow-up period. The question may then arise—and did arise in the DRS—whether thc observed early benefit of treatment may be offset at some time in the future by the subsequent development of harmful treatment effects. If this question raises serious concerns, then the investigators are faced with a dilemma. If the trial is stopped because of the observed early treatment benefit and the treatment is administered to the untreated control group as well as to patients outside the study and if the treatment is later found to have deleterious effects, then it may ultimately do more harm than good to patients. Moreover, the fact that the treatment is harmful may never become known. If, on the other hand, the trial is not stopped and the treatment proves to have no deleterious effects, then the control group and patients outside the study would be harmed because the treatment was withheld. We show how, in the DRS, this very problem was formulated and resolved. First, a severe, delayed harmful treatment effect was postulated. Projections based on this postulation showed that the early gains were so great that they were unlikely to be offset—ever. Based in part on these projections, the following decisions were made. (1) the study protocol would be changed so as to allow treatment of the untreated control group, and (2) patients would continue to be followed in order to make possible the detection of late, harmful treatment effects, should they develop.

10. Diabetic Retinopathy Study Research Group: Factors influencing the development of visual loss in advanced diabetic retinopathy. DRS Report Number 10. *Invest Ophthalmol Vis Sci.* 1985;26:983–991. Copyright 1985, Association for Research in Vision and Ophthalmology. Reprinted with permission.

Abstract Natural history data from the DRS were examined by multivariate methods to determine which baseline characteristics could predict the occurrence of severe visual loss (SVL) in eyes originally assigned to no treatment. The presence and extent of new blood vessels on the optic disc (NVD) (neovascularization of the disc) had the strongest association with severe visual loss (SVL). Several other ocular characteristics also were strongly associated with visual outcome. In the absence of new blood vessels on the optic disc (NVD) at baseline, the degree of intraretinal hemorrhages and microaneurysms (HMA) had the strongest association with development of SVL. Macular edema was a factor in determining visual loss to 20/200 but not SVL (less than 5/200). Among systemic characteristics, urinary protein was the best predictor of visual outcome, but none were as good as the major ocular variables.

11. Diabetic Retinopathy Study Research Group: Intraocular pressure following panretinal photocoagulation for diabetic retinopathy. DRS Report Number 11. *Arch Ophthalmol.* 1987;105:807–809. Copyright 1987, American Medical Association. Reprinted with permission.

Abstract Data collected during the first 5 years after randomization in the DRS were analyzed to determine the effect of panretinal photocoagulation on intraocular pressure (IOP). At each follow-up visit, median IOP was identical for the treated and untreated eyes. Mean IOP rose slightly in each group. The proportion of untreated eyes with IOP above 30 mmHg at two consecutive visits was twice that of the treated eyes (2% versus 1%). These data show that panretinal photocoagulation reduces the risk of subsequent intraocular hypertension, apparently by preventing the development of neovascular glaucoma.

12. Diabetic Retinopathy Study Research Group: Macular edema in Diabetic Retinopathy Study patients. DRS Report Number 12. *Ophthalmology*. 1987;94:754–760. Courtesy of *Ophthalmology*.

Abstract Results from the DRS demonstrate that scatter photocoagulation is associated with some loss of visual acuity soon after treatment. The visual loss is especially prominent in the eyes with preexisting macular edema. It is also associated with the intensity of treatment. Reducing macular edema by focal photocoagulation before initiating scatter treatment and dividing scatter treatment into multiple sessions with less intense burns may decrease the risk of the visual loss associated with photocoagulation.

13. Diabetic Retinopathy Study Research Group: Factors associated with visual outcome after photocoagulation for diabetic retinopathy. DRS Report Number 13. *Invest Ophthalmol Vis Sci*. 1989;30:23–28. Copyright 1989, Association for Research in Vision and Ophthalmology. Reprinted with permission.

Abstract Six risk factors for severe visual loss despite panretinal (scatter) photocoagulation were identified by analyzing data collected during the first 5 years after randomization in the DRS. Proportional hazards regression revealed NVD (neovascularization on/around the optic disc) to be the most important risk factor. The risk of severe visual loss rose with increasing NVD, hemorrhages, microaneurysms, retinal elevation, proteinuria, and hypoglycemia and fell with increasing "treatment density." These results are similar to previous DRS findings on untreated eyes. The importance of "treatment density" as an independent predictor of visual outcome is a new finding and lends support to the common clinical practice of repeating photocoagulation if initial treatment does not reduce or stabilize retinal neovascularization.

14. Diabetic Retinopathy Study Research Group: Indications for photocoagulation treatment of diabetic retinopathy. DRS Report Number 14. *Int Ophthalmol Clin*. 1987;27:239–253. Courtesy of Lippincott-Raven Publishes.

Conclusions When photocoagulation is to be undertaken in the hope of reducing the risk of severe visual loss, the principal factor influencing the decision between prompt treatment and deferral of treatment with continued careful follow-up is the presence of DRS high-risk characteristics. The situation is particularly urgent when there is a threat that dispersion or recurrence of vitreous hemorrhage may soon preclude treatment or when new vessels in the anterior chamber angle pose the threat of neovascular glaucoma. Intraretinal changes should also be considered; when they are severe in both eyes, prompt initiation of treatment in one is attractive. When macular edema is present in an eye needing scatter photocoagulation, it may be desirable to treat the edema with focal or grid photocoagulation first, if scatter treatment is not urgent.

A-2

EARLY TREATMENT DIABETIC RETINOPATHY STUDY (ETDRS)

1. Early Treatment Diabetic Retinopathy Study Research Group: Photocoagulation for diabetic macular edema. ETDRS Report Number 1. *Arch Ophthalmol* 1985;103:1796–1806. Copyright 1985, American Medical Association. Reprinted with permission.

Abstract Data from the ETDRS show that focal photocoagulation of "clinically significant" diabetic macular edema substantially reduces the risk of visual loss. Focal treatment also increases the chance of visual improvement, decreases the frequency of persistent macular edema, and causes only minor visual field losses. In this randomized clinical trial, which was supported by the National Eye Institute, 754 eyes that had macular edema and mild-to-moderate diabetic retinopathy were randomly assigned to focal argon laser photocoagulation, while 1490 such eyes were randomly assigned to deferral of photocoagulation. The beneficial effects of treatment demonstrated in this trial suggest that all eyes with clinically significant diabetic macular edema should be considered for focal photocoagulation. Clinically significant macular edema is defined as retinal thickening that involves or threatens the center of the macula (even if visual acuity is not yet reduced) and is assessed by stereoscopic contact lens biomicroscopy or stereoscopic photography. Follow-up of all ETDRS patients continues without other modifications in the study protocol.

2. Early Treatment Diabetic Retinopathy Study Research Group: Treatment techniques and clinical guidelines for photocoagulation of diabetic macular edema. ETDRS Report Number 2. *Ophthalmology.* 1987;94:761–774. Courtesy of *Ophthalmology.*

Abstract The ETDRS has recently shown that argon laser photocoagulation treatment is beneficial in reducing the risk of visual loss from clinically significant diabetic macular edema. The ETDRS treatment consisted of a combination of focal treatment to individual leaking microaneurysms and grid treatment to areas of diffuse leakage and capillary nonperfusion. These techniques are described in detail and the concepts of "clinically significant macular edema" and "treatable lesions" are defined. Guidelines for the application of ETDRS findings to clinical practice are discussed.

3. Early Treatment Diabetic Retinopathy Study Research Group: Techniques for scatter and local photocoagulation treatment of diabetic retinopathy. ETDRS Report Number 3. *Int Ophthalmol Clin.* 1987;27:254–264. Courtesy of Lippincott-Raven Publishers.

Comments ETDRS techniques for scatter and local photocoagulation evolved from those of the DRS (Diabetic Retinopathy Study), which were based on those of many previous investigators. The full scatter and local protocols presented here are, we believe, suitable whenever photocoagulation is undertaken for PDR (proliferative diabetic retinopathy). We believe that follow-up treatment is important and that the clinical guidelines outlined in the protocol are suitable for widespread application.

4. Early Treatment Diabetic Retinopathy Study Research Group: Photocoagulation for diabetic macular edema. ETDRS Report Number 4. *Int Ophthalmol Clin.* 1987;27:265–272. Courtesy of Lippincott-Raven Publishers.

Comments The combination of focal and grid photocoagulation used in the ETDRS led to a reduction in the occurrence of visual acuity decrease (doubling of the visual angle) by approximately 50% to 70% in eyes with retinal thickening or associated hard exudate involving or threatening the center of the macular and visual acuity of 20/200 or better. ETDRS photocoagulation for macular edema emphasized focal treatment, with attempts to close larger microaneurysms directly, and follow-up treatment. In applying these results to clinical practice, it is important to remember that the comparisons presented are between prompt photocoagulation and indefinite deferral of photocoagulation, regardless of the course followed. In clinical practice, the decision is between prompt photocoagulation and deferral with careful follow-up, with reconsideration of this decision at each visit. Factors to be taken into account include the degree to which the center of the macula is involved or threatened by thickening or hard exudate, the proximity of focal leaks requiring treatment to the center and visual acuity.

4a. Early Treatment Diabetic Retinopathy Study Research Group: Case Reports to Accompany Early Treatment Diabetic Retinopathy Study Reports 3 and 4. *Int Ophthalmol Clin.* 1987;27:273–333. Courtesy of Lippincott-Raven Publishers.

Summary The principals exemplified by the proceeding case reports are summarized below. (1) Although the presence of DRS (Diabetic Retinopathy Study) high-risk characteristics is the single most important indication for initiating scatter photocoagulation, intraretinal lesions suggesting ischemia (soft exudates), IRMA [intraretinal microvascular abnormalities], venous beading, arteriolar abnormalities, and moderately severe hemorrhages and/or microaneurysms) are also important. When these lesions are severe, rapid progression is likely, and initiation of scatter photocoagulation should be considered for at least one eye even when new vessels are absent or mild (Cases 3, 5, 9, and 11). Both eyes should be followed carefully, whether treated or not, and special attention to blood pressure and renal status may be important. When these intraretinal lesions are mostly absent or mild, progression of PDR [proliferative diabetic retinopathy] may be very slow (Cases 1, 6, and 7). (2) NVD [neovascularization of the disc] is the single most important prognostic feature of diabetic retinopathy, and when it is well established (i.e., greater than or equal to DRS standard photograph 10A), the indication for initiation of scatter photocoagulation is strong (Cases 7, 8, 10, and 11). (3) NVE [neovascularization elsewhere] in the absence of vitreous or preretinal hemorrhage or the severe intraretinal lesions listed in item 1 are a weaker indication for photocoagulation, and careful observation of such eyes is a reasonable alternative to prompt treatment. (4) The *initial* vitreous or preretinal hemorrhage in eyes with PDR is rarely so large that photocoagulation cannot be carried out before a subsequent larger hemorrhage occurs, *provided patients report symptoms and are examined promptly.* In such cases, it is prudent to treat the lower quadrants first, if possible, before they become obscured by hemorrhage (Cases 3 to 7 and 9 to 11). (5) Even after full scatter photocoagulation, with burns placed no more than one half burn diameter apart, there is ample room for additional treatment between scars, and this often seems to be effective in encouraging regression of new vessels that remain or recur after the completion of the initial treatment. Such additional scatter treatment may be concentrated in the areas of NVE (Cases 2 and 5) or applied throughout the fundus (Cases 4 and 9–11). Extension of scatter photocoagulation in the posterior pole also appears to be effective sometimes (Case 8). (6) Knowledge of the tendency for new vessels to follow a cycle proliferation and regression is important when considering additional scatter treatment when new vessels fail to regress or recur after initial scatter treatment. With this tendency in mind, the goal of photocoagulation set for such eyes can be the more realistic one of retaining new vessels rather than completely eliminating them (Cases 2, 4, and 10). With such a goal, it is less likely that peripheral field will be destroyed. (7) Familiarity with the typical course followed by posterior vitreous detachment in eyes with PDR is also important. Prior to posterior vitreous detachment, proliferation of new vessels is paralleled by increasing vitreoretinal adhesions, but this is not the case when new vessels grow along the detached posterior vitreous surface or arise from the retina in areas where the vitreous is detached. Only occasionally do sheets of new vessels in fibrous tissue capable of causing retinal distortion secondary to their contraction proliferate on the retinal surface after posterior vitreous detachment. An eye in which new vessels and fibrous proliferations are limited mostly to the detached posterior vitreous surface is at little risk of traction retinal detachment and, if severe vitreous hemorrhage occurs, is a good candidate for vitrectomy (Cases 2, 10, and 11). Small patches of new vessels are sometimes avulsed completely from the retina, and the vitreous hemorrhage accompanying this event frequently is the last to occur (Cases 5–7). (8) Elevated new vessels seem less easily influenced by scatter photocoagulation than those on the surface of the retina (Cases 2, 10, and 11). (9) Because the size of photocoagulation burns is influenced not only by spot size setting, but also by strength of the burns (dependent on both power and duration as well as clarity of the media), the total number of scattered burns at a specified setting is not a satisfactory measure of the amount of treatment applied (Cases 4, 5, and 8). (10) Narrowing of retinal vessels frequently accompanies quiescence of retinopathy (Cases 4, 5, and 7–9). (11) Strong local confluent photocoagulation of NVE may cause noticeable scotomas, including nerve fiber bundle defects (Cases 3 and 7). (12) There is no doubt that photocoagulation improves the outlook for maintaining visual acuity in eyes with diabetic macular edema and that, for eyes with clinically significant macular edema, prompt treatment is preferable to permanent non treatment. But progression often is slow (Case 14, left eye), and occasionally

spontaneous improvement occurs (Cases 3, 11, 16 [right eye], and 18), so that deferral of treatment and careful follow-up may often be a useful strategy, particularly
when thickening of the center of the macula is absent or equivocal or lesions to be
treated are close to it (Cases 17, 18, and 20). (13) In view of the adverse effect that
scatter photocoagulation often has, at least temporarily, on macular edema, it may
be desirable in eyes needing such treatment to carry out focal or grid treatment for
macular edema before (or at least concurrently with) scatter treatment (Cases 3 and
11). Note that case 12 did well with no treatment for macular edema. (14) Hard
exudates not infrequently increase temporarily when macular edema decreases
(spontaneously or after grid or focal treatment), and this may threaten the center
of the macula (Cases 11 and 16). (15) The ETDRS protocol emphasized careful
follow-up after initial treatment for macular edema, with retreatment whenever
clinically significant macular edema and treatable lesions were present (Case 15).
(16) Fluorescein leakage without retinal thickening *does not constitute* macular
edema (Case 19). [Emphases in original.]

5. Kinyoun J, Barton F, Fisher M, et al.: Detection of diabetic macular edema:
ophthalmoscopy vs. photography. ETDRS Report Number 5. *Ophthalmology.*
1989;96:746–751. Courtesy of *Ophthalmology.*

Abstract Clinical and photographic methods were used to assess retinopathy during the examination of diabetic patients enrolled in the ETDRS. In analyzing
available data from eyes randomly selected for deferral of treatment, the authors
compare the clinical detection (including contact lens biomicroscopy) with photographic detection (30 degrees stereoscopic fundus photographs) of diabetic macular edema. Based on clinical detection, 53% (1778 patients) had hard exudates
within 1 disc diameter (DD) of the center of the macula, 56% (1868 patients) had
retinal thickening within this region, and 31% (1027 patients) had thickening at
the center of the macula. These analyses show agreements of 83%, 78%, and
83% between retinal specialists and photographic graders when assessing these
three characteristics, respectively. Agreement was 81% in the detection of macular edema for which treatment is indicated (clinically significant macular edema).
Each method has its advantages, but in general there was close agreement between
these methods, particularly for clinically significant macular edema, which supports the reliability of each method.

6. Early Treatment Diabetic Retinopathy Study Research Group: C-peptide in
the classification of diabetes mellitus patients in the Early Treatment Diabetic
Retinopathy Study. ETDRS Report Number 6. *Ann Epidemiol.* 1993;3:9–17.
Copyright 1993. Reprinted with permission from Elsevier Science.

Abstract The ETDRS, conducted at 22 clinical studies during the period of 1980–
1989, collected baseline data on C-peptide levels after ingestion of Sustacal in 582
patients with diabetes mellitus, prior to enrollment in the trial. Data on several
clinical factors associated with diabetes were also collected from all 3711 enrolled
patients. C-peptide data were used to develop sets of clinical criteria for the classification of ETDRS patients and to compare and contrast definitions of type of

diabetes used in previous studies. The distribution of C-peptide levels was strikingly bimodal, suggesting a division of study participants into two groups—those with levels at 80 pmol/L or less and those with more than 80 pmol/L of C-peptide after Sustacal ingestion. Constellations of clinical characteristics that could serve as proxies for C-peptide level were ascertained. The result was two sets of clinically developed definitions for type of diabetes in the ETDRS. According to the more restrictive set of definitions, three groups were identified, compared to two groups using the "broad" set of definitions. Discriminant analysis was also used to classify ETDRS patients, yielding similar results. A comparison of definitions of type of diabetes used in the ETDRS and in previous studies revealed that even in the absence of C-peptide data, clinically derived definitions provided good discrimination between type I and type II diabetes.

7. Early Treatment Diabetic Retinopathy Study Group: Early Treatment Diabetic Retinopathy Study design and baseline patient characteristics. ETDRS Report Number 7. *Ophthalmology*. 1991;98:741–756. Courtesy of *Ophthalmology*.

Abstract The ETDRS, a multicenter collaborative clinical trial supported by the National Eye Institute, was designed to assess whether argon laser photocoagulation or aspirin treatment can reduce the risk of visual loss or slow the progression of diabetic retinopathy in patients with mild to severe nonproliferative or early proliferative diabetic retinopathy. The 3711 patients enrolled in the ETDRS were assigned randomly to either aspirin (650 mg per day) or placebo. One eye of each patient was assigned randomly to early argon laser photocoagulation, and the other to deferral of photocoagulation. Both eyes were to be examined at least every four months and photocoagulation was to be initiated in eyes assigned to deferral as soon as high risk proliferative retinopathy was detected. Examination of a large number of baseline ocular and patient characteristics indicated that there were no important differences between randomized treatment groups at baseline.

8. Early Treatment Diabetic Retinopathy Study Research Group: Effects of aspirin treatment on diabetic retinopathy. ETDRS Report Number 8. *Ophthalmology*. 1991;98:757–765. Courtesy of *Ophthalmology*.

Abstract Aspirin treatment did not alter the course of diabetic retinopathy in patients enrolled in the ETDRS. In the randomized clinical trial supported by the National Eye Institute, 3711 patients with mild to severe nonproliferative or early proliferative diabetic retinopathy were assigned randomly to either aspirin (650 mg per day) or placebo. Aspirin did not prevent the development of proliferative retinopathy and did not reduce the risk of visual loss, nor did it increase the risk of vitreous hemorrhage. This was true both for eyes assigned randomly to deferral of photocoagulation and for eyes assigned randomly to early argon laser photocoagulation. The ETDRS results indicate that for patients with mild to severe nonproliferative or early proliferative diabetic retinopathy, it is likely that aspirin has no clinically important beneficial effects on the progression of retinopathy. The data also show that aspirin 650 mg per day had no clinically important harmful effects for diabetic patients with retinopathy. These findings suggest there are no ocular contraindications to aspirin when required for cardiovascular disease or other medical indications.

9. Early Treatment Diabetic Retinopathy Study Research Group: Early photocoagulation for diabetic retinopathy. ETDRS Report Number 9. *Ophthalmology*. 1991;98:766–785. Courtesy of *Ophthalmology*.

Abstract The ETDRS enrolled 3711 patients with mild to severe nonproliferative or early proliferative diabetic retinopathy in both eyes. One eye of each patient was assigned randomly to early photocoagulation, and the other to deferral of photocoagulation. Follow-up examinations were scheduled at least every four months, and photocoagulation was initiated in eyes assigned to deferral as soon as high risk proliferative retinopathy was detected. Eyes selected for early photocoagulation received one of four different combinations of scatter (panretinal) and focal treatment. This early treatment, compared with deferral of photocoagulation, was associated with a small reduction in the incidence of severe visual loss (visual acuity less than 5/200 at two consecutive visits), but five year rates were low in both the early treatment and the deferral groups (2.6% and 3.7%, respectively). Adverse effects of scatter photocoagulation on visual acuity and visual field were also observed. These adverse effects were most evident in the months immediately following treatment and were less in eyes assigned to less extensive scatter photocoagulation. Provided careful follow-up can be maintained, scatter photocoagulation is not recommended for eyes with mild to moderate nonproliferative diabetic retinopathy. When retinopathy is more severe, scatter photocoagulation should be considered and usually should not be delayed if the eye has reached the high risk proliferative stage. The ETDRS results demonstrate that, for eyes with macular edema, focal photocoagulation is effective in reducing the risk in moderate visual loss, but that scatter photocoagulation is not. Focal treatment also increases the chance of visual improvement, decreases the frequency of persistent macular edema, and causes only minor visual field losses. Focal treatment should be considered for eyes with macular edema that involves or threatens the center of the macula.

10. Early Treatment Diabetic Retinopathy Study Research Group: Grading diabetic retinopathy from stereoscopic color fundus photographs: an extension of the modified Airlie House classification. ETDRS Report Number 10. *Ophthalmology*. 1991;98:786–806. Courtesy of *Ophthalmology*.

Abstract The modified Airlie House classification of diabetic retinopathy has been extended for the use in ETDRS. The revised classification provides additional steps in the grading scale from some characteristics, separates other characteristics previously combined, expands the section on macular edema, and adds several characteristics not previously graded. The classification is described and illustrated, and its reproducibility between graders is assessed by calculating percentages of agreement and kappa statistics for duplicate gradings of baseline color nonsimultaneous stereoscopic fundus photos. For retinal hemorrhages and/or microaneurysms, hard exudates, new vessels, fibrous proliferations, and macular edema, agreement was substantial (weighted kappa: 0.61–0.80). For soft exudates, intraretinal micro-vascular abnormalities, and venous beading, agreement was moderate (weighted kappa: 0.41–0.60). A double grading system, with adjudication of disagreements of two or more steps between duplicate gradings, led to some improvement in reproducibility for most characteristics.

11. Early Treatment Diabetic Retinopathy Study Research Group: Classification of diabetic retinopathy from fluorescein angiograms. ETDRS Report Number 11. *Ophthalmology.* 1991;98:807–822. Courtesy of *Ophthalmology.*

Abstract The ETDRS included use of nonsimultaneous stereoscopic fluorescein angiography to assess severity of characteristics such as capillary loss and fluo-rescein leakage and to guide treatment of macular edema. Two 30 degree pho-tographic fields were taken, extending along the horizontal meridian from about 25 degrees nasal to the disc to about 20 degrees temporal to the macula, and the classification system was constructed to allow assessment of the selected charac-teristics. This classification system relies on comparisons with standard example photographs to evaluate the presence and severity of capillary loss and dilation, arteriolar abnormalities, leakage of fluorescein dye (including characterization of source), abnormalities of the retinal pigment epithelium, cystoid changes, and several other features. The classification is described and illustrated, and its repro-ducibility between graders assessed by calculating percentages of agreement and kappa statistics for duplicate gradings of baseline angiograms. Agreement was substantial (weighted kappa: 0.61–0.80) for severity of fluorescein leakage and cystoid spaces and moderate (weighted kappa: 0.41–0.60) for capillary loss, cap-illary dilation, narrowing/pruning of arteriolar branches, staining of arteriolar walls, and source of fluorescein leakage (microaneurysms vs. diffusely leaking capillaries).

12. Early Treatment Diabetic Retinopathy Study Research Group: Fundus pho-tographic risk factors for progression of diabetic retinopathy. ETDRS Report Number 12. *Ophthalmology.* 1991;98:823–833. Courtesy of *Ophthalmology.*

Abstract In the ETDRS, a randomized clinical trial sponsored by the National Eye Institute, one eye of each patient was assigned to early photocoagulation and the other to deferral of photocoagulation (i.e., careful follow-up and initiation of pho-tocoagulation only if high-risk proliferative retinopathy developed). This design allowed observation of the natural course of diabetic retinopathy in the initially untreated eye. Gradings of baseline stereoscopic fundus photographs of eyes with nonproliferative retinopathy assigned to deferral of photocoagulation were used to examine the power of various abnormalities and combinations of abnormalities to predict progression to proliferative retinopathy in photographs taken at the 1-, 3-, and 5-year follow-up visits. Severity of intraretinal microvascular abnormal-ities, hemorrhages, and/or microaneurysms, and venous beading were found to be the most important factors in predicting progression. On the basis of these anal-yses and other considerations, a retinopathy severity scale was developed. This scale, which divides diabetic retinopathy into 13 levels ranging from absence of retinopathy to severe vitreous hemorrhage, can be used to describe overall retinopathy severity and change in severity over time.

13. Early Treatment Diabetic Retinopathy Study Research Group: Fluorescein angiographic risk factors for progression of diabetic retinopathy. ETDRS Report Number 13. *Ophthalmology.* 1991;98:834–840. Courtesy of *Ophthalmology.*

Abstract In the ETDRS, a multicenter clinical trial sponsored by the National Eye Institute, one eye of each patient was assigned randomly to early photocoagulation and the other to deferral of photocoagulation (i.e., careful follow-up and initiation of photocoagulation only if high-risk proliferative retinopathy developed). This design allowed observation of the natural course of diabetic retinopathy in the initially untreated eye. Gradings of baseline stereoscopic fluorescein angiograms of these eyes were used to examine relationships of angiographic characteristics with each other, with retinopathy severity level and macular edema status graded from color photographs, and with risk of progression for nonproliferative to proliferative retinopathy during 1 to 5 years of follow-up. Fluorescein leakage (particularly diffuse), capillary loss and dilation, and various arteriolar abnormalities were associated with retinopathy severity and with the likelihood of progression to proliferative retinopathy during follow-up. Severity of fluorescein leakage was strongly associated with macular edema.

14. Early Treatment Diabetic Retinopathy Study Research Group: Aspirin effects on mortality and morbidity in patients with diabetes mellitus. ETDRS Report Number 14. *J Am Med Assn.* 1992; 268: 1292–1300. Copyright 1992, American Medical Association. Reprinted with permission.

Abstract *Objectives*: This report presents information on the effects of aspirin on mortality, the occurrence of cardiovascular events, and the incidence of kidney disease in the patients enrolled in the ETDRS. *Study design:* This multicenter, randomized clinical trial of aspirin versus placebo was sponsored by the National Eye Institute. *Patients:* Patients (N = 3711) were enrolled in 22 clinical centers between April 1980 and July 1985. Men and women between the ages of 18 and 70 years with a clinical diagnosis of diabetes mellitus were eligible. Approximately 30% of all patients were considered to have type I diabetes mellitus, 31% type 2, and 39% type 1 or 2 could not be determined definitely. *Intervention:* Patients were randomly assigned to aspirin or placebo (two 325-mg tablets once per day). *Main outcome measures:* Mortality from all causes was specified as the primary outcome measure for assessing the systemic effects of aspirin. Other outcome variables included cause-specific mortality and cardiovascular events. *Results:* The estimate of relative risk for total mortality for aspirin-treated patients compared with placebo-treated patients for the entire study period was 0.91 (99% confidence interval: 0.75 to 1.11). Larger differences were noted for the occurrence of fatal and nonfatal myocardial infarction: the estimate of relative risk was 0.83 for the entire follow-up period (99% confidence interval: 0.66 to 1.04). *Conclusions:* The effects of aspirin on any of the cardiovascular events considered in the ETDRS were not substantially different from the effects observed in other studies that included mainly nondiabetic persons. Furthermore, there was no evidence of harmful effects of aspirin. Aspirin has been recommended previously for persons at risk for cardio-vascular disease. The ETDRS results support application of this recommendation to those persons with diabetes at increased risk of cardiovascular disease.

15. Early Treatment Diabetic Retinopathy Study Research Group: Impaired color vision associated with diabetic retinopathy. ETDRS Report Number 15. *Am J Ophthalmol.* 1999;128:612–617. Copyright 1999. Reprinted with permission from Elsevier Science.

Abstract *Purpose*: To report color vision abnormalities associated with diabetic retinopathy. *Methods:* Color vision function was measured at baseline in 2701 patients enrolled in the ETDRS, a randomized trial investigating photocoagulation and aspirin in the treatment of diabetic retinopathy. Hue discrimination was measured by the Farnsworth-Munsell 100-Hue test, and errors in color vision were reported as the square root of the total 100-Hue (SQRT 100-Hue) score. *Results:* Approximately 50% of the ETDRS population had color vision scores (SQRT 100-Hue score) worse than 95% of the normal population reported by Verriest and associates. The factors most strongly associated with impaired hue discrimination were macular edema severity, age, and presence of new vessels. A tritan-like defect was prominent and increased in magnitude with increasing severity of macular edema. However, many patients had color discrimination impairment without macular edema. *Conclusions:* Impaired color vision is a common observation among participants enrolled the ETDRS. Compared with published data on normal subjects, approximately 50% of the patients in the ETDRS had abnormal hue discrimination. Macular edema severity, age, and presence of new vessels were the factors most strongly associated with impaired color discrimination. A tritan-like defect was prominent and increased in magnitude with increasing severity of macular edema. Impaired color vision should be considered in the evaluation and counseling of patients with diabetic retinopathy.

16. Early Treatment Diabetic Retinopathy Study Research Group: Aspirin effects on the development of cataracts in patients with diabetes mellitus. ETDRS Report Number 16. *Arch Ophthalmol.* 1992;110:339–342. Copyright 1992, American Medical Association. Reprinted with permission.

Abstract The ETDRS, a randomized clinical trial supported by the National Eye Institute, was designed to assess the effect of photocoagulation and aspirin in 3711 patients with mild-to-severe nonproliferative or early proliferative diabetic retinopathy. Although the primary goal of the study was to evaluate the effect of photocoagulation and aspirin on diabetic retinopathy, the study also provided an opportunity to evaluate the effects of aspirin on the development of cataract. No evidence showed that aspirin use reduced the risk of development of cataract requiring extraction (4.1% versus 4.3% in patients assigned to aspirin or placebo treatment, respectively; Mantel-Cox $P = .77$; relative risk 1.05; 99% confidence interval: 0.73 to 1.51). Aspirin use also did not reduce the risk of less extensive but visually significant lens opacities developing (29.6% versus 28.3 %; Mantel-Cox

$P = .76$; relative risk: 0.99; 99% confidence interval: 0.85 to 1.15). ETDRS results do not support the hypothesis that aspirin (at a dose of 650 mg per day) reduces the risk of cataract development in this diabetic population.

17. Early Treatment Diabetic Retinopathy Study Research Group: Pars plana vitrectomy in the Early Treatment Diabetic Retinopathy Study. ETDRS Report Number 17. *Ophthalmology.* 1992;99:1351–1357. Courtesy of *Ophthalmology.*

Abstract *Background:* The ETDRS enrolled 3711 patients with mild-to-severe nonproliferative or early proliferative diabetic retinopathy in both eyes. Patients were randomly assigned to aspirin 650 mg per day or placebo. One eye of each patient was assigned randomly to early photocoagulation, and the other to deferral of photocoagulation. Follow-up examinations were scheduled at least every 4 months, and photocoagulation was initiated in eyes assigned to deferral as soon as high-risk proliferative retinopathy was detected. Aspirin was not found to have an effect on retinopathy progression or rates of vitreous hemorrhage. The risk of a combined end point, severe visual loss or vitrectomy, was low in eyes assigned to deferral (6% at 5 years) and was reduced by early photocoagulation (4% at 5 years). Vitrectomy was carried out in 208 patients during the 9 years of the study. This report presents baseline and previtrectomy characteristics and visual outcome in these patients. *Methods:* Information collected at baseline and during follow-up as part of the ETDRS protocol was supplemented by review of clinical charts for visual acuity and ocular status immediately before vitrectomy. *Results:* Vitrectomy was performed in 208 (5.6%) of the 3711 patients (243 eyes) enrolled in the ETDRS. The 5-year vitrectomy rates for eyes grouped by their initial photocoagulation assignment were as follows: 2.1% in the early full scatter photocoagulation group, 2.5% in the early mild scatter group, and 4.0% in the deferral group. The 5-year rates of vitrectomy (in one or both eyes) were 5.4% in patients assigned to aspirin and 5.2% in patients assigned to placebo. The indications for vitrectomy were either vitreous hemorrhage (53.9%) or retinal detachment with or without vitreous hemorrhage (46.1%). Before vitrectomy, visual acuity was 5/200 or worse in 66.7% of eyes and better than 20/100 in 6.2%. One year after vitrectomy, the visual acuity was 20/100 or better in 47.6% of eyes, including 24.0% with visual acuity of 20/40 or better. *Conclusions:* With frequent follow-up examinations and timely scatter (panretinal) photocoagulation, the 5-year cumulative rate of pars plana vitrectomy in ETDRS patients was 5.3%. Aspirin use did not influence the rate of vitrectomy.

18. Early Treatment Diabetic Retinopathy Study Research Group: Risk factors for high-risk proliferative diabetic retinopathy and severe visual loss. ETDRS Report Number 18. *Invest Ophthalmol Vis Sci.* 1998;39:233–252. Copyright 1998, Association for Research in Vision and Ophthalmology. Reprinted with permission.

Abstract *Purpose:* To identify risk factors for the development of high-risk proliferative diabetic retinopathy (PDR) and for the development of severe visual loss or vitrectomy (SVLV) in eyes assigned to deferral of photocoagulation in the ETDRS.

Methods: Multivariable Cox models were constructed to evaluate the strength and statistical significance of baseline risk factors for development of high-risk PDR and of SVLV. *Results:* The baseline characteristics identified as risk factors for high-risk PDR were increased severity of retinopathy, decreased visual acuity (or increased extent of macular edema), higher glycosylated hemoglobin, history of diabetic neuropathy, lower hematocrit, elevated triglycerides, lower serum albumin, and, in persons with mild-to-moderate nonproliferative retinopathy, younger age (or type I diabetes). The predominant risk factor for development of SVLV was the prior development of high-risk PDR. The only other clearly significant factor was decreased visual acuity at baseline. In the eyes that developed SVLV before high-risk proliferative diabetic retinopathy was observed, baseline risk factors were decreased visual acuity (or increased extent of macular edema), older age (or type 2 diabetes), and female gender. *Conclusions:* These analyses supported the view that retinopathy-inhibiting effect of better glycemic control extends across all ages, both diabetes types, and all stages of retinopathy up to and including the severe nonproliferative and early proliferative stages and the possibility that reducing the elevated blood lipids and treating anemia slow the progression of retinopathy.

19. Early Treatment Diabetic Retinopathy Study Research Group: Focal photocoagulation treatment of diabetic macular edema: relationship of treatment effect to fluorescein angiographic and other retinal characteristics at baseline. ETDRS Report Number 19. *Arch Ophthalmol.* 1995;113:1144–1155. Copyright 1995, American Medical Association. Reprinted with permission.

Abstract *Objective*: To determine whether the efficacy of photocoagulation treatment of diabetic macular edema may be influenced by degree of capillary closure, severity of source of fluorescein leakage, extent of retinal edema, presence of cystoid changes, or severity of hard exudates. *Patients:* Patients with mild-to-moderate nonproliferative diabetic retinopathy and macular edema definitely or questionably involving the center of the macula. *Design:* One eye of each patient was assigned to early photocoagulation; the other was assigned to deferral of photocoagulation, with follow-up visits scheduled every 4 months and photocoagulation to be carried out promptly if high-risk proliferative retinopathy developed. In this report, the beneficial effect of photocoagulation was examined in subgroups defined by severity of the characteristics specified above. *Results:* We found no subgroup in which eyes that were assigned to immediate focal treatment had a less favorable visual acuity outcome than those that were assigned to deferral (i.e., no qualitative interaction). *Conclusions:* Focal photocoagulation should be considered for eyes with clinically significant macular edema, particularly when the center of the macula is involved or imminently threatened. Trends for treatment effect to be less in eyes with less extensive retinal thickening and less thickening at the center of the macula support our previous recommendation that, for such eyes, an initial period of close observation may be preferable to immediate treatment, particularly when most of the leakage to be treated arises close to the center of the macula, increasing the risk of damage to it from direct treatment or subsequent migration of treatment scars.

20. Early Treatment Diabetic Retinopathy Study Research Group: Effects of aspirin on vitreous/preretinal hemorrhage in patients with diabetes mellitus. ETDRS Report Number 20. *Arch Ophthalmol*. 1995;113:52–55. Copyright 1995, American Medical Association. Reprinted with permission.

Abstract *Objective*: To assess whether the use of aspirin exacerbates the severity or duration of vitreous/preretinal hemorrhages in patients with diabetic retinopathy. *Design*: The ETDRS, a multicenter randomized clinical trial, was designed to assess the effect of photocoagulation and aspirin on 3711 patients with mild-to-severe nonproliferative or early proliferative diabetic retinopathy. *Intervention*: Patients were randomly assigned to either an aspirin (650 mg per day) or a placebo group. One eye of each patient was randomly assigned to early photocoagulation, and the other to deferral of photocoagulation. *Main outcome measures*: The severity and duration of the vitreous/preretinal hemorrhages were determined from gradings from the annual, seven standard stereoscopic field, fundus photographs. Clinical examinations scheduled every 4 months also provided information on the presence and duration of hemorrhages. *Results*: Annual fundus photographs of eyes assigned to deferral of photocoagulation revealed vitreous/preretinal hemorrhages at some time during follow-up in 564 patients (30%) assigned to the placebo group and 585 patients (32%) assigned to the aspirin group ($P = .48$). Based on gradings of fundus photographs, there were no statistical differences in the severity of vitreous/preretinal hemorrhages ($P = .11$) or their rate of resolution ($P = .86$) between the groups. Clinical examination of eyes assigned to deferral of photocoagulation revealed that 721 eyes (37%) assigned to the placebo group had vitreous/preretinal hemorrhages during the course of the study ($P = .30$). Again, no statistically significant difference was found between the rates of resolution, as assessed clinically, between the two treatment groups ($P = .43$). *Conclusions*: As previously reported, the use of aspirin did not increase the occurrence of vitreous/preretinal hemorrhages in patients enrolled in the ETDRS. The data presented in this report demonstrate that the severity and duration of these hemorrhages were not significantly affected by the use of aspirin and that there were no ocular contraindications to its use (650 mg per day) in persons with diabetes who require it for treatment of cardiovascular disease or for other medical indications.

21. Early Treatment Diabetic Retinopathy Study Research Group: Accommodative amplitudes in the Early Treatment Diabetic Retinopathy Study. ETDRS Report Number 21. *Retina*. 1995;15:275–281. Courtesy of Lippincott-Raven Publishers.

Abstract *Purpose*: Accommodative amplitude in persons with diabetes was investigated using data collected as part of the ETDRS. *Methods*: Accommodative amplitude was measured at the baseline visit in 1058 patients who had good visual acuity and who were less than 46 years old. Risk factors for low accommodative amplitude at baseline were evaluated using multivariable linear regression. Change in accommodative amplitude after photocoagulation was evaluated using paired *t* tests and repeated measures analysis of variance for the 578 patients who underwent follow-up measurements at the 4-month visit. *Results*: Accommodative amplitudes in ETDRS patients were lower than normal accommodative amplitudes. Older age

($P = < 0.001$) and increased duration of diabetes ($P < 0.001$) were risk factors associated with low amplitudes of accommodation in the ETDRS. Full scatter photocoagulation was associated with an apparently transient additional reduction in accommodative amplitude; a one-third diopter loss in accommodative amplitude was demonstrated only at the 4-month visit ($P < 0.001$). *Conclusion:* This study demonstrates that diabetes and duration of diabetes, along with age, are important factors for reduced accommodative amplitude. These factors, along with an apparently transient decrease in accommodative amplitude following scatter photocoagulation, should be considered when assessing the accommodative needs of patients with diabetes and when discussing side effects of full scatter photocoagulation.

22. Early Treatment Diabetic Retinopathy Study Research Group: Association of elevated serum lipid levels with retinal hard exudate in diabetic retinopathy. ETDRS Report Number 22. *Arch Ophthalmol.* 1996;114:1079–1084. Copyright 1996, American Medical Association. Reprinted with permission.

Abstract *Objective*: To evaluate the relationship between serum lipid levels, retinal hard exudate, and visual acuity in patients with diabetic retinopathy. *Design:* Observational data from the ETDRS. *Participants:* Of the 3711 patients enrolled in the ETDRS, the first 2709 enrolled had serum lipid levels measured. *Main outcome measures:* Baseline fasting serum lipid level, best-corrected visual acuity, and assessment of retinal thickening and hard exudate from stereoscopic macular photographs. *Results:* Patients with elevated total serum cholesterol levels or serum low-density lipoprotein cholesterol levels at baseline were twice as likely to have retinal hard exudates as patients with normal levels. These patients were also at higher risk of developing hard exudate during the course of the study. The risk of losing visual acuity was associated with the extent of hard exudate even after adjusting for the extent of macular edema. *Conclusions:* These data demonstrate that elevated serum lipid levels are associated with an increased risk of retinal hard exudate in persons with diabetic retinopathy. Although retinal hard exudate accompanies diabetic macular edema, increasing amounts of exudate appear to be independently associated with an increased risk of visual impairment. Lowering elevated serum lipid levels has been shown to decrease the risk of cardiovascular morbidity. The observational data from the ETDRS suggest that lipid lowering may also decrease the risk of hard exudate formation and associated vision loss in patients with diabetic retinopathy. Preservation of vision may be an additional motivating factor for lowering serum lipid levels in persons with diabetic retinopathy and elevated serum lipid levels.

23. Early Treatment Diabetic Retinopathy Study Research Group: Subretinal fibrosis in diabetic macular edema. ETDRS Report Number 23. *Arch Ophthalmol.* 1997;115:873–877. Copyright 1997. American Medical Association. Reprinted with permission.

Abstract *Objective*: To describe the characteristics of and risk factors for subretinal fibrosis (SRF) in patients with diabetic macular edema. *Patients and methods:* A total of 109 eyes (in 96 persons) with SRF, defined as a mound or sheet of gray-to-white tissue beneath the retina at or near the center of the macula, were identified during the ETDRS, which is a randomized clinical trial of photocoagulation and aspirin treatment in patients with mild-to-severe nonproliferative or early proliferative diabetic retinopathy. The patients and the ocular characteristics of these 109 eyes, all of which had clinically significant macular edema, were compared with those of 5653 eyes in which clinically significant macular edema, but not SRF, was observed during the trial. *Results:* In 9 of 109 eyes, the development of SRF may have been directly related to focal photocoagulation. Seventy-four percent of the eyes in which SRF developed had very severe hard exudates in the macula prior to the development of SRF, while this level of hard exudates was seen in only 2.5% of the eyes with clinically significant macular edema in which SRF did not develop ($P < .001$). Of the 254 eyes with this level of hard exudates at baseline (N = 29) or during follow-up (N = 235), SRF developed in 30.7% of the eyes, while this complication developed in only 0.05% of 5498 eyes with clinically significant macular edema without this level of hard exudates. *Conclusions:* Subretinal fibrosis is an infrequent complication of diabetic macular edema. Although it has been reported to be associated with photocoagulation burn intensity, in only 9 of 109 eyes in which SRF developed was it located adjacent to a photocoagulation-related scar (among 4823 eyes that received focal photocoagulation for treatment of macular edema). The strongest risk factor for the development of SRF is very severe hard exudate.

24. Early Treatment Diabetic Retinopathy Study Research Group: Causes of severe visual loss in the Early Treatment Diabetic Retinopathy Study. ETDRS Report Number 24. *Am J Ophthalmol.* 1999;127:137–141. Copyright 1999. Reprinted with permission from Elsevier Science.

Abstract *Purpose:* To describe the causes of and risk factors for persistent severe visual loss occurring in the ETDRS. *Methods:* The ETDRS was a randomized clinical trial investigating photocoagulation and aspirin in 3711 persons with mild-to-severe nonproliferative or early proliferative diabetic retinopathy. Severe visual loss, defined as best-corrected visual acuity of less than 5/200 on at least two consecutive 4-month follow-up visits, developed in 257 eyes (219 persons). Of these 257 eyes, 149 (127 persons) did not recover to 5/200 or better at any visit (persistent severe visual loss). Ocular characteristics of these eyes were compared with those of eyes with severe visual loss that improved to 5/200 or better at any subsequent visit. Characteristics of patients with severe visual loss that did and did not improve and those without severe visual loss were also compared. *Results:* Severe visual loss that persisted developed in 149 eyes of 127 persons. In order of decreasing frequency, reasons recorded for persistent visual loss included vitreous or preretinal hemorrhage, macular edema or macular pigmentary changes related to macular edema, macular or retinal detachment, and neovascular glaucoma. Compared with all patients without persistent severe visual loss, patients with persistent severe visual loss had higher mean levels of hemoglobin A1C (10.4% versus 9.7 %; $P = .001$) and higher levels of cholesterol (244.1 versus 228.5 mg/dL; $P = .0081$) at baseline. Otherwise, patients with persistent severe visual loss were similar to patients with severe visual loss that improved and to those without severe visual loss. *Conclusions:* Persistent severe visual loss was an infrequent occurrence in the ETDRS. Its leading cause was vitreous or preretinal hemorrhage, followed by macular edema or macular pigmentary changes related to macular edema and retinal detachment. The low frequency of persistent severe visual loss in the ETDRS is most likely related to the nearly universal intervention with scatter photocoagulation (either before or soon after high-risk proliferative diabetic retinopathy developed) and the intervention with vitreous surgery when clinically indicated.

25. Chew EY, Benson WE, Remaley NA, et al.: Results after lens extraction in patients with diabetic retinopathy. ETDRS Report Number 25. *Arch Ophthalmol.* 1999;117:1600–1606. Reprinted with permission of the American Medical Association.

Abstract *Objective*: To assess the visual results after surgical lens removal in patients with diabetic retinopathy. *Design:* A multicenter randomized clinical trial designed to assess the effect of photocoagulation and aspirin in patients with mild to severe nonproliferative or early proliferative diabetic retinopathy and/or macular edema. *Participants:* Of the 3711 patients enrolled in the Early Treatment Diabetic Retinopathy Study, lens surgery was performed on 205 patients (270 eyes) during follow-up that ranged from 4 to 9 years. *Outcome Measurements:* Visual acuity, macular edema status, and degree of diabetic retinopathy. In addition, risk factors associated with lens extraction and with poor postoperative visual acuity (worse than 20/100) were assessed. *Results:* The risk of lens extraction increased with increasing age, female sex, and baseline proteinuria. Ocular variables associated with increased risk of lens surgery included poor baseline visual acuity and vitrectomy performed during the course of the study. At 1 year after lens surgery, visual acuity improvement of 2 or more lines from preoperative levels occurred in 64.3% of the operated-on eyes assigned to early photocoagulation and 59.3% of eyes assigned to deferral of photocoagulation. In eyes assigned to early photocoagulation, 46% of eyes achieved visual acuity better than 20/40; 73%, better than 20/100; and 8%, 5/200 or worse at 1 year after surgery. Visual acuity results for eyes assigned to deferral of laser photocoagulation at 1 year were not as favorable; 36% achieved visual acuity better than 20/40; 55%, better than 20/100; and 17%, 5/200 or worse at 1 year after surgery. Evaluation of 1-year postoperative visual acuities for all eyes with mild to moderate nonproliferative diabetic retinopathy at the annual visit before lens surgery showed that 53% were better than 20/40; 90%, better than 20/100; and 1%, 5/200 or worse. However, for eyes with severe nonproliferative or worse retinopathy at the annual visit before lens surgery, only 25% were better than 20/40; 42%, better than 20/100; and 22%, 5/200 or worse at 1 year after lens surgery. There was little change in visual acuity between 1 and 2 years postoperatively. Increased severity of retinopathy and poor visual acuity before surgery were associated with visual acuity of worse than 20/100 at 1 year after surgery. Lens surgery was associated with a borderline statistically significant increased risk of progression of diabetic retinopathy in the adjusted analyses (P = .03). No statistically significant long-term increased risk of macular edema was documented after lens surgery. *Conclusions:* Visual acuity results after lens surgery in patients in the Early Treatment Diabetic Retinopathy Study were better than published results for similar patients. This may be because of more intensive photocoagulation for lesions of diabetic retinopathy in the Early Treatment Diabetic Retinopathy Study than in previously reported studies. Although patients with severe nonproliferative retinopathy or worse before lens surgery had poorer visual results, visual improvement was seen in 55% of these patients at 1-year follow-up. The main causes of poor visual results in eyes after lens surgery were complications of proliferative retinopathy and/or macular edema.

26. Chew EY, Ferris FL III, Csaky KG, et al.: The long-term effects of laser photocoagulation treatment in patients with diabetic retinopathy. The Early Treatment Diabetic Retinopathy Follow-up Study. *Ophthalmology*. 2003;110:1683–1689. Courtesy of Ophthalmology.

Abstract *Objectives*: To evaluate the long-term natural history and effects of laser photocoagulation treatment in patients with diabetic retinopathy. *Design*: Follow-up study of the 214 surviving patients enrolled originally at the Johns Hopkins Clinical Center for the Early Treatment Diabetic Retinopathy Study (ETDRS), which was a clinical trial designed to evaluate the role of laser photocoagulation and aspirin treatment in patients with diabetic retinopathy. *Methods*: Early Treatment Diabetic Retinopathy Study patients enrolled in the Johns Hopkins Clinical Center had complete eye examinations, including best-corrected visual acuity measurements, fundus photographs, and medical questionnaires throughout the 7-year study. They had the same examinations at the final long-term follow-up visit at the National Eye Institute, National Institutes of Health, 13 to 19.5 years after the initial laser photocoagulation (median, 16.7 years). *Main Outcome Measures*: The major outcomes were mortality and the rates of moderate and severe vision loss. The secondary outcomes were progression of diabetic retinopathy and need for other eye surgery. *Results*: Of the 214 patients who were alive at the end of the original ETDRS in 1989, 130 (61%) were deceased at the time of the re-examination. Of the 84 who were alive, 71 (85%) were examined at their long-term follow-up visit at the National Institutes of Health. At the long-term follow-up examination, 42% had visual acuity of 20/20 or better, and 84% had visual acuity of 20/40 or better in the better eye. Compared with baseline, 20% of patients had moderate vision loss (loss of 3 lines or more vision) in the better eye at follow-up. Only one patient had visual acuity of 20/200 bilaterally. He had visual acuity loss secondary to age-related macular degeneration. No patient had severe vision loss (worse than 5/200). All the initially untreated eyes of patients who had severe nonproliferative diabetic retinopathy or worse by the time of the ETDRS closeout visit of the original study received scatter photocoagulation treatment. Focal photocoagulation was performed in 43% bilaterally and 2% unilaterally. Cataract surgery was performed in 31% of the patients, vitrectomy in 17%, and glaucoma surgery in one patient. *Conclusions*: As previously reported, the mortality rate of patients with diabetic retinopathy is much higher than that of the general population. For those who survived, aggressive follow-up, with treatment when indicated, seems to be associated with maintenance of good long-term visual acuity for most patients. The need for laser scatter photocoagulation with long-term follow-up seems to be high.

A-3

DIABETIC RETINOPATHY VITRECTOMY STUDY (DRVS)

1. Diabetic Retinopathy Vitrectomy Study Research Group: Two-year course of visual acuity in severe proliferative diabetic retinopathy with conventional management. DRVS Report Number 1. *Ophthalmology*. 1985;92:492–502. Courtesy of *Ophthalmology*.

Abstract Seven hundred forty-four eyes with very severe proliferative diabetic retinopathy (PDR) were followed with conventional management over a 2-year period. Decreases in visual acuity were more frequent during the first year of follow-up than during the second, and were related to baseline visual acuity level and retinopathy severity. After 2 years, visual acuity was less than 5/200 in 45% of eyes with more than 4 disc areas of new vessels and visual acuity of 10/30 to 10/50 at baseline, but in only 14% of eyes with traction retinal detachment not involving the center of the macula and without active new vessels or fresh vitreous hemorrhage at baseline. Vitrectomy, which was undertaken only if retinal detachment involving the center of the macula occurred or if severe vitreous hemorrhage failed to clear after a 1-year waiting period, had been carried out in 25% of eyes after 2 years of follow-up.

2. Diabetic Retinopathy Vitrectomy Study Research Group: Early vitrectomy for severe vitreous hemorrhage in diabetic retinopathy: two-year results of a randomized trial. DRVS Report Number 2. *Arch Ophthalmol*. 1985;103:1644–1652. Copyright 1985, American Medical Association. Reprinted with permission.

Abstract Six hundred sixteen eyes with recent severe diabetic vitreous hemorrhage reducing visual acuity to 5/200 or less for at least 1 month were randomly assigned to either early vitrectomy or deferral or vitrectomy for 1 year. After 2 years of follow-up, 25% of the early vitrectomy group had visual acuity of 10/20 or better compared with 15% in the deferral group (*P* = .01). In patients with type I diabetes, who were on the average younger and had more severe proliferative retinopathy, there was a clear-cut advantage for early vitrectomy, as reflected in the percentage of eyes recovering visual acuity of 10/20 or better (36% versus 12% in the deferral group, *P* = .0001. No such advantage was found in the type 2 diabetes group (16% in the early group versus 18% in the deferral group), but evidence that this advantage differed by diabetes type was of borderline significance.

3. Diabetic Retinopathy Vitrectomy Study Research Group: Early vitrectomy for severe proliferative diabetic retinopathy in eyes with useful vision: results of a randomized trial. DRVS Report Number 3. *Ophthalmology*. 1985;95:1307–1320. Courtesy of *Ophthalmology*.

Abstract Three hundred seventy eyes with advanced, active, proliferative diabetic retinopathy (PDR) and visual acuity of 10/200 or better were randomly assigned to either vitrectomy or conventional management. After 4 years of follow-up, the percentage of eyes with a visual acuity of 10/20 or better was 44% in the early vitrectomy group and 28% in the conventional management group. The proportion with very poor visual outcome was similar in the two groups. The advantage of early vitrectomy tended to increase with increasing severity of new vessels. In the group with the least severe new vessels, no advantage of early vitrectomy was apparent.

4. Diabetic Retinopathy Vitrectomy Study Research Group: Early vitrectomy for severe proliferative diabetic retinopathy in eyes with useful vision: clinical application of results of a randomized trial. DRVS Report Number 4. *Ophthalmology.* 1998;95:1321–1334. Courtesy of *Ophthalmology.*

Abstract Six patients are described, each of whom underwent early vitrectomy for advanced, active, proliferative diabetic retinopathy (PDR) in an eye with useful vision. These cases were selected to illustrate the spectrum of retinopathy severity for which early vitrectomy should be considered and the favorable outcome that can follow this procedure. None of the eyes that had an unfavorable result after early vitrectomy is presented. The eyes most suitable for early vitrectomy are those in which both fibrous proliferations and at least moderately severe new vessels are present, and in which extensive scatter photocoagulation has already been carried out or is precluded by vitreous hemorrhage.

5. Diabetic Retinopathy Vitrectomy Study Research Group: Early vitrectomy for severe vitreous hemorrhage in diabetic retinopathy: four-year results of a randomized trial. DRVS Report Number 5. *Arch Ophthalmol.* 1990;108:958–964. Published erratum appears in *Arch Ophthalmol.* 1990;108:1452. Copyright 1990, American Medical Association. Reprinted with permission.

Abstract Six hundred sixteen eyes with recent severe diabetic vitreous hemorrhage reducing visual acuity to 5/200 or less for at least 1 month were randomly assigned to either early vitrectomy or deferral of vitrectomy for 1 year. The proportion of eyes with visual acuity of 10/20 or better was higher in the early vitrectomy group than in the deferral group throughout the 4-year follow-up period. Up to the 18-month visit, the early group had a higher proportion of eyes with visual acuity to no light perception. An increased chance of obtaining good vision with early vitrectomy was clearly present in the type 1 diabetes group, particularly in patients who developed severe vitreous hemorrhage after less than 20 years of diabetes, a patient group tending to have more severe proliferative retinopathy. This advantage was not found in the type 2 diabetes group, in which patients were older and tended to have less severe retinopathy. The findings of this and previous DRVS reports support early vitrectomy in eyes known or suspected to have very severe proliferative diabetic retinopathy as a means of increasing the chance of restoring or maintaining good vision.

A-4

DIABETES CONTROL AND COMPLICATIONS TRIAL (DCCT)

1. Diabetes Control and Complications Trial Research Group: Color photography vs. fluorescein angiography in the detection of diabetic retinopathy in Diabetes

Control and Complications Trial. *Arch Ophthalmol*. 1987;105:1344–1351. Copyright 1987. American Medical Association. Reprinted with permission.

Abstract During eligibility screening for the DCCT, we compared stereoscopic color fundus photography and stereoscopic fluorescein angiography in the detection of diabetic retinopathy in 320 patients (mean age: 24 years [SD:8 years]) with insulin-dependent diabetes (mean duration: 7 years [SD: 4 years]) and no or mild diabetic retinopathy. Of 153 patients classified as having no retinopathy according to color photographs of seven standard 30° fields of both eyes, 21% of the patients had evidence of retinopathy (mostly one or two microaneurysms in one eye) on review of fluorescein angiograms, including two standard 30° fields in each eye. Of those patients with no retinopathy detected on angiograms, 19% had retinopathy on review of color photographs. When used in conjunction with color photography, angiography allows a modest increase in sensitivity to the earliest signs of retinopathy, a gain potentially useful in some research applications, although not of demonstrated value in patient management.

2. Diabetic Control and Complications Trial Research Group: The effect of intensive treatment of diabetes on the development and progression of long-term complications in insulin-dependent diabetes mellitus. *N Engl J Med*. 1993;329:977–986. Copyright © 1993, Massachusetts Medical Society. All rights reserved.

Abstract *Background*: Long-term microvascular and neurologic complications cause major morbidity and mortality in patients with insulin-dependent diabetes mellitus (IDDM). We examined whether intensive treatment with the goal of maintaining blood glucose concentrations close to the normal range could decrease the frequency and severity of these complications. *Methods:* A total of 1441 patients with IDDM – 726 with no retinopathy at baseline (the primary-prevention cohort) and 715 with mild retinopathy (the secondary-intervention cohort) – were randomly assigned to intensive therapy administered either with an external insulin pump or by three or more daily insulin injections and guided by frequent blood glucose monitoring or to conventional therapy with one or two daily insulin injections. The patients were followed for a mean of 6.5 years, and the appearance and progression of retinopathy and other complications were assessed regularly. *Results:* In the primary-prevention cohort, intensive therapy reduced the adjusted mean risk for the development of retinopathy by 76% (95% confidence interval: 62% to 85%), as compared with conventional therapy. In the secondary-intervention cohort, intensive therapy slowed the progression of retinopathy by 54% (95% confidence interval: 39% to 66%) and reduced the development of proliferative or severe nonproliferative retinopathy by 47% (95% confidence interval: 14% to 67%). In the two cohorts combined, intensive therapy reduced the occurrence of microalbuminuria (urinary albumin excretion of ≥40 mg per 24 hours) by 39% (95% confidence interval: 21% to 52%), that of albuminuria (urinary albumin excretion of ≥300 mg per 24 hours) by 54% (95% confidence interval: 19% to 74%), and that of clinical neuropathy by 60% (95% confidence interval: 38% to 74%). The chief adverse event associated with intensive therapy was a two to three-fold increase in severe hypoglycemia. *Conclusions:* Intensive therapy effectively delays the onset and slows the progression of diabetic retinopathy, nephropathy, and neuropathy in patients with IDDM.

3. Diabetes Control and Complications Trial Research Group: Effect of intensive diabetes treatment on the development and progression of long-term complications in adolescents with insulin-dependent diabetes mellitus: Diabetes Control and Complications Trial. *J Pediatr.* 1994;125:177–188. Reproduced with permission from Mosby Year Book, Inc.

Abstract The DCCT has demonstrated that intensive diabetes treatment delays the onset and slows the progression of diabetic complications in subjects with insulin-dependent diabetes mellitus from 13 to 39 years of age. We examined whether the effects of such treatment also occurred in the subset of young diabetic subjects (13 to 17 years of age at entry) in the DCCT. One hundred twenty-five adolescent subjects with insulin-dependent diabetes mellitus but with no retinopathy at baseline (primary-prevention cohort) and 70 adolescent subjects with mild retinopathy (secondary-intervention cohort) were randomly assigned to receive either (1) intensive therapy with an external insulin pump or at least three daily insulin injections, together with frequent daily blood-glucose monitoring, or (2) conventional therapy with one or two daily insulin injections and once-daily monitoring. Subjects were followed for a mean of 7.4 years (4 to 9 years). In the primary-prevention cohort, intensive therapy decreased the risk of having retinopathy by 53% (95% confidence interval: 1% to 78%; $P = 0.048$) in comparison with conventional therapy. In the secondary-intervention cohort, intensive therapy decreased the risk of retinopathy progression by 70% (95% confidence interval: 25% to 88%; $P = 0.010$) and the occurrence of microalbuminuria by 55% (95% confidence interval: 3% to 79%; $P = 0.042$). Motor and sensory nerve conduction velocities were faster in intensively treated subjects. The major adverse event with intensive therapy was a nearly a three-fold increase of severe hypoglycemia. We conclude that intensive therapy effectively delays the onset and slows the progression of diabetic retinopathy and nephropathy when initiated in adolescent subjects; the benefits outweigh the increased risk of hypoglycemia that accompanies such treatment.

4. Diabetes Control and Complications Trial Research Group: The effect of intensive diabetes treatment on progression of diabetic retinopathy in insulin-dependent diabetes mellitus. *Arch Ophthalmol.* 1995;113:36–51. Copyright 1995, American Medical Association. Reprinted with permission.

Abstract *Objective*: To determine the magnitude of the decrease in the risk of retinopathy progression observed with intensive treatment and its relationship to baseline retinopathy severity and duration of follow-up. *Design:* Randomized clinical trial, with 3 to 9 years of follow-up. *Setting and patients:* Between 1983 and 1989, 29 centers enrolled 1441 patients with insulin-dependent diabetes mellitus aged 13 to 39 years, including 726 patients with no retinopathy and a duration of diabetes of 1 to 5 years (primary-prevention cohort) and 715 patients with very mild to moderate nonproliferative diabetic retinopathy and a duration of diabetes of 1 to 15 years (secondary-intervention cohort). Ninety-five percent of all scheduled examinations were completed. *Interventions:* Intensive treatment consisted of the administration of insulin at least three times a day by injection or pump, with doses adjusted based on self-blood glucose monitoring and with the goal of normo-glycemia. Conventional treatment consisted of one or two daily insulin injections. *Outcome measures:* Change between and follow-up visits on the Early Treatment Diabetic Retinopathy Study retinopathy severity scale, assessed with masked grad-ings of stereoscopic color fundus photographs obtained every 6 months. *Results:* Cumulative 8.5-year rates of retinopathy progression by three or more steps at two consecutive visits were 54.1% with conventional treatment and 11.5% with intensive treatment in the primary-prevention cohort and 49.2% and 17.1% in the secondary-intervention cohort. At the 6- and 12-month visits, a small adverse effect of intensive treatment was noted ("early worsening"), followed by a benefi-cial effect that increased in magnitude with time. Beyond 3.5 years of followup, the risk of progression was five or more times lower with intensive treatment than with conventional treatment. Once progression occurred, subsequent recovery was at least two times more likely with intensive treatment than with conventional treatment. Treatment effects were similar in all baseline retinopathy severity sub-groups. *Conclusion:* The results of the DCCT strongly support the recommen-dation that most patients with insulin-dependent diabetes mellitus use intensive treatment, aiming for levels of glycemia as close to the nondiabetic range as is safely possible.

5. Diabetic Control and Complications Trial Research Group: Progression of ret-inopathy with intensive versus conventional treatment in the Diabetes Control and Complications Trial. *Ophthalmology.* 1995;102:647–661. Courtesy of *Ophthalmology.*

Abstract *Purpose*: To answer the following questions regarding the effect of inten-sive diabetes management on retinopathy in insulin-dependent diabetes mellitus (IDDM). (1) Does intensive therapy completely prevent the development of reti-nopathy? (2) Are some states of retinopathy too advanced to benefit from intensive therapy? (3) Are the retinopathy end points in the DCCT clinically important? and (4) What other factors influence the effectiveness of therapy? *Methods:* A total of 1441 patients, ranging in age from 13 to 39 years and with IDDM of 1 to 5 years' duration and no retinopathy at baseline (primary-prevention cohort) or with 1 to 15 years' duration and minimal-to-moderate nonproliferative retinopathy (secondary-intervention cohort), were assigned randomly to either intensive or conventional diabetes therapy. Intensive therapy, aimed at achieving glycemic levels as close to the normal range as possible, included three or more daily insulin injections or con-tinuous subcutaneous insulin infusion, guided by four or more glucose tests daily. Conventional therapy included one or two daily injections. Seven-field stereoscopic fundus photography was performed every 6 months, for a mean follow-up of 6.5 years (range: 4 to 9 years). *Results:* Intensive therapy reduced the risk of any ret-inopathy (≥ 1 microaneurysm) developing in the primary-prevention cohort (70% of intensive versus 90% of conventional treatment group; $P = 0.002$) by 27%. It reduced the risk of retinopathy developing or progressing to the clinically signifi-cant degrees by 34% to 76%. Intensive therapy was most effective when initiated early in the course of IDDM. It had a substantial beneficial effect over the entire spectrum of retinopathy studied in the DCCT and, with rare exceptions, in all patient subgroups. *Conclusion:* Although intensive therapy does not prevent retinopathy completely, it has a beneficial effect that begins after 3 years of therapy on all levels of retinopathy studied on the DCCT. The reduction in risk observed in the study is translatable directly into reduced need for laser treatment and saved sight. Intensive therapy should form the backbone of any healthcare strategy aimed at reducing the risk of visual loss from diabetic retinopathy.

6. Diabetes Control and Complications Trial Research Group: The relationship of glycemic exposure (HbA1C) to the risk of development and progression of retinopathy in the Diabetes Control and Complications Trial. *Diabetes.* 1995;44:968–983. Reprinted with permission of the American Diabetes Association.

Abstract The DCCT demonstrated that a regimen of intensive therapy aimed at maintaining near-normal blood glucose values markedly reduces the risks of development or progression of retinopathy and other complications of insulin-dependent diabetes mellitus (IDDM) when compared with a conventional treatment regimen. This report presents an epidemiological assessment of the association between levels of glycemic exposure (HbA1C) before and during the DCCT with the risk of retinopathy progression within each treatment group. The initial level of HbA1C observed at eligibility screening as an index of pre-DCCT glycemia and the duration of IDDM on entry were the dominant baseline predictors of the risk of progression. The shorter the duration of IDDM on entry, the greater were the benefits of intensive therapy. In each treatment group, the mean HbA1C during the trial was the dominant predictor of retinopathy progression, and the risk gradients were similar in the two groups; a 10% lower HbA1C (eg, 8% versus 7.2%) is associated with a 43% lower risk in the intensive group and a 45% lower risk in the conventional group. These risk gradients applied over the observed range of HbA1C values and were unaffected by adjustment for other covariates. Over the range of HbA1C achieved by DCCT intensive therapy, there does not appear to be a level of glycemia below which the risks of retinopathy progression are eliminated. The change in risk over time, however, differed significantly between the treatment groups, the risk increasing with time in the study in the conventional group but remaining relatively constant in the intensive group. The risks were compounded by a multiplicative effect of the level of HbA1C with the duration of exposure (time in study). Total glycemic exposure was the dominant factor associated with the risk of retinopathy progression. When examined simultaneously within each treatment group, each of the components of pre-DCCT glycemic exposure (screening HbA1C value and IDDM duration) and glycemic exposure during the DCCT (mean HbA1c, time in study, and their interaction) were significantly associated with the risk of retinopathy progression. Similar results also apply to other retinopathic, nephropathic, and neuropathic outcomes. The recommendation of the DCCT remains that intensive therapy with the goal of achieving near-normal glycemia should be implemented as early as possible in as many IDDM patients as is safely possible.

7. Diabetes Control and Complications Trial Research Group: Early worsening of diabetic retinopathy in the Diabetes Control and Complications Trial. *Arch*

Abstract *Objectives*: To document the frequency, importance of, and risk factors for "early worsening" of diabetic retinopathy in the DCCT. *Methods:* The DCCT was a multicenter, randomized clinical trial comparing intensive versus conventional treatment in insulin-dependent diabetic patients who had no-to-moderate nonproliferative retinopathy. Retinopathy severity was assessed in 7-field stereoscopic fundus photographs taken at baseline and every 6 months. For this study, worsening was defined as progression of three steps or more on the ETDRS final scale, as the development of soft exudates and/or intraretinal microvascular abnormalities, as the development of clinically important retinopathy, or as any of the above, and was considered "early" if it occurred between baseline and 12-month follow-up visits. *Results:* Early worsening was observed at the 6- and/or 12-month visit in 13.1% of 711 patients assigned to intensive treatment and in 7.6% of 728 patients assigned to conventional treatment (odds ratio: 2.06; $P = 0.001$); recovery had occurred at the 18-month visit in 51% and 55% of these groups, respectively ($P = 0.39$). The risk of three-step or greater progression from the retinopathy level present 18 months after entry into the trial was greater in patients who previously had had early worsening than in those who had not. However, the large long-term risk reduction with intensive treatment was such that outcomes in intensively treated patients who had early worsening were similar to or more favorable than outcomes in conventionally treated patients who had not. The most important risk factors for early worsening were higher hemoglobin A1C level at screening and reduction of this level during the first 6 months after randomization. We found no evidence to suggest that more gradual reduction of glycemia might be associated with less risk of early worsening. Early worsening led to high risk proliferative retinopathy in 2 patients and to clinically significant macular edema in 3; all responded well to treatment. *Conclusions:* In the DCCT trial, the long-term benefits of intensive insulin treatment greatly outweighed the risk of early worsening. Although no case of early worsening was associated with serious visual loss, our results are consistent with previous reports of sight-threatening worsening when intensive treatment is initiated in patients with long-standing poor glycemic control, particularly if retinopathy is at or past the moderate nonproliferative stage. Ophthalmologic monitoring before initiation of intensive treatment and at 3-month intervals for 6 to 12 months thereafter seems appropriate for such patients. In patients whose retinopathy is already approaching the high-risk stage, it may be prudent to delay the initiation of intensive treatment until photocoagulation can be completed, particularly if hemoglobin A1C is high.

A-5

SORBINIL RETINOPATHY TRIAL (SRT)

1. Sorbinil Retinopathy Trial Research Group: A randomized trial of sorbinil, an aldose reductase inhibitor, in diabetic retinopathy. *Arch Ophthalmol.* 1990;108:1234–1244. Copyright 1990, American Medical Association. Reprinted with permission.

Abstract A total of 497 patients aged 18 to 56 years with insulin-dependent diabetes mellitus for 1 to 15 years were randomly assigned to take oral sorbinil or placebo and followed up for a median of 41 months. The percentage of patients whose retinopathy severity grade at maximum follow-up had worsened by two or more levels was not significantly different between the two treatment groups (28% in the sorbinil group and 32% in the placebo group, $P = .344$). The number of microaneurysms increased at a slightly slower rate in the sorbinil group than in the placebo group, with statistically significant differences at 21 ($P - .046$) and 30 ($P - .039$) months but not at the maximum follow-up ($P = .156$). About 7% of the patients assigned to take sorbinil developed a hypersensitivity reaction in the first 3 months. On the basis of these results, it is unlikely that sorbinil administered at a dosage of 250 mg daily for 3 years has a clinically important effect on the course of retinopathy in adults with insulin-dependent diabetes of moderate duration. Our data are consistent, however, with a slightly slower progression rate in the microaneurysm count among patients assigned to take sorbinil, a finding of uncertain clinical importance.

A-6

UNITED KINGDOM PROSPECTIVE DIABETES STUDY (UKPDS)

1. United Kingdom Prospective Diabetes Study Group: Intensive blood-glucose control with sulphonylureas or insulin compared with conventional treatment and risk of complications in patients with type 2 diabetes. UKPDS 33. *Lancet.* 1998;352:837–853. Reprinted with permission of The Lancet.

Summary *Background*: Improved blood-glucose control decreases the progression of diabetic microvascular disease, but the effect on macrovascular complications is unknown. There is concern that sulphonylureas may increase cardiovascular mortality in patients with type 2 diabetes and that high insulin concentrations may enhance atheroma formation. We compared the effects of intensive blood-glucose control with either sulphonylurea or insulin and conventional treatment on the risk of microvascular and macrovascular complications in patients with type 2 diabetes in a randomized control trial. *Methods:* 3867 newly diagnosed patients with type 2 diabetes, median age 54 years (IQR [interquartile range] 48 to 60 years), who after 3 months' diet treatment had a mean of two fasting plasma glucose (FPG) concentrations of 6.1 to 15.0 mmol/L were randomly assigned intensive policy with a sulphonylurea (chlorpropamide, glibenclamide, or glipizide) or with insulin, or conventional policy with diet. The aim in the intensive group was FPG less than 6 mmol/L. In the conventional group, the aim was the best achievable FPG with diet alone; drugs were added only if there were hyperglycemic symptoms or FPG greater than 15 mmol/L. Three aggregate end points were used to assess differences between conventional and intensive treatment: (1) any diabetes-related end point (sudden death, death from hyperglycemia or hypoglycemia, fatal or nonfatal myocardial infarction, angina, heart failure, stroke, renal failure, amputation [of at least one digit], vitreous hemorrhage, retinopathy requiring photocoagulation, blindness in one eye, or cataract extraction); (2) diabetes-related death (death from myocardial infarction, stroke, peripheral vascular disease, renal disease, hyperglycemia or hypoglycemia, and sudden death); (3) all-cause mortality. Single clinical end points and surrogate subclinical end points were also assessed. All analyses were by intention to treat, and frequency of hypoglycemia was also analyzed by actual therapy. *Findings:* Over 10 years, hemoglobin A1C (HbA1C) was 7.0% (.2 to 8.2) in the intensive group compared with 7.9 % (6.9 to 8.8) in the conventional group-an 11% reduction. There was no difference in HbA1C among agents in the intensive group. Compared with the conventional group, the risk in the intensive group was 12% lower (95% confidence interval: 1 to 21; $P = 0.029$) for any diabetes-related end point; 10% lower (–11 to 27; $P = 0.34$) for any diabetes-related death; and 6% lower (–10 to 20; $P = 0.44$) for all cause mortality. Most of the risk reduction in the any diabetes-related aggregate end point was due to a 25% risk reduction (7 to 40; $P = 40$; $P = 0.0099$) in microvascular end points, including the need for retinal photocoagulation. There was no difference for any of the three aggressive end points between the three intensive agents (chlorpropamide, glibenclamide, or insulin). Patients in the intensive group had more hypoglycemic episodes than those in the conventional group on both types of analysis (both $P < 0.0001$). The rates of major hypoglycemic episodes per year were 0.7% with conventional treatment, 1% with chlorpropamide, 1.4% with glibenclamide, and 1.8% with insulin. Weight gain was significantly higher in the intensive group (mean 2.9 kg) than in the conventional group ($P < 0.001$), and patients assigned insulin had a greater gain in weight (4.0 kg) than those assigned chlorpropamide (2.6 kg) or glibenclamide (1.7 kg). *Interpretation:* Intensive blood-glucose control by either sulphonylureas or insulin substantially decreases the risk of microvascular complications, but not macrovascular disease in patients with type 2 diabetes. None of the individual drugs had an adverse effect on cardiovascular outcomes. All intensive treatment increased the risk of hypoglycemia.

2. United Kingdom Prospective Diabetes Study Group: Tight blood pressure control and risk of macrovascular and microvascular complications in type 2 diabetes. UKPDS 38. *Br Med J.* 1998;317:703–713. This abstract was first published in the *British Medical Journal* and is reproduced by permission of the BMJ Publishing Group.

Abstract *Objective*: To determine whether tight control of blood pressure prevents macrovascular and microvascular complications in patients with type 2 diabetes. *Design:* Randomized controlled trial comparing tight control of blood pressure aiming at the blood pressure of <150/85 mmHg (with the use of an angiotensin-converting enzyme inhibitor, captopril, or a beta blocker, atenolol, as main treatment), with less tight control aiming at a blood pressure of <180/105 mmHg. *Setting:* 20 hospital-based clinics in England, Scotland, and Northern Ireland. *Subjects:* 1148 hypertensive patients with type 2 diabetes (mean age: 56, mean blood pressure at entry 160/94 mmHg); 758 patients were allocated to tight control of blood pressure, and 390 patients to less tight control with a median follow-up of 8.4 years. *Main outcome measures:* Predefined clinical end points, fatal and nonfatal, related to diabetes, deaths related to diabetes, and all-cause mortality. Surrogate measures of microvascular disease included urinary albumin excretion and retinal photography. *Results:* Mean blood pressure during follow-up was significantly reduced in the group assigned to tight blood pressure control (144/82 mmHg; compared with the $P < 0.0001$). Reductions in risk in the group assigned to tight control compared with that assigned to less tight control were 24% in diabetes-related end points (95% confidence interval: 8% to 38%; $P = 0.0046$), 32% in deaths related to diabetes (6% to 51%; $P = 0.019$), 44% in strokes (11% to 65%; $P = 0.013$), and 37% in microvascular end points (11% to 56%; $P = 0.0092$), predominately owing to a reduced risk of retinal photocoagulation. There was nonsignificant reduction in all-cause mortality. After 9 years of follow-up, the group assigned to tight blood pressure control also had a 34% reduction in risk in the proportion of patients with deterioration of retinopathy by two steps (99% confidence interval: 11% to 50%; $P = 0.004$) and a 47% reduced risk (7% to 70%; $P = 0.004$) of deterioration in visual acuity by three lines of the Early Treatment of Diabetic Retinopathy Study (ETDRS) chart. After 9 years of follow-up, 29% of patients in the group assigned to tight control required three or more treatments to lower blood pressure to achieve target blood pressures. *Conclusion:* Tight blood pressure control in patients with hypertension and type 2 diabetes achieves a clinically important reduction in the risk of deaths related to diabetes, complications related to diabetes, progression of diabetic retinopathy, and deterioration in visual acuity.

3. United Kingdom Prospective Diabetes Study Group: Glycemic control with diet, sulfonylurea, metformin, or insulin in patients with type 2 diabetes mellitus: progressive requirement for multiple therapies. UKPDS 49. *J Am Med Assoc.* 1999;281:2005–2012. Copyright 1999, American Medical Association. Reprinted with permission.

Abstract *Context:* Treatment with diet alone, insulin, sulfonylurea, or metformin is known to improve glycemia in patients with type 2 diabetes mellitus, but which treatment most frequently attains target fasting plasma glucose (FPG) concentration of less than 7.8 mmol/L (140 mg/dL) or glycosylated hemoglobin A1C (HbA1C) below 7% is unknown. *Objective:* To assess how often each therapy can achieve the glycemic control target levels set by the American Diabetes Association. *Design:* Randomized controlled trial conducted between 1977 and 1997. Patients were recruited between 1977 and 1991 and followed up every 3 months for 3, 6, and 9 years after enrollment. *Setting:* Outpatient diabetes clinics in 15 UK hospitals. *Patients:* A total of 4075 patients newly diagnosed as having type 2 diabetes ranged in age between 25 and 65 years and had a median (interquartile range) FPG concentration of 11.5 (9.0 to 14.4) mmol/L [207 162 to 259) mg/dL], HbA1C levels of 9.1% (7.5% to 10.7%), and a mean (SD) body mass index of 29 (6) kg/m². *Interventions:* After 3 months on a low-fat, high-carbohydrate, high-fiber diet, patients were randomized to therapy with diet alone, insulin, sulfonylurea, or metformin. *Main outcome measures:* Fasting plasma glucose and HbA1C levels, and the proportion of patients who achieved target levels below 7% HbA1C or less than 7.8 mmol/L (140 mg/dL) FPG at 3, 6, and 9 years following diagnosis. *Results:* The proportion of patients who maintained target glycemic levels declined markedly over 9 years of follow-up. After 9 years of monotherapy with diet, insulin, or sulfonylurea, 8%, 42%, and 24%, respectively, achieved FPG levels of less than 7.8 mmol/L (140 mg/dL) and 9%, 28%, and 24% achieved HbA1C levels below 7%. In obese patients randomized to metformin, 18% attained FPG levels of less than 7.8 mmol/L (140 mg/dL) and 13% attained HbA1C levels below 7%. Patients less likely to achieve target levels were younger, more obese, or more hyperglycemic than other patients. *Conclusions:* Each therapeutic agent, as monotherapy, increased two to three-fold the proportion of patients who attained HbA1C below 7% compared with diet alone. However, the progressive deterioration of diabetes control was such that after 3 years, approximately 50% of patients could attain this goal with monotherapy, and by 9 years, this declined to approximately 25%. The majority of patients need multiple therapies to attain these glycemic target levels in the longer term.

A-7

PROTEIN KINASE C BETA INHIBITOR DIABETIC RETINOPATHY STUDY (PKC-DRS)

1. The PKC-DRS Study Group: The effect of ruboxistaurin on visual loss in patients with moderately severe to very severe nonproliferative diabetic retinopathy: initial results of the Protein Kinase C beta Inhibitor Diabetic Retinopathy Study (PKC-DRS) multicenter randomized clinical trial. *Diabetes.* 2005;54(7):2188–2197. Reprinted with permission of the American Diabetes Association.

Abstract The purpose of this study was to evaluate the safety and efficacy of the orally administered protein kinase C (PKC) β isoform-selective inhibitor ruboxistaurin (RBX) in subjects with moderately severe to very severe nonproliferative diabetic retinopathy (NPDR). In this multicenter, double-masked, randomized, placebo-controlled study, 252 subjects received placebo or RBX (8, 16, or 32 mg/day) for 36–46 months. Patients had an Early Treatment Diabetic Retinopathy Study (ETDRS) retinopathy severity level between 47B and 53E inclusive, an ETDRS visual acuity of 20/125 or better, and no history of scatter (panretinal) photocoagulation. Efficacy measures included progression of DR, moderate visual loss (MVL) (doubling of the visual angle), and sustained MVL (SMVL). RBX was well tolerated without significant adverse effects but had no significant effect on the progression of DR. Compared with placebo, 32 mg/day RBX was associated with a delayed occurrence of MVL (log rank, $P = 0.038$) and of SMVL ($P = 0.226$). RBX reduction of SMVL was evident only in eyes with definite diabetic macular edema at baseline (10% 32 mg/day RBX vs. 25% placebo, $P = 0.017$). In multivariable Cox proportional hazard analysis, 32 mg/day RBX significantly reduced the risk of MVL compared with placebo (hazard ratio 0.37 [95% CI 0.17–0.80], $P = 0.012$). In this clinical trial, RBX was well tolerated and reduced the risk of visual loss but did not prevent DR progression.

2. The PKC-DMES Study Group: Effect of ruboxistaurin in patients with diabetic macular edema. Thirty-month results of the randomized PKC-DMES Clinical Trial. *Arch Ophthalmol.* 2007;125:318–324. Reprinted with permission of the American Medical Association.

Abstract *Objective*: To evaluate the safety and efficacy of orally administered ruboxistaurin (RBX) as a mesylate salt in patients with diabetic macular edema (DME). *Design:* Multicenter, double-masked, randomized, placebo-controlled study of 686 patients receiving placebo or RBX orally (4, 16, or 32 mg/d) for 30 months. At baseline, patients had DME farther than 300 μm from the center of the macula, an Early Treatment Diabetic Retinopathy Study retinopathy severity level from 20 to 47A without prior photocoagulation, and an Early Treatment Diabetic Retinopathy Study visual acuity of 75 or more letters in the study eye. The primary study outcome was progression to sight-threatening DME or application of focal/grid photocoagulation for DME. *Main Outcome Measure:* Masked grading of stereoscopic fundus photographs. *Results:* The delay in progression to the primary outcome was not statistically significant (32 mg of RBX vs. placebo, P=.14 [unadjusted]; Cox proportional hazards model adjusted for covariates, hazards ratio = 0.73; 95% confidence interval, 0.53–1.0; P=.06). However, application of focal/grid photocoagulation prior to progression to sight-threatening DME varied by site, and a secondary analysis of progression to sight-threatening DME alone showed that 32 mg of RBX per day reduced progression, compared with placebo (P=.054 [unadjusted]; Cox proportional hazards model, hazards ratio = 0.66; 95% confidence interval, 0.47–0.93; P= .02). *Conclusions:* Although progression to the primary outcome was not delayed, daily oral administration of RBX may delay progression of DME to a sight-threatening stage. Ruboxistaurin was well tolerated in this study.

3. Davis MD, Sheetz MJ, Aiello LP, et al.: Effect of ruboxistaurin on the visual acuity decline associated with long-standing diabetic macular edema. *Invest Ophthalmol Vis Sci.* 2009;50:1–4. Reprinted courtesy of the Association for Research in Vision and Ophthalmology.

Abstract *Purpose*: To compare relationships between severity and duration of diabetic macular edema (DME) and visual acuity (VA) observed in the PKC-DRS2 with those from the Early Treatment Diabetic Retinopathy Study (ETDRS) and to assess the effect of the orally administered PKC β inhibitor ruboxistaurin (RBX) on these parameters. *Methods:* In the PKC-DRS2, patients with moderately severe to very severe nonproliferative diabetic retinopathy ($n = 685$) were randomly assigned to 32 mg/d RBX or placebo and followed up for 36 months with ETDRS VA measurements and fundus photographs (FP) every 3 to 6 months. Mean VA was calculated across all FP visits for eyes in each level of the ETDRS DME severity scale at those visits. For eyes with baseline VA ≥ 20/40, relationships between change in VA from baseline to last visit and duration of severe DME were analyzed with linear regression. *Results:* Mean VA decreased by approximately 22 letters between the mildest and most severe levels of the DME scale in the PKC-DRS2, compared with 27 letters in the ETDRS. In the placebo group, the rate of decrease in VA over time associated with duration of severe DME was 0.67 letters per month (24 letters over 36 months, compared with 20 letters over 28–36 months in the ETDRS). This rate was 30% less in the RBX group (0.47 letter per month, $P = 0.022$). *Conclusions:* The VA decrease in the PKC-DRS2 associated with long-standing DME agrees well with estimates from the ETDRS. RBX appears to ameliorate this decrease, an effect that could be important clinically. (ClinicalTrials.gov number, NCT00604383.)

A-8

DIABETIC RETINOPATHY CLINICAL RESEARCH (DRCR) NETWORK STUDIES

1. Diabetic Retinopathy Clinical Research Network: Diurnal variation in retinal thickening measurement by OCT in center-involved diabetic macular edema. *Arch Ophthalmol*. 2006;124:1701–1707. Reprinted with permission of American Medical Association.

Abstract *Objective*: To evaluate diurnal variation in Optical Coherence Tomography (OCT)-measured retinal thickness in patients with center-involved diabetic macular edema (DME). *Methods:* Serial OCT3 measurements were performed in 156 eyes of 96 subjects with clinically-diagnosed DME and OCT central subfield retinal thickness ≥225 microns at 8 a.m. Central subfield thickness was measured from OCT3 retinal thickness maps at 6 time points over a single day between 8 a.m. and 4 p.m. A change in central subfield thickening (observed thickness minus mean normal thickness) of at least 25% and of at least 50 microns at two consecutive time points or between 8 a.m. and 4 p.m. was considered to have met the composite outcome threshold. *Results:* At 8 a.m., the mean central subfield thickness was 368 microns and the mean visual acuity was 66 letters (approximately 20/50). The mean change in relative central subfield retinal thickening between 8 a.m. and 4 p.m. was a decrease of 6% (95% CI –9% to –3%) and the mean absolute change was a decrease of 13 microns (95% CI –17 to –8). The absolute change was significantly greater in retinas that were thicker at 8 a.m. ($P <0.001$) but the relative change was not (P=0.14). The composite threshold of reduction in central subfield thickening (as defined above) was observed in 5 eyes of 4 subjects (3% of eyes, 95% CI, 1% to 8%) while 2 eyes of 2 subjects (1%, 95% CI, 0% to 5%) had an increase in central subfield thickening of this same magnitude. The maximum decrease was observed at 4 p.m. in all 5 eyes. *Conclusions:* Although on average there are slight decreases in retinal thickening during the day, most eyes with DME have little meaningful change in OCT central subfield thickening between 8 a.m. and 4 p.m.

2. Diabetic Retinopathy Clinical Research Network: The relationship between OCT-measured central retinal thickness and visual acuity in diabetic macular edema. *Ophthalmology*. 2007;114:525–536. Courtesy of *Ophthalmology*.

Abstract *Objective*: To compare optical coherence tomography (OCT)-measured retinal thickness and visual acuity in eyes with diabetic macular edema (DME) both before and after macular laser photocoagulation. *Design:* Cross-sectional and longitudinal study. *Participants:* 210 subjects (251 eyes) with DME enrolled in a randomized clinical trial of laser techniques. *Methods:* Retinal thickness was measured with OCT and visual acuity was measured with the electronic-ETDRS procedure. *Main Outcome Measures:* OCT-measured center point thickness and visual acuity *Results:* The correlation coefficients for visual acuity versus OCT center point thickness were 0.52 at baseline and 0.49, 0.36, and 0.38 at 3.5, 8, and 12 months post-laser photocoagulation. The slope of the best fit line to the baseline data was approximately 4.4 letters (95% C.I.: 3.5, 5.3) better visual acuity for every 100 microns decrease in center point thickness at baseline with no important difference at follow-up visits. Approximately one-third of the variation in visual acuity could be predicted by a linear regression model that incorporated OCT center point thickness, age, hemoglobin A1C, and severity of fluorescein leakage in the center and inner subfields. The correlation between change in visual acuity and change in OCT center point thickening 3.5 months after laser treatment was 0.44 with no important difference at the other follow-up times. A subset of eyes showed paradoxical improvements in visual acuity with increased center point thickening (7–17% at the three time points) or paradoxical worsening of visual acuity with a decrease in center point thickening (18–26 at the three time points). *Conclusions:* There is modest correlation between OCT-measured center point thickness and visual acuity, and modest correlation of changes in retinal thickening and visual acuity following focal laser treatment for DME. However, a wide range of visual acuity may be observed for a given degree of retinal edema and paradoxical increases in center point thickening with increases in visual acuity as well as paradoxical decreases in center point thickening with decreases in visual acuity were not uncommon. Thus, although OCT measurements of retinal thickness represent an important tool in clinical evaluation, they cannot reliably substitute as a surrogate for visual acuity at a given point in time. This study does not address whether short-term changes on OCT are predictive of long-term effects on visual acuity.

3. Diabetic Retinopathy Clinical Research Network: Comparison of modified-ETDRS and mild macular grid laser photocoagulation strategies for diabetic macular edema. *Arch Ophthalmol.* 2007;125:469–480. Reprinted with permission of the American Medical Association.

Abstract *Purpose*: To compare two laser photocoagulation techniques for treatment of diabetic macular edema (DME): modified-ETDRS direct/grid photocoagulation (mETDRS) and a, potentially milder, but potentially more extensive, mild macular grid (MMG) laser technique in which small mild burns are placed throughout the macula, whether or not edema is present, and microaneurysms are not treated directly. *Methods:* 263 subjects (mean age 59 years) with previously untreated DME were randomly assigned to receive laser photocoagulation by mETDRS (N=162 eyes) or MMG (N=161 eyes) technique. Visual acuity, fundus photographs and OCT measurements were obtained at baseline and after 3.5, 8, and 12 months. Treatment was repeated if DME persisted. *Main Outcome Measure:* Change in OCT measures at 12-months follow up. *Results:* From baseline to 12 months, among eyes with baseline central subfield thickness ≥250 microns, central subfield thickening decreased by an average of 88 microns in the mETDRS group and decreased by 49 microns in the MMG group (adjusted mean difference: 33 microns, 95% confidence interval 5 to 61 microns, $P = 0.02$). Weighted inner zone thickening by OCT decreased by 42 and 28 microns, respectively (adjusted mean difference: 14 microns, 95% confidence interval 1 to 27 microns, $P=0.04$), maximum retinal thickening (maximum of the central and four inner subfields) decreased by 66 and 39 microns, respectively (adjusted mean difference: 27 microns, 95% confidence interval 6 to 47 microns, $P=0.01$), and retinal volume decreased by 0.8 and 0.4 mm³, respectively (adjusted mean difference: 0.3 mm³, 95% confidence interval 0.02 to 0.53 mm³, $P=0.03$). At 12 months, the mean change in visual acuity was 0 letters in the mETDRS group and 2 letters worse in thc MMG group (adjusted mean difference: 2 letters, 95% confidence interval −0.5 to 5 letters, $P=0.10$). *Conclusions:* At 12 months after treatment, the MMG technique is less effective at reducing OCT measured retinal thickening than the more extensively evaluated current mETDRS laser photocoagulation approach. However, the visual acuity outcome with both approaches is not substantially different. Given these findings, a larger long-term trial of the MMG technique is not justified. *Application to Clinical Practice:* Modified ETDRS focal photocoagulation should continue as a standard approach for treating diabetic macular edema.

4. Diabetic Retinopathy Clinical Research Network: Randomized trial of peribulbar triamcinolone acetonide with and without focal photocoagulation for mild diabetic macular edema: a pilot study. *Ophthalmology.* 2007;114:1190–1196. Courtesy of *Ophthalmology.*

Abstract *Objective*: To provide pilot data on the safety and efficacy of anterior and posterior sub-Tenon injections of triamcinolone either alone or in combination with focal photocoagulation in the treatment of mild diabetic macular edema (DME). *Design*: Prospective, phase II, multicenter, randomized clinical trial. *Participants*: One hundred nine patients (129 eyes) with mild DME and visual acuity 20/40 or better. *Methods*: The participants were assigned randomly to receive either focal photocoagulation (n = 38), a 20-mg anterior sub-Tenon injection of triamcinolone (n = 23), a 20-mg anterior sub-Tenon injection followed by focal photocoagulation after 4 weeks (n = 25), a 40-mg posterior sub-Tenon injection of triamcinolone (n = 21), or a 40-mg posterior sub-Tenon injection followed by focal photocoagulation after 4 weeks (n = 22). Follow-up visits were performed at 4, 8, 17, and 34 weeks. *Main Outcome Measures*: Change in visual acuity and retinal thickness measured with optical coherence tomography (OCT). *Results*: At baseline, mean visual acuity in the study eyes was 20/25 and mean OCT central subfield thickness was 328 μm. Changes in retinal thickening and in visual acuity were not significantly different among the 5 groups at 34 weeks (P = 0.46 and P = 0.94, respectively). There was a suggestion of a greater proportion of eyes having a central subfield thickness less than 250 μm at 17 weeks when the peribulbar triamcinolone was combined with focal photocoagulation. Elevated intraocular pressure and ptosis were adverse effects attributable to the injections. *Conclusions*: In cases of DME with good visual acuity, peribulbar triamcinolone, with or without focal photocoagulation, is unlikely to be of substantial benefit. Based on these results, a phase III trial to evaluate the benefit of these treatments for mild DME is not warranted.

5. Diabetic Retinopathy Clinical Research Network: Reproducibility of macular thickness and volume using Zeiss optical coherence tomography in patients with diabetic macular edema. *Ophthalmology.* 2007;114:1520–1525. Courtesy of *Ophthalmology.*

Abstract *Purpose*: To evaluate optical coherence tomography (OCT) reproducibility in patients with diabetic macular edema (DME). *Design:* Prospective 1-day observational study. *Participants:* Two hundred twelve eyes of 107 patients with DME involving the macular center by clinical exam and OCT central subfield thickness ≥ 225 microns. *Methods:* Retinal thickness was measured with the OCT3 system, and scans were evaluated by a reading center. Reproducibility of retinal thickness measurements was assessed, and 95% confidence intervals (CIs) for a change in thickness were estimated. *Main Outcome Measures:* Reproducibility of OCT-measured central subfield thickness. *Results:* Reproducibility was better for central subfield thickness than for center point thickness (half-width of the 95% CI for absolute change, 38 vs. 50 μm, and for relative change, 11% vs. 17%, respectively; P<0.001). The median absolute difference between replicate measurements of the central subfield was 7 μm (2%). Half-widths of the 95% CI for a change in central subfield thickness were 22, 23, 33, and 56 μm for scans with central subfield thicknesses of <200, 200 to <250, 250 to <400 and ≥400 μm, respectively. When expressed as percentage differences between 2 measurements, half-widths of the 95% CI for a change in central subfield thickness were 10%, 10%, 10%, and 13% for scans with central subfield thicknesses of <200, 200 to <250, 250 to <400 and ≥400 μm, respectively. We were unable to identify an effect on reproducibility of central subfield measurements with respect to the presence of cystoid abnormalities, subretinal fluid, vitreomacular traction, or reduced visual acuity. Reproducibility was better when both scans had a standard deviation (SD) of the center point <10.0% (half-width of the 95% CI for change, 33 vs. 56 μm; *P* < 0.001). *Conclusions:* Reproducibility is better for central subfield thickness measurements than for center point measurements, and variability is less with retinal thickness when expressed as a percent change than when expressed as an absolute change. A change in central subfield thickness exceeding 11% is likely to be real. Scans with an SD of the center point of ≥10.0% are less reproducible and should be viewed with caution when assessing the validity of an observed change in retinal thickness in patients with DME.

6. Bhavsar AR, Ip MS, Glassman AR, DRCRnet, the SCORE Study Groups: The risk of endophthalmitis following intravitreal triamcinolone injection in the DRCRnet and SCORE clinical trials. *Am J Ophthalmol.* 2007;144:454–456. Reprinted with permission of Elsevier.

Abstract *Purpose*: To report the incidence of endophthalmitis following intravitreal injection using a standardized injection procedure.*Design:* Two randomized clinical trials. *Methods:* Nonpreserved intravitreal triamcinolone acetonide in prefilled syringes (Allergan, Inc, Irvine, California, USA) was injected intravitreally in the Diabetic Retinopathy Clinical Research Network (DRCR net) and the Standard Care vs COrticosteroid for REtinal Vein Occlusion (SCORE) clinical trials. The standardized injection procedure did not include the use of topical antibiotics during the days prior to the injection. *Results:* As of December 31, 2006, 1,378 intravitreal injections (538 eyes) have been administered in the Diabetic Retinopathy Clinical Research Network Diabetic Macular Edema trial and 631 injections (301 eyes) in Standard Care vs COrticosteroid for REtinal Vein Occlusion. There was one case of endophthalmitis in the 2009 injections to date (0.05%, 95% confidence interval 0.001% to 0.277%). *Conclusions:* A low rate of endophthalmitis is achievable using a standardized procedure for intravitreal injection without prescribing antibiotic prophylaxis on the days prior to the injection.

7. Diabetic Retinopathy Clinical Research Network, Scott IU, Edwards AR, et al.: A phase II randomized clinical trial of intravitreal bevacizumab for diabetic macular edema. *Ophthalmology.* 2007;114:1860–1867. Courtesy of *Ophthalmology.*

Abstract *Objective*: To provide data on the short-term effect of intravitreal bevacizumab for diabetic macular edema (DME). *Design:* Randomized phase II clinical trial. *Participants:* One hundred twenty-one eyes of 121 subjects (109 eligible for analysis) with DME and Snellen acuity equivalent ranging from 20/32 to 20/320. *Interventions:* Random assignment to 1 of 5 groups: (A) focal photocoagulation at baseline (n = 19), (B) intravitreal injection of 1.25 mg of bevacizumab at baseline and 6 weeks (n = 22), (C) intravitreal injection of 2.5 mg of bevacizumab at baseline and 6 weeks (n = 24), (D) intravitreal injection of 1.25 mg of bevacizumab at baseline and sham injection at 6 weeks (n = 22), or (E) intravitreal injection of 1.25 mg of bevacizumab at baseline and 6 weeks with photocoagulation at 3 weeks (n = 22). *Main Outcome Measures:* Central subfield thickness (CST) on optical coherence tomography and best-corrected visual acuity (VA) were measured at baseline and after 3, 6, 9, 12, 18, and 24 weeks. *Results:* At baseline, median CST was 411 μm and median Snellen VA equivalent was 20/50. Compared with group A, groups B and C had a greater reduction in CST at 3 weeks and about 1 line better median VA over 12 weeks. There were no meaningful differences between groups B and C in CST reduction or VA improvement. A CST reduction > 11% (reliability limit) was present at 3 weeks in 36 of 84 (43%) bevacizumab-treated eyes and 5 of 18 (28%) eyes treated with laser alone, and at 6 weeks in 31 of 84 (37%) and 9 of 18 (50%) eyes, respectively. Combining focal photocoagulation with bevacizumab resulted in no apparent short-term benefit or adverse outcomes. Endophthalmitis developed in 1 eye. The following events occurred during the first 24 weeks in subjects treated with bevacizumab without attributing cause to the drug: myocardial infarction (n = 2), congestive heart failure (n = 1), elevated blood pressure (n = 3), and worsened renal function (n = 3). *Conclusion:* These results demonstrate that intravitreal bevacizumab can reduce DME in some eyes, but the study was not designed to determine whether treatment is beneficial. A phase III trial would be needed for that purpose.

8. Scott IU, Bressler NM, Bressler SB, et al.: Agreement between clinician and reading center gradings of diabetic retinopathy severity level at baseline in a phase 2 study of intravitreal bevacizumab for diabetic macular edema. *Retina.* 2008;28:36–40. Reprinted with permission of Lippincott Williams & Wilkins.

Abstract *Purpose*: To evaluate agreement in diabetic retinopathy severity classification by retina specialists performing ophthalmoscopy versus reading center (RC) grading of seven-field stereoscopic fundus photographs in a phase 2 clinical trial of intravitreal bevacizumab for center-involved diabetic macular edema. *Methods:* Clinicians' grading scale used four levels: microaneurysms only, mild/moderate nonproliferative diabetic retinopathy (NPDR), severe NPDR, and proliferative diabetic retinopathy (PDR) or prior panretinal photocoagulation (PRP) or both. The RC scale used eight levels: microaneurysms only, mild NPDR, moderate NPDR, moderately severe NPDR, severe NPDR, mild PDR, moderate PDR, and high-risk PDR. Percent agreement and kappa statistic were defined by collapsing RC categories to match those used by clinicians. *Results:* There was agreement in 89/118 eyes (75%) with kappa = 0.55 (95% confidence interval [0.41, 0.68]). In six eyes, disagreements were of potential substantial clinical importance: five eyes with subtle retinal neovascularization and one with a small preretinal hemorrhage identified only in photographs. *Conclusions:* Clinician grading of retinopathy severity had moderate agreement with RC grading and might be useful for placing eyes into broad baseline categories.

9. Davis MD, Bressler SB, Aiello LP, et al.: Comparison of time-domain OCT and fundus photographic assessments of retinal thickening in eyes with diabetic macular edema. *Invest Ophthalmol Vis Sci.* 2008;49:1745–1752. Reprinted courtesy of the Association for Research in Vision and Ophthalmology.

Abstract *Purpose*: To explore the correlation between optical coherence Tomography (OCT) and stereoscopic fundus photographs (FP) for the assessment of retinal thickening (RT) in diabetic macular edema (DME) within a clinical trial. *Methods:* OCT, FP, and best corrected visual acuity (VA) measurements were obtained in both eyes of 263 participants in a trial comparing two photocoagulation techniques for DME. Correlation coefficients (r) were calculated comparing RT measured by OCT, RT estimated from FP, and VA. Principal variables were central subfield retinal thickness (CSRT) obtained from the OCT fast macular map and DME severity assessed by a reading center using a seven-step photographic scale combining the area of thickened retina within 1 disc diameter of the foveal center and thickening at the center. *Results:* Medians (quartiles) for retinal thickness within the center subfield by OCT at baseline increased from 236 (214, 264) μm in the lowest level of the photographic scale to 517 (455, 598) μm in the highest level (r = 0.67). However, CSRT interquartile ranges were broad and overlapping between FP scale levels, and there were many outliers. Correlations between either modality and VA were weaker (r = 0.57 for CSRT, and r = 0.47 for the FP scale). OCT appeared to be more reproducible and more sensitive to change in RT between baseline and 1 year than was FP. *Conclusions:* There was a moderate correlation between OCT and FP assessments of RT in patients with DME and slightly less correlation of either measure with VA. OCT and FP provide complementary information but neither is a reliable surrogate for VA. (ClinicalTrials.gov number, NCT00071773.)

10. Bressler NM, Edwards AR, Antoszyk AN, et al.: Retinal thickness on Stratus optical coherence tomography in people with diabetes and minimal or no diabetic retinopathy. *Am J Ophthalmol.* 2008;145:894–901. Reprinted with permission of Elsevier.

Abstract *Purpose:* To evaluate optical coherence tomography (OCT) thickness of the macula in people with diabetes but minimal or no retinopathy and to compare these findings with published normative data in the literature from subjects reported to have no retinal disease. *Design:* Cross-sectional study. *Methods:* In a multicenter community- and university-based practices setting, 97 subjects with diabetes with no or minimal diabetic retinopathy and no central retinal thickening on clinical examination and a center point thickness of 225 μm or less on OCT (Stratus OCT; Carl Zeiss Meditec, Dublin, California, USA) were recruited. Electronic Early Treatment of Diabetic Retinopathy Study best-corrected visual acuity, seven-field stereoscopic color fundus photographs, and Stratus OCT fast macular scan were noted. Main outcome measures were central subfield (CSF) thickness measured on Stratus OCT. *Results*: On average, CSF thickness was 201 ± 22 μm. CSF thickness was significantly greater in retinas from men than retinas from women (mean ± standard deviation, 209 ± 18 μm vs. 194 ± 23 μm; $P < 0.001$). After adjusting for gender, no additional factors were found to be associated significantly with CSF thickness ($P > .10$). *Conclusion:* CSF thicknesses on Stratus OCT in people with diabetes and minimal or no retinopathy are similar to thicknesses reported from a normative database of people without diabetes. CSF thickness is greater in men than in women, consistent with many, but not all, previous reports. Studies involving comparisons of retinal thickness with expected norms should consider different mean values for women and men.

11. Ip MS, Bressler SB, Antoszyk AN, et al.: A randomized trial comparing intravitreal triamcinolone and focal/grid photocoagulation for diabetic macular edema: baseline features. *Retina.* 2008;28:919–930. Reprinted with permission of Lippincott Williams & Wilkins.

Abstract *Purpose*: To compare baseline demographic, systemic, and ocular characteristics within age and racial subgroups among participants in this Diabetic Retinopathy Clinical Research Network clinical trial and to compare this cohort with other cohorts enrolled in phase 3 clinical trials for diabetic retinopathy. *Methods:* Thirty-six month, randomized, controlled, multicenter clinical trial of 693 participants with diabetic macular edema enrolled at 88 clinical sites in the United States. Participants were categorized into self-reported race/ethnicity subgroups and into one of three age groups: 18 to <60, 60 to <70, and 70 and older. *Results:* Mean age of participants was 63 years, 72% were white, and median visual acuity letter score was 62 (approximately 20/63). No substantial difference was identified between racial subgroups for any baseline variable. Older participants were more likely to have type 2 diabetes mellitus and longer duration disease. The most frequent levels of diabetic retinopathy among 840 study eyes were moderate (level 43) to moderately severe (level 47) nonproliferative disease. *Conclusion:* While the racial composition of this cohort does not differ from other cohorts in large phase 3 trials that have evaluated participants with diabetic retinopathy, the inclusion of many subjects over age 70 and a better level of glycemic control are distinguishing features.

12. Diabetic Retinopathy Clinical Research Network: A Randomized Trial Comparing Intravitreal Triamcinolone Acetonide and Focal/Grid Photocoagulation for Diabetic Macular Edema. *Ophthalmology.* 2008;115:1447–1459. Courtesy of *Ophthalmology.*

Abstract *Objective*: To evaluate the efficacy and safety of 1-mg and 4-mg doses of preservative-free intravitreal triamcinolone in comparison with focal/grid photocoagulation for the treatment of diabetic macular edema (DME). *Design:* Multicenter, randomized clinical trial. *Participants:* Eight hundred forty study eyes of 693 subjects with DME involving the fovea and with visual acuity of 20/40 to 20/320. *Methods:* Eyes were randomized to focal/grid photocoagulation (n = 330), 1 mg intravitreal triamcinolone (n = 256), or 4 mg intravitreal triamcinolone (n = 254). Re-treatment was given for persistent or new edema at 4-month intervals. The primary outcome was evaluated at 2 years. *Main Outcome Measures:* Visual acuity measured with the Electronic Early Treatment Diabetic Retinopathy Study method (primary), optical coherence tomography-measured retinal thickness (secondary), and safety. *Results:* At 4 months, mean visual acuity was better in the 4-mg triamcinolone group than in either the laser group ($P<0.001$) or the 1-mg triamcinolone group ($P = 0.001$). By 1 year, there were no significant differences among groups in mean visual acuity. At the 16-month visit and extending through the primary outcome visit at 2 years, mean visual acuity was better in the laser group than in the other 2 groups (at 2 years, $P = 0.02$ comparing the laser and 1-mg groups, $P = 0.002$ comparing the laser and 4-mg groups, and $P = 0.49$ comparing the 1-mg and 4-mg groups). Treatment group differences in the visual acuity outcome could not be attributed solely to cataract formation. Optical coherence tomography results generally paralleled the visual acuity results. Intraocular pressure increased from baseline by 10 mmHg or more at any visit in 4%, 16%, and 33% of eyes in the 3 treatment groups, respectively, and cataract surgery was performed in 13%, 23%, and 51% of eyes in the 3 treatment groups, respectively. *Conclusions:* Over a 2-year period, focal/grid photocoagulation is more effective and has fewer side effects than 1-mg or 4-mg doses of preservative-free intravitreal triamcinolone for most patients with DME who have characteristics similar to the cohort in this clinical trial. The results of this study also support that focal/grid photocoagulation currently should be the benchmark against which other treatments are compared in clinical trials of DME.

13. Browning DJ, Glassman AR, Aiello LP, et al.: Optical coherence tomography measurements and analysis methods in optical coherence tomography studies of diabetic macular edema. *Ophthalmology.* 2008;115:1366–1371. Courtesy of *Ophthalmology.*

Abstract *Objective*: To evaluate optical coherence tomography (OCT) measurements and methods of analysis of OCT data in studies of diabetic macular edema (DME). *Design:* Associations of pairs of OCT variables and results of 3 analysis methods using data from 2 studies of DME. *Participants:* Two hundred sixty-three subjects from a study of modified Early Treatment of Diabetic Retinopathy Study (mETDRS) versus modified macular grid (MMG) photocoagulation for DME and 96 subjects from a study of diurnal variation of DME. *Methods:* Correlations were calculated for pairs of OCT variables at baseline and for changes in the variables over time. Distribution of OCT measurement changes, predictive factors for OCT measurement changes, and treatment group outcomes were compared when 3 measures of change in macular thickness were analyzed: absolute change in retinal thickness, relative change in retinal thickness, and relative change in retinal thickening. *Main Outcome Measures:* Concordance of results using different OCT variables and analysis methods. *Results:* Center point thickness correlated highly with central subfield mean thickness (CSMT) at baseline (0.98–0.99). The distributions of changes in CSMT were approximately normally distributed for absolute change in retinal thickness and relative change in retinal thickness, but not for relative change in retinal thickening. Macular thinning in the mETDRS group was significantly greater than in the MMG group when absolute change in retinal thickness was used, but not when relative change in thickness and relative change in thickening were used. Relative change in macular thickening provides unstable data in eyes with mild degrees of baseline thickening, unlike the situation with absolute or relative change in retinal thickness. *Conclusions:* Central subfield mean thickness is the preferred OCT measurement for the central macula because of its higher reproducibility and correlation with other measurements of the central macula. Total macular volume may be preferred when the central macula is less important. Absolute change in retinal thickness is the preferred analysis method in studies involving eyes with mild macular thickening. Relative change in thickening may be preferable when retinal thickening is more severe.

14. Browning DJ, Altaweel MM, Bressler NM, Bressler SB, Scott IU, on behalf of the Diabetic Retinopathy Clinical Research Network: Diabetic macular edema: what is focal and what is diffuse? *Am J Ophthalmol.* 2008;146:649–655. Reprinted with permission of Elsevier.

Abstract *Purpose:* To review the available information on classification of diabetic macular edema (DME) as focal or diffuse. *Design:* Interpretive essay. *Methods:* Literature review and interpretation. *Results:* The terms focal diabetic macular edema and diffuse diabetic macular edema frequently are used without clear definitions. Published definitions often use different examination methods and often are inconsistent. Evaluating published information on the prevalence of focal and diffuse DME, the responses of focal and diffuse DME to treatments, and the importance of focal and diffuse DME in assessing prognosis is hindered because the terms are used inconsistently. A newer vocabulary may be more constructive, one that describes discrete components of the concepts such as extent and location of macular thickening, involvement of the center of the macula, quantity and pattern of lipid exudates, source of fluorescein leakage, and regional variation in macular thickening and that distinguishes these terms from the use of the term focal when describing one type of photocoagulation technique. Developing methods for assessing component variables that can be used in clinical practice and establishing reproducibility of the methods are important tasks. *Conclusions:* Little evidence exists that characteristics of DME described by the terms focal and diffuse help to explain variation in visual acuity or response to treatment. It is unresolved whether a concept of focal and diffuse DME will prove clinically useful despite frequent use of the terms when describing management of DME. Further studies to address the issues are needed.

15. Glassman AR, Beck RW, Browning DJ, Danis RP, Kollman C for the Diabetic Retinopathy Clinical Research Network Study Group: Comparison of optical coherence tomography retinal thickness measurements in diabetic macular edema with and without reading center manual grading from a clinical trials perspective. *Invest Ophthalmol Vis Sci.* 2009;50:560–566. Reprinted courtesy of the Association for Research in Vision and Ophthalmology.

Abstract *Purpose:* To analyze the value of reading center error correction in automated optical coherence tomography (OCT; Stratus; Carl Zeiss Meditec, Inc., Dublin, CA) retinal thickness measurements in eyes with diabetic macular edema (DME).

Methods: OCT scans (n=6522) obtained in seven Diabetic Retinopathy Clinical Research Network (DRCR.net) studies were analyzed. The reading center evaluated whether the automated center point measurement appeared correct, and when it did not, measured it manually with calipers. Center point standard deviation (SD) as a percentage of thickness, center point thickness, signal strength, and analysis confidence were evaluated for their association with an automated measurement error (manual measurement needed and exceeded 12% of automated thickness). Curves were constructed for each factor by plotting the error rate against the proportion of scans sent to the reading center. The impact of measurement error on interpretation of clinical trial results and statistical power was also assessed. *Results:* SD was the best predictor of an automated measurement error. The other three variables did not augment the ability to predict an error using SD alone. Based on SD, an error rate of 5% or less could be achieved by sending only 33% of scans to the reading center (those with an SD >or= 5%). Correcting automated errors had no appreciable effect on the interpretation of results from a completed randomized trial and had little impact on a trial's statistical power. *Conclusions:* In DME clinical trials, the error involved with using automated Stratus OCT center point measurements is sufficiently small that results are not likely to be affected if scans are not routinely sent to a reading center, provided adequate quality control measures are in place.

16. Diabetic Retinopathy Clinical Research Network: An observational study of the development of diabetic macular edema following panretinal (scatter) photocoagulation (PRP) given in 1 or 4 sittings. *Arch Ophthalmol.* 2009;127:132–140. Reprinted with permission of the American Medical Association.

Abstract *Objective:* To compare the effects of single-sitting vs 4-sitting panretinal photocoagulation (PRP) on macular edema in subjects with severe nonproliferative or early proliferative diabetic retinopathy with relatively good visual acuity and no or mild center-involved macular edema. *Methods:* Subjects were treated with 1 sitting or 4 sittings of PRP in a nonrandomized, prospective, multicentered clinical trial. *Main Outcome Measure:* Central subfield thickness on optical coherence tomography (OCT). *Results:* Central subfield thickness was slightly greater in the 1-sitting group (n = 84) than in the 4-sitting group (n = 71) at the 3-day (P = .01) and 4-week visits (P = .003). At the 34-week primary outcome visit, the slight differences had reversed, with the thickness being slightly greater in the 4-sitting group than in the 1-sitting group (P = .06). Visual acuity differences paralleled OCT differences. *Conclusions:* Our results suggest that clinically meaningful differences are unlikely in OCT thickness or visual acuity following application of PRP in 1 sitting compared with 4 sittings in subjects in this cohort. More definitive results would require a large randomized trial. *Application to Clinical Practice:* These results suggest PRP costs to some patients in terms of travel and lost productivity as well as to eye care providers could be reduced.

17. Diabetic Retinopathy Clinical Research Network: Three-year follow-up of a randomized trial comparing focal/grid photocoagulation and intravitreal triamcinolone for diabetic macular edema. *Arch Ophthalmol* 2009;127(3):245–251. Reprinted with permission of the American Medical Association.

Abstract *Objective:* To report 3-year outcomes of patients who participated in a randomized trial evaluating 1-mg and 4-mg doses of preservative-free intravitreal triamcinolone compared with focal/grid photocoagulation for treatment of diabetic macular edema. *Methods:* Eyes with diabetic macular edema and visual acuities of 20/40 to 20/320 were randomly assigned to focal/grid photocoagulation or 1 or 4 mg of triamcinolone. At the conclusion of the trial, 3-year follow-up data were available in 306 eyes. *Results:* Between 2 years (time of the primary outcome) and 3 years, more eyes improved than worsened in all three treatment groups. Change in visual acuity letter score from baseline to 3 years was +5 in the laser group and 0 in each triamcinolone group. The cumulative probability of cataract surgery by 3 years was 31%, 46%, and 83% in the laser and 1-mg and 4-mg triamcinolone groups, respectively. Intraocular pressure increased by more than 10 mm Hg at any visit in 4%, 18%, and 33% of eyes, respectively. *Conclusions:* Results in a subset of randomized subjects who completed the 3-year follow-up are consistent with previously published 2-year results and do not indicate a long-term benefit of intravitreal triamcinolone relative to focal/grid photocoagulation in patients with diabetic macular edema similar to those studied in this clinical trial. Most eyes receiving 4 mg of triamcinolone as given in this study are likely to require cataract surgery.

18. Browning DJ, Apte RS, Bressler SB, et al.: Association of the extent of diabetic macular edema as assessed by optical coherence tomography with visual acuity and retinal outcome variables. *Retina* 2009;29(3):300–305. Reprinted with permission of Lippincott Williams & Wilkins.

Abstract *Purpose:* To determine whether the extensiveness of diabetic macular edema using a 10-step scale based on optical coherence tomography explains pretreatment variation in visual acuity and predicts change in macular thickness or visual acuity after laser photocoagulation. *Methods:* Three hundred twenty-three eyes from a randomized clinical trial of two methods of laser photocoagulation for diabetic macular edema were studied. Baseline number of thickened optical coherence tomography subfields was used to characterize diabetic macular edema on a 10-step scale from 0 to 9. Associations were explored between baseline number of thickened subfields and baseline fundus photographic variables, visual acuity, central subfield mean thickness (CSMT), and total macular volume. Associations were also examined between baseline number of thickened subfields and changes in visual acuity, CSMT, and total macular volume at 3.5 and 12 months after laser photocoagulation. *Results:* For baseline visual acuity, the number of thickened subfields explained no more variation than did CSMT, age and fluorescein leakage. A greater number of thickened subfields was associated with a greater baseline CSMT, total macular volume, area of retinal thickening, and degree of thickening at the center of the macula ($r = 0.64, 0.77, 0.61$–0.63, and 0.45, respectively) and with a lower baseline visual acuity ($r = 0.38$). Baseline number of thickened subfields showed no association with change in visual acuity ($r \leq 0.01$–0.08) and weak associations with change in CSMT and total macular volume (r from 0.11 to 0.35). *Conclusion:* This optical coherence tomography based assessment of the extensiveness of diabetic macular edema did not explain additional variation in baseline visual acuity above that explained by other known important variables nor predict changes in macular thickness or visual acuity after laser photocoagulation.

19. Sun JK, Aiello LP, Stockman M, et al.: Effects of dilation on electronic-ETDRS visual acuity in diabetic patients. *Invest Ophthalmol Vis Sci.* 2009;50:1580–1584. Reprinted courtesy of the Association for Research in Vision and Ophthalmology.

Abstract *Purpose*: To evaluate the effect of pupillary dilation on electronic-ETDRS visual acuity (EVA) in diabetic subjects and to assess postdilation EVA as a surrogate for predilation VA. Methods: DRCR.net-protocol refraction and EVA were measured before and after dilation in diabetic subjects by independent, masked examiners. Results: In 129 eyes of 66 subjects, the median (25th, 75th percentiles) predilation EVA score was 69 (54, 86) (Snellen-equivalent 20/40-1 [20/80-1, 20/20+1]). Predilation VA was >20/20, <20/20 to 20/40, <20/40 to 20/80, and <20/80 in 29%, 19% 26%, and 26% of eyes, respectively. Median EVA change postdilation was -3 letters (-7, 0). The absolute change in EVA score was >15 letters (>3 ETDRS lines) in 9% of eyes and >10 letters (>2 ETDRS lines) in 19% of eyes. Extent of change (range +12 to -25 letters) was associated with baseline VA. No relationship was identified between EVA change and gender, race, lens status, refractive error, DR severity, or primary cause of vision loss. Conclusions: In an optimized clinical trial setting, there is a decline in best corrected EVA after dilation in diabetic subjects. The large range and magnitude of VA change preclude using postdilation EVA as a surrogate for undilated VA.

20. Scott IU, Danis RP, Bressler SB, et al. Effect of focal/grid photocoagulation on visual acuity and retinal thickening in eyes with non-center-involved diabetic macular edema. *Retina* 2009;29:613–617. Reprinted with permission of Lippincott Williams and Wilkins.

Abstract *Purpose*: To report visual acuity and anatomic changes from baseline to 12 months after modified Early Treatment Diabetic Retinopathy Study (ETDRS)-style (focal/grid) photocoagulation in eyes with non-center-involved (non-CI) clinically significant macular edema. *Methods*: Visual acuity, optical coherence tomography, fluorescein angiography, and fundus photography data were analyzed from eyes with non-CI clinically significant macular edema treated with modified ETDRS-style (focal/grid) photocoagulation in a Diabetic Retinopathy Clinical Research Network trial. *Results*: Among the 22 eyes (of 22 patients) with 12-month follow-up, median visual acuity letter score remained within 1 letter of baseline over 12 months. The median central subfield retinal thickness decreased by 10 μm, median total macular volume decreased by 0.2 mm^3, and median fluorescein leakage area within the grid decreased by 0.7 disk areas. *Conclusion*: We are unaware of any other systematic evaluation of eyes with non-CI clinically significant macular edema since the ETDRS. Focal/grid laser in these non-CI eyes was associated with relatively stable visual acuity and retinal thickness measurements, and decreased fluorescein leakage area at 1 year. One-year visual acuity results are consistent with those published by the ETDRS, despite the intervening significant differences in the management of diabetes. Although this was a small study without a concurrent control group, the ETDRS recommendation to consider focal/grid laser in eyes with non-CI clinically significant macular edema still seems appropriate.

Glossary

INGRID U. SCOTT, MD, MPH,
AND HARRY W. FLYNN, JR., MD

Clinically significant macular edema (CSME): Retinal thickening at or within 500 microns of the center of the macula; and/or hard exudates at or within 500 microns of the center of the macula, if associated with thickening of the adjacent retina; and/or a zone or zones of retinal thickening 1 disc area in size, any part of which is within 1 disc diameter of the center of the macula.

DCCT: Diabetes Control and Complications Trial.

Diabetes mellitus: According to the American Diabetes Association expert committee, the criteria for the diagnosis of diabetes mellitus are as follows:

Symptoms of diabetes plus casual plasma glucose concentration equal to or exceeding 200 mg/dL (11.1 mmol/L). "Casual" is defined as any time of day without regard to time since last meal. The classic symptoms of diabetes include polyuria, polydipsia, and unexplained weight loss;
or

Fasting plasma glucose equal to or exceeding 126 mg/dL (7.0 mmol/L). Fasting is defined as no caloric intake for at least 8 h;
or

A plasma glucose measurement at 2 h postload equal to or exceeding 200 mg/dL (11.1 mmol/L) during an oral glucose tolerance test. The test is to be performed as described by the World Health Organization, using a glucose lead containing the equivalent of 75 g anhydrous glucose dissolved in water. However, the expert committee has recommended against oral glucose tolerance testing for routine clinical use.

Diabetes type: Type 1, previously called juvenile-onset or insulin-dependent diabetes, is characterized by beta-cell destruction and usually leads to absolute insulin deficiency. Type 2, previously called adult-onset or noninsulin-dependent diabetes, is characterized by insulin resistance with an insulin secretory defect that leads to relative insulin deficiency. (Source: Report of the Expert Committee on the Diagnosis and Classification of Diabetes Mellitus. *Diabetes Care*. 2003;26[Suppl 1]:S5–S20.)

DRCR: Diabetic Retinopathy Clinical Research network.

DRS: Diabetic Retinopathy Study.

DRVS: Diabetic Retinopathy Vitrectomy Study.

Early proliferative diabetic retinopathy (i.e., proliferative retinopathy without DRS high-risk characteristics): New vessels not meeting the criteria of high-risk proliferative retinopathy.

EDIC: Epidemiology of Diabetes Interventions and Complications study.

ETDRS: Early Treatment Diabetic Retinopathy Study.

Focal photocoagulation: A laser technique directed to abnormal blood vessels with specific areas of focal leakage (i.e., microaneurysms) to reduce chronic fluid leakage in patients with macular edema.

Grid photocoagulation: A laser technique in which a grid pattern of scatter burns is applied in areas of diffuse macular edema and nonperfusion. Typically, fluorescein angiograms of these areas show a diffuse pattern rather than focal leakage.

Hard exudates: Protein and lipid accumulation within the retina.

High-risk proliferative diabetic retinopathy: New vessels on or within 1 disc diameter of the optic disc equaling or exceeding standard photograph 10A (about 1/4–1/3 disc area), with or without vitreous or preretinal hemorrhage; or vitreous and/or preretinal hemorrhage accompanied by new vessels either on the optic disc less than standard photograph 10A or elsewhere equaling or exceeding ½ disc area.

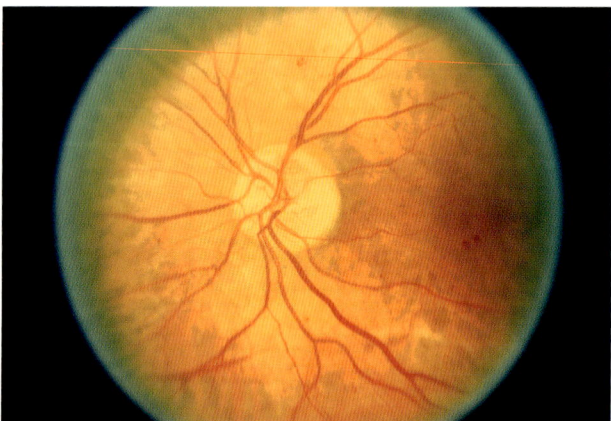

Diabetic Retinopathy Study standard photograph 10A demonstrating definite disc neovascularization. (Source: Published with permission form Diabetic Retinopathy Study Research Group: Photocoagulation treatment of proliferative diabetic retinopathy: the second report of Diabetic Retinopathy Study findings. *Ophthalmology*. 1978;85:82–106.)

Intraretinal microvascular abnormalities (IRMA): Tortuous intraretinal vascular segments, varying in caliber from barely visible to 31 microns in diameter

(1/4 the width of a major vein at the disc margin); they occasionally can be larger. IRMA may be difficult to distinguish from neovascularization.

Local photocoagulation: A laser technique in which small, flat NVE is treated with confluent, moderately intense burns. This technique alone has little role in current clinical practice.

Macular edema: Thickening of the retina within 1 or 2 disc diameters of the center of the macula.

Mild macular grid: 360-degree treatment around the center of the macular with no attempt to treat specific microaneurysms.

Mild nonproliferative diabetic retinopathy: At least one microaneurysm and less than moderate nonproliferative diabetic retinopathy.

Moderate nonproliferative diabetic retinopathy: Hemorrhages and/or microaneurysms greater than standard photograph 2A, and/or soft exudates, venous beading, or intraretinal microvascular abnormalities present but less than severe nonproliferative retinopathy.

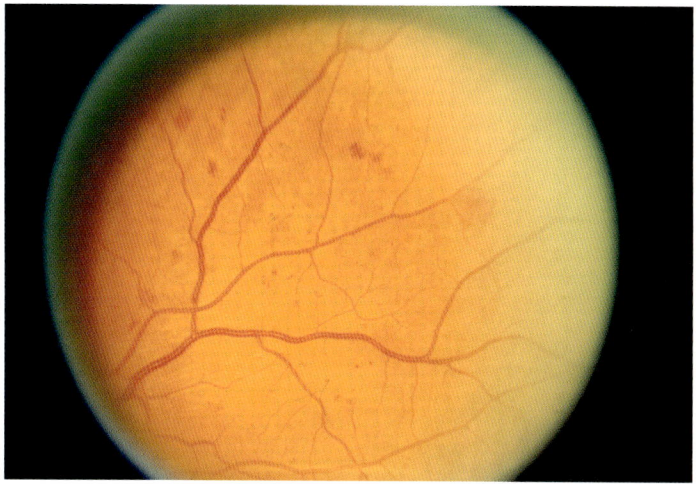

Early Treatment Diabetic Retinopathy Study standard photograph 2A. Hemorrhages and/or microaneurysms equaling or exceeding this severity in 4 quadrants indicates "Severe NPDR." (Source: Reprinted with permission from the Fundus Reading Center, Dept of Ophthalmology and Visual Sciences, University of Wisconsin, Madison, Wisconsin.)

Moderate visual loss: The loss of 15 or more letters on the ETDRS visual acuity chart, or doubling of the visual angle (e.g., 20/20–20/40, or 20/50–20/100).

Modified ETDRS grid: Light intensity, treating only areas of leakage.

Nonproliferative diabetic retinopathy (NPDR): The phases of diabetic retinopathy with no evidence of retinal neovascularization.

NPDR: Nonproliferative diabetic retinopathy.

NVD: Neovascularization on or within 1 disc diameter of the optic disc.

NVE: Neovascularization elsewhere in the retina and greater than 1 disc diameter from the optic disc margin.

NVI: Neovascularization of the iris.

PDR: Proliferative diabetic retinopathy.

Proliferative diabetic retinopathy (PDR): Advanced disease characterized by NVD and/or NVE.

Scatter (panretinal) photocoagulation: A type of laser surgery used for patients with proliferative diabetic retinopathy. The surgery is delivered in a scatter pattern throughout the peripheral fundus and is intended to lead to a regression of neovascularization.

Severe nonproliferative diabetic retinopathy: Using the 4–2-1 rule, the presence of at least one of the following features: (1) severe intraretinal hemorrhages and microaneurysms, equaling or exceeding standard photograph 2A, present in four quadrants; (2) venous beading in two or more quadrants; or (3) moderate intraretinal microvascular abnormalities equaling or exceeding standard photograph 8A in one or more quadrants.

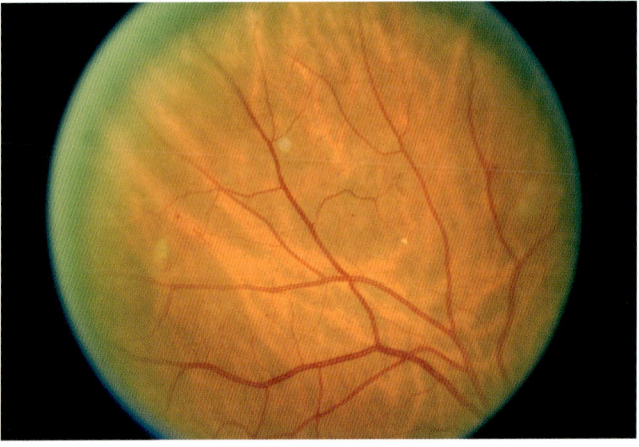

Early Treatment Diabetic Retinopathy Study standard photograph 8A. Intraretinal microvascular abnormalities equaling or exceeding this severity in one or more quadrants indicates "Severe NPDR." (Source: Reprinted with permission from the Fundus Reading Center, Dept of Ophthalmology and Visual Sciences, University of Wisconsin, Madison, Wisconsin.)

Severe visual loss: Occurrence of visual acuity worse than 5/200 at any two consecutive visits, scheduled at 4-month intervals.

UKPDS: United Kingdom Prospective Diabetes Study.

VEGF: Vascular endothelial growth factor.

Very severe nonproliferative diabetic retinopathy: Presence of two or more of the features described in the definition of severe nonproliferative diabetic retinopathy.

Index

NOTE: Page references in italics refers to illustrations and tables.